COLONIC DISEASES

COLONIC DISEASES

Edited by

TIMOTHY R. KOCH, MD

Medical College of Wisconsin,
Milwaukee, WI

Foreword by

JOSEPH B. KIRSNER, MD, PhD, DSci (Hon)

The Louis Block Distinguished Service Professor of Medicine, Department of Medicine,
The University of Chicago Pritzker School of Medicine, Chicago, IL

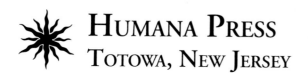

HUMANA PRESS
TOTOWA, NEW JERSEY

© 2003 Humana Press Inc.
999 Riverview Drive, Suite 208
Totowa, New Jersey 07512

www.humanapress.com

The content and opinions expressed in this book are the sole work of the authors and editors, who have warranted due diligence in the creation and issuance of their work. The publisher, editors, and authors are not responsible for errors or omissions or for any conequences arising fom the information or opinions presented in this book and make no warranty, express or implied, with respect to its contents.

Cover illustrations: Fig. 1A from Chapter 16, "Colonoscopy," by Donald G. Seibert; Fig. 6 from Chapter 17, "Interpretation of Colonic Biopsies in Patients with Diarrhea," by Sarah M. Dry, Galen R. Cortina, and Klaus J. Lewin; Figs. 2C and 3E from Chapter 22, "Cross-Sectional Imaging of the Large Bowel," by Diego R. Martin, Ming Yang, and Paul Hamilton; Fig. 1 from Chapter 24, "Acute Megacolon, Acquired Megacolon, and Volvulus," by Marc Stauffer and Timothy R. Koch; and Fig 4. from Chapter 31, "Ischemic Colitis," by Peter Grübel and David R. Cave.

Production Editor: Tracy Catanese
Cover design by Patricia F. Cleary.

For additional copies, pricing for bulk purchases, and/or information about other Humana titles, contact Humana at the above address or at any of the following numbers: Tel: 973-256-1699; Fax: 973-256-8341; E-mail: humana@humanapr.com or visit our website at http://www.humanapress.com

Due diligence has been taken by the publishers, editors, and authors of this book to assure the accuracy of the information published and to describe generally accepted practices. The contributors herein have carefully checked to ensure that the drug selections and dosages set forth in this text are accurate and in accord with the standards accepted at the time of publication. Notwithstanding, as new research, changes in government regulations, and knowledge from clinical experience relating to drug therapy and drug reactions constantly occurs, the reader is advised to check the product information provided by the manufacturer of each drug for any change in dosages or for additional warnings and contraindications. This is of utmost importance when the recommended drug herein is a new or infrequently used drug. It is the responsibility of the treating physician to determine dosages and treatment strategies for individual patients. Further it is the responsibility of the health care provider to ascertain the Food and Drug Administration status of each drug or device used in their clinical practice. The publisher, editors, and authors are not responsible for errors or omissions or for any consequences from the application of the information presented in this book and make no warranty, express or implied, with respect to the contents in this publication.

This publication is printed on acid-free paper. ∞
ANSI Z39.48-1984 (American National Standards Institute)
Permanence of Paper for Printed Library Materials.

Printed in the United States of America.   10 9 8 7 6 5 4 3 2 1

Library of Congress Cataloging-in-Publication Data

Main entry under title:

Colonic diseases / edited by Timothy R. Koch.
        p. ; cm.
     Includes bibliographical references and index.
     ISBN 0-89603-961-7 (alk. paper); 1-59259-314-3 (e-book)
     1. Colon (Anatomy)--Diseases. 2. Colon (Anatomy)--Pathophysiology. I. Koch, Timothy R.
     [DNLM: 1. Colonic Diseases. 2. Rectal Diseases. 3. Colon--physiology. 4. Rectum--physiology. WI 520 C7177 2003]
     RC860 .C656 2003
     616.3'4--dc21   2002032857

Foreword

The Scientification of Gastroenterology During the 20th Century[*]

Science contributes to medicine in three ways: It provides a body of relatively secure knowledge. Some of that knowledge has been applied to develop technologies which have had a major impact upon the practice and effectiveness of medicine. Last, science offers to medicine a way of thinking.

— J. McCormick
[(1993) The Contribution of Science to Medicine. *Perspect. Biol. Med.* **16,** 315.]

Awareness of the digestive system began with the dawn of civilization, when man, observing the feeding habits of animals in the surrounding environment, experimented with foods, edible and inedible. Identity came with discoveries of the digestive organs during the 16th and 17th centuries. Function was revealed by physiologic studies of digestion, absorption and secretion, metabolism, and motility during the 18th and 19th centuries. Diagnostic access improved with the technological advances of the 20th century. Understanding of gastrointestinal (GI) disease followed the growth of the basic sciences and gastroenterology's involvement in scientific research during the latter half of the 20th century.

Early in the 20th century, gastroenterology was yet an undefined activity without clinical or scientific guidelines. Diagnostic approach to the digestive tract was minimal. Valid concepts of disease were lacking. Visceroptosis, sitophobia, and "colonic autointoxication" were common "diagnoses." Therapeutic resources were scarce.

The scientification of medicine began during the latter part of the 19th century with the discovery of bacterial causes of disease, and when the dogma of the past began to yield to perceptive observation and investigation. Additional impetus came from A. Flexner's 1910 report on Medical Education, documenting the necessity for a scientific foundation in medicine. Funds for gastroenterologic investigation remained small, but research was in progress in the physiology laboratories of academic medical centers.

During the 1920s, organized clinical gastroenterology programs, led by outstanding physicians (J. Friedenwald, W. L. Palmer, H. L. Bockus, C. M. Jones, G. Eusterman), were established at several institutions. The entry of scientifically oriented young physicians into gastroenterology during the 1930s and 1940s energized laboratory and clinical research. Specialization in medicine was underway in the United States, and in 1940 Gastroenterology was certified as a medical and academic specialty. Further progress was interrupted by World War II (1941–1945).

Post-World War II was the most productive period in history for the basic and biomedical sciences. Wartime discoveries had demonstrated the unlimited potential of research and motivated the public, charitable foundations, and government to support "basic research."

---

[*]Based in part on 100 Years of American Gastroenterology (1900–2000). Medscape Gastroenterology January 4, 2000. Available at Website: http://www.medscape.com/medscape/gastro/journal/2000/v02.n01/mge0103.kirs/mge0103.kirs-0l.html

This trend was accelerated at the end of World War II (August 1945), when the office of Scientific Research and Development (US War Department) transferred 44 military-oriented research contracts with universities to the National Institutes of Health (NIH). The General Medicine Study Section of the National Institute of Arthritis and Metabolic Diseases (NIH), established in 1955, became a major support of research and training in medicine and in gastroenterology. During the 1960s, 1970s, and 1980s, university medical center faculties enlarged, training programs proliferated, and research activities increased, creating new technologies and new disciplines. Because science represented knowledge and prestige, Gastroenterology sought to become more "scientific," incorporating basic science into its research.

By 1980, gastrointestinal etiopathogenetic concepts had advanced significantly. Because *Colonic Diseases* deals with the colon, the following selected observations relate to this area of GI. Innovative research on CNS–neurohumoral and neuroimmune interactions of the GI tract, mediating colonic motility, and visceral sensitivity replaced psychogenic hypotheses of the irritable bowel. Physiologic studies modified the process of colon diverticular formation from pulsion by intraluminal gases to sustained colonic musculature contraction, compartmentalizing the colon into high-pressure segments and forcing mucosa through weaknesses in the bowel wall. Studies of gastrointestinal immunology, including the gut mucosal immune system and the molecular mechanisms of inflammation, generated new etiologic concepts and therapeutic resources in IBD. Advancing fiberoptic methodology expanded access to the GI tract, including the colon. Laser-scanning confocal microscopy enabled study of epithelial cells and intracellular protein processing. Microbiological and chromatographic studies of the enteric flora facilitated the diagnosis of bacterial overgrowth responsive to antibacterial therapy. Gas chromatographic techniques, breath H_2 excretion, and measurement of colonic CH_4 and CO_2 production elevated the study of intestinal gas to a scientific discipline.

Quantitative measurements of GI blood flow including laser Doppler velocimetry and the Stromuhr blood-flow technique facilitated recognition of colonic vascular impairment. Neurogastroenterology introduced methods of electrophysiology and cellular neurophysiology, identified the enteric nervous system as a "minibrain with intelligent circuits," and provided new understanding of "physiologic" GI disorders. Transgenic methodology created innovative animal models, enabling multidisciplinary studies of intestinal inflammation. Molecular genetics established the genetic basis of colorectal cancer, identified a colorectal cancer marker among Ashkenazi Jews, and demonstrated the possible prevention of colorectal cancer via the modulation of APC gene function.

Many favoring circumstances converged to bring gastroenterology into the mainstream of advancing scientific thought:

1. An enlarging body of basic scientific knowledge and its translation to clinical problems.
2. Technological advances permitting safer and more precise human studies.
3. Public, pharmaceutical, and governmental support of research.
4. The adoption of controlled studies.
5. The contribution of philanthropic organizations (e.g., Rockefeller).
6. The growth and influence of academic medical centers.
7. NIH-supported research and training.
8. The impact of research-oriented societies (e.g., AGA, Gastroenterology Research Group).
9. The enlarging global scientific communication network (journals, databases, and electronic and computer systems).
10. Increasing awareness of the significant health problems represented in digestive diseases.

Karl Popper said "The more we learn...and the deeper is our learning, the more conscious, specific and articulate will be our knowledge of what we do not know." Gastroenterology's scientific progress notwithstanding, the etiology and pathogenesis of colonic diseases remain incompletely understood and stand as challenges for the 21st century. The expanding frontiers of gastroenterologic research now include the immunogenetic biology of the intestinal epithelium and the molecular disciplines (microbiology, cell biology, immunology, genetics) mediating colonic physiology and the expression of disease, as reflected in Timothy Koch's well-designed and authoritative book. These remarkable resources form the basis of our optimism for the future.

Joseph B. Kirsner, MD, PhD, DSci (Hon)
The Louis Block Distinguished Service Professor of Medicine
Department of Medicine
The University of Chicago Pritzker School of Medicine, Chicago, IL

Preface

Colorectal disorders are common diseases that are often chronic in nature. We are now working with an increasingly older population. This population trend increases the number of individuals with colorectal neoplasia, inflammatory bowel disease, diverticular disease, and constipation. We therefore thought that the beginning of the new millennium was an extremely relevant and timely period to prepare a new book about colorectal disorders.

The purpose of *Colonic Diseases* is to provide a bridge between basic and clinical research and the present clinical care of individuals with colonic disorders. *Colonic Diseases* examines the origins and treatment of common colorectal disorders, and it blends new outcomes and epidemiological research with molecular mechanisms of disease to improve our present and future understanding of colonic diseases and their management.

Colonic Diseases has been divided into three parts: Colorectal Physiology, Investigation of Disease Processes, and Colorectal Disease. Part I provides an extensive overview of normal colonic physiology. Part II utilizes the expertise of active investigators who are studying the pathophysiology of colonic disorders, and includes a survey of techniques that are used in clinical research of colonic diseases. Understanding the mechanisms of disease development may provide important clues for future therapy. In Part III potential symptoms, pathological and radiological findings, the differential diagnosis, presently recommended evaluation and therapy, and potential future alternative therapies for common colorectal diseases are reviewed.

Colonic Diseases is intended for gastroenterologists, gastrointestinal fellows, and scientists in gastrointestinal research who are interested in bridging basic and clinical research and diseases processes. This book will be a useful reference resource for primary care physicians who care for patients with chronic colonic disorders, and may also prove of interest to colorectal surgeons, although it is not designed to be a textbook for the performance of colorectal surgery.

I wish to dedicate this book to Dr. Joseph B. Kirsner, who inspired our great interest in colonic diseases at the University of Chicago, and to Dr. Joseph Szurszewski, who promoted a strong quantitative approach to basic colonic physiology at the Mayo Clinic in Rochester.

I would like to acknowledge the great patience of my wife, Nancy, and my daughter, Kristina, during the preparation of this book. I wish to thank Ms. Debbie Williams for her excellent secretarial and managerial assistance.

Timothy R. Koch, MD

Contents

PART I. COLORECTAL PHYSIOLOGY

PART II. INVESTIGATION OF DISEASE PROCESSES

PART III. COLORECTAL DISEASE

Contributors

CAROL LYNN BERSETH, MD, *Director, Medical Affairs, North America, Mead Johnson Nutritionals, Evansville, IN*

THOMAS J. BORODY, MD, *Centre for Digestive Diseases, Sydney, Australia*

MICHAEL CAMILLERI, MD, *Professor of Medicine and Physiology, Division of Gastroenterology, Mayo Clinic and Foundation, Rochester, MN*

DAVID R. CAVE, MD, *Chief of Gastroenterology, St. Elizabeth Medical Center, Brighton, MA*

YANG K. CHEN, MD, *Professor of Medicine, Division of Gastroenterology and Hepatology, University of Colorado Health Sciences Center, Denver, CO*

CAROLYN E. COLE, MSN, MM, *Associate Director, Colon Cancer Prevention Program, University of Wisconsin, Madison, WI*

PATRICIA L. CONWAY, MSC, PhD, *School of Microbiology and Immunology, University of New South Wales, Sydney, Australia*

GALEN R. CORTINA, MD, PhD, *Department of Pathology and Laboratory Medicine, UCLA Center for the Health Sciences, Los Angeles, CA*

MICHAEL D. CROWELL, PhD, *Senior Director of Scientific Affairs, Novartis Pharmaceuticals Corporation, East Hanover, NJ; and Marvin M. Schuster Center for Digestive and Motility Disorders, The Johns Hopkins University School of Medicine, Baltimore, MD*

CHRISTOPHER F. CUFF, PhD, *Department of Microbiology, Immunology, and Cell Biology, Robert C. Byrd Health Science Center, West Virginia University, Morgantown, WV*

CYNTHIA A. CUNNINGHAM, PhD, *Department of Microbiology, Immunology, and Cell Biology, Robert C. Byrd Health Science Center, West Virginia University, Morgantown, WV*

SEBASTIAN G. DE LA FUENTE, MD, *Fellow, Gastrointestinal Surgery Research, Duke University Medical Center, Durham NC*

SARAH M. DRY, MD, *Department of Pathology and Laboratory Medicine, UCLA Center for the Health Sciences, Los Angeles, CA*

PRADEEP K. DUDEJA, PhD, *Associate Professor of Physiology in Medicine, Department of Medicine, Chicago Westside Veterans Affairs System, University of Illinois at Chicago, Chicago, IL*

JONATHAN R. FULTON, PhD, *Department of Microbiology and Immunobiology, Robert C. Byrd Health Science Center, West Virginia University, Morgantown, WV*

LISA M. GANGAROSA, MD, *Division of Digestive Diseases, University of North Carolina at Chapel Hill, Chapel Hill, NC*

RAVINDER GILL, PhD, *Research Associate, Department of Medicine, Chicago Westside Veterans Affairs System, University of Illinois at Chicago, Chicago, IL*

PETER GRÜBEL, MD, *Division of Gastroenterology, New England Medical Center, Boston, MA*

PAUL HAMILTON, MD, *Sunnybrook and Women's College of Health Sciences Center, University of Toronto, Toronto, Canada*

STEPHEN B. HANAUER, MD, *Chief, Division of Gastroenterology, University of Chicago, Chicago, IL*

SAMUEL B. HO, MD, *Gastroenterology Division, Department of Medicine, Veterans Affairs Medical Center and University of Minnesota, Minneapolis, MN*

WALTER J. HOGAN, MD, *Professor of Medicine and Radiology, Division of Gastroenterology and Hepatology, Medical College of Wisconsin, Milwaukee, WI*

RUSSELL F. JACOBY, MD, *Associate Professor of Medicine, and Director, Colon Cancer Prevention Program, University of Wisconsin Medical School, Madison, WI*

JOHN F. JOHANSON, MD, MSC, *Clinical Associate Professor of Medicine, Rockford Gastroenterology Associates, Rockford, IL*

MOHAMMED M. H. KALAN, MD, MS, *Assistant Professor of Surgery, Georgetown University Hospital, Washington, DC*

JOSEPH B. KIRSNER, MD, PhD, *The Louis Block Professor of Medicine, Department of Medicine, The Joseph B. Kirsner Center for the Study of Digestive Diseases, University of Chicago, Chicago, IL*

TIMOTHY R. KOCH, MD, *Division of Gastroenterology and Hepatology, Medical College of Wisconsin, Milwaukee, WI*

BRIAN E. LACY, MD, PhD, *Marvin M. Schuster Center for Digestive and Motility Disorders, The John Hopkins Bayview Medical Center, The John Hopkins University School of Medicine, Baltimore, MD*

BRET A. LASHNER, MD, MPH, *Center for Inflammatory Bowel Disease, Department of Gastroenterology, Cleveland Clinic Foundation, Cleveland, OH*

KLAUS J. LEWIN, MD, FRCPATH *Department of Pathology and Laboratory Medicine, UCLA Center for the Health Sciences, Los Angeles, CA*

VINCENT H. S. LOW, FRANZCR, *Clinical Associate Professor and Head, Department of Radiology, Sir Charles Gairdner Hospital, Nedlands, Western Australia*

ANNE LUTZ-VORDERBRUEGGE, MD, *Gastroenterologische Gemeinschaftspraxis, Mainz, Germany*

CHRISTOPHER R. MANTYH, MD, *Assistant Professor of Surgery, Duke University Medical Center, Durham, NC*

DIEGO R. MARTIN, MD, PhD, *Associate Professor of Radiology and Director of MRI, Robert C. Byrd Health Science Center, West Virginia University, Morgantown, WV*

JOSEPH P. MULDOON, MD, *Assistant Clinical Professor of Surgery, Northwestern University Medical School, Evanston Hospital, Evanston, IL*

EMMANUEL C. OPARA, PhD, *Department of Surgery, Baker House, Duke South Hospital, Duke University Medical Center, Durham, NC*

BRUCE A. ORKIN, MD, FACS, FASCRS, *Professor of Surgery, and Director, Division of Colon and Rectal Surgery, George Washington University, Washington, DC*

MARY F. OTTERSON, MD, MS, *Associate Professor, Department of Surgery and Physiology, Zablocki VA Medical Center, Medical College of Wisconsin, Milwaukee, WI*

THEODORE N. PAPPAS, MD, *Professor of Surgery, Department of Surgery, Duke University Medical Center, Durham, NC*

DEVANG N. PRAJAPATI, MD, *Fellow in Gastroenterology, Medical College of Wisconsin, Milwaukee, WI*

K. RAMASWAMY, PhD, *Professor of Physiology in Medicine, Department of Medicine, Chicago Westside Veterans Affairs System, University of Illinois at Chicago, Chicago, IL*

KENTON M. SANDERS, PhD, *Professor and Chairman, Department of Physiology and Cell Biology, University of Nevada School of Medicine, Reno, NV*

ARND SCHULTE-BOCKHOLT, MD, *Gastroenterologische Schwerpunktpraxis, Karlsruhe, Germany*

DONALD G. SEIBERT, MD, *GI Consultants, SW Virginia Carilion Medical Center, Roanoke, VA*

AMIT G. SHAH, MD, *Senior Fellow in Gastroenterology, University of Chicago, Chicago, IL*

LAURIE L. SHEKELS, PhD, *Gastroenterology Division, Department of Medicine, Veterans Affairs Medical Center and University of Minnesota, Minneapolis, MN*

TERENCE K. SMITH, PhD, *Professor, Department of Physiology and Cell Biology, University of Nevada School of Medicine, Reno, NV*

WILLIAM J. SNAPE, JR., MD, *Medical Director Gastrointestinal Motility Service, California Pacific Medical Center, San Francisco, CA*

MARC STAUFFER, MD, *Resident in Internal Medicine, Department of Medicine, West Virginia University, Morgantown, WV*

STEVEN J. STRYKER, MD, *Associate Professor of Clinical Surgery, Department of Surgery, Northwestern University, Chicago, IL*

GORDON L. TELFORD, MD, *Professor of Surgery, Department of Surgery, Medical College of Wisconsin, Milwaukee, WI*

SUSAN W. TELFORD, PhD, *Assistant Professor, Department of Anesthesia, Medical College of Wisconsin, Milwaukee, WI*

MELANIE B. THOMAS, MD, *Assistant Professor of Medicine, Department of Gastrointestinal Medical Oncology, M.D. Anderson Cancer Center, University of Texas, Houston, TX*

STACEY A. WEILAND, MD, *Division of Gastroenterology and Hepatology, University of Colorado Health Sciences Center, Denver, CO*

ROBERT A. WOLFF, MD, *Assistant Professor of Medicine, Department of Gastrointestinal Medical Oncology and Digestive Diseases, M.D. Anderson Cancer Center, University of Texas, Houston, TX*

MING YANG, MD, *Department of Radiology, West Virginia University, Robert C. Byrd Health Science Center, Morgantown, WV*

Color Plates

Color photography supported by an unrestricted educational grant from AstraZeneca.

I COLORECTAL PHYSIOLOGY

1

Absorption–Secretion and Epithelial Cell Function

Pradeep K. Dudeja, Ravinder Gill, and K. Ramaswamy

1. INTRODUCTION

Under normal physiological conditions, the mammalian colon absorbs Na^+, Cl^-, and water and secretes K^+ and HCO_3^-. In diarrheal disorders, disturbances in ion transport result in excessive secretion of electrolytes and water. In recent years, a number of reviews have addressed the mechanisms of ion transport in mammalian intestine. Also, the recent molecular cloning of several electrolyte transporters has dramatically advanced our knowledge of molecular mechanisms of the electrolyte transport in the mammalian intestine. This chapter reviews the role of various absorptive and secretory processes in colonic physiology with special emphasis on the human colon. Current advances in molecular mechanisms of absorption of Na^+, Cl^-, short chain fatty acids (SCFA), H_2O, sulfate, oxalate, and bacterially synthesized water soluble vitamins, as well as mechanisms of secretion of Cl^-, HCO_3^- and K^+ are discussed. Lastly, the regulation of these transporters under physiological and pathophysiological conditions and the importance of these transport mechanisms to the colonocyte integrity and function is evaluated.

1.1. Electrolyte Transport Pathways

Intestinal electrolyte transport processes that operate between the gut lumen and blood can be categorized into two major pathways: transcellular and paracellular (1,2). The transcellular process is mostly active in nature and involves movement of ions through the antipodal plasma membranes and cytosol of the polarized epithelial cell. In contrast, paracellular transport is generally passive and involves movement of the ions via the intercellular tight junctions. The presence of transporters on apical and basolateral plasma membranes of the polarized epithelial cells determines the selectivity of the epithelial cells for the

From: *Colonic Diseases*
Edited by: T. R. Koch © Humana Press Inc., Totowa, NJ

vectorial transport of specific ions. The ions are transported by a combination of both the active and passive transport processes. The Na^+-K^+ adenosine triphosphatase (ATPase) localized on the epithelial cell basolateral membrane plays a central role in all active ion transport processes. The ion gradients generated by this transporter mostly provide the driving force for other ion and nutrient movement across plasma membranes and are, therefore, termed as secondary active transport processes. Additionally, the transport processes can either be electroneutral (no net movement of charges across the membrane, e.g., Na^+-H^+ and Cl^--HCO_3^- exchangers) or electrogenic (involving net movement of charge across the membranes, e.g., Na^+, K^+, and Cl^- channels, sodium-glucose cotransporters [SGLTs] or sodium bicarbonate co-transporters [NBCs].

1.2. Types of Transport

Transport pathways can be mainly grouped into diffusion and carrier-mediated transport. Diffusion can be defined as passive movement of molecules down the concentration gradient (from high to low concentration) and continues until the steady state equilibrium across the membrane is achieved. Diffusion can occur through the lipid bilayer (e.g. for oxygen, carbon dioxide, lipid soluble substances and small ions); through ion-specific protein channels (e.g., for Na^+, K^+, Cl^- and Ca^{2+}), which mediate the passive movement of ions down the electrochemical gradient of ions across the membrane. Osmosis is another mechanism of passive diffusion for water down its concentration gradient. Cell membranes consisting of lipid cores are impermeable to a variety of polar solutes and ions. Therefore, specialized carrier proteins are needed for such polar substances to cross cell membranes. These specialized transport proteins are inserted into the plasma membranes to mediate and regulate transport. The transport process utilizing these carriers is termed as carrier-mediated transport. Carrier-mediated transport systems exhibit specificity and saturability of the carrier for the substrate. This transport can be further divided into three main categories: (i) primary active; (ii) secondary active; and (iii) facilitated diffusion. Primary active transport involves movement of ions or substrates against their concentration gradient (i.e., from low to high concentration) at the expense of high-energy molecules, e.g., adenosine triphosphate (ATP). The best example of such a transporter is the epithelial cell basolateral membrane (BLM) Na^+-K^+ ATPase, which pumps 3 ions of Na^+ out of the cell in exchange for two K^+ ions, deriving energy from hydrolysis of 1 molecule of ATP. Secondary active transport processes, on the other hand, are the most common in polarized epithelial cells and also involve transport of substrates against their concentration gradient (uphill transport), but the driving force for these transporters is set up by the primary active transporters, e.g., Na^+-K^+ ATPase generating the needed ion gradients. Transport of a wide variety of nutrients and ions through either exchangers or co-transporters predominantly involves a secondary active transport process. In contrast to the primary and secondary active transporters, the facilitated diffusion process (e.g., the uptake of fructose by the enterocytes) is also a carrier-mediated process, but involves the transport of substrates down the concentration gradient, however, exhibits specificity and saturability of the carrier. Other modes of transports include vesicular transport, e.g., endocytosis or exocytosis. These pathways require ATP. Endocytosis could be either via pinocytosis (transport of small volumes of fluid or proteins) or phagocytosis (uptake of particulate materials, e.g., bacteria or cellular debris). Recently, the role of caveolae (cavelike indentations on the plasma membranes) in membrane transport into the cells and in signal transduction has also been identified (3). The transport via caveole has been termed as potocytosis, which is believed to be a mechanism for the uptake of selected small molecules and ions. For example, the uptake of folic acid into some cells has been shown to involve caveolae (3).

2. ABSORPTIVE MECHANISMS:
2.1. Sodium Absorption

Although, sodium is absorbed efficiently throughout the mammalian intestine, its mechanisms of transport exhibit regional and species differences (4). In general, the predominant mechanisms of sodium absorption in the mammalian small intestine have been shown to be via either solute (sugars and amino acids)-dependent co-transport; Na^+-H^+ exchangers (in jejunum) or coupled Na^+-H^+ and Cl^--HCO_3^- exchangers in the ileum. In the mammalian proximal colon, it has been shown to be via a coupled Na^+-H^+ and Cl^--HCO_3^- exchangers mediating electroneutral NaCl absorption, whereas in the distal colon it has been suggested to involve both the electroneutral as well as electrogenic processes involving amiloride-sensitive sodium channels (4).

Although, the transport mechanisms of electrolytes in the intestine of rat, guinea pig, or rabbit have been extensively investigated (1,4), very limited studies were available until recently with respect to direct investigation of the electrolyte transport in the human intestine. Recent advancements with respect to development of techniques for the isolation and purification of the antipodal plasma membranes from the human small intestine and colon from organ donor mucosal tissues and molecular expression and cloning studies of the human-specific electrolyte transporters have greatly advanced our knowledge in this area (5–11). The need for direct investigations in the human intestine was warranted from a number of studies indicating that observations from the animal species could not be simply extrapolated to understand human intestinal electrolyte transport due to observed differences not only in the mechanisms of basal transport or regional variations, but also due to their differential hormonal regulation (6–8,12).

2.1.1. Na^+ Absorption in the Human Colon

Previous studies performed in the human colon employed either in vivo steady state perfusion techniques (13–16) or in vitro preparations of intact mucosa using short circuit current method (17–21). Findings of these previous studies in the human colon can be briefly summarized as follows: (i) the human colon in vivo absorbs Na^+, Cl^-, and H_2O and secretes K^+ and HCO_3^- and (ii) studies employing short circuit current technique (12,17–21) or in vivo perfusion (22) to measure amiloride inhibition and/or spontaneous potential, report conflicting results in relation to Na^+ transport mechanism(s) in the proximal and distal human colon (12,17–22). For example, a number of studies suggested that Na^+ absorption in proximal human colon appears to occur by a predominantly electroneutral process (12,20,21), whereas in the distal colon it was suggested to occur predominantly by an electrogenic process based on an amiloride (10^{-6} M) sensitive short circuit current (17–21). In contrast, in vivo steady state perfusion studies (22) and in vitro studies of Sellin and DeSoigne (12) utilizing short-circuited human colon indicated the presence of almost equivalent components of electroneutral and electrogenic Na^+ absorption in both the proximal and distal human colon. Detailed studies of these electroneutral processes had not been conducted and the mechanisms of coupling of Na^+ had not been investigated. Also, the mechanism(s) of Na^+ exit across the BLM domain of human colonocytes were not known.

The above pattern of Na^+ transport in the human colon is different from the rat colon but somewhat similar to the rabbit colon (4). For example, Na^+ transport in the rat colon has been shown to occur by a chloride independent electroneutral Na^+-H^+ exchange process in both the proximal and distal colonic segments (4). Electrogenic sodium uptake, while present in the proximal colon, is almost absent in the rat distal colon (4). The rabbit colon (23,24) appears to behave more like the human colon in vitro (17–21), in that it was shown to exhibit predominantly electroneutral NaCl absorption in the proximal colon and electrogenic Na^+ absorption in the distal colon in vitro (23,24). Recent studies directly performed with purified human colonic apical membrane vesicles, however, demonstrated the presence of almost equivalent proportions of electroneutral and conductive pathways for Na^+ absorption in both the proximal and distal human colon (6,7). The human colonic electroneutral sodium absorption is via coupled activity of both the Na^+-H^+ and Cl^--HCO_3^- exchangers in proximal and distal human colon (25,26). Both segments of the human colon demonstrated conductive or electrogenic sodium transport as well (6,7).

2.1.2. MOLECULAR BIOLOGY OF Na^+-H^+ EXCHANGERS

Until recently, the molecular nature and regulation of these transporters was not well understood. A number of studies from a variety of polarized epithelial cell types, e.g., rat distal colonocytes (27), rabbit ileal villus cells (28) and LLC-PK1 (a porcine kidney cell line) (29), and human colonic epithelial cells (6,7,30) have shown the presence of distinct forms of Na^+-H^+ exchangers in apical and basolateral membrane domains. These Na^+-H^+ exchangers exhibit differences in amiloride sensitivity and regulation (31–35). Studies have suggested that in a variety of epithelial cells, the Na^+-H^+ antiporter of the basolateral membrane may represent a "housekeeping" antiporter involved in maintenance of intracellular pH, volume regulation, and cell proliferation, whereas the apical membrane Na^+-H^+ antiporter(s) may be involved in transepithelial (vectorial) transport of Na^+ (31,32).

Recent studies have identified a family of six functionally and structurally related isoforms of Na^+-H^+ exchangers (NHEs) termed NHE1 to NHE6 (32,34,36). NHE isoforms have been divided into N-terminal and C-terminal regions. N-terminal regions have been predicted to contain 10–12 transmembrane domains, involved in Na^+-H^+ exchange, amiloride inhibition and containing a H^+ modifier site. This region of NHEs also shows maximal homology between different isoforms as well in different species. In contrast, the C-terminal region is cytosolic in nature and is the most divergent between different isoforms. It has been shown to be important in regulation of NHEs by various signal transduction mechanisms. Several regions of this domain have been shown to be important for mediating the effects of calcium, calmodulin, cyclic adenosine 5'-monophosphate (cAMP) and different growth factors. The cytoplasmic regulatory factors and cytoskeletal proteins have also been shown to be involved in second messenger regulation of these transporters (33,35,37–40).

Mammalian intestine (small and large) has been shown to express the NHE1, 2 and 3 isoforms (8,31,32), and these three have been the ones most characterized with respect to their molecular biology and regulation. NHE4 isoform has been shown to be expressed in the stomach. The NHE1 isoform of Na^+-H^+ exchangers is considered to be ubiquitously expressed, and its protein product is localized to the basolateral membranes of polarized epithelial cells (31,32). NHE-3 isoform has been suggested to represent the antiporter localized on the apical surface of intestinal and kidney epithelial cells and involved in vectorial Na^+ absorption (31,32). Tissue distribution studies in the rabbit intestine showed that the mRNA for NHE3 was abundant in rabbit ileum and ascending colon, but it was absent from duodenum and descending colon, where neutral NaCl absorption is absent (41). Tissue distribution of NHE3 message in rat intestine, however, does not necessarily parallel the presence of neutral NaCl absorption patterns. For example, the NHE3 mRNA was abundant in proximal colon and stomach, but was almost absent from rat duodenum and ileum (42). These findings suggest that specificity of expression of NHE isoforms may vary from species to species and also in various segments of intestine. Tissue distribution studies of the NHE isoforms in the human intestine showed that NHE1, 2, and 3 isoforms were expressed throughout the human intestine (8). The relative

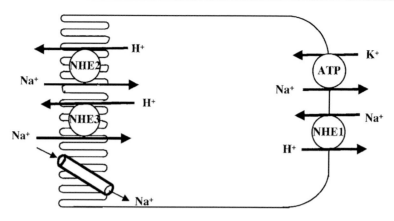

Fig. 1. Model of Na$^+$ absorption in the human colon.

abundance of NHE1 mRNA was unchanged throughout the human gastrointestinal tract. In contrast, the expression of NHE3 mRNA was the highest in the ileum, whereas the NHE2 expression was the highest in the colon. Surface–crypt axis expression studies showed that in the human colon, NHE3 was localized to the surface epithelial cells, whereas NHE2 expression was observed throughout the surface–crypt axis *(8)*. Studies have also shown that in rat, rabbit, as well as in the human intestine, NHE2 and 3 were localized to the luminal membrane *(43,44)*, whereas NHE1 was localized to BLM *(30,43,45)*. Studies examining the role of sodium uptake in rabbit intestine under basal conditions indicated that both NHE2 and NHE3 equally contributed to basal Na$^+$ uptake *(46)*. Preliminary studies utilizing purified apical membranes form the jejunum, ileum, proximal and distal colon from organ donors, and inhibitors to differentiate between NHE2 and NHE3 activity (HOE694 and EIPA) have shown that, in the human intestine, NHE3 was the predominant isoform involved in sodium uptake in the jejunum and ileum, whereas NHE2 was more important for sodium uptake in the colon (Dudeja, Tyagi, Gill, and Ramaswamy, unpublished observations). Based on the above studies, a proposed model of sodium absorption in the human colon is presented in Fig. 1.

2.1.3. REGULATION OF INTESTINAL NHEs

Intestinal luminal sodium uptake mediated via NHE activity has been shown to be inhibited by an increase in intracellular cAMP and Ca^{2+} *(47,48)*. In general, NHEs have been shown to be regulated by variety of second messenger cascades. For example, intracellular calcium, cAMP, cytoskeletal proteins, membrane physical state, nitric oxide, and various protein kinases have been shown to modulate NHE activities involving multiple mechanisms *(33,35,37,49–51)*. One of the important mechanisms has been shown to be via alterations in the rate of insertion of transporter molecules into the plasma membrane or retrieval from the membrane *(52)*. Recently, there have been intensive studies to investigate the signal transduction pathways involved in these regulatory cascades. For example, a number of regulatory factors (e.g. NHERF, E3KARP) and cytoskeletal proteins have been shown to be involved in cAMP-mediated regulation of NHE3 activity *(33,37)*. However, very little is known about the transcriptional regulation of the NHEs. In this regard, although promoters for the rat *(53)*, mouse *(54)*, pig *(55)*, rabbit NHE1 *(56)*, rat NHE2 *(57)* and rat NHE3 *(58)*, and the human NHE1 *(59)* and human NHE2 *(11)* have recently been cloned and partially characterized, limited information is available with respect to promoter sequences for the human NHE3*(10)*. Glucocorticoids *(60)* and thyroid hormones *(61)* have been shown to transcriptionally activate the NHE3 . Mitogenic stimulation has been shown to stimulate NHE1 promoter activity *(62)*. Recently, the *cis*-elements for the osmotic activation of the rat NHE2 were identified *(63)*. Transcriptional regulation of NHEs has also been shown to play an important role in their tissue-specific expression and developmental regulation *(64)*. Future detailed studies focusing on the mechanisms of transcriptional regulation of the human NHEs should yield crucial information concerning molecular regulation of sodium absorption in the human intestine.

2.1.4. SODIUM CHANNELS

Electrogenic sodium transport in many distal colonic epithelia has been shown to be mediated by epithelial sodium channels (ENaCs) *(4)*. The rate of electrogenic sodium absorption across the epithelium depends upon the entry at the apical domain (via EnaC) and exit from the basolateral domain via a Na^+-K^+ ATPase pump (Fig. 1). Electrogenic sodium transport has been shown to be present in distal colon of rabbit, pig, turtle, toad, and human *(4)*. In contrast, electrogenic sodium transport has been shown to be absent in normal distal colon of the rat *(4)*. In this regard, recent membrane vesicle studies, utilizing voltage clamping, as well as inhibition by amiloride analogs benzamil and phenamil, have indicated the presence of both the conductive (presumably mediated by ENaC) as well as electroneutral sodium uptake (mediated by NHE) mechanisms in the human ileum, proximal colon and distal colon *(5–7)* (Fig. 1).

Epithelial sodium channels are highly selective for Na^+ and are inhibited by micromolar concentrations of amiloride and its analogs, e.g., phenamil and benzamil *(65,66)*. In contrast, inhibition of Na^+-H^+ exchangers usually requires relatively higher concentrations of amiloride for inhibition. These channels are inwardly rectifying, i.e., they are more effective in carrying out Na^+ influx compared to Na^+ efflux from epithelial cells *(65,66)*. The ENaC is comprised of three subunits: α, β, and γ *(65,66)*. The subunits share about 35% homology. Each subunit is predicted to be an integral membrane protein. Expression of α-subunit alone has been shown to produce channels with characteristics of the native protein with respect to inhibition by amiloride or voltage-current relationship. Expression of all subunits, however, is required for optimal targeting and functioning of the channel *(65,66)*.

The permeability of Na^+ through these channels has been shown to be regulated *(4)*. For example, mucosal sodium concentration, intracellular sodium concentration as well as hyperaldosteronism secondary to salt depletion or in response to exogenous aldosterone treatment, have been shown to regulate sodium entry (mediated by ENaC) through the apical membrane. An increase in mucosal sodium concentration results in a decrease in sodium permeability. Conversely, a decrease in mucosal sodium concentration results in an increase in sodium permeability. Similarly, the cellular sodium concentration has also been shown to be inversely related to the apical membrane sodium permeability. Aldosterone increases electrogenic Na^+ absorption in the colon via an increase in the expression of both the apical membrane ENaC and BLM Na^+-K^+ ATPase *(4)*.

2.2. Chloride Absorption

Mammalian colon absorbs chloride by two major pathways: passive and active. Passive chloride absorption is secondary to the electrical potential generated by electrogenic sodium absorption. Active chloride absorption occurs in exchange for bicarbonate, which is secreted in the lumen parallel to the decrease in luminal chloride concentration. This active chloride absorption has been shown to be mediated by a sodium-independent Cl^--HCO_3^- exchange process localized to the apical membrane *(4)*. This active chloride transport process

rat distal colon is partially ouabain-sensitive, but is not substantially inhibited by either omeprazole or Sch 28080 (126).

H^+-K^+ ATPase is a member of the gene family of P-type ATPases also called nongastric ATPases (128). This transmembrane protein consists of a catalytic α-subunit with 10 membrane spanning segments and a glycosylated β-subunit. Several species variants of the α-subunits of nongastric H^+-K^+ ATPase, have been cloned. These include rat colonic H^+-K^+ ATPase, human H^+-K^+ ATPase (ATP1AL1), and the guinea pig and rabbit colonic H^+-K^+ ATPase (128). A β-subunit has recently been cloned from rat colon (129). Recently, Sangan et al. (130) reported that the β-subunit of both H^+-K^+ ATPase and Na^+-K^+ATPase proteins can form a functional enzyme complex with the α-subunit of H^+-K^+ ATPase protein in human embryonic kidney (HEK)-293 cells and results in the expression of ouabain-insensitive H^+-K^+ ATPase activity and ^{86}Rb uptake.

Active potassium absorption has been shown to be enhanced under different experimental conditions: dietary potassium depletion, dietary lithium feeding and increased aldosterone levels (but only when aldosterone-induced potassium secretion is inhibited) (126). The increase in activity of this exchange by high levels of aldosterone may help in the recycling of K^+ expelled by apical channels during acute Na^+ retention (131).

2.5. Water Absorption

The intestine possesses a tremendous capacity to absorb water. About 7–10 L of water entering the gastrointestinal tract during a 24-h period is absorbed by the small intestine. The colon plays an important role in the desiccation of stool by absorbing an additional 2 L of fluid. In fact, the colon absorbs more water per unit of luminal surface area, if the differences in length and luminal surface area are also considered (132). Several conditions causing malabsorption of solutes and water in the small intestine can increase the fluid entering the colon to overwhelm its absorptive capacity and hence lead to diarrhea.

The small intestine contains a leaky epithelium with low electric resistance and low reflection co-efficients for small solutes. Water generally moves in the gastrointestinal tract secondary to hydrostatic pressure and osmotic differences created by active electrolyte transport. A paracellular pathway for rapid water movement in small intestine has been suggested. Various studies have proposed that sodium, glucose, and other sodium-coupled transporters can serve as active water transporters. Wright and Loo (133) recently demonstrated that water is co-transported along with Na^+ and sugar through SGLT1 and involves a combination of two processes: the co-transport of 2 Na^+, 1 glucose, and 210 water molecules, and the passive component through SGLT1 water channel. There is also the existence of aquaporins (AQP) on the enterocyte plasma membrane, which can form a pore and act as water channels. Recent data indicate the expression of AQP-4 on the BLM of deep glands of small intestine and AQP-8 to the villus epithelium (132).

Colon, on the other hand is a tight epithelium with high electric resistance and probably much lower paracellular water permeability. Water must move out of the lumen despite the high effective osmolarity of feces, and yet under some conditions, colon secretes fluid in large quantities. The colonic epithelium is generally compartmentalized with respect to absorptive and secretory functions. The absorption is believed to be a function of villus cells whereas secretion is a function of crypt cells. Some studies have shown colonic crypts to be the sites of both absorption and secretion (134). Naftalin and Pedley (135) demonstrated a role of crypt cells in water absorption. The model proposed suggests that the movement of the solutes that are actively transported out of the crypt lumen across a relatively water impermeable crypt barrier creates the hypertonic interstitial space and builds up a negative pressure in the crypt. This creates a vacuum that extracts water from fecal matter. Recent studies in mouse colon suggest the role of AQP-4, which is localized to colonic surface epithelium, in colonic water permeability *(132)*. The role of other AQP, e.g., AQP-8, also expressed in colon is still not clear.

2.6. Absorption of Water Soluble Vitamins in the Human Colon

Recent studies utilizing purified plasma membrane vesicles from the organ donor colons as well as studies utilizing NCM460 (primary human colonocytes in culture) or Caco-2 cells, have provided evidence for the existence of transporters for the uptake of bacterially synthesized water soluble vitamins on the colonocyte plasma membranes *(136–140)*. For example, a pH sensitive, DIDS inhibitable folate transporter has been identified on the apical, as well as BLM domains of the human colonocyte *(136,137)*. This transporter was shown to be regulated via a protein tyrosine kinase-mediated mechanism *(138)*. Specific carrier proteins for thiamine (Dudeja and Said, unpublished observations) and biotin *(140)* on the human colonic luminal membrane vesicles have also been identified. These transporters may play an important role in the event of massive small intestinal disease or in maintaining localized epithelial nutrition. Additional studies are required to define physiological role for these transporters.

3. SECRETORY MECHANISMS
3.1. Chloride Secretion

Diarrhea caused by infectious agents results in massive secretion of fluid and electrolytes by the small intestine. The role of active chloride secretion in pathophysiology of diarrhea was originally identified in studies of cholera enterotoxin in rabbit ileum *(141,142)*. The enterotoxins (e.g., cholera toxin or heat stable enterotoxin [Sta]) cause fluid secretion into the intestinal lumen secondary to a stimulation of active chloride secretion. Subsequent studies in rat and rabbit colon established that secretagogues, such as acetylcholine, vasoactive intestinal peptide, and locally liberated autacoids, such as prostaglandins and guanylin, can also induce chloride secretion *(141,142)*.

Electrogenic chloride secretion represents the major determinant of mucosal hydration in all the segments of the gastrointestinal tract. The general mechanism of chloride secretion in colon entails both discrete basolateral chloride entry steps into the cell and its exit across the apical membrane. Uptake of Cl across the BLM occurs through the electroneutral Na^+-K^+-$2Cl^-$ co-transporter (NKCC1) sensitive to loop-diuretic. Sodium entering with Cl returns to the serosal interstitial space via the ouabain-sensitive Na^+-K^+ ATPase pump. Basolateral K^+ channels open to recycle K^+ across this membrane, causing hyperpolarization of the cell, thus providing the driving force for Cl exit. Thus, Cl accumulates intracellularly above its electrochemical gradient and then exits through specific Cl channels, down its electrochemical gradient across the apical membranes *(141,142)*.

3.1.1. CFTR: An Apical Chloride Channel

The Cl channel responsible for major portion of chloride movement across the apical membrane is the product of the cystic fibrosis (CF) gene (CFTR) *(143)*. The normal CFTR is cAMP-activated, nonrectifying, or linear (i.e., it conducts ions with equal efficiency in either an inward or outward direction), with a permselectivity of $Cl^- > Br^- > I^-$. Recently, however, the presence of calcium-activated chloride channels (CaCC) that mediate Cl secretion in response to agonists that increase intracellular Ca^{2+} has also been suggested in the apical membranes of intestinal epithelial cells *(141)*. Molecular studies have also revealed a number of other voltage-gated Cl channels, such as CLC2 *(144)* and CLC5. CLC5 is expressed mainly in kidney and colon *(145)* with a permselectivity of $I^- > Cl^-$ but is not activated by cAMP. However, the role of these channels needs to be substantiated by furthur studies in the small intestine and colon.

CFTR acts not only as a cAMP-activated chloride channel but can perform additional roles. These vary from being a transporter for HCO_3^-, ATP, and water, to being a regulator of other ion channels, such as inactivation of ENaC and the regulation of outwardly rectifying large conductance Cl channel *(146,147)*. Recently, a role of CFTR in regulating the apical Cl^--HCO_3^- exchange *(148)* and DRA has also been defined *(149)*. CFTR is associated with two major human diseases: (i) CF, a common autosomal recessive disorder results from mutational inactivation of CFTR, which is characterized by severe obstructive lung pathology and abnormal intestinal tract functions *(150)*; and (ii) secretory diarrhea, a fluid and electrolyte disorder caused by increased Cl secretion in the gut *(151)*.

The intestine of CF patients does not exhibit Cl and fluid secretion, even in response to agonists such as cAMP, Ca^{2+} or acetylcholine. Additionally, in the absence of CFTR-induced inactivation of ENAC in the CF colon, absorption of NaCl and water continues, contributing to the concentration of mucus. This results in meconium ileus in approx 10% of newborns with CF and obstructive gut disease in adults. The development of transgenic CF mouse models suggested the ileocecum and colon as the primary sites of intestinal blockade, whereas jejunal obstructions occur less frequently *(152)*.

3.1.2. Regulation of Chloride Secretion

The primary points for regulation of the Cl secretory mechanism are the apical chloride channels (CFTR), basolateral K channels, and the NKCC1 transporter *(141)*. Regulation of Cl secretion can also occur through cellular factors such as Ca^{2+}, which can act on both basolateral potassium and apical chloride channels to increase their open probability *(141)*.

CFTR can be regulated through covalent modification, such as phosphorylation of the regulatory domain. CFTR is a large protein comprising of 12 transmembrane segments that are presumed to form the pore of the channel, two nucleotide binding folds as well as a large regulatory domain that contains consensus sequences for phosphorylation by several protein kinases *(141)*. CFTR is regulated in a two-step process that involves covalent modification of the regulatory domain by cAMP-dependent protein kinase A (PKA), followed by nucleotide binding and hydrolysis in the nucleotide binding domains *(141)*. Both these steps are required for opening of the channel. CFTR activation by cAMP in the colon does not appear to involve detectable exocytosis, which can increase the channel density on apical membrane *(147)*. Regulation of CFTR by other protein kinases, for example protein kinase C (PKC)ε has also been proposed *(142)*. There is an evidence that PKC-specific phosphorylation is required for continued activation of CFTR by PKA *(153)*. Vaandrager at al. *(154)* demonstrated that cyclic guanosine 5'-monophosphate (cGMP) via cGMP-regulated (G) protein kinase II (PKG II) mediates the effect of Sta (*Escherichia coli*, heat stable enterotoxin) in increasing chloride secretion.

Active chloride secretion has been postulated to be localized to crypt, but not surface epithelial cells, which correlates with the observation that expression of transport proteins such as CFTR and NKCC1, both essential for eliciting Cl secretion, appears most often to be restricted to cells located in the crypt *(154)*.

3.2. K⁺ Secretion

In parallel to chloride secretion, the colonic epithelium is able to secrete K^+. Active K^+ secretion has been demonstrated in all portions of mammalian colon including humans *(4)*. Intake of low salt diet, which leads to an increase in plasma levels of aldosterone, is known to enhance K⁺ secretion *(4)*. Epithelia in distal portions of nephron and colon adapt to chronic dietary potassium loading by increasing the rates of K secretion and thus protecting against the lethal effects of hyperkalemia *(155)*. K⁺ secretion can also be stimulated by cAMP-dependent secretagogues and appears to occur concomitantly with Cl⁻ secretion *(156)*. The cellular paradigm for K⁺ secretion is similar to that proposed for Cl secretion. Potassium is accumulated in the cell and then leaves across an apical K⁺ conductance when K⁺ secretion is stimulated. Aldosterone-induced K⁺ secretion is inhibited by removal of either Na or Cl from serosal medium or by bumetanide, suggesting the involvement of the NKCC1 in the uptake of K across the BLM *(157)*. K⁺ secretion is also linked to Na⁺-K⁺ pump as serosal addition of ouabain inhibits K⁺ secretion. Besides its role in establishing driving gradients for K⁺ secretion, there have been reports that the Na⁺-K⁺ pump can also supply the secreted K⁺ instead of NKCC1 *(1)*. K⁺ secretion is sensitive to inhibition by classical K⁺ channel blockers, e.g., barium and tetraethylammonium ion, applied luminally.

3.3. HCO$_3^-$ Secretion

HCO$_3^-$ secretion is a key function that occurs in the stomach, pancreas, and small and large intestine. HCO$_3^-$ secretion is particularly important in the duodenum to protect the mucosa against acidic effluents from the stomach *(158)*. In the ileum and colon, HCO$_3^-$ secretion is suggested to be an important means of chloride conservation by the apical Cl⁻-HCO$_3^-$ exchange. Additionally, HCO$_3^-$ secretion may be needed for maintaining the pH in the luminal membrane microenvironment through out the length of the intestine.

Trans-epithelial secretion of HCO$_3^-$ may involve more than one mechanism. The likely source of secreted HCO$_3^-$ may involve either the carrier-mediated uptake of HCO$_3^-$ across the BLM (Na⁺-HCO$_3^-$ co-transporter) and/or production of HCO$_3^-$ by intracellular carbonic anhydrase activity. The HCO$_3^-$ exit across the apical membrane has both electrogenic and electroneutral components.

Electrogenic HCO$_3^-$ secretion is stimulated by an increase in intracellular concentrations of second messengers, cAMP, cGMP or Ca^{2+} *(159)*. CFTR is known to be permeable to HCO$_3^-$, [HCO$_3^-$ to Cl⁻ permeability ratios range from 1:8–1:4] making it a suitable candidate for an electrogenic HCO$_3^-$ secretory component *(159)*. In vivo perfusion studies with CFTR knock-out mice showed marked impairment in both basal and stimulated HCO$_3^-$ secretion *(160)*. Similarly, Clarke et al. *(161)* demonstrated that CFTR participates in cAMP-stimulated HCO$_3^-$ secretion across the murine duodenum and the absence of CFTR caused a reduction in this response. These studies demonstrate a central role of CFTR in HCO$_3^-$ secretion and exclude the possibility that there are separate HCO$_3^-$ channels mediating this secretion in the intestine, although, the hypothesis that CFTR can conduct both Cl⁻ and HCO$_3^-$ is complicated by the anomalous mole fraction behavior of channel *(162)*, i.e., channel conductance of a less permeable ion is greatly reduced in the presence of a more permeable ion. Recently, Pratha et al. *(163)* identified a key role for CFTR in the maintenance of normal human duodenal bicarbonate secretion and also suggested the existence of a cGMP-Ca^{2+}-sensitive HCO$_3^-$ channel, which can compensate for dysfunctional CFTR in duodenal epithelium from patients with CF.

Studies with CF mouse have established that CFTR is required for cAMP stimulation of Cl⁻-HCO$_3^-$ exchange *(161)*. In an electroneutral mechanism, HCO$_3^-$ is exchanged for intralumenal Cl⁻ provided by the cAMP-stimulated Cl⁻ channel, CFTR, by means of an apical Cl⁻-HCO$_3^-$ exchange. Both electrogenic and electroneutral mechanisms may operate concomitantly, however the relative contribution of each can differ depending on the luminal environment and the activity of basolateral mechanism(s) of HCO$_3^-$ uptake *(164)*.

In summary, the absorptive and secretory pathways of the colonic epithelial cells are crucial for the maintenance of electrolyte homeostasis of the body, health and integrity of the epithelium, as well as the health of colonocytes. Recent expansion of our knowledge with respect to the molecular identity and structure–function studies of a number of these transporters has greatly helped our understanding of the physiology and molecular basis of the diseases of the colon. Future studies, focusing on the molecular identity of the other uncharacterized transporters reviewed here, as well as the molecular regulation of the transporters presented in this review, will be of great benefit for a better understanding of the colonic pathophysiology.

REFERENCES

1. Montrose MH, Keely SJ, Barrett KE. Electrolyte secretion and absorption: small intestine and colon. In *Textbook of Gastroenterology, 3rd ed.* Yamada T, Alpers DH, Laine L, Owyang C, Powell DW (eds.), Lippincott Williams & Wilkins, Philadelphia, PA, 1999, pp. 320–355.
2. Rao M. Absorption and secretion of water and electrolytes. In *Small Bowel Disorders.* Ratricke RN, (ed.), Arnold Press, London, UK, 2000, pp. 116–133.
3. Fujimoto T. Cell biology of caveolae and its implication for clinical medicine. *Nagoya J. Med. Sci.*, **63** (2000) 9–18.
4. Binder HJ, Sandle GI. Electrolyte transport in the mammalian colon. In *Physiology of the Gastrontestinal Tract,* 3rd ed., Johnson LR (ed.), Raven Press, New York, NY, 1994, pp. 2133–2171.
5. Ramaswamy K, Harig JM, Kleinman JG, Harris MS. Characteristics of Na^+/H^+ and Cl^-/HCO_3^- antiport systems in human ileal brush border membrane vesicles. *NY Acad. Sci.*, **574** (1989) 128–130.
6. Dudeja PK, Harig JM, Baldwin ML, Cragoe JEJ, Ramaswamy K, Brasitus TA. Na^+ transport in human proximal colonic apical membrane vesicles. *Gastroenterology*, **106** (1994) 125–133.
7. Dudeja PK, Baldwin ML, Harig JM, Cragoe EJ Jr, Ramaswamy K, Brasitus TA. Mechanisms of Na^+ transport in human distal colonic apical membrane vesicles. *Biochim. Biophys. Acta*, **1193** (1994) 67–76.
8. Dudeja PK, Rao DD, Syed I, et al. Intestinal distribution of human Na^+/H^+ exchanger isoforms NHE1, NHE2, and NHE3 mRNA. *Am. J. Physiol. Gastrointest. Liver Physiol.*, **271** (1996) G483–G493.
9. Malakooti J, Dahdal RY, Schmidt L, Layden TJ, Dudeja PK, Ramaswamy K. Molecular cloning, tissue distribution, and functional expression of the human $Na^{(+)}/H^{(+)}$ exchanger NHE2. *Am. J. Physiol.*, **277** (1999) G383– G390.
10. Malakooti J, Memark VC, Dudeja PK, Ramaswamy K. Transcriptional regulation of the human Na+/H+ exchanger NHE3 isoform. *Gastroenterology*, **118** (2000) A607.
11. Malakooti J, Dahdal RY, Dudeja PK, Layden TJ, Ramaswamy K. The human $Na^{(+)}/H^{(+)}$ exchanger NHE2 gene: genomic organization and promoter characterization. *Am. J. Physiol. Gastrointest. Liver Physiol.*, **280** (2001) G763–G773.
12. Sellin JH, De Soignie R. Ion transport in human colon in vitro. *Gastroenterology*, **93** (1987) 441–448.
13. Devroede GJ, Phillips SF. Conservation of sodium, chloride, and water by the human colon. *Gastroenterology*, **56** (1969) 101–109.
14. Devroede GJ, Phillips SF, Code CF, Lind JF. Regional differences in rates of insorption of sodium and water from the human large intestine. *Can. J. Physiol. Pharmacol.*, **49** (1971) 1023–1029.
15. Edmonds CJ, Godfrey RC. Measurement of electrical potentials of the human rectum and pelvic colon in normal and aldosterone-treated patients. *Gut*, **11** (1970) 330–337.
16. Levitan R, Fordtran JS, Burrows BA, Ingelfinger FJ. Water and salt absorption in the human colon. *J. Clin. Invest.*, **41** (1962) 1754–1759.
17. Grady GF, Duhamel RC, Moore EW. Active transport of sodium by human colon in vitro. *Gastroenterology*, **59** (1972) 583–588.
18. Hawker PC, Mashiter KE, Turnberg LA. Mechanisms of transport of Na^+, Cl^- and K^+ in the human colon. *Gastroenterology*, **74** (1978) 1241–1247.
19. Rask-Madsen J, Hjelt K. Effect of amiloride on electrical activity and electrolyte transport in human colon. *Scand. J. Gastroenterol.*, **12** (1977) 1–6.
20. Sandle GI, Wills NK, Alles W, Binder HJ. Electrophysiology of the human colon: evidence of segmental heterogeneity. *Gut*, **27** (1986) 999–1005.

21. Sandle GI, Mcglone F. Segmental variability of membrane conductances in rat and human colonic epithelia. *Pflugers Arch.*, **410** (1987) 173–180.
22. Schiller LR, Santa Ana CA, Morawski SG, Fordtran JS. Effect of amiloride on sodium transport in the proximal, distal, and entire human colon in vivo. *Dig. Dis. Sci.*, **33** (1988) 969–976.
23. Frizzell RA, Koch MJ, Schultz SG. Ion transport by rabbit colon. I. Active and passive components. *J. Membr. Biol.*, **27** (1976) 297–316.
24. Schultz SG. A cellular model for active sodium absorption by mammalian colon. *Annu. Rev. Physiol.*, **46** (1984) 435–451.
25. Mahajan RJ, Baldwin ML, Harig JM, Ramaswamy K, Dudeja PK. Chloride transport in human proximal colonic apical membrane vesicles. *Biochim. Biophys. Acta*, **1280** (1996) 12–18.
26. Dudeja PK, Harig JM, Ramswamy K, Prell M, Brasitus TA. Evidence for a carrier mediated Cl^-/HCO_3^- exchange process in human distal colonic apical membrane vesicles. *Gastroenterology*, **102** (1992) A208.
27. Dudeja PK, Foster ES, Brasitus TA. Na^+/H^+ antiporter of rat colonic basolateral membrane vesicles. *Am. J. Physiol.*, **257** (1989) G624–G632.
28. Knickelbein RG, Aronson PS, Dobbins JW. Membrane distribution of sodium-hydrogen and chloride-bicarbonate exchangers in crypt and villus cell membranes from rabbit ileum. *J. Clin. Invest.*, **82** (1988) 2158–2163.
29. Haggerty JG, Agarwal N, Reilly RF, Adelberg EA, Slayman CW. Pharmacologically different Na^+/H^+ antiporters on the apical and basolateral surfaces of cultured porcine kidney cells (LLC-PK1). *Proc. Natl. Acad. Sci. USA*, **85** (1988) 6797–6801.
30. Tyagi S, Joshi V, Alrefai WA, Gill RA, Ramaswamy K, Dudeja PK. Evidence for a Na^+-H^+ exchange across human colonic basolateral plasma membranes purified from organ donor colons. *Dig. Dis. Sci.*, **45** (2000) 2282–2289.
31. Yun CHC, Tse CM, Nath SK, Levine SK, Brant SR, Donowitz M. Mammalian Na^+-H^+ exchanger gene family: structure and function studies. *Am. J. Physiol.*, **269** (1995) G1–G11.
32. Orlowski J, Grinstein S. Na^+/H^+ Exchangers of Mammalian Cells. *J. Biol. Chem.*, **272** (1997) 22,373–22,376.
33. Szaszi K, Grinstein S, Orlowski J, Kapus A. Regulation of the epithelial $Na^{(+)}/H^{(+)}$ exchanger isoform by the cytoskeleton. *Cell Physiol. Biochem.*, **10** (2000) 265–272.
34. Counillon L, Pouyssegur J. The expanding family of eucaryotic $Na^{(+)}/H^{(+)}$ exchangers. *J. Biol. Chem.*, **275** (2000) 1–4.
35. Noel J, Pouyssegur J. Hormonal regulation, pharmacology, and membrane sorting of vertebrate Na^+/H^+ exchanger isoforms. *Am. J. Physiol.*, **268** (1995) C283–C296.
36. Baird NR, Orlowski J, Szabo EZ, et al. Molecular cloning, genomic organization, and functional expression of Na^+/H^+ exchanger isoform 5 (NHE5) from human brain. *J. Biol. Chem.*, **274** (1999) 4377–4382.
37. Donowitz M, Janecki A, Akhter S, et al. Short-term regulation of NHE3 by EGF and protein kinase C but not protein kinase A involves vesicle trafficking in epithelial cells and fibroblasts. *Ann. NY Acad. Sci.*, **915** (2000) 30–42.
38. Minkoff C, Shenolikar S, Weinman EJ. Assembly of signaling complexes by the sodium-hydrogen exchanger regulatory factor family of PDZ-containing proteins. *Curr. Opin. Nephrol. Hypertens.*, **8**(1999) 603–608.
39. Shenolikar S, Weinman EJ. NHERF: targeting and trafficking membrane proteins. *Am. J. Physiol. Renal Physiol.*, **280** (2001) F389–F395.
40. Khurana S. Role of actin cytoskeleton in regulation of ion transport: examples from epithelial cells. *J. Membr. Biol.*, **178** (2000) 73–87.
41. Tse CM, Brant SR, Walker MS, Pouyssegur J, Donowitz M. Cloning and sequencing of a rabbit cDNA encoding an intestinal and kidney-specific Na^+/H^+ exchanger isoform (NHE3). *J. Biol. Chem.*, **267** (1992) 9340–9346.
42. Orlowski J, Kandasamy RA, Shull GE. Molecular cloning of putative members of the Na^+/H^+ exchanger gene family. *J. Biol. Chem.*, **267** (1992) 9331–9339.
43. Bookstein C, DePaoli AM, Xie Y, et al. Na^+/H^+ exchangers, NHE1 and NHE3, of rat intestine. Expression and localization. *J. Clin. Invest.*, **93** (1994) 106–113.
44. Hoogerwerf S, Tsao SC, Devuyst O, et al. NHE2 and NHE3 are human and rabbit intestinal brush-border proteins. *Am. J. Physiol.*, **270** (1996) G29–G41.
45. Tse CM, Ma AI, Yang VW, et al. Molecular cloning and expression of a cDNA encoding the rabbit ileal villus cell basolateral membrane Na^+/H^+ exchanger. *EMBO J.*, **10** (1991) 1957–1967.
46. Wormmeester L, Sanchez de Medina F, Kokke F, et al. Quantitative contribution of NHE2 and NHE3 to rabbit ileal brush-border Na^+/H^+ exchange. *Am. J. Physiol.*, **274** (1998) C1261–C1272.
47. Donowitz M. Ca^{2+} in the control of active intestinal Na and Cl transport and involvement of neurohumoral action. *Am. J. Physiol.*, **245** (1983) G165–G177.

48. Donowitz M, Welsh MJ. Ca^{2+} and cyclic AMP in regulation of intestinal Na, K and Cl transport. *Annu. Rev. Physiol.*, **48** (1986) 135–150.

49. Pouyssegur J. Molecular biology and hormonal regulation of vertebrate Na^+/H^+ exchanger isoforms. *Renal Physiol. Biochem.*, **17** (1994) 190–203.

50. Bookstein C, Musch MW, Dudeja PK, et al. Inverse relationship between membrane lipid fluidity and activity of Na^+-H^+ exchangers, NHE1 and NHE3, in transfected fibroblasts. *J. Membr. Biol.*, **160** (1997) 183–192.

51. Gill R, Tyagi S, Syed I, et al. Regulation of NHE3 by nitric oxide in Caco-2 cells. *Am. J. Physiol. Gastrointest. Liver Physiol.*, **283** (2002) G747–G756.

52. Janecki AJ, Montrose MH, Zimniak P, et al. Subcellular redistribution is involved in acute regulation of the brush border Na^+/H^+ exchanger isoform 3 in human colon adenocarcinoma cell line Caco-2. *J. Biol. Chem.*, **273** (1998) 8790–8798.

53. Yang W, Dyck JR, Fliegel L. Regulation of NHE1 expression in L6 muscle cells. *Biochim. Biophys. Acta*, **1306** (1996) 107–113.

54. Wang H, Singh D, Yang W, Dyck JR, Fliegel L. Structure and analysis of the mouse Na^+/H^+ exchanger (NHE1) gene: homology and conservation of splice sites. *Mol. Cell. Biochem.*, **165** (1996) 155–159.

55. Facanha AL, dos Reis MC, Montero-Lomeli M. Structural study of the porcine Na^+/H^+ exchanger NHE1 gene and its 5'- flanking region. *Mol. Cell. Biochem.*, **210** (2000) 91–99.

56. Blaurock MC, Reboucas NA, Kusnezov JL, Igarashi P. Phylogenetically conserved sequences in the promoter of the rabbit sodium-hydrogen exchanger isoform 1 gene (NHE1/SLC9A1). *Biochim. Biophy. Acta*, **1262** (1995) 159–163.

57. Muller YL, Collins JF, Bai L, Xu H, Ghishan FK. Molecular cloning and characterization of the rat NHE2 gene promoter. *Biochim. Biophy. Acta*, **1442**(1998) 314–319.

58. Cano A. Characterization of the rat NHE3 promoter. *Am. J. Physiol.*, **271** (1996) F629–F636.

59. Miller RT, Counillon L, Pages G, Lifton RP, Sardet C, Pouyssegur J. Structure of the 5'-flanking regulatory region and gene for the human growth factor-activatable Na/H exchanger NHE-1. *J. Biol. Chem.*, **266** (1991) 10,813–10,819.

60. Kandasamy RA, Orlowski J. Genomic organization and glucocorticoid transcriptional activation of the rat Na^+/H^+ exchanger NHE3 gene. *J. Biol. Chem.*, **271** (1996) 10,551–10,559.

61. Cano A, Baum M, Moe OW. Thyroid hormone stimulates the renal Na/H exchanger NHE3 by transcriptional activation [in process citation]. *Am. J. Physiol.*, **276** (1999) C102–C108.

62. Besson P, Fernandez-Rachubinski F, Yang W, Fliegel L. Regulation of Na^+/H^+ exchanger gene expression: mitogenic stimulation increases NHE1 promoter activity. *Am. J. Physiol.*, **274** (1998) C831–C839.

63. Bai L, Collins JF, Muller YL, Xu H, Kiela PR, Ghishan FK. Characterization of cis-elements required for osmotic response of rat $Na^{(+)}/H^{(+)}$ exchanger-2 (NHE2) gene. *Am. J. Physiol.*, **277** (1999) R1112–R1119.

64. Kiela PR, Guner YS, Xu H, Collins JF, Ghishan FK. Age- and tissue-specific induction of NHE3 by gluco-corticoids in the rat small intestine. *Am. J. Physiol. Cell Physiol.*, **278** (2000) C629–C637.

65. Alvarez de la Rosa D, Canessa CM, Fyfe GK, Zhang P. Structure and regulation of amiloride-sensitive sodium channels. *Annu. Rev. Physiol.*, **62** (2000) 573–594.

66. Benos DJ, Stanton BA. Functional domains within the degenerin/epithelial sodium channel (Deg/ENaC) superfamily of ion channels. *J. Physiol.*, **520** (1999) 631–644.

67. Tyagi S, Ramaswamy K, Dudeja PK. Evidence for the existence of a Cl^--HCO_3^- exchange process in the human colonic basolateral membrane vesicles. *Gastroenterology*, **110** (1996) A369.

68. Rajendran VM, Binder HJ. Cl^--HCO_3 and Cl^--OH exchanges mediate Cl uptake in apical membrane vesicles of rat distal colon. *Am. J. Physiol.*, **264** (1993) G874–G879.

69. Lohi H, Kujala M, Kerkela E, Saarialho-Kere U, Kestila M, Kere J. Mapping of five new putative anion transporter genes in human and characterization of SLC26A6, a candidate gene for pancreatic anion exchanger. *Genomics*, **70** (2000) 102–112.

70. Waldegger S, Moschen I, Ramirez A, et al. Cloning and characterization of slc26a6, a novel member of the solute carrier 26 gene family. *Genomics*, **72** (2001) 43–50.

71. Alper SL. The band 3-related AE anion exchanger gene family. *Cell Physiol. Biochem.*, **4** (1994) 265–281.

72. Tsuganezawa H, Kobayashi K, Iyori M, et al. A new member of the HCO_3^- transporter superfamily is an apical anion exchanger of beta-intercalated cells in the kidney. *J. Biol. Chem.*, **1** (2000) 1.

73. Kopito RR. Molecular Biology of the anion exchanger gene family. *Int. Rev. Cytol.*, **123** (1990) 177–199.

74. Chow A, Zhou W, Jacobson R. Regulation of AE2 Cl^-/HCO_3^- exchanger during intestinal development. *Am. J. Physiol.*, **271** (1996) G330–G337.

75. Cox KH, Adair-Kirk TL, Cox JV. Variant AE2 anion exchanger transcripts accumulate in multiple cell types in the chicken gastric epithelium. *J. Biol. Chem.*, **271** (1996) 8895–8902.

76. Medina JF, Lecanda J, Acin A, Ciesielczyk P, Prieto J. Tissue-specific N-terminal isoforms from overlapping alternate promoters of the human AE2 anion exchanger gene. *Biochem. Biophys. Res. Commun.*, **267** (2000) 228–235.

77. Alrefai WA, Tyagi S, Nazir TM, et al. Human intestinal anion exchanger isoforms: expression, distribution, and membrane localization. *Biochim. Biophys. Acta*, **1511** (2001) 17–27.

78. Chow A, Dobbins JW, Aronson PS, Igarashi P. cDNA cloning and localization of a band 3 related protein from ileum. *Am. J. Physiol.*, **263** (1992) G345–G352.

79. Stuart-Tilley AK, Shmukler BE, Brown D, Alper SL. Immunolocalization and tissue-specific splicing of AE2 anion exchanger in mouse kidney [in process citation]. *J. Am. Soc. Nephrol.*, **9** (1998) 946–959.

80. Alper SL, Rossmann H, Wilhelm S, Stuart-Tilley AK, Shmukler BE, Seidler U. Expression of AE2 anion exchanger in mouse intestine. *Am. J. Physiol.*, **277** (1999) G321–G32.

81. Lubman RL, Danto SI, Chao DC, Fricks CE, Crandall ED. Cl⁻-HCO₃⁻exchanger isoform AE2 is restricted to the basolateral surface of alveolar epithelial cell monolayers. *Am. J. Respir. Cell Mol. Biol.*, **12** (1995) 211–219.

82. Stuart-Tilley A, Sardet C, Pouyssegur J, Schwartz MA, Brown D, Alper SL. Immunolocalization of anion exchanger AE2 and cation exchanger NHE1 in distinct adjacent cells of gastric mucosa. *Am. J. Physiol.*, **266** (1994) C559–C568.

83. Rossmann H, Nader M, Seidler U, Classen M, Alper S. Basolateral membrane localization of the AE2 isoform of the anion exchanger family in both stomach and ileum. *Gastroenterology*, **108** (1995) A319.

84. Kere J, Lohi H, Hoglund P. Genetic disorder of membrane transport III. Congenital chloride diarrhea. *Am. J. Physiol.*, **276** (1999) G7–G13.

85. Moseley RH, Hoglund P, Wu GD, et al. Downregulated in adenoma gene encodes a chloride transporter defective in congenital chloride diarrhea. *Am. J. Physiol.*, **267** (1999) G185–G192.

86. Bieberdorf FA, Gordon P, Fordtran JS. Pathogenesis of congenital alkalosis with diarrhea: implications for the physiology of normal ileal electrolyte absorption and secretion. *J. Clin. Invest.*, **51** (1972) 1958–1968.

87. Silberg DG, Wang W, Moseley RH, Traber PG. The down-regulated in adenoma (dra) gene encodes an intestine-specific membrane sulfate transport protein. *J. Biol. Chem.*, **270** (1995) 11,897–11,902.

88. Melvin JE, Park K, Richardson L, Schultheis PJ, Shull GE. Mouse down-regulated in adenoma (DRA) is an intestinal Cl(⁻)/HCO(3)(⁻) exchanger and is up-regulated in colon of mice lacking the NHE3 Na(⁺)/H(⁺) exchanger. *J. Biol. Chem.*, **274** (1999) 22,855–22,861.

89. Rajendran VM, Binder HJ. Characterization and molecular localization of anion transporters in colonic epithelial cells. *Ann. NY Acad. Sci.*, **915** (2000) 15–29.

90. Rajendran VM, Black J, Ardito TA, et al. Regulation of DRA and AE1 in rat colon by dietary Na depletion. *Am. J. Physiol. Gastrointest. Liver Physiol.*, **279** (2000) G931–G942.

91. Alrefai WA, Tyagi S, Mansour F, et al. Sulfate and chloride transport in Caco-2 cells: differential regulation by thyroxine and the possible role of DRA gene. *Am. J. Physiol. Gastrointest. Liver Physiol.*, **280** (2001) G603–G613.

92. Hadjiagapiou C, Hausman A, Schmidt L, et al. Developmental and tissue distribution studies of anion exchanger AE2 in the human intestine. *Gastroenterology*, **111** (1997) A367.

93. Fejes-Toth G, Rusvai E, Cleaveland ES, Naray-Fejes-Toth A. Regulation of AE2 mRNA expression in the cortical collecting duct by acid/base balance. *Am. J. Physiol.*, **274** (1998) F596–F601.

94. Humphreys BD, Jiang L, Chernova MN, Alper SL. Hypertonic activation of AE2 anion exchanger in xenopus oocytes via NHE-mediated intracellular alkalization. *Am. J. Physiol.*, **268** (1995) C201–C209.

95. Saksena S, Gill R, Tyagi S, et al. Modulation of Cl⁻/OH–exchange activity in Caco-2 cells by nitric oxide. *Am. J. Physiol. Gastrointest. Liver Physiol.*, **283** (2002) G626–G633.

96. Saksena, S., Gill, R.K., Syed, I.A., et al. Inhibition of the apical Cl—OH- exchange activity in Caco2 cells by phorbol esters is mediated by protein kinase Cε. *Am. J. Physiol—Cell Physiol.* **283** (2002) C1492–C1500.

97. Cook SI, Sellin JH. Review article: short chain fatty acids in health and disease. Aliment *Pharmacol. Ther.*, **12** (1998) 499–507.

98. Ramakrishna BS, Mathan VI. Colonic dysfunction in acute diarrhoea: the role of luminal short chain fatty acids. *Gut*, **34** (1993) 1215–1218.

99. Velazquez OC, Lederer HM, Rombeau JL. Butyrate and the colonocyte. Production, absorption, metabolism, and therapeutic implications. *Adv. Exp. Med. Biol.*, **427** (1997) 123–134.

100. von Engelhardt W, Bartels J, Kirschberger S, Meyer zu Duttingdorf HD, Busche R. Role of short-chain fatty acids in the hind gut. *Vet. Q.*, **20(Suppl 3)** (1998) S52–S59.

101. Zhang J, Lupton JR. Dietary fibers stimulate colonic cell proliferation by different mechanisms at different sites. *Nutr. Cancer*, **22** (1994) 267–276.

102. Breuer RI, Soergel KH, Lashner BA, et al. Short chain fatty acid rectal irrigation for left-sided ulcerative colitis: a randomised, placebo controlled trial. *Gut*, **40** (1997) 485–491.

103. Kim YI. Short-chain fatty acids in ulcerative colitis. *Nutr. Rev.*, **56** (1998) 17–24.

104. Pouillart PR. Role of butyric acid and its derivatives in the treatment of colorectal cancer and hemoglobino-pathies. *Life Sci.*, **63** (1998) 1739–1760.

105. Bugaut M. Occurrence, absorption and metabolism of short chain fatty acids in the digestive tract of mammals. *Comp. Biochem. Physiol.*, **86B** (1987) 439–472.

106. Mortensen PB, Clausen MR. Short-chain fatty acids in the human colon: relation to gastrointestinal health and disease. *Scand. J. Gastroenterol. Suppl.*, **216** (1996) 132–148.

107. Harig JM, Soergel KH, Barry JA, Ramaswamy K. Transport of propionate by human ileal brush-border membrane vesicles. *Am. J. Physiol.*, **260** (1991) G776– G782.

108. Harig JM, NG EK, Dudeja PK, Brasitus TA, Ramaswamy K. Transport of n-butyrate into human colonic luminal membrane vesicles. *Am. J. Physiol.*, **271** (1996) G415–G422.

109. Charney AN, Micic L, Egnor RW. Nonionic diffusion of short-chain fatty acids across rat colon. *Am. J. Physiol.*, **274** (1998) G518–G524.

110. Chu S, Montrose MH. Non-ionic diffusion and carrier-mediated transport drive extracellular pH regulation of mouse colonic crypts. *J. Physiol. (Lond)*, **494** (1996) 783–793.

111. von Engelhardt W, Gros G, Burmester M, Hansen K, Becker G, Rechkemmer G. Functional role of bicarbon-ate in propionate transport across guinea-pig isolated caecum and proximal colon. *J. Physiol. (Lond)*, **477** (1994) 365–371.

112. Reynolds DA, Rajendran VM, Binder HJ. Bicarbonate-stimulated [^{14}C]butyrate uptake in basolateral mem-brane vesicles of rat distal colon. *Gastroenterology*, **105** (1993) 725–732.

113. Venugopalakrishnan J, Tyagi S, Ramaswamy K, Dudeja PK. Mechanism of n-butyrate transport across the human colonic basolateral membrane. *Gastroenterology*, **116** (1999) A941.

114. Musch MW, Bookstein C, Xie Y, Sellin JH, Chang EB. SCFA increase intestinal Na absorption by induction of NHE3 in rat colon and human intestinal C2/bbe cells. *Am. J. Physiol. Gastrointest. Liver Physiol.*, **280** (2001) G687–G693.

115. Hadjiagapiou C, Schmidt L, Dudeja PK, Layden TJ, Ramaswamy K. Mechanism(s) of butyrate transport in caco-2 cells: role of monocarboxylate transporter 1. *Am. J. Physiol. Gastrointest. Liver Physiol.*, **279** (2000) G775–G780.

116. Ritzhaupt A, Wood IS, Ellis A, Hosie KB, Shirazi-Beechey SP. Identification and characterization of a monocarboxylate transporter (MCT1) in pig and human colon: its potential to transport L-lactate as well as butyrate. *J. Physiol. (Lond)*, **513** (1998) 719–732.

117. Stein J, Zores M, Schroder O. Short-chain fatty acid (SCFA) uptake into Caco-2 cells by a pH-dependent and carrier mediated transport mechanism. *Eur. J. Nutr.*, **39** (2000) 121–125.

118. Alrefai WA, Tyagi S, Gill R, et al. Regulation of butyrate uptake in Caco2 cells: involvement of monocarboxylate transporter MCT1. *Gastroenterology*, **120** (2001) A528.

119. Halestrap AP, Price NT. The proton-linked monocarboxylate transporter (MCT) family: structure, function and regulation. *Biochem. J.*, **343** (1999) 281–299.

120. Price NT, Jackson VN, Halestrap AP. Cloning and sequencing of four new mammalian monocarboxylate transporter (MCT) homologues confirms the existence of a transporter family with an ancient past. *Biochem .J.*, **329** (1998) 321–328.

121. Tiruppathi C, Balkovetz DF, Ganapathy V, Miyamoto Y, Leibach FH. A proton gradient, not a sodium gradient, is the driving force for active transport of lactate in rabbit intestinal brush-border membrane vesicles. *Biochem. J.*, **256** (1988) 219–223.

122. Lamers JM. Some characteristics of monocarboxylic acid transfer across the cell membrane of epithelial cells from rat small intestine. *Biochim. Biophys. Acta*, **413** (1975) 465–476.

123. Foster ES, Jones WJ, Hayslett JP, Binder HJ. Role of aldosterone and dietary potassium in potassium adap-tation in the distal colon of the rat. *Gastroenterology*, **88** (1985) 41–46.

124. Agarwal R, Afzalpurkar R, Fordtran JS. Pathophysiology of potassium absorption and secretion by the human intestine. *Gastroenterology*, **107** (1994) 548–571.

125. Binder HJ, Sandle GI, Rajenderan VM. Colonic fluid and electrolyte transport in health and disease. In *The Large Intestine: Physiology, Pathophysiology, and Disease.* Phillips SF (ed.), Raven, New York, NY, 1991, pp. 141–168.

126. Binder HJ, Sangan P, Rajendran VM. Physiological and molecular studies of colonic H$^+$/K$^+$ ATPase. *Semin. Nephrol.*, **19** (1999) 405–414.

127. Gill R, Kunhiraman BP, Saksena S, Tyagi S, Dudeja PK. Expression of K$^+$-activated ATPase in apical membranes of the human distal colon. *Gastroenterology*, **120** (2001) A531.

128. Frederic J, Ahmed TB. The nongastric H$^+$-/K$^+$-ATPases: molecular and functional properties. *Am. J. Physiol.*, **276** (1999) F812–F824.

129. Sangan P, Kolla SS, Rajendran VM, Kashgarian M, Binder HJ. Colonic H-K-ATPase beta-subunit: identification in apical membranes and regulation by dietary K depletion. *Am. J. Physiol.*, **276** (1999) C350–C360.

130. Sangan P, Thevananther S, Sangan S, Rajendran VM, Binder HJ. Colonic H-K-ATPase alpha- and beta-subunits express ouabain-insensitive H-K-ATPase. *Am. J. Physiol. Cell Physiol.*, **279** (2000) C182–C189.

131. Pandiyan V, Rajendran VM, Binder HJ. Mucosal ouabain and Na^+ inhibit active $Rb^+(K^+)$ absorption in normal and sodium-depleted rat distal colon. *Gastroenterology*, **102** (1992) 1846–1853.

132. Wang KS, Ma T, Filiz F, Verkman AS, Bastidas JA. Colon water transport in transgenic mice lacking aquaporin-4 water channels. *Am. J. Physiol. Gastrointest. Liver Physiol.*, **279** (2000) G463–G470.

133. Wright EM, Loo DD. Coupling between Na^+, sugar, and water transport across the intestine. *Ann. NY Acad. Sci.*, **915** (2000) 54–66.

134. Ma T, Verkman AS. Aquaporin water channels in gastrointestinal physiology. *J. Physiol.*, **517** (1999) 317–326.

135. Naftalin RJ, Pedley KC. Regional crypt function in rat large intestine in relation to fluid absorption and growth of the pericryptal sheath. *J. Physiol.*, **514** (1999) 211–227.

136. Dudeja PK, Torania SA, Said HM. Evidence for a pH-dependent, DIDS-sensitive carrier mediated folate uptake mechanism in the human colonic luminal membrane vesicles. *Am. J. Physiol.*, **272** (1997) G1408–G1415.

137. Dudeja PK, Kode A, Alnounou M, Tyagi S, Torania S, Said HM. Mechanism of folate transport in the human colonic basolateral membranes. *Am. J. Physiol. Gastrointest. Liver Physiol.*, **281** (2001) G54–G60.

138. Kumar CK, Moyer MP, Dudeja PK, Said HM. A protein tyrosine kinase regulated, pH dependent, carrier-mediated uptake system for folate in human normal colonic epithelial cell line. *J. Biol. Chem.*, **272** (1997) 6226–6231.

139. Said HM, Rose R, Seetharam B. *Intestinal Absorption of Water Soluble Vitamins: Cellular and Molecular Aspects*. Academic Press, New York, NY, 2000.

140. Dudeja PK, Tyagi S, Jhandiya F, Said HM. Existence of a carrier mediated biotin uptake process in the human colonic apical membrane vesicles. *FASEB J.*, **10** (1996) A121.

141. Barrett KE, Keely SJ. Chloride secretion by the intestinal epithelium: molecular basis and regulatory aspects. *Annu. Rev. Physiol.*, **62** (2000) 535–572.

142. Morris AP. The regulation of epithelial cell cAMP- and calcium-dependent chloride channels. *Adv. Pharmacol.*, **46** (1999) 209–251.

143. Trezise AE, Buchwald M. In vivo cell-specific expression of the cystic fibrosis transmembrane conductance regulator. *Nature*, **353** (1991) 434–437.

144. Kirk KL. Chloride channels and tight junctions. Focus on "Expression of the chloride channel ClC-2 in the murine small intestine epithelium". *Am. J. Physiol. Cell Physiol.*, **279** (2000) C1675–C1676.

145. Vandewalle A, Cluzeaud F, Peng KC, et al. Tissue distribution and subcellular localization of the ClC-5 chloride channel in rat intestinal cells. *Am. J. Physiol. Cell Physiol.*, **280** (2001) C373–C381.

146. Greger R, Mall M, Bleich M, et al. Regulation of epithelial ion channels by the cystic fibrosis transmembrane conductance regulator. *J. Mol. Med.*, **74** (1996) 527–534.

147. Greger R. Role of CFTR in the colon. *Annu. Rev. Physiol.*, **62** (2000) 467–491.

148. Lee MG, Wigley WC, Zeng W, et al. Regulation of Cl^-/HCO_3^- exchange by cystic fibrosis transmembrane conductance regulator expressed in NIH 3T3 and HEK 293 cells. *J. Biol. Chem.*, **274** (1999) 3414–3421.

149. Wheat VJ, Shumaker H, Burnham C, Shull GE, Yankaskas JR, Soleimani M. CFTR induces the expression of DRA along with $Cl^-/HCO(3)^-$ exchange activity in tracheal epithelial cells. *Am. J. Physiol. Cell Physiol.*, **279** (2000) C62–C71.

150. Welsh MJ, Smith AE. Molecular mechanisms of CFTR chloride channel dysfunction in cystic fibrosis. *Cell*, **73** (1993) 1251–1254.

151. Gabriel SE, Brigman KN, Koller BH, Boucher RC, Stutts MJ. Cystic fibrosis heterozygote resistance to cholera toxin in the cystic fibrosis mouse model. *Science*, **266** (1994) 107–109.

152. Rozmahel R, Gyomorey K, Plyte S, et al. Incomplete rescue of cystic fibrosis transmembrane conductance regulator deficient mice by the human CFTR cDNA. *Hum. Mol. Genet.*, **6** (1997) 1153–1162.

153. Jia Y, Mathews CJ, Hanrahan JW. Phosphorylation by protein kinase C is required for acute activation of cystic fibrosis transmembrane conductance regulator by protein kinase A. *J. Biol. Chem.*, **272** (1997) 4978–4984.

154. Vaandrager AB, Bot AG, Ruth P, Pfeifer A, Hofmann F, De Jonge HR. Differential role of cyclic GMP-dependent protein kinase II in ion transport in murine small intestine and colon. *Gastroenterology*, **118** (2000) 108–114.

155. Hayslett JP, Binder HJ. Mechanism of potassium adaptation. *Am. J. Physiol.*, **243** (1982) F103–F112.

156. Edmonds CJ, Willis CL. The effect of dietary sodium and potassium intake on potassium secretion and kinetics in rat distal colon. *J. Physiol.*, **424** (1990) 317–327.

157. Halm DR, Halm ST. Aldosterone stimulates K secretion prior to onset of Na absorption in guinea pig distal colon. *Am. J. Physiol.*, **266** (1994) C552–C558.

158. Quigley EM, Turnberg LA. pH of the microclimate lining human gastric and duodenal mucosa in vivo. Studies in control subjects and in duodenal ulcer patients. *Gastroenterology*, **92** (1987) 1876–1884.
159. Illek B, Fischer H, Machen TE. Genetic disorders of membrane transport. II. Regulation of CFTR by small molecules including HCO_3. *Am. J. Physiol.*, **275** (1998) G1221–G1226.
160. Hogan DL, Crombie DL, Isenberg JI, Svendsen P, Schaffalitzky de Muckadell OB, Ainsworth MA. CFTR mediates cAMP- and Ca^{2+}-activated duodenal epithelial HCO_3^- secretion. *Am. J. Physiol.*, **272** (1997) G872–G878.
161. Clarke LL, Harline MC. Dual role of CFTR in cAMP-stimulated HCO_3^- secretion across murine duodenum. *Am. J. Physiol.*, **274** (1998) G718–G726.
162. Tabcharani JA, Rommens JM, Hou YX, et al. Multi-ion pore behaviour in the CFTR chloride channel. *Nature*, **366** (1993) 79–82.
163. Pratha VS, Hogan DL, Martensson BA, Bernard J, Zhou R, Isenberg JI. Identification of transport abnormalities in duodenal mucosa and duodenal enterocytes from patients with cystic fibrosis. *Gastroenterology*, **118** (2000) 1051–1060.
164. Isenberg JI, Ljungstrom M, Safsten B, Flemstrom G. Proximal duodenal enterocyte transport: evidence for $Na^{(+)}$-H^+ and $Cl^{(-)}$- HCO_3^- exchange and $NaHCO_3$ cotransport. *Am. J. Physiol.*, **265** (1993) G677–G685.

2

Normal Motility and Smooth Muscle Function

Mary Francis Otterson

1. INTRODUCTION

The gastrointestinal tract normally functions to move ingested food, in an organized fashion, from the oropharynx, through the stomach, small intestine and colon and into the rectum, from which it can be expelled. The primary function of the colon is to absorb water and electrolytes from the chyme delivered and, thus, determine the frequency, consistency, and volume of stools eliminated. The colon (i) mixes luminal contents so that they are optimally exposed to the absorptive mucosal surface; (ii) slowly propels feces caudally to allow adequate time for the absorption of water, electrolytes, and metabolic products of bacterial degradation; (iii) allows storage of feces; and (iv) rapidly and efficiently propels feces during defecation. Transit time through the colon is significantly slower than through the proximal bowel and is achieved through contractions that are less coordinated. The discoordination is due to highly variable frequency and phase unlocking of electrical activity within the colon.

From: *Colonic Diseases*
Edited by: T. R. Koch © Humana Press Inc., Totowa, NJ

2. INDIVIDUAL PHASIC CONTRACTIONS

The colon exhibits both short and long duration contractions (Fig. 1). This is in contrast to the stomach and small intestine, where only short duration contractions are observed. In both humans and dogs, short duration contractions last less than 15 s and occur at a frequency of 2–13/min. The frequency of the long duration is 0.5–2/min. The short and long duration contractions may occur independently of one another, or the short duration contractions may be superimposed upon the long duration contractions. The long duration contractions may occasionally propagate in either an orad or caudad direction, however, the short duration contractions rarely appear to propagate. The viscosity of fecal contents may necessitate the longer duration contractions for efficient propulsion of contents. Both types of colonic phasic contractions are under myogenic, neural, and chemical control (1).

3. MYOGENIC CONTROL

The interior of the smooth muscle cell is maintained electronegative relative to the extracellular fluid. This negative potential is called the resting membrane potential. The resting membrane potential depolarizes periodically and this is termed electrical control activity (ECA) or slow waves (Fig. 2). When neural or chemical stimulation is present, the amplitude of depolarization may exceed an excitation threshold potential. This causes voltage-sensitive calcium channels to open and produces an inward calcium current. Alternately, internal calcium stores may be mobilized. A burst of rapid electrical oscillations called electrical response activity (ERA), spikebursts, or action potentials (2–5) results. ERA has a one-to-one relationship with individual phasic contractions (Fig. 2). Because ERA can only occur during the depolarization phase of ECA, the frequency of individual phasic contractions is determined by and limited to the frequency of ECA. Beyond this myogenic control, it must be understood that neural and chemical stimulation may not be present during every cycle of ECA and, thus, contractions do not occur at maximal frequency (Fig. 2).

The frequency of human colonic ECA ranges from 2–13 cycles/min. Within the ascending and sigmoid colon, 2–9 cycles/min is the dominant frequency. This narrows to a range of 9–13 cycles/min in the transverse and descending colon (6).

Long duration contractions within the colon are controlled by intermittent bursts of membrane potential oscillations called contractile electrical complexes (CECs) (7). The frequency of membrane potential oscillations within a CEC occur in the range of 25–40 cycles/min. These oscillations generally exceed the contractile excitation threshold and produce a long duration contraction of the colon that has duration equal to that of the CEC. The oscillations of ERA associated with a CEC have been called continuous ERA, because the activity persists throughout the duration of several ECA cycles. CECs and the long duration contractions they represent most frequently propagate in a caudal direction, but occasionally propagate in an orad direction.

4. NEURAL CONTROL

Control of colonic contractile activity rests within the enteric, autonomic, and central nervous system. Just as within the rest of the gastrointestinal tract, the enteric nervous system plays a prominent role in the moment-to-moment control of contractile activity. The autonomic nervous system, both sympathetic and parasympathetic, exerts significant influences and may play a role in pathologic states, such as irritable bowel syndrome. Finally, because of the ability of animals and humans to willfully control the timing of the voluntary release of feces, the central nervous system plays a critical role in colonic contractile function.

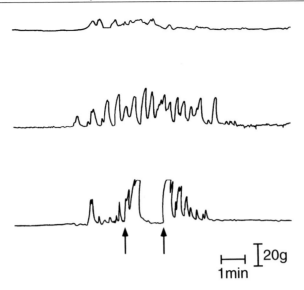

Fig. 1. The topmost tracing demonstrates long duration contractions in the proximal colon of the dog approx 5 cm distal to the ileocolonic junction. The second tracing is short duration colonic contractions at the same recording site. The final tracing shows two GMCs of the proximal colon. Note the suppression of contractile activity often the first GMC. Within the small intestine, GMCs have a specific electrical recording that is distinct from other contractions. This is not true in the colon.

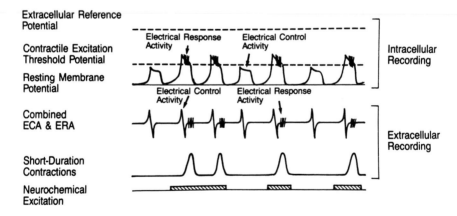

Fig. 2. The top tracings demonstrate the relationship between intracellularly recorded myoelectric activity, neurochemical excitation, and contractions. Resting membrane potential is negative with respect to the extracellular reference potential. In the absence of neurochemical excitation, the ECA depolarizations do not exceed the excitation threshold potential. Therefore, no ERA burst occurs nor contraction occurs. In contrast, during the second, third, fifth, and seventh ECA cycle, neurochemical excitation occurs, ECA depolarization exceeds the excitation threshold, an ERA burst occurs, and the muscle contracts. The lower electrical tracings demonstrate the relationship to extracellular myoelectric activity. Extracellular electrodes record from a large number of smooth muscle cells. The shape of the electrical recording depends upon whether the electrode is bipolar or monopolar and the distance between the poles of the recording device. (Reproduced from ref. 2 with permission)

5. ENTERIC NEURAL CONTROL

The enteric nervous system within the colon is organized in to two plexuses, the myenteric and the submucosal. The myenteric neurons are located between the circular and longitudinal muscle layers, and the submucosal plexus can be found within the muscularis propria. Nerve cell bodies within each plexus are organized and grouped into ganglia that range in size from several to 40 distinct soma. The neurons thought to be responsible for the control of colonic contractile activity consist of motor neurons, sensory neurons, and interganglionic and interplexus neurons.

Enteric motor neurons project axons to both the circular and longitudinal muscle layers. Each enteric neuron affects several smooth muscle cells. These neurons may be either excitatory or inhibitory. The excitatory neurotransmitter is acetylcholine and, in vivo, all spontaneous colonic contractile activity can be inhibited with atropine. There is some evidence that glutamate may also act as an excitatory neurotransmitter, much as what has been described within the central nervous system. The precise identification of the inhibitory neurotransmitter is more controversial. These nonadrenergic noncholinergic (NANC) neurons have several putative inhibitory neurotransmitters. These include nitric oxide, adenosine triphosphate (ATP) and vasoactive intestinal polypeptide (VIP) *(1,8–13)*. Both the excitatory and inhibitory motor neurons of the gut receive input from other enteric neurons as well as sympathetic and parasympathetic extrinsic neurons.

In addition to the cholinergic excitatory and NANC inhibitory neurons, a variety of peptidergic neurons have been mapped within the gut wall using immunohistochemistry. There is directionality to these neurons. For example, within the guinea pig small intestine, myenteric substance P and enkephalin-containing neurons project in an orad direction, and neuropeptide Y and gastrin-releasing peptide project in a caudad direction. The precise role of these peptidergic neurons in the control of human in vivo contractile activity has yet to be determined. It is possible that the role of these neurotransmitters may be elucidated with novel molecular techniques that allow the over expression or deletion of these peptides from the enteric nervous system.

Sensory neurons perceive mechanical and chemical stimulation from the luminal contents of the gut and project onto enteric as well as prevertebral and higher centers. This neural input provides the signal for both local enteric reflexes as well as higher reflexes. Substance P is one of the substances found within these sensory neurons. Sensory neurons synapse upon both the inhibitory and excitatory motor neurons and may act by stimulation or inhibition of spontaneous contractions.

Interganglionic neurons provide pathways to allow communication within the ganglia, while interplexus neurons project from one plexus to another. These neurons are critical for the coordination of colonic motor activity as well as epithelial transport.

6. AUTONOMIC NEURAL CONTROL

Sympathetic neural control of the colon occurs through the lumbar, splanchnic, and hypogastric nerves. The parasympathetic neural control occurs through the vagal and pelvic (sacral) nerves. A surprising large proportion of these extrinsic nerves, particularly the vagus, consist of sensory afferent fibers *(14,15)*. Each projection of these autonomic nerves may affect a number of enteric ganglia *(16)*. The autonomic nerves can be thought of as providing the conduit for central nervous system input to the reflexes that occur throughout and between the different regions of the colon. The autonomic nervous system also provides a pathway for the reflexive interactions between the colon and other organs.

7. CENTRAL NEURAL CONTROL

Under normal circumstances, the central nervous system does not regulate the moment-to-moment control of the colon. We do not voluntarily control the passage of feces through our colon. However, the CNS is capable of modulating colonic contractile activity during situations such as voluntary defecation and during involuntary situations, such as extreme stress *(17–22)*. Signals to and from the central nervous system take place through the autonomic nervous system and, eventually, the enteric nervous system.

8. CHEMICAL CONTROL

Chemical control of the contractile activity of the colon refers to regulation via chemicals or hormones released from endocrine or paracrine cells or glands. These chemicals may affect colonic motility through actions upon the smooth muscle, enteric neurons, sympathetic or parasympathetic neurons, or the central nervous system. One example of how endocrine substances may influence colonic motility is hypothyroidism. When a patient is hypothyroid, the colonic transit time may be profoundly slowed. In contrast, hyperthyroidism accelerates transit time.

Chemical control of the colon may be physiologic, pathologic, or pharmacological. Physiologic control of motility is exerted by endogenous substances released in normal amounts that control the normal contractile patterns of the colon during the fasted and fed state. Pathologic control refers to the control exerted by the abnormal release of substances during a disease process. Examples include substances released by carcinoid tumors, the response to injury or surgery (ileus), or the ill-defined effects of stress upon colonic motility. When substances, such as therapeutic drugs are administered, they may exert pharmacological control of colonic motility. These substances may be synthesized within living systems. Erythromycin and opioids are two substances that exert a pharmocologic effect upon the colon's contractile activity.

9. MOLECULAR BASIS OF ELECTRICAL AND CONTRACTILE RHYTHMICITY

Enzymatically dispersed smooth muscle cells have been used extensively to identify specific ionic components within colonic tissue. Some functional effects of specific ionic channels can be inferred from the vast work accomplished in this area.

There is wide diversity in the molecular confiiguation of voltage-dependant K^+ channels. The responses of smooth muscle cells to slow wave depolarization depend, in large part, on the extent to which these various types of K^+ channels are expressed *(23)*. Inhibitory regulation of smooth muscle may act through activation of these channels.

While both the α- and β- subunits of Ca^{2+}-activated K^+ channels have been cloned from colonic smooth muscle, their role is less clear. These Ca^{2+}-activated K^+ channels are also referred to as BK channels. The negative membrane potential of gastrointestinal smooth muscle makes activation of this channel less than optimal. It has been postulated that BK channels may serve as a brake on excitatory activity *(24)*.

There are also inward rectifier and ATP-sensitive K^+ channels that may act to repolarize smooth muscle, thus preserving phasic electrical and mechanical activity.

The predominant Ca^{2+} channel in smooth muscle is an L-type channel. Blockade of Ca^{2+} channels reduces the duration and amplitude of electrical slow waves. It should be noted that L-type channel blockade does not eliminate ECA or the slow wave.

The final type of channel discussed in this chapter is the Cl⁻ channel. These have not been studied as extensively, but are thought to be an important component of the acetyl choline response in tissue. Because of the importance of cholinergic excitatory input to colonic motility, these channels may prove to be quite influential *(24)*.

10. INTERSTITIAL CELLS OF CAJAL

By light microscopy, the best marker for interstitial cells of cajal (ICC) appeared to be immunoreactivity for c-kit. Ultrastructurally, ICCs are characterized by the presence of many mitochondria, bundles of intermediate filaments, and gap junctions, which linked ICC with each other. However, ICC are morphologically heterogeneous and have unique features, depending on their tissue and organ location, as well as species. ICC in the deep muscular plexus of the small intestine and in the submuscular plexus of the colon are the most like smooth muscle cells and have a distinct basal lamina and numerous caveolae. In contrast, ICC of Auerbach's plexus at all levels of the gastrointestinal tract are the least like smooth muscle cells. They most closely resemble unremarkable fibroblasts. ICCs within the circular muscle layer appear intermediate in form *(25)*. Isolation of the ICCs for use in in vitro experiments has been extremely difficult. Many experts in this field believe that contamination with fibroblasts led to early confusion regarding the role and characteristics of the ICC.

Increasing evidence has suggested that the ICCs act as pacemaker cells and possess unique ionic conductances, which may trigger slow wave or ECA within the smooth muscle cells of the bowel *(24)*. Clearly, the conductance of both smooth muscle cells and ICCs affect one another and the total electrical activity displayed. The electrical responses generated from this complex array of electrically active and coupled cells cannot be modeled and predicted from studies either on isolated myocytes or ICCs. In addition, previous studies on the electrical behavior of smooth muscle cells have grouped all myocytes together. Evidence now suggests that the activities of the circular and longitudinal muscle cells can vary widely and that the electrical activity of myocytes within a given muscle layer can be widely different *(25–27)*. This suggests a level of fine control that develops sequentially region by region within an organ such as the colon *(28)*.

11. ORGANIZED GROUPS OF CONTRACTIONS

In most species, including humans, individual contractions of the colon are organized into groups separated from one another by quiescent states. In many species, colonic contractile states propagate primarily in a caudal direction. Occasionally, they may propagate in an orad direction. This facilitates the mixing and absorptive function of the colon. Within the colon, when colonic contractile states propagate more than half of the length of the colon in either direction, they have been defined as colonic migrating motor complexes (MMC) (Fig. 3) *(29–31)*. This definition is arbitrary but helps to classify and interpret in vivo manometric, electrical and contractile tracings. In contrast to the MMC, which is seen in the small intestine, colonic MMCs are not disrupted by a meal, although the frequency of the MMCs and their characteristics may be altered, depending upon the size and content of the meal *(30,31)*.

Rectal motor complexes are intermittent periods of contractile activity that occur in the fasted state and after feeding and have not been associated with proximal intestinal motility or the rapid eye movement (REM) stage of sleep *(32)*.

12. SPECIAL SITUATION CONTRACTIONS

Giant migrating contractions (GMCs) of the colon have been recorded from humans as well as animal models of contractile activity. GMCs of the proximal colon are associated with mass

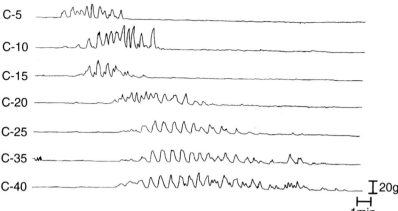

Fig. 3. This group of colonic contractile states migrates from the proximal to distal colon over greater than half of the length of the colon and can be described as a colonic MMC. The letter C to the left of the tracings represents colon. The numbers following C are the distance from the ileocolonic junction in centimeters. These recordings were performed in a canine model.

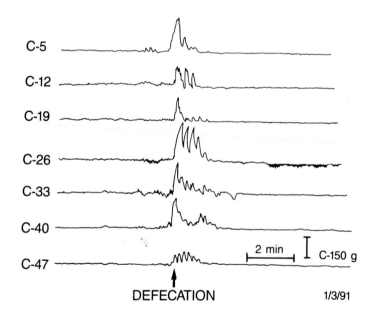

Fig. 4. GMCs of the colon are powerful high amplitude long duration contractions that are associated with mass movements in the proximal colon and defecation when they occur within the distal colon. When increased in frequency, GMCs can be associated with uncontrollable diarrhea. See Fig. 3 for details.

movements of feces (Figs. 1 and 4). When these specialized contractions occur within the distal colon, they are associated with defecation (Fig. 4). With increased frequency of GMCs, semi-liquid stool may be delivered into the distal colon and result in diarrhea that may be difficult to control. There is no discrete electrical activity that has been identified that represents the GMC. Rather, these impressive contractile events appear as a burst of ERA, indistinguishable from another phasic contraction within the colon.

During individual phasic contractions of the small intestine, longitudinal muscle lengthens while circular muscle contracts. In contrast, when longitudinal muscle contracts, circular muscle lengthens. It is impossible to determine, using strain gauge technology, whether the increase in length of the muscles is passive or active. In comparison, during special situation contractions, such as GMCs, there is a period of overlap when both the circular and longitudinal muscle layers contract. Presumably, there is a similar effect in the colon, although this has not been proven. Thus, during a GMCs, when both the circular and longitudinal muscles contract, there is foreshortening and contraction of the bowel to effectively propel intestinal contents forward.

The enteric neural control of GMCs is unclear. They are increased in frequency during inflammatory states, including enteric infections. Abdominal exposure to ionizing radiation also increases the frequency of GMCs *(33)*.

13. COORDINATION OF COLONIC MOTOR ACTIVITY WITH THE DISTAL SMALL INTESTINE

Colonic MMCs are not coordinated within the small intestine *(31)*. However, colonic GMCs, particularly within the proximal colon, are frequently directly related to those that occur within the ileum *(33)*. In normal animals, approx 50% of these contractions propagate from the small intestine into the proximal colon. In pathologic states, such as following irradiation when the frequency of GMCs is dramatically increased, the proportion of GMCs coordinated across the ileocolonic junction is also increased. These contractions effectively move enteric contents from the small bowel, across the ileum, and into the colon. This contributes to diarrhea due to insufficient time allowed for the reabsorption of bile salts.

14. SUMMARY

Normal colonic contractile activity occurs primarily through local regional control with higher central nervous system influences. These motor functions of the colon allow the animal optimal absorption of water and electrolytes and controlled expulsion of waste. As we understand more of the normal physiology of the colon, we have begun to appreciate normal variants and also the hallmarks of disease or disrupted function. The vocabulary of contractile events produced by the colon remains relatively limited, and pathologic contractile disturbances can be catagorized into excess or insufficient frequency of normal contractile events. Thus, a keen understanding of normal physiology and the control mechanisms remains important to the understanding of disease processes that affect motility.

REFERENCES

1. Sarna SK. Colonic motor activity. *Surg. Clin. N. Am.*, **73** (1993) 1201–1223.
2. Sarna SK. In vivo myoelectric activity: methods, analysis and interpretation. In *Handbook of Physiology: Gastrointestinal Motility and Circulation*. Wood JD (ed.), American Physiology Society, Bethesda, MD, 1989, pp. 817–863.
3. Sethi AK, Sarna SK. Relationship between colonic motor activity and transit [abstract]. *Gastroenterology*, **100** (1991) A841.
4. Wade PR, Wood JD. Synaptic behavior of myenteric neurons in guinea pig distal colon. *Am. J. Physiol.*, **254** (1988) G184–G190.
5. Sarna SK, Bardakjian BL, Waterfall WE, Lind JF. Human colonic electrical activity (ECA). *Gastroenterology*, **90** (1980) 1197–1204.
6. Sarna SK, Latimer P, Campbell D, Waterfall WE. Electrical and contractile activities of the human rectosigmoid. *Gut*, **23** (1982) 698–705.

7. Burleigh DE. Ng-nitro-L-arginine reduces nonadrenergic, noncholinergic relaxations of human gut. *Gastroenterology*, **102** (1992) 679–683.

8. Burnstock G. Purinergic nerves. *Pharmacol. Rev.*, **24** (1972) 509–581.

9. Rattan S, Shah R. Influence of purinoreceptors' agonists and antagonists on opossum internal and sphincter. *Am. J. Physiol.*, **255** (1988) G394.

10. Burnstock G, Campbell G, Satchell D, Smythe A. Evidence that adenosine triphosphate or a related nucleotide is the transmitter substance released by non-adrenergic nerves in the gut. *Br. J. Pharmacol.*, **40** (1970) 668–688.

11. Fahrenkrug J. Vasoactive intestinal polypeptide: measurement, distribution and putative neurotransmitter function. *Digestion*, **19** (1979) 149–169.

12. Gabella G. Innervation of the gastrointestinal tract. *Int. Rev. Cytol.*, **59** (1979) 129–193.

13. Grider JR, Makhlouf GM. Colonic peristaltic reflex: identification of vasoactive intestinal peptide as mediator of descending relaxation. *Am. J. Physiol.*, **251** (1986) G40–G45.

14. Agostoni E, Chinnock JE, Daly MD, et a. Functional and histological studies of the vagus nerve and its branches to the heart, lungs and abdominal viscera in the cat. *J. Physiol. (Lond)*, **135** (1975) 182–205.

15. Evans DHL, Murray JG. Histological and functional studies on the fibre composition of the vagus nerve of the rabbit. *J. Anat.*, **88** (1954) 320–337.

16. Christensen J, Rick GA, Robison BA, Stiles MJ, Wix MA. Arrangement of the myenteric plexus throughout the gastrointestinal tract of the opossum. *Gastroenterology*, **85** (1983) 890–899.

17. Bueno L, Fioramonti J. Effects of corticotropin-releasing factor corticotropin and cortisol on gastrointestinal motility in dogs. *Peptides*, **7** (1986) 73–77.

18. Gue M, Fioramonti J, Frexinos J, Alvinerie M, Bueno L. Influence of acoustic stress by noise on gastrointestinal motility in dogs. *Dig. Dis. Sci.*, **32** (1987) 1411–1417.

19. Narducci F, Snape WJ Jr, Battle WM, London RL, Cohen S. Increased colonic motility during exposure to a stressful situation. *Dig. Dis. Sci.*, **30** (1985) 40–44.

20. Schang JC, Hemond MG, Herbert M, Pilote M. Myoelectrical activity and intraluminal flow in human sigmoid colon. *Dig. Dis. Sci.*, **31** (1986) 1331–1337.

21. Tache Y, Garrick T, Raybould H. Central nervous system action of peptides to influence gastrointestinal motor function. *Gastroenterology*, **98** (1990) 517–528.

22. Williams C, Peterson J, Villar R, Burks TF. Corticotropin-releasing factor directly mediates colonic responses to stress. *Am. J. Physiol.*, **253** (1987) G582–G586.

23. Horowitz B, Ward SM, Sanders KM. Cellular and molecular basis for electrical rhythmicity in gastrointestinal muscles. *Annu. Rev. Physiol.*, **61** (1999) 19–43.

24. Sanders KM. A case for interstitial cells of Cajal as pacemakers and dediators of neurotransmission in the gastrointestinal tract. *Gastroenterology*, **111** (1996) 492–515.

25. Komuro T. Comparative morphology of interstitial cells of Cajal: ultrastructural characterization. *Microsc? Res. Technol.*, **47** (1999) 267–285.

26. Smith TK, Reed JB, Sanders KM. Interaction of two electrical pacemakers in muscularis of canine proximal colon. *Am. J. Physiol.*, **252** (1987) C290–C299.

27. Smith TK, Reed JB, Sanders KM. Origin and propagation of electrical slow waves in circular smooth muscle of canine proximal colon. *Am. J. Physiol.*, **252** (1987) C215–C224.

28. Xiong Z, Sperelakis N, Noffsinger A, Fenoglio-Preiser C. Changes in calcium channel current densities in rat colonic smooth muscle cells during development and aging. *Am. J. Physiol.*, **265** (1993) C617–C625.

29. Flouri B, Phillips S, Richter HI: Cyclic motility in canine colon: responses to feeding and perfusion. *Dig. Dis. Sci.*, **34** (1989) 1185–1192.

30. Gioramonti J, Bueno L: Diurnal changes in colonic motor profile in conscious dogs. *Dig. Dis. Sci.*, **28** (1983) 257–264.

31. Sarna SK, Lang IM: Colonic motor response to a meal in dogs. *Am. J. Physiol.*, **257** (1989) G830–G835.

32. Shibata C, Sasaki I, Matsuno E, et al. Characterization of colonic motor activity in conscious dogs. *J. Gastrointest. Motility*, **5** (1993) 9–16.

33. Otterson MF, Sarna Sk, Leming SC, Moulder JE, Fink J. Effects of fractionated doses of ionizing radiation on colonic motor activity. *Am. J. Physiol.*, **263** (1992) G518–G526.

3

Neural Regulation
of Colonic Motor Function

Kenton M. Sanders and Terence K. Smith

1. INTRODUCTION

Colonic motility is complex, consisting of storage, mixing, and propulsive functions. The tunica muscularis of the colon consists of a longitudinal muscle layer at the serosal aspect and a circular muscle layer at the submucosal aspect. The longitudinal muscle layer in the human is primarily organized into three muscular cables known as the taenia coli. These are spaced at equal intervals around the colon, and between the taenia is a thin layer of muscle cells arranged in the longitudinal direction. The taenia converge towards the end of the sigmoid colon to form the continuous longitudinal muscle coat of the rectum and internal anal sphincter (IAS). The circular muscle layer is continuous along the length of the colon and near the anus to form the IAS. The smooth muscle layers, by the actions of pacemaker cells and by intrinsic excitability of smooth muscle cells can generate spontaneous mechanical activity. However, this activity could not accomplish the tasks necessary for productive colonic motility without the superimposition of enteric neural activity, which, in turn, is modulated by the autonomic nervous system. Together these nerves control, to a large extent, the contractile behavior of muscles and produce normal motility. In this chapter, the basic anatomy and physiology of the neurons and postjunctional mechanisms that regulate colonic motor function are described.

2. THE ENTERIC NERVOUS SYSTEM IN THE LARGE INTESTINE

The enteric nervous system in the colon is similar in many features to the organization of enteric neurons in other regions of the gastrointestinal (GI) tract (*1–4*). The myenteric

From: *Colonic Diseases*
Edited by: T. R. Koch © Humana Press Inc., Totowa, NJ

plexus forms an extensive network of ganglia, cell bodies, and interconnecting nerve fibers in the region between the circular and longitudinal muscle layers. A less extensive plexus is also present in the submucosa and along the inner surface of the circular muscle layer. There are several types of neurons in the myenteric plexus, including: (i) primary sensory neurons, which are both mechano- and chemosensitive; (ii) interneurons, which carry information in the oral and anal directions; (iii) motor neurons, which carry excitatory or inhibitory signals to the muscle layers; and (iv) intestinofugal neurons, which project to superior and inferior mesenteric ganglia. The submucous plexus contains neurons that regulate secretory and/or absorptive activities of the mucosa (secretomotor neurons) and the contractile activity of the muscularis mucosa. The submucosal plexus is divided into two regions in larger mammals; ganglia lying adjacent to the circular muscle layer have been referred to as Schabadasch's or Henle's plexus, and ganglia within the submucosa are referred to as Meissner's plexus. Neurons arising from Meissner's plexus are the secretomotor neurons and motor neurons that regulate the muscularis mucosa, and neurons from Henle's plexus provide motor input to the pacemaker region along the submucosal surface of the circular muscle layer (1,2,59).

2.1. Electrophysiological and Morphological Characteristics of Myenteric Neurons

Many of the electrophysiological features of colonic neurons are similar to the neurons of the small intestine (4–9). Both S (for spiking) and AH (for after-hyperpolarization) neurons have been noted in the proximal, distal colon, and rectum of several species, including humans. When intracellular dyes (biocytin or lucifer yellow) are injected during electrophysiological recording, the morphology of cells with specific electrophysiological properties can be ascertained. S neurons in the small and large intestine have mainly a Dogiel type I morphology. They have one main axon and a variety of somal shapes and dendritic processes. The projection of S neurons within the myenteric plexus is either oral or anal or they leave the myenteric plexus and project to the circular or longitudinal muscle layers. Within the class of S neurons are the ascending and descending interneurons and the excitatory and inhibitory motor neurons. S neurons are characterized by the fact that they receive fast synaptic inputs (fast excitatory postsynaptic potentials [FEPSPs], duration 10–20 ms). FEPSPs result from the release of acetylcholine (ACh) or adenosine triphosphate (ATP) from presynaptic neurons. Postjunctional responses in S neurons result from activation of nicotinic receptors by ACh and P_2X receptors by ATP on S cell dendrites or somas.

Dogiel type II/AH neurons, which have projections into the villi of the mucosa, are likely to serve as intrinsic primary afferent neurons (IPANS) or intrinsic sensory neurons (6,8,10–13). These cells have multiple axonal projections oriented within a circumferential plane and do not receive FEPSPs (6). However, FEPSPs can be elicited in a subset of neurons that have characteristics similar to AH neurons are ascending interneurons (4,7).

Both AH neurons and some S neurons exhibit slow excitatory postsynaptic potentials (SEPSPs) (6,9). These events are sustained depolarizations of postjunctional neurons that last up to 60 s depending upon intensity of stimulation. SEPSPs produce long lasting excitability of the postjunctional cell. Transmitters for these events include substance P (acting on neurokinin 3 [NK3] receptors), 5-hydroxytryptamine [5-HT] (acting on 5-HT_{1P} receptors), vasoactive intestinal peptide (VIP), and somatostatin. These substances are present in subpopulations of ascending or descending interneurons and AH neurons (1–3).

S neurons have variable patterns of action potential (AP) in response to intracellular current injection (4,5,7–9,12). In some cells, APs fire repeatedly throughout depolarizing current pulses. These cells are referred to as tonic neurons or slowly adapting neurons. In other S neurons, one or two APs fire at the beginning of depolarizing pulse. These cells are called phasic neurons or rapidly adapting neurons. AH neurons are always phasic or rapidly adapting. Depolarization results in a few APs and these events are followed by a prolonged AH. The rising phase of S neuron APs is due to tetrodotoxin-sensitive Na^+ channels, whereas both Na^+ and Ca^{2+} currents contribute to the APs in AH cells. In AH neurons, the influx of a small amount of Ca^{2+} during the action potential causes the release of more Ca^{2+} (calcium-induced calcium release or CICR) from internal ryanodine-sensitive calcium stores that activates Ca^{2+}-dependent K^+ conductances, which contribute to the AH *(14)*. There is a good correlation between the amplitude and duration of the rise in internal Ca^{2+} following an AP and the AH (12, 14). During the AH, the excitability of AH neurons is greatly reduced; therefore, enhancing the activity of these cells (e.g., SEPSPs) is associated with blocking the conductances responsible for the AH *(9,14,15)*.

2.2. Extrinsic Nerves that Regulate the Function of the Colon

Efferent innervation of the colon comes from the parasympathetic and sympathetic nerves *(16)*. Parasympathetic nerves come from opposite ends of the spinal cord, and fibers from both the vagus and pelvic nerves nerves innervate the colon. Fibers of the vagus, with cell bodies in the dorsal motor nucleus of the brainstem, innervate the proximal colon and the proximal third of the transverse colon. Vagal fibers make synaptic connections with neurons of the myenteric plexus. Fibers of the pelvic nerves (pelvic splanchnic nerves), with cell bodies in the sacral spinal cord (S2 to S4), enter the pelvis and converge with postganglionic neurons of the pelvic or inferior hypogastric plexus. These fibers enter the colon at the rectosigmoid junction and ascend within the region of the myenteric plexus and descend into the anal canal in shunt fasicles. Pelvic fibers innervate myenteric neurons along these routes. In the transverse colon, innervation by fibers from vagus and pelvic nerves overlap.

Preganglionic sympathetic fibers supplying the large intestine have their cell bodies in the spinal cord (mainly T5 to L2). These fibers converge and form the greater and lesser splanchnic nerves and the lumbar-splanchnic nerves and synapse with postganglionic sympathetic neurons with cell bodies in the celiac ganglia and the superior and inferior mesenteric ganglia (SMG and IMG, respectively). Mesenteric nerves carry postganglionic sympathetic axons to the proximal colon from the SMG, and the lumbarcolonic nerves carry postganglionic fibers to the distal colon from the IMG. Axons of these neurons typically terminate within the myenteric ganglia, but in larger mammals, sympathetic fibers also innervate the muscle layers.

Extrinsic afferent fibers run within the parasympathetic (vagal, pelvic, and pudendal nerves) and sympathetic nerves to the colon. These fibers carry sensory information to the central nervous system (CNS), including the sensations of fullness and pain, if the colon is overly distended. Parasympathetic afferents in these reflex pathways travel in the pelvic nerves with cell bodies in dorsal root ganglia mainly at the level of S1 and S2. Sympathetic afferents travel via the colonic nerves to the splanchnic nerves with cell bodies in dorsal root ganglia mainly in L3 and L5. The lower anal canal is lined with squamous epithelium that is richly innervated by sensory fibers. These somatic afferents, which regulate the tone of the external anal sphincter (EAS), travel in the pudendal nerves.

The skeletal muscles that comprise the EAS, which surround the visceral tube, are innervated by somatic efferents in the pudendal nerves that arise from S2 and S3. Somatic nerves originating in S4 also supply the voluntary muscles of the pelvic floor, the levator muscles, which includes the puborectus muscle.

3. NEUROMUSCULAR JUNCTION
AND POSTJUNCTIONAL RESPONSES
3.1. Postjunctional Responses to Enteric
Neurotransmitters in Smooth Muscle Cells

The motility of colonic muscles is controlled by both excitatory and inhibitory neurotransmitters. That is, both propulsion-generating contractions and relaxations are active processes controlled by specific populations of motor neurons. Studies of neural regulation have evaluated the pharmacology of postjunctional electrical and mechanical responses and developed a list of candidate neurotransmitters and receptors that mediate these effects. Standard tests to determine whether a particular substance qualifies as an enteric neurotransmitter have been performed on a variety of mammalian colonic muscles and cells, including human. These studies have concluded that, in general, enteric motor neurons utilize ACh and substance P or NKA as excitatory transmitters and nitric oxide (NO), ATP, and VIP or pituitary adenylate cyclase-activating polypeptide (PACAP) as inhibitory transmitters in colonic muscles. Receptors utilized for postjunctional effects include: muscarinic receptors (M_2 and M_3 for ACh); (NK1 and NK2 receptors for substance P and NKA); soluble guanylyl cyclase (for NO), P_2Y receptors [isoform(s) unknown, for ATP], and VIP-specific receptors and PAC1 receptors (for VIP and PACAP). Many postjunctional pathways are involved in responses, and space in this short review permits only a brief description of major mechanisms. The reader is directed to specific reviews on mechanisms of neurotransmitter action in smooth muscles *(17,18)*.

The goal of excitatory neurotransmission is to generate contraction, and since colonic muscles tend to be spontaneously contractile the goal is really to increase contractile frequency and amplitude. Ultimately, there are three major approaches to obtaining more forceful contractions in smooth muscles: (i) enhancing Ca^{2+} entry; (ii) increasing release of Ca^{2+} from intracellular stores; and (iii) adjusting the sensitivity of the contractile apparatus to Ca^{2+}. The major excitatory neurotransmitters can accomplish each of these functions to varying degrees. ACh and NKs (including substance P) activate nonselective cation channels in smooth muscle cells. The molecular nature of these channels is not yet understood, but the current that is generated tends to depolarize muscle cells and increase the openings of voltage-dependent Ca^{2+} channels (L-type Ca^{2+} channels). This increases Ca^{2+} flux and generates more forceful and more frequent contractions. Coupling of M_3 receptors and NK receptors to Gq species of G proteins causes activation of phopholipase C upon receptor activation and the generation of inositol triphosphate (IP_3) and diacylglycerol (DAG). IP_3 can stimulate Ca^{2+} release from internal stores, and DAG, via activation of protein kinase C, can increase the Ca^{2+} sensitivity of the contractile apparatus. Thus, a cascade of events after stimulation by ACh and NKs results in enhanced frequency and force of contractions in colonic muscles.

Inhibitory neurotransmission results in an inhibition of spontaneous contractile activity and contributes to receptive relaxation during colonic reflexes. Active relaxation is also critical to sphincteric function during colonic filling through the ileocolonic sphinter) and during the defecation reflex via the IAS. The 3 classes of inhibitory neurotransmitters function by different mechanisms to produce inhibitory effects. All of the inhibitory transmitters work by enhancing the openings of K^+ channels. This tends to hyperpolarize (or stabilize) resting potential and reduce the opening of L-type Ca^{2+} channels. Thus, activating K^+ channels tends to reduce the amount of Ca^{2+} that enters smooth muscle cells. NO, the dominant inhibitory neurotransmitter, works via binding to guanylyl cyclase, production of cyclic guanosine 5'-monophosphate (cGMP), and stimulation of protein kinase G (PKG) to activate at least 3 types of K^+ channels. One of these channels is a stretch-dependent K^+ channel (TREK) that also helps the colon accommodate to filling and distension *(19)*. PKG-dependent mechanisms also directly inhibit L-type Ca^{2+} channels. The mechanism utilized by ATP to accomplish inhibition is rather unexpected. ATP works via P_2Y receptors that are coupled to production of IP_3 in colonic smooth muscle cells. However, instead of producing a global increase in Ca^{2+}, Ca^{2+} released by this mechanism is highly localized and directed to activation of small conductance Ca^{2+}-activated K^+ channels in the plasma membrane *(20)*. These channels are blocked by the bee venom, apamin. VIP activates delayed rectifier K^+ channels, K_{ATP} channels, and large-conductance Ca^{2+}-activated K^+ channels. Interestingly, mechanisms activated by both ATP and VIP (production of DAG and cyclic adenosine 5'-monophosphate [cAMP], respectively) tend to have stimulatory effects on L-type Ca^{2+} channels, but activation of K^+ channels is more potent, and the hyperpolarization responses or inhibition of APs caused by activation of K^+ channels supercedes the direct stimulatory effects on L-type Ca^{2+} channels. Finally, NO and VIP also tend to reduce the sensitivity of the contractile apparatus to Ca^{2+} via cGMP- and cAMP-dependent mechanisms.

3.2. Role of Interstitial Cells of Cajal
In Mediating Inputs from the Enteric Nervous System

Although most of the mechanistic work describing the actions of enteric neurotransmitters in GI muscles has been performed on smooth muscle cells, it is possible that these cells are not the primary targets for motor neurotransmission in the GI tract. Long ago, Ramon y Cajal noted that interstitial cells often made close contacts with the nerve terminals of autonomic nerves (see ref. *21*). When electronmicroscopy was later performed on GI muscles it was discovered that a very close relationship (<20 nm) was common between enteric motor nerve terminals and interstitial cells of Cajal (ICC), throughout the gut (see ref. *22*). The specific associations between motor nerve terminals, ICC and smooth muscle cells in the guinea pig colon have been studied with immunochemical techniques and electron microscopy *(23)*. Intramuscular ICC (IC-IM) are in close anatomical association motor nerve fibers labeled with antibodies for nitric oxide synthase (NOS) to label inhibitor fibers or ACh vesicular transporter (vAChT) to label excitatory fibers. The nerve fibers come in close contact with multiple IC-IM. Electron microscopy showed that the apparent close contacts are indeed very close (i.e. <20 nM) and synaptic-like structures are apparent between these cells with both pre- and postjunctional densifications. Contacts like this also occurred between motor neurons and smooth muscle cells, but these contacts are far more rare than contacts between nerve terminals and IC-IM. Processes of the IC-IM are closely associated with neighboring smooth muscle fibers and form gap junctions with these cells. Immuno-electron microscopy demonstrated that both excitatory and inhibitory nerve terminals form very close associations with IC-IM, suggesting that ICC may be involved in mediation of both types of neural regulation in the colon. These anatomical observations suggest a central role for ICC, in the neural control of colonic muscles. While there may be parallel innervation of both ICC and smooth muscle cells, the main focus of innervation may be between motor neurons and IC-IM, and neural regulation of smooth muscle cells may be mediated by flow of current between ICC and smooth muscle cells. The same morphological relations between motor neurons, ICC and smooth muscle cells exist in the human GI tract, however, the role of ICC in enteric neurotransmission has not been rigorously tested yet in these tissues.

4. INTEGRATION AND NEURAL REGULATION OF COLONIC FUNCTION
4.1. Antiperistaltic and Peristaltic Waves

Fluid from the ileum is emptied into the cecum, which contracts periodically to drive its contents into the proximal colon. The proximal colon is characterized by antiperistaltic waves that often appear to originate near the "pacemaker zone", which is a region of high contractility where fecal pellets are produced between the proximal and distal colon (16,24–26). Antiperistaltic waves do not generally occlude the lumen and likely promote mixing and retention of contents for absorption of water and electrolytes. Reflux of contents from the proximal colon back into the ileum is prevented by the activation of intrinsic excitatory nervous reflex pathways, which contract the ileocecal sphincter as the proximal colon is distended. The rhythmic mixing or segmental contractions of the colon are manifest as haustra, which are in part anatomical and part driven by neural inputs.

Occasionally, peristaltic waves occur in the proximal colon (16,24–26). These events are mediated by neural reflexes and usually start near the cecum and sweep (at about 8 mm/s in the guineapig) (26) along the length of the proximal colon. Peristaltic waves are triggered by the movement of material from the cecum into the proximal colon and by luminal distension of the proximal colon. Peristaltic waves are sometimes luminally occlusive and drive the contents of the proximal colon toward the pacemaker zone. The ratio of peristaltic to antiperistaltic waves depends in part on the fluid volume or luminal distension of the proximal colon.

The distal colon exhibits mainly neurally mediated orthograde waves of contraction (25–29). These consist mainly of two types: strong fast (1.6 mm/s; guineapig distal colon) peristaltic waves, which are generated by the distension caused by a fecal pellet, and slow (0.3 mm/s; guineapig distal colon) shallow spontaneous waves of contraction that originate at the oral end of an isolated empty segment of distal colon (26,27,29). Both types of contraction are dependent on the enteric nervous system, since they are blocked by atropine, hexamethonium, and tetradotoxin (TTX) and occur in isolated segments of colon.

4.2. Spontaneous Complexes and Propulsion

The spontaneous slowly propagating descending waves of excitation that occur in an isolated empty segment of guineapig distal colon may be a second mechanism in addition to local reflexes aiding fecal pellet propulsion (26,27). Such spontaneous complexes have been recorded in the large intestine of a number of species. These have been described using a variety of terminologies that include colonic migrating myoelectrical complexes in the dog (30); migrating spike bursts in the cat (31); colonic migrating motor complexes (CMMCs), migrating contractile complexes, and neurogenic slow depolarizations in the mouse (32–34), and high amplitude propagating contractions in humans (35). Wood et al. (36) provided evidence that pellet propulsion in the murine colon was associated with the occurrence of a spontaneous myoelectric complex.

In the isolated murine large intestine, CMMCs (duration approx 31 s), which occur every 3.5 min, usually originate in the proximal colon and appear to spread slowly (3.5 mm/s) down the colon (32). A contractile complex occurring in the proximal colon is closely followed by the development of a complex in the distal colon. A relaxation (or hyperpolarization) sometimes precedes the contractile (depolarizing) phase of the CMMC in the distal colon (Fig. 1) (32–34). Therefore, the CMMC involves the activation of both descending inhibitory and excitatory nervous pathways. The CMMC can also propagate orally to promote retention or mixing of contents, and therefore, the CMMC must also utilize ascending excitatory nervous pathways must also be utilized. As the CMMC is abolished by hexamethonium, both the inhibitory and excitatory phases of the complex are activated by fast (nicotinic-FEPSPs)

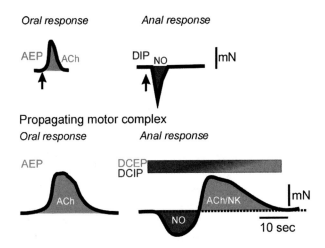

Fig. 1. Local responses to mucosal stimulation. Mechanical stimulation of the colonic mucosa or distension evokes a transient oral contraction and an anal relaxation in both the longitudinal muscle (LM) and circular muscle (CM). The ascending excitatory pathway (AEP) mediating these responses is largely cholinergic (i.e., reduced by hexamethonium), and the descending inhibitory pathway (DIP) is noncholinergic (unaffected by hexamethonium). The oral contraction is largely due to the release of ACh from motor neurons onto muscarinic receptors in the muscle since it is reduced by atropine. The anal relaxation is largely due to release of NO from inhibitory motor neurons. Both responses are largely mediated by the action of neurotransmitters on ICC and conveyed to the muscle cells via electrical coupling. Propagating motor complex. Spontaneous motor complexes utilize some of the same nervous pathways as local responses. Spontaneous motor complexes usually arise in the proximal colon and appear to migrate anally. The oral complex is a monotonic excitatory response. The oral complex depends upon the activation of an ascending cholinergic excitatory nervous pathway (AEP). The anal response is preceded by a prolonged relaxation (mainly due to release of NO from inhibitory motor neurons) and followed by a prolonged contraction (largely due to ACh released from excitatory motor neurons) of the LM and CM. Inhibitory or excitatory motor neurons to both muscles are activated at the same time. Initially, the inhibitory response exceeds the excitatory response (blue tone of bar at onset of descending cholinergic inhibitory pathway [DCIP]), and then the excitatory component becomes dominant (red tone of bar as descending cholinergic excitatory pathway [DCEP] becomes predominant). The cholinergic interneurons underlying the anal complex are inhibited by hexamethonium, NO and sympathetic nerve stimulation (see color figure in insert following page 238).

neurotransmission along descending and ascending cholinergic interneurons. The distal recruitment of descending inhibitory pathways (DIPs) is likely responsible for the distally increasing phase delay in the contraction, which gives the complex an apparent slow conduction velocity. Therefore, the CMMC most likely involves the simultaneous neural activation of large regions of colon, rather than the slow spread of excitability from one region to another. CMMCs occur in isolated segments of murine intestine and are sensitive to 5-HT3 antagonists, suggesting that they may be driven by spontaneous 5-HT release from enterochromaffin cells (ECCs) activating the endings of intrinsic sensory neurons projecting to the mucosa or via descending seroternergic interneurons (37).

Another form of neurally mediated migrating motor activity, which is highly propulsive, is the giant migrating contraction (GMC), observed in the canine large intestine (38). GMCs occur infrequently (twice daily), are of long duration (approx 3–5 min), large amplitude (2.5x larger than CMMCs), and propagate quickly (2–30 mm/s) anally over long lengths of colon. GMCs are not associated with the propulsion of inflated intraluminal balloons; however, they do appear to cause mass movements of fecal material, and their occurrence in the distal colon is associated with defecation. GMC frequency is increased during inflammation and may be responsible for explosive diarrhea.

4.3. Complex Actions of NO

NO seems to be very important in regulating the CMMC. After inhibiting NO synthesis with N omega-nitro-L-arginine (L-NA), the frequency of CMMC increases, propagation direction frequently changes, and the relaxation (or muscle hyperpolarization) preceding the contraction (or muscle depolarization) is substantially reduced *(39,40)*. Because the smooth muscle depolarizes following L-NA in the murine colon, it has been hypothesized that the depolarizing phase of the CMMC is not only due to the activation of cholinergic motor neurons but also to the turning off of inhibitory motor neurons (i.e., disinhibition) that maintain the muscle in a hyperpolarized state. Also, mucosal stimulation following blockade of NO synthesis in interneurons generates a complex *(41,42)*. Therefore, NO also depresses neuroneuronal transmission within chains of descending cholinergic interneurons by inhibiting the release of ACh that excites both the descending inhibitory and excitatory phases of the CMMC (Fig. 1).

4.4. Peristaltic Reflexes in the Large Intestine

Peristaltic waves in the large intestine are dependent upon the activation of intrinsic neural reflexes *(24–29,41–43)*. Distension of the proximal colon by accumulating viscous chyme in the proximal colon and by fecal pellets in the distal colon activates these reflexes, which are modified in turn by extrinsic neural reflexes and hormones. Local reflex stimulation (mechanical stimulation of the mucosa or distension) of the colon leads to the activation of IPANS, which excite ascending excitatory and descending inhibitory reflexes to the circular and longitudinal muscle *(27,41–42)*. Interneurons, in turn, excite excitatory motor neurons to the circular and longitudinal muscle above and inhibitory motor neurons to the circular and longitudinal muscle below the stimulus (Fig. 1).

4.5. Descending Excitation

Alvarez (1940) *(44)* criticized the concept of descending inhibition advocated by Bayliss and Starling for both the small and large intestine *(45,46)*. A number of investigators had observed not only contraction oral but also contraction anal to a local stimulus, or a contraction in front of a moving bolus. Alvarez believed that any distension of the gut ahead of a peristaltic wave was not due to active inhibition but to passive distension by the column of fluid ahead of a propagating contraction. With reference to the propulsion of a fecal pellet in the rabbit colon recorded with a camera, Alvarez observed: "..but instead of distending inhibition, there is a contraction, and the bowel does not widen until the ball is forced into it." Costa & Furness *(27)* did, however, measure a relaxation in front of a moving fecal pellet in guineapig distal colon. When electrical recordings are made from the serosal surface of the large intestine, distension is found to evoke a transient inhibitory junction potential (IJP) in the proximal colon and a prolonged burst of IJPs superimposed on a slow hyperpolarization anal to the site of stimulation in the guineapig and rabbit distal colon *(47,48)*. Therefore, the robustness of descending inhibitory responses appears to depend on colonic content, namely fluid in the proximal colon vs pellets in the distal colon. However, the descending inhibitory response in the colon is occasionally followed by periodic bursts of APs superimposed on excitatory junction potentials (EJPs) or a prolonged contraction (descending excitation) anal to the stimulus *(41–42,47,48)*, as it is in the small intestine *(49,50)*. In fact, in response to a peristaltic wave the initial relaxation (descending inhibition) response is interrupted by a prolonged contraction (descending excitation) in the distal colon *(43)*. Interestingly, these descending responses resemble a spontaneous CMMC, suggesting that both events use the same reflex pathways. These results suggest that strong stimulation unleashes not only descending inhibitory but also descending excitatory nervous pathways as well. Presumably, prolonged or intense stimulation of the large intestine overcomes the ongoing nitrergic inhibition that normally suppresses the descending cholinergic interneurons involved in descending excitation *(41,42)*. These complex descending inhibitory and excitatory contractile and electrical responses occur at the same time in both the longitudinal and circular muscle layers. Thus, descending excitation likely adds to the propulsive force by contracting both muscle layers oral and relaxing both muscle layers anal to a bolus.

4.6. Synchronous Vs Reciprocal Activation of the Two Muscle Layers

It is surprising to find that both muscle layers contract and relax together during reflex stimulation and peristalsis, because the relative movements of the two muscles have been a subject of controversy for over 100 yr. Bayliss and Starling *(45,46)* presented evidence that both muscle layers of the intestine contract and relax together during peristalsis and relax together during sympathetic nerve stimulation. Later investigators reached different conclusions and suggested that the muscles sometimes move synchronously, sometimes independently, or are constrained by intrinsic neural circuits and anatomy to move 180° out of phase with each other *(44,52)*. In particular, studies of the relative movements of the two muscle layers during peristalsis in the guineapig ileum led initially to the idea that the two muscles contracted independently and, later, to the concept described in many textbooks as reciprocal innervation. Reciprocal innervation postulates that the longitudinal and circular muscles of the intestine are opposing muscles and are neuronally wired in such a way that when one muscle is excited, the other is inhibited *(51)*. In support of this, it has been suggested that the longitudinal and circular muscles are, by their anatomical arrangement opposing muscles and that passive mechanical interactions, independent of nerves, occur so that when one muscle contracts the other must by necessity elongate *(52)*. Recent studies, however, do not support the idea of reciprocal innervation or that the two muscles oppose each other either in the small or large intestine. An examination of the reflex responses of the two muscle layers in the ileum and colon, using special dissection techniques to isolate the reflex responses of the longitudinal muscle from those of the circular muscle, and simultaneous calcium imaging of the two muscle layers, demonstrated that the two muscle layers receive similar synchronous ascending excitatory (oral) and descending inhibitory (anal) neuromuscular inputs during reflex stimulation and during peristaltic waves *(41–43;50,53,55)*. These studies were confirmed by simultaneous intracellular electrophysiological recordings from both muscle layers (<200 µm apart) during spontaneous electrical activity in the canine colon *(55)* and during reflex stimulation of the guineapig distal colon *(56)*. Rhythmic oscillations in membrane potential (approx 17/min) called myenteric potential oscillations (MPO) (canine colon) are synchronized in both the longitudinal and circular muscle layers near the myenteric border *(55)*. However, action potential firing on the crest of MPOs is unsynchronized across the two muscles suggesting this may be a reason why they often appear independent during spontaneous movements. Most convincingly, following the initiation of enteric reflexes of the guineapig distal colon, it was observed that EJPs (ascending excitation) and IJPs (descending inhibition) occur at the same time in the longitudinal and circular muscle oral and anal to the stimulus, respectively *(56)*. Therefore, even though the muscles appear to act somewhat independently during spontaneous synchronously movements, their respective inhibitory or excitatory motor neurons are likely to be activated by common interneurons during the peristaltic reflex. Studies in the human esophagus using ultrasonography suggest that both muscle layers thicken orally and thin anally during ascending excitatory and descending inhibitory reflex stimulation, respectively, and that the thickness of the muscularis is proportional to the pressure generated (57). Previous studies that examined the passive interactions of the two muscles had ignored changes in muscle thickness and had just concentrated on changes in muscle area. The combined thickening of the two muscles during excitation, where high pressures are generated, and thinning of the two muscles, where lower pressures are generated, is consistent with Laplace's Law, since it ensures that stress is uniform across the muscularis despite the large loads placed on the gut musculature during a peristaltic wave (57).

Further confirmation of the synchronous activation of both muscle layers of the colon via common interneurons came from studies of the effects of extrinsic nerve stimulation on intrinsic reflex responses to both muscle layers (42). Sympathetic nerve stimulation suppresses intrinsic reflex responses at the same time in both the longitudinal and circular muscle layer by presynaptic inhibition (activation of adrenergic $\alpha2$-receptors) of ACh release from common ascending and descending cholinergic interneurons. As a note, activation of sympathetic fibers directly innervating the muscle layers is also synchronous, since stimulation of these nerves directly relaxes both the longitudinal and circular muscle via activation of postjunctional β-receptors. Earlier, it had been shown, using special pinning techniques in an attempt to minimize interactions between the two muscles, that pelvic nerve stimulation contracts both muscle layers of the colon at the same time (58). It is possible that parasympathetic nerves may activate peristalsis by releasing ACh to stimulate enteric interneurons that supply motor neurons to both muscle layers.

In summary, the intrinsic neural circuitry of the colon is complex, but is simplified by the fact that the different excitatory or inhibitory motor neurons to each layer can be activated at the same time by common interneurons. This ensures that, during peristalsis, maximum force is produced by the contraction of both muscles behind a bolus and that tone is removed from both muscles below the bolus.

4.7. Effect of Reflexes on Slow Waves

Excitatory nerves increase the amplitude, duration, and frequency of slow waves, whereas inhibitory nerves reduce their amplitude and frequency (59–61). When electrical slow waves are present in the guineapig distal colon, distension of the lumen causes a slow wave to occur prematurely in its cycle oral to the site of stimulation (48). The premature slow wave, which is induced by cholinergic nerve activity (i.e., blocked by atropine), often reaches threshold to elicit an AP (ascending excitation). Anal to the site of stimulation, distension causes membrane hyperpolarization, which reduces the amplitude of slow waves.

4.8. Responses of Myenteric Neurons During Enteric Reflexes

Both stretch and mechanical stimulation of the mucosa (pressure applied to the mucosa with a sponge or a stroke with a brush) evokes bursts of FEPSPs and APs in myenteric S interneurons and motor neurons located oral (ascending pathway) or anal (descending pathway) of the site of stimulation in the distal colon of the guineapig. AP rates of 20–30 Hz, with instantaneous frequencies of up to a 100 Hz, can be evoked in S cells by reflex stimulation (62,63). The responses to stimulation are attenuated by hexamethonium, suggesting ACh acting on nicotinic receptors is a major neuroneuronal transmitter. In contrast, AH neurons in the distal colon do not respond to either stimulus applied more than 10 mm either oral or anal to the recording site. This observation suggests that these cells may be IPANS, which are only activated at the site of stimulation. In fact, AH neurons in the guinea pig proximal colon have been shown to respond with bursts of antidromic APs and proximal process potentials when puffs of 5-HT are applied to the mucosa suggesting they do indeed have a sensory function (10,11). However, it is premature to say that they are the only intrinsic sensory neuron, since AH neurons are quiescent in stretched preparations of distal colon where muscle movement has been paralyzed with nicardipine (activity in IPANS is critically dependent upon muscle tension) (see ref. 64), which still exhibits ongoing reflex activity (spontaneous oral EJPs coordinated with anal IJPs) (63). It is possible that other neurons, probably S type interneurons, are also stretch sensitive.

4.9. Calcium Waves and Enteric Reflexes

Calcium is a critical second messenger regulating motility since a rise in intracellular Ca^{2+} ($[Ca^{2+}]_i$) triggers smooth muscle contraction. The level of $[Ca^{2+}]_i$ is a direct measure of muscle excitability that can be measured in muscle cells in intact tissues using calcium fluorescent indicators (Fig. 2) (53,54). Such studies reveal that the longitudinal muscle (and sometimes the circular muscle) in both the small and large intestine exhibit continuous waves of intercellular calcium, which propagate along and across (1000 × 200 µm) many smooth muscle cells producing local contractions that create muscle tone and mix intestinal contents (Fig. 2). Calcium waves are caused by calcium influx during AP propagation. L-type Ca^{2+} channel antagonists, such as nifedipine or nicardipine, block APs and calcium waves. Calcium waves, like APs, are limited in their extent of propagation by collisions with other calcium waves, which leads to their annihilation and often confines the excitability of the longitudinal muscle to small zones (approx 200–500 µm wide × 1000 µm long) of activity. Ascending and descending excitatory reflexes produce calcium waves at the same time in both the longitudinal and circular muscle around the intestine and are the basis for contractile responses. Descending inhibitory reflexes block both the initiation and propagation of calcium waves into the inhibited zone leading to intestinal accommodation.

Calcium fluorescent imaging of the tunica muscularis provides a reliable tool to study the spread of excitability within GI smooth muscle layers during mixing and propulsive movements.

4.10. Pharmacology of Enteric Reflexes

The pharmacology of enteric reflexes at motor terminals confirms that the transmitters identified from in vitro experiments mediate the motor responses observed during reflexes. EJPs, calcium waves, or contractions evoked in both the longitudinal and circular muscle by activation of ascending excitatory and descending excitatory reflexes, peristalsis, and the CMMC are substantially reduced, if not abolished, by muscarinic antagonists, suggesting that ACh is the major excitatory neurotransmitter to both muscles in the large intestine (27,29,32,33,40,41,42,53–56). At higher grades of stretch, oral reflex contractions are only partially reduced by muscarinic antagonists, suggesting that noncholinergic excitatory neurotransmitters such as tachykinins (substance P and NKA), are also released from excitatory motor neurons onto NK1 and NK2 receptors on the muscle (65,66). These substances, along with ACh are probably released from the same excitatory motor neurons innervating each muscle, with the proportions of different transmitters depending on the frequency of AP firing in excitatory motor neurons, which in turn depends on the strength of activation of neural reflex pathways. IJPs, inhibition of calcium waves, and relaxation of longitudinal and circular muscle of the distal colon (guineapig and rat) produced by activation of descending inhibitory nervous reflexes are substantially reduced or blocked by inhibitors of NO production (41–43,54,56). Blocking NO synthesis, which in large part most likely removes the relaxation ahead of a bolus, reduces or abolishes peristalsis in the colon (28). The evoked IJP

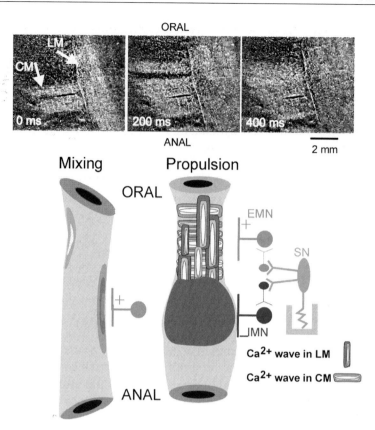

Fig. 2. Calcium waves appear independently and spontaneously in both the LM and CM of the colo
These calcium waves cause localized contractions and produce muscle tone and mixing. They sprea
rapidly (approx 80 mm/s) along the muscle fibers and more slowly (approx 8 mm/s) perpendicular to th
muscle fibers (video images at top). During mixing, these waves can occur spontaneously or be gener
ated by ACh release from excitatory motor neurons (leftmost colonic segment). During peristalsis an
propulsion there is a simultaneous firing of excitatory motor neurons (EMN) above (ascending excit
tion) the mucosal stimulus (conveyed by sensory neurons to the mucosa; SN) which induces multipl
calcium waves at the same time in both the LM and CM (rightmost colonic segment). This generates
uniform contraction of both muscle layers. During excitation, the spread of calcium waves in bo
muscle layers is restricted due to collisions between waves in neighboring bundles of muscle. Activatic
of descending inhibitory motor neurons (IMN) blocks generation and propagation of calcium waves
the inhibited zone. This leads to receptive relaxation below the site of mucosal stimulation. Upper pane
the LM has been removed from the left hand side of the preparation to reveal more clearly calcium wav
propagating slowly in the underlying CM.

in the circular muscle is also reduced by the bee venom apamin, which blocks small conduc
tance K^+ (S_K) channels on the muscle opened by ATP *(56)*. In contrast, the IJP in longitudina
muscle is largely unaffected by apamin, but blocked by inhibitors of NO synthesi
(42,43,54,56). Other inhibitory neurotransmitters in addition to NO (longitudinal and circu
lar muscle) and ATP (circular muscle), such as VIP and PACAP, may also contribute t
muscle relaxation (see above) *(67,68)*.

In summary, colonic motility is complex, since slow waves (circular muscle) and APs o
MPOs (longitudinal and circular muscle) regulate rhythmic contractions, and at least thre
mechanisms may underlie propulsion in the distal colon: (i) spontaneous CMMCs; (ii) lon

lasting complex peristaltic responses generated by a pellet, which resemble a CMMC; and (iii) phasic ongoing oral EJPs and anal IJPs induced by stretch by a pellet. It is hardly surprising that colonic motility can be dramatically affected by drugs such as: (i) L-type Ca^{2+} channel antagonists, which block AP generation in the muscle and reduce the plateau phase of the slow wave; (ii) muscarinic and NK antagonists, which reduce the effect of excitatory transmitters on the muscle; (iii) NO synthesis inhibitors, such as L-NA, which interfere with peristalsis by blocking descending inhibition of the smooth muscle ahead of a bolus, and interfere with neuroneuronal cholinergic transmission by increasing ACh release; (iv) nicotinic antagonists and NK3 antagonists, which block fast (interneurons to interneurons; interneurons to inhibitory and excitatory motor neurons; parasympathetic neurons to enteric neurons) and slow (IPANS to IPANS; IPANS to interneurons) synaptic transmission respectively; (v) 5-HT antagonists which block the activation of IPANS by 5-HT released from ECCs in the mucosa; and (vi) sympathetic $\alpha 2$- and β-agonists to reduce motility and $\alpha 2$- and β-antagonists to increase motility. For example, discomfort in ulcerative colitis patients appears to be associated with increases in both motility and tone in the sigmoid colon. Nicotine can reduce both motility and tone and alleviate symptoms by exciting inhibitory motor neurons to release NO and relax the muscle *(69)*.

5. COMPLEX NEURONAL PATHWAYS IN THE DISTAL COLON

Figure 3 is a neural circuit diagram that attempts to clarify aspects of the intricate nerve pathways underlying synchronous activation and inhibition of both the longitudinal and circular muscle during activation of local enteric reflexes, peristalsis, and the CMMC in the colon. Local mucosal stimulation or distension activates ascending excitatory nerve pathways (AEPs) and descending inhibitory pathways (DIPs) that produce the transient oral contraction and transient anal relaxation, respectively, of both muscles. The AEPs are cholinergic, since they are blocked by hexamethonium. The DIPs are noncholinergic, since they are insensitive to hexamethonium, but inhibited by low Ca^{2+}/high Mg^{2+} solutions that block synaptic transmission. However, in response to a peristaltic wave, CMMC, or to a mucosal stimulus following blockade of NO synthesis in interneurons, a prolonged anal relaxation, followed by a prolonged contraction, is observed. This complex resulting from activation of descending cholinergic inhibitory pathways (DCIPs) and descending cholinergic excitatory pathways (DCEPs) is the motor response underlying pellet propulsion and the CMMC. Presumably, release of NO inhibits the output of ACh in DCIPs and DCEPs *(41,42)*. ACh could either be co-localized with nitric oxide synthase (NOS) in these interneurons, or NO may be released from a separate population of descending interneurons *(3)*. NO is likely to act as an inhibitory neuromodulator that reduces the output of ACh from nerve terminals or directly reduces the soma excitability of interneurons in these pathways. Most interestingly, sympathetic nerve stimulation blocks both the ascending contraction and the descending complex, but not the early noncholinergic relaxation evoked by mucosal stimulation. Sympathetic nerve stimulation reduces the output of ACh by activating presynaptic α-receptors on the terminals of cholinergic interneurons, thereby extinguishing the excitatory motor drive at the same time to both muscles. In contrast, sympathetic nerve stimulation has no effect on the evoked early transient relaxation; this suggests that noncholinergic activation of inhibitory motor neurons can facilitate the inhibition of motility produced by sympathetic nerve stimulation. Descending cholinergic interneurons also synapse with intestinofugal neurons, which activate extrinsic sympathetic reflexes *(5)*. Therefore, the possibility exists that extrinsic inhibitory feedback through prevertebral ganglia occurs because stimulation of intestinofugal neurons by increases in colonic motility leads to the inhibition of the cholinergic interneurons *(42)*, which, in turn, excite the intestinofugal neurons.

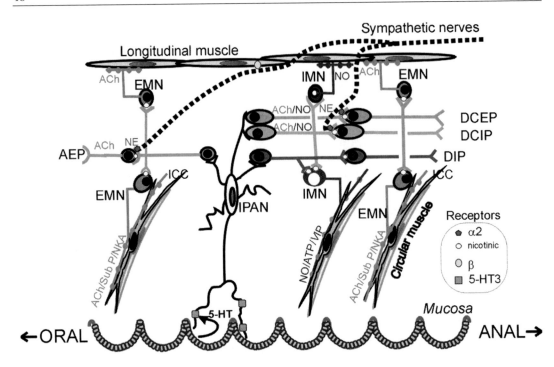

Fig. 3. Neural circuits underlying regulation of LM and CM layers during local reflexes and migrating motor complexes. EMNs and IMNs innervate the LM and CM. Excitatory or inhibitory motor neurons to both the LM and CM are activated by common interneurons. Activation of these interneurons during local stimulation leads to simultaneous contraction of the LM and CM oral to the site of mucosal stimulation and simultaneous relaxation of LM and CM anal to the stimulus. During a migrating motor complex or peristaltic wave, DCEP and DCIP are activated leading to relaxation of both muscles, followed by contraction of both muscles (see Fig. 1). EMN release mainly ACh; IMN release mainly NO. Signals from EMN and IMN are transduced through IC-IM.

6. NEURAL CONTROL OF THE IAS AND THE DEFECATION REFLEX

6.1. Rectum and anal canal

Another zone of high contractile activity and pressure appears to exist in the upper rectum at the junction with the sigmoid colon (15). Its function may be to prevent the untimely progression of fecal masses into the rectum, which remains empty for long periods and fills only intermittently. The anal canal is normally empty and exhibits a high degree of tone accompanied by rhythmic contractions that result mainly from the myogenic activity in the IAS. The rhythmic contractions in the anal canal are faster more distally. This contractile gradient ensures that feces are forced back into the rectum. Even though the rectum remains empty for long periods and only fills intermittently, the longitudinal and circular smooth muscle of IAS and skeletal muscle of the EAS are normally contracted. The contracted state of the longitudinal smooth muscle shortens the anal canal. Roughly 85% of the basal pressure in the anus results from the tone in the circular smooth muscle of the IAS, since local anesthesia of the pudendal nerve to block somatic afferents and efferents lowers the resting pressure by only 15%. The tone in the circular smooth muscle of the IAS is maintained in large part by its intrinsic myogenic electrical activity, which has a frequency between 10–24 cpm.

6.2. Continence

Activity in lumber sympathetic nerves also promotes retention of feces, closing off the large intestine, by relaxing the colon and contracting the IAS. The colonic muscle is both inhibited by reducing the outflow of ACh from myenteric neurons via presynaptic α-receptors and by sympathetic activation of β-receptors on the muscle. In contrast, the IAS is contracted by sympathetic activation of α-receptors on the smooth muscle. Tone in the EAS is also maintained by extrinsic somatic reflexes. The somatic efferents contract the EAS by releasing ACh onto nicotinic receptors onto the endplates of the skeletal muscle fibers of the EAS. Continence is also facilitated by contraction of the puboerectus muscle, which arches around the upper part of the anal canal and pulls the anal canal forward so that it makes a right angle with the rectum.

6.3. Defecation

The propulsion of colonic contents into the rectum during a mass movement causes rectal distension, which activates intrinsic and extrinsic neural reflexes, called the rectosphincteric reflex *(15)*. Distension of the rectum relaxes the IAS, but contracts the EAS. The relaxation of the IAS is transient in response to maintained distension. However, repeated brief distensions of the rectum are more effective in maintaining relaxation of the IAS. The IAS is relaxed by stretch activation of the descending inhibitory reflex pathways which stimulate intrinsic inhibitory motor neurons to release VIP and NO to relax the circular smooth muscle. Filling of the rectum is associated with the sensation to void. If the time is inconvenient, then voluntary contractions of the EAS can overcome the reflex. The IAS regains tone, because relaxation of the IAS is transient owing to the accommodation of the sensory receptors in the rectal wall to distension. The rectum then accommodates the fecal matter until another mass movement further increases distension of the rectum and again signals the urge to defecate. If defecation is suppressed there is a retrograde movement of colonic contents. Reverse peristalsis has been shown to occur whenever the intestine is obstructed. Squeezing the rabbit colon causes its contents to reverse direction, as does the tight aganglionic segment in the Hirschsprung's mouse *(70)*.

If defecation is convenient, then the effects of rectal distension are facilitated by parasympathetic reflexes, which can initiate a peristaltic rush that sweeps the contents down the descending colon towards the anal canal, where there occurs a coordinated relaxation of the IAS. Pelvic nerves contract the colon by stimulating myenteric excitatory motor neurons and relax the IAS by stimulating intrinsic inhibitory motor neurons. At the same time, there is a reduction in efferent activity to the EAS. These involuntary movements are aided by voluntary acts, such as flexing the hips for the normal defecation posture and contracting the abdominal wall muscles against a closed glottis, which result in an increase in abdominal pressure. Descent of the pelvic floor results from an active relaxation of the pelvic floor muscles and the increase in abdominal pressure. The anorectal angle is abolished during defecation, facilitating the passage of feces.

At the end of defecation there is a rebound of increased excitation in the EAS, which is the closing reflex. Along with contraction of the EAS, there is a contraction of the muscles of the pelvic floor, which are returned to their resting condition.

ACKNOWLEDGMENTS

This chapter was supported by grants from the National Institutes of Health, DK 41315 to K.M.S. and T.K.S.; and DK 45713 to T.K.S.

REFERENCES

1. Barbiers M, Timmermans JP, Adriansen D, De Groodt-Lasseel MH, Scheuermann DW. Projections of neurochemically specified neurons in the porcine colon. *Histochem. Cell Biol.*, **1039** (1995) 115–126.
2. Domoto T, Bishop AE, Oki M, Polak JM. An in vitro study of the projections of the enteric vasoactive intestinal polypeptide immunoreactive neurons in the human colon. *Gastroenterology*, **98** (1990) 819–827.
3. Lomax AE, Furness JB. Neurochemical classification of enteric neurons in the guineapig distal colon. *Cell Tissue Res.* , **302** (2000) 59–72.
4. Lomax AE, Sharkey KA, Bertrand PP, Low AM, Bornstein JC, Furness JB. Correlation of morphology, electrophysiology and chemistry of neurons in the myenteric plexus of the guineapig distal colon. *J. Auton. Nerv. Syst.* , **76** (1999) 45–61.
5. Lomax AE, Zhang JY, Furness JB. Origins of cholinergic inputs to the cell bodies of intestinofugal neurons in the guinea pig distal colon. *J. Comp. Neurol.* , **416** (2000) 451–460.
6. Neunlist M, Dobreva G, Schemann M. Characteristics of mucosally projecting myenteric neurons in the guineapig proximal colon. *J. Physiol. (Lond)*, **517** (1999) 533–546.
7. Tamura K, Ito H, Wade PR. Morphology, electrophysiology, and calbindin immunoreactivity of myenteric neurons in the guinea pig distal colon. *J. Comp. Neurol.*, **437** (2001) 423–437.
8. Brookes SJH, Ewart WR, Wingate DL. Intracellular recordings from myenteric neurones in the human colon. *J. Physiol. (Lond)* , **390** (1987) 305–318.
9. Furukawa K, Taylor GS, Bywater RAR. An intracellular study of myenteric neurons in the mouse colon. *J. Neurophys.*, **55** (1986) 1395–1406.
10. Smith TK. Myenteric AH neurons are sensory neurons in the guineapig proximal colon: an electrophysiological analysis in intact preparations. *Gastroenterology*, **862** (1994) A–216.
11. Smith TK. An electrophysiological identification of intrinsic sensory neurons responsive to 5-HT applied to the mucosa that underlie peristalsis in the guineapig proximal colon. *J. Physiol. (Lond)*, **495** (1996) 102.
12. Vogalis F, Hillsley K, Smith TK. Recording ionic events from cultured, DiI-labelled myenteric neurons in the guineapig proximal colon. *J. Neurosci. Methods*, **96** (2000) 25–34.
13. Furness JB, Kunze WA, Bertrand PP, Clerc N, Bornstein JC. Intrinsic primary afferent neurons of the intestine. *Prog. Neurobiol.*, **54** (1998) 1–18.
14. Hillsley K, Kenyon JL, Smith TK. Ryanodine-sensitive stores regulate the excitability of AH neurons in the myenteric plexus of guineapig ileum. *J. Neurophysiol.*, **84** (2000) 2777–2785.
15. Alex G, Kunze WA, Furness JB, Clerc N. Comparison of the effects of neurokinin-3 receptor blockade on two forms of slow synaptic transmission in myenteric AH neurons. *Neuroscience*, **104** (2001) 263–269.
16. Smith TK, Sanders KM. Motility of the large intestine. In *Textbook of Gastroenterology I.* Yamada T, Alpers DH, Owyang C, Powell DW, Silverstein FE. (eds.) JB Lippincott Co., Philadelphia, PA, 1994, 234–261.
17. Sanders KM. G protein-coupled receptors in gastrointestinal physiology. IV. Neural regulation of gastrointestinal smooth muscle. *Am. J. Physiol.*, **275(1)** (1998) 1:G1–G7.
18. Shuttleworth CW, Keef KD. Roles of peptides in enteric neuromuscular transmission. *Regul. Pept.*, **56** (1995) 101–120
19. Koh SD, Sanders KM. Stretch-dependent potassium channels in murine colonic smooth muscle cells. *J. Physiol.*, **533** (2001) 155–163.
20. Bayguinov O, Hagen B, Bonev AD, Nelson MT, Sanders KM. Intracellular calcium events activated by ATP in murine colonic myocytes. *Am. J. Physiol. Cell Physiol.*, **279** (2000) C126–C135.
21. Ward SM, Sanders KM. Interstitial cells of Cajal: primary targets of enteric motor innervation. *Anat. Rec.*, **262** (2001) 125–135
22. Daniel EE, Posey-Daniel V. Neuromuscular structures in opossum esophagus: role of interstitial cells of Cajal. *Am. J. Physiol.*, **246** (1984) G305–G315.
23. Wang XY, Sanders KM, Ward SM. Relationship between interstitial cells of Cajal and enteric motor neurons in the murine proximal colon. *Cell Tissue Res.*, **302** (2000) 331–342.
24. Costa M, Furness JB. Nervous control of motility. In *Mediators and Drugs in Gastrointestinal Motility I.* Bertaccini G (ed.), Springer-Verlag, Berlin, Germany, 1981, pp. 279–306.
25. Elliott TR, Barclay-Smith E. Antiperistalsis and other muscular activities of the colon. *J. Physiol. (Lond)*, **31** (1904) 272–304.
26. D'Antona G, Hennig GW, Costa M, Humphreys CM, Brookes SJ. Analysis of motor patterns in the isolated guineapig large intestine by spatio-temporal maps. *Neurogastroenterol Motil.*, **13** (2001) 483–492.
27. Costa M, Furness JB. The peristaltic reflex: an analysis of the nerve pathways and their pharmacology. *Naunyn Schmiedeberg's Arch. Pharmacol.*, **294** (1976) 47–60.

28. Foxx-Orenstein AE & Grider JR Regulation of colonic propulsion by enteric excitatory and inhibitory neurotransmitters. *Am. J. Physiol.*, **271** (1996) G433–G437.
29. Mackenna BR, McKirdy HC. Peristalsis in the rabbit distal colon. *J. Physiol. (Lond)*, **220** (1972) 33–54.
30. Sarna SK. Myoelectric correlates of colonic motor complexes and contractile activity. *Am. J. Physiol.*, **250** (1986) G213–220.
31. Christensen J, Anuras S, Hauser RL. Migrating spike bursts and electrical slow waves in the cat colon: effect of sectioning. *Gastroenterology*, **66** (1974) 240–247.
32. Bush TG, Spencer NJ, Watters N, Sanders KM, Smith, TK. Spontaneous migrating motor complexes occur in both the terminal ileum and colon of the C57BL/6 mouse in vitro. *Auton. Neurosci.*, **84** (2000) 162–168.
33. Bywater RA, Small RC, Taylor GS Neurogenic slow depolarizations and rapid oscillations in the membrane potential of circular muscle of mouse colon. *J. Physiol. (Lond)*, **413** (1989) 505–519.
34. Bywater RA, Spencer NJ, Fida R, Taylor GS. Second-, minute- and hour-metronomes of intestinal pacemakers. *Clin. Exp. Pharmacol. Physiol.*, **25** (1998) 857–861.
35. Basotti G, Gaburri M. Manometric investigation of high-amplitude propagated contractile activity of the human colon. *Am. J. Physiol.*, **255** (1988) G660–G664.
36. Wood JD, Brann LR, Vermillion DL Electrical and contractile behaviour of large intestinal musculature of piebald mouse model for hirschsprung's disease. *Dig. Dis. Sci.*, **31** (1986) 638–650.
37. Bush TG, Spencer NJ, Watters N, Sanders KM, Smith TK Effects of alosetron on spontaneous migrating motor complexes in murine small and large bowel in vitro. *Amer. J. Physiol.*, **281** (2001) G974–G983.
38. Karaus M, Sarna SK. Giant migrating contractions during defecation in the dog colon. *Gastroenterology*, **92** (1987) 925–933.
39. Powell AK, Bywater RA. Endogenous nitric oxide release modulates the direction and frequency of colonic migrating motor complexes in the isolated mouse colon. *Neurogastroenterol. Motil.*, **13** (2001) 221–228.
40. Spencer NJ, Bywater RAR, Taylor GS Disinhibition during myoelectric complexes in the mouse colon. *J. Auton. Nerv. Syst.*, **71** (1998) 37–47.
41. Smith TK, McCarron S Nitric oxide modulates cholinergic reflex pathways to the longitudinal and circular muscle in the isolated guineapig distal colon. *J. Physiol. (Lond)*, **512** (1998) 893–906.
42. Spencer N, McCarron SL, Smith TK Sympathetic inhibition of ascending and descending interneurons during the peristaltic reflex in the isolated guineapig distal colon. *J. Physiol. (Lond)*, **519** (1999) 539–550.
43. Smith TK, Robertson WJ. Synchronous movements of the longitudinal and circular muscle during peristalsis in the guineapig distal colon. *J. Physiol. (Lond)*, **506** (1998) 563–577.
44. Alvarez WC. Ch. 1, In *An Introduction to Gastro-enterology*, 3rd ed., Wm. Heinmann, London, UK, 1940, pp. 28–30.
45. Bayliss W, Starling EH The movements and innervation of the small intestine. *J. Physiol. (Lond)*, **24** (1899) 99–143.
46. Bayliss W, Starling EH. The movements and innervation of the large intestine. *J. Physiol. (Lond)*, **26** (1900) 107–118.
47. Jule Y Nerve mediated descending inhibition in the proximal colon of the rabbit. *J. Physiol. (Lond)*, **309** (1980) 487–498.
48. Smith TK, Bywater RAR, Holman ME, Taylor GS. Electrical responses of the muscularis externa to distension of the isolated guineapig distal colon. *J. Gastrointest. Motil.*, **4** (1992) 145–156.
49. Hirst GDS, Holman ME & McKirdy HC Two descending nerve pathways activated by distension of guineapig small intestine. *J. Physiol. (Lond)*, **244** (1975) 113–127.
50. Spencer N, Walsh M, Smith TK Purinergic and cholinergic neuro-neuronal transmission underlying reflexes evoked by mucosal stimulation in the guineapig small intestine. *J. Physiol. (Lond)*, **522** (2000) 321–31.
51. Kottegoda SR An analysis of the possible nervous mechanisms involved in the peristaltic reflex. *J. Physiol. (Lond)*, **200** (1969) 687–712.
52. Wood JD Mixing and moving in the gut. *Gut*, **45** (1999) 333–334.
53. Stevens RJ, Publicover NG, Smith TK Propagation and neural regulation of calcium waves in circular and longitudinal muscle layers of guineapig small intestine. *Gastroenterology*, **118** (2000) 1–15.
54. Stevens RJ, Publicover NG, Smith TK Induction and regulation of Ca^{2+} waves by enteric neural reflexes. *Nature*, **399** (1999) 62–66.
55. Smith TK, Reed JB, Sanders KM Interaction of two electrical pacemakers in the circular muscle of the canine proximal colon. *Am. J. Physiol.*, **252** (1987) C290–C299.
56. Spencer N, Smith TK Simultaneous intracellular recordings from longitudinal and circular muscle during the peristaltic reflex in guineapig colon. *J. Physiol. (Lond)*, **533** (2001) 787–799.
57. Pehlivanov N, Liu J, Kassab GS, Puckett JL, Mittal RK. Relationship between esophageal muscle thickness and intraluminal pressure: an ultrasonographic study. *Am. J. Physiol.*, **280** (2001) G1093–G1098.

58. McKirdy HC Functional relationship of longitudinal and circular layers of the muscularis externa of the rabbit large intestine. *J. Physiol. (Lond)*, **227** (1972) 839–853.
59. Sanders KM, Smith TK. Motor neurons of the submucous plexus regulate electrical activity of the circular muscle of the canine proximal colon. *J. Physiol. (Lond)*, **380** (1986) 293–310.
60. Sanders KM, Smith TK (1986). Enteric neural regulation of slow waves in the circular muscle of the canine proximal colon. *J. Physiol. (Lond)*, **377** (1986) 297–313.
61. Smith TK, Reed JB, Sanders KM. Electrical pacemakers of the canine proximal colon are functionally innervated by inhibitory motor neurons. *Am. J. Physiol.*, **256** (1989) C466–C477.
62. Spencer NJ, Smith TK Electrical reflex responses of myenteric neurons, longitudinal and circular muscle to mucosal stimulation in the isolated guineapig distal colon. *Gastroenterology*, **118** (2000) 3664.
63. Spence NJ, Smith TK. Simultaneous intracellular recordings from myenteric neurons and circular muscle cells during spontaneously discharging peristaltic reflex pathways in guineapig colon. *Neurogastroenterol. Motil.*, **13** (2001) 433.
64. Kunze WAA, Furness JB, Bertrand PP, Bornstein, JC Intracellular recording from myenteric neurons that respond to stretch. *J. Physiol. (Lond)*, **506** (1998) 827–842.
65. Grider JR. Tachykinins as transmitters of the ascending contractile component of the peristaltic reflex. *Am. J. Physiol.*, **257** (1989) G709–G714.
66. Grider JR, Makhlouf GM. Regulation of the peristaltic reflex by peptides of the myenteric plexus. *Arch Int. Pharmacodyn. Ther.*, **303** (1990) 232–251.
67. Grider JR, Makhlouf GM. Colonic peristalsis: identification of vasoactive intestinal peptide as a mediator of descending relaxation. *Am. J. Physiol.*, **253** (1987) G7.
68. Grider JR, Makhlouf GM. Colonic peristalsis: identification of vasoactive intestinal peptide as a mediator of descending relaxation. *Am. J. Physiol.*, **251** (1987) G40–G45.
69. Green JT, Richardson C, Marshall RW, Rhodes J, McKirdy HC, Thomas GA, Williams GT. Nitric oxide mediates a therapeutic effect of nicotine in ulcerative colitis. *Aliment. Pharmacol. Ther.*, **14** (2000) 1429–1434.
70. Brann L, Wood JD. Motility of the large intestine of piebald-lethal mice. *Dig. Dis. Sci.*, **21** (1976) 633–640.

4

Mucin and Goblet Cell Function

Samuel B. Ho and Laurie L. Shekels

CONTENTS

1. INTRODUCTION

The intestine and colon are coated by a protective mucous gel. The mucous gel consists of a variety of large mucin glycoproteins, trefoil factors (TFF), defensins, secreted immunoglobulins (Ig), electrolytes, sloughed epithelial cells, phospholipids, commensal bacteria, and other components. These factors form a dynamic barrier that protects epithelial surfaces from toxins, harmful bacteria, parasites, and digestive chemicals. Mucous gel components are largely derived from the secretory products of goblet cells. The protective functions of goblet cell products make them an integral part of the innate immune response of the gut. This review will focus on recent insights into the function of intestinal goblet cells and their secretory products that contribute to the protective mucous layer.

2. GOBLET CELL PHYSIOLOGY AND SECRETION

2.1. Goblet Cell Morphology

Goblet cells have a distinctive appearance characterized by a basolateral nucleus and a large supranuclear region in which can be found a rough endoplasmic reticulum, a large Golgi apparatus, and condensing vacuoles *(1)*. There is a prominant apical accumulation of storage granules containing mucin and other glycoproteins, which are surrounded by a cytokeratin-rich theca. Goblet cells are found in many epithelial tissues that are exposed to the environment, including conjuntiva, respiratory, cervix, and digestive tract epitheium. Within the intestine and colon, goblet cells arise from pluripotent stem cells located toward the crypt base *(2)*. An early form of the goblet cell is the oligomucous cell located in the lower crypts. These cells continue to differentiate as they migrate to the villus or surface epithelium and are subsequently

From: *Colonic Diseases*
Edited by: T. R. Koch © Humana Press Inc., Totowa, NJ

sloughed into the lumen *(3)*. The density of goblet cells increases distally from the duodenum to the ileum in the small intestine. The colon contains the largest concentration of goblet cells, the density of which also increases aborally from the cecum to the rectum. Intestinal cell populations exhibit a rapid turnover; occurring every 2 to 3 d in rodents and every 3–8 d in humans *(4)*.

2.2. Goblet Cell Secretion

Constitutive secretion from goblet cells maintains the protective mucous coat of intestinal tissues. This coat is sparse in the small intestine but is readily recognized in histologic studies of colon mucosa. Akamatsu et al. and Matsuo et al. have shown that the surface mucous gel layer in the rectum consists of histologically distinct inner and outer layers *(5,6)*. These investigators used frozen sections or sections fixed in Carnoy's fixative, which provides preservation of the surface mucous coat with less shrinkage than other methods of fixation. Histochemical stains showed that the inner layer consisted of a thin layer intimately attached to the surface epithelium, with a obliquely striped appearance. The outer layer was thicker and consisted of a lateral striped pattern, except in the cecum, where this layer was a homogeneous thin band. Cell debris, food residues and bacteria were observed sandwiched between the laminated arrays of the outer layer. In Carnoy-fixed paraffin sections, these layers were noted to be thinner in the cecum and thickest in the rectum. The inner and outer layers measured 5.6 $\pm$ 0.2 μM and 31.1 $\pm$ 7.2 μM in the cecum, respectively; and 12.7 $\pm$ 6.0 μM and 88.8 $\pm$ 80.1 μM in the rectum, respectively. On frozen sections, these layers appear approximately twice as thick as in Carnoy's-fixed sections due to shrinkage caused by fixation *(7)*. Histochemical stains indicate that the inner layer consists primarily of nonsulfated sialomucins, whereas the outer layer consists of heterogeneous layers of nonsulfated sialomucins and sulfated mucins. The multilaminated structure found in the outer layer may reflect different chemical properties of mucins secreted simultaneously from the same goblet cell or separately from the goblet cells lining the different levels of the crypts.

Baseline secretion of mucin is accomplished by periodic exocytosis of mucin granules. Radiolabeling studies of mucin carbohydrate indicate that turnover of granules along the periphery of the theca is faster than centrally-located granules within the goblet cell vacuole. Microtubules direct granule migration to the cell apex and actin filaments play a role in controlling contact of the mucin granules with the apical plasma membrane *(1,3)*. Rapid secretion occurs by fusion of contiguous mucin granules with the apical plasma membrane, a process known as compound exocytosis. Granule secretion has been shown to progress through central and peripheral granules, resulting in cavitation of the total apical granule mass *(3)*. Rat colon goblet cell cavitation occurs rapidly in the midcrypt regions, with the volume of intracellular mucous granules decreasing to 61% of control granules within 5 min of carbachol stimulation. Mucin granule stores recover to 94% of control levels by 4 h after stimulation *(8)*.

Secretion of goblet cell mucin can be stimulated by a variety of both chemical and mechanical agents *(1)*. These include neurotransmitter cholinergic stimulation, intestinal anaphylaxis, and chemical and physical irritation. Nonspecific release of neurotransmitters by electrical stimulation of rat intestinal sheets mounted in Ussing chambers causes crypt goblet cell secretion. This is partially inhibited by atropine and totally inhibited by blocking nerve sodium channels with tetrodotoxin. Muscarinic receptors have been shown to be present in rat colon epithelial cells. Acetylcholine and carbachol directly stimulate goblet cell secretion, but again, only in goblet cells located in the crypts of the small intestine and colon, with no effect on goblet cells located in intestinal villi and colon surface epithelium. The cholinergic stimulation of mucin in the HT29-18N2 intestinal goblet cell line occurs through noncompound exocytosis independent of protein kinase C (PKC). However, stimulation of PKC increased mucin secretion by a compound exocytotic pathway (9).

A variety of gut hormones and neurotransmitters, including cholecystokinin (CCK), gastrin, secretin, vasoactive intestinal polypeptide, substance P, neurotensin, and somatostatin, have been shown to have no effect on basal and acetylcholine-stimulated goblet cell secretion in rabbit colon organ cultures (10). Immobilization stress of rat intestines causes increased mucin release involving neurotensin (11) The release of mucin by neurotensin requires intracellular calicium mobilization. This is in contrast to carbachol-induced mucin release, which depends on both the release of calcium from intracellular stores and an influx of extracellular calcium (12). Mast cell and inflammatory mediators, such as histamine, prostaglandins and leukotrienes, and immune complexes, have been implicated in goblet cell secretion (1).

Luminal chemicals, lectins, and toxins may cause secretion of goblet cell mucins. Nonspecific membrane damage by mustard oils or alcohol may cause surface cell exfoliation and indirect mucin release. Cholera toxin elicits active mucin secretion by goblet cells, which is independent of cyclic adenosine 5'-monophosphate (cAMP) and is mediated in part by activation of a 5-hydroxytryptamine (5-HT)-like receptor. Mucin secretion in response to exogenous 5-HT occurs in two differing pathways: one is mediated by a 5-HT4-like receptor and is capsaicin-sensitive and tetrodotoxin-insensitive, and one that is sensitive to tetrodotoxin, but lacks the capsaicin-sensitive 5-HT4-mediated response. Both pathways converge to a common cholinergic pathway (13). These data indicate that there exists multiple independent and interconnecting pathways that elicit a stimulated mucin release.

2.3. Mucous Layer and Intestinal Bacteria

The mucous layer serves as an environmental niche for commensal intestinal bacteria and serves as a substrate for bacterial degradative enzymes. In mouse ileum, only a small proportion of intestinal flora actually contact and adhere to epithelial surfaces (14). Poulson et al. have shown that commensal Escherichia coli in mouse large intestine inhabit the adherent mucin layer rather than bind to the epithelial cells (15). Thus, the mucous layer appears to physically trap bacteria, viruses and other lumenal content. Mucin oligosaccharides may mimic membrane receptors for microbes and preferentially adhere to them. For example, oligomannosides of mucin N-glycans bind type 1 pili of some E. coli 0157:H7 bacteria, fucose(Fuc)-containing structures are recognition sites for Salmonella typhimurium, and Gal-GalNAc are receptors for Enatamoeba histolytica (16–18). Mucins have been shown to act as competitive inhibitors of E. coli, Yersinia enterocolitica, and E. histolytica binding to intestinal epithelium (19–20). Intestinal mucins have also been shown to inhibit rotavirus replication in an oligosaccharide-dependent manner (22). Mucins are closely associated with IgA, which contributes to the antimicrobial properties of the mucous gel (23). IgA-coated bacteria remain trapped in the mucous layers and subsequent turnover of the mucous layer and peristalsis allow for disposal of the bacteria. Probiotic bacteria, such as Lactobacillus species, have been shown to stimulate mucin production, which may be a mechanism for their protective effects in the colon (24).

Hooper et al. used DNA microarray techniques to compare ileal gene expression in age-matched germ-free mice and mice colonized with the intestinal commensal Bacteroides thetaiotaomicron (25). Commensal bacteria in the ileum modulated the expression of genes involved in nutrient absorption, glycoprotein fucosylation, mucosal barrier function, xenobiotic metabolism, and angiogenesis. Colonized mice exhibited the up-regulation of the CRP-ductin gene encoding both a cell surface and mucous layer protein (MUCLIN) and a putative receptor for trefoil peptides. B. thetaiotaomicron have also been shown to use a repressor, FucR, as a molecular sensor of L-Fuc availability in the intestine (26). FucR coordinates expression of an

Table 1
Human Mucin Genes

Designation	Source	Type[a]	No. aa in tandem repeat	Chromosomal location	Tandem repeat aa sequence	Reference
MUC1	Mammary, pancreatic	mem	20	1q21q24	GSTAPPAHGVTSAPDTRPAP	(123)
MUC2	Intestinal	sec	23	11p15	PTTTPITTTTTVTPTPTPTGTQT	(124)
MUC3	Intestinal	mem	17	7q22	HSTPSFTSSITTTETTS	(38,125)
MUC4	Tracheal	mem	16	3q29	(T)SS(A)ST(GHA)T(P)L(P)VT(D)[b]	(126)
MUC5AC	Tracheal, gastric	sec	8	11p15	TTSTTSAP	(127)
MUC5B	Tracheal, gallbladder, cervix	sec	29	11p15	SSTPGTAHTHTEQTTTATTPTATGTT ATP[c]	(49,50,128)
MUC6	Gastric	sec	169	11p15	SPFSSTGPMTATSFQTTTTYPTPSH PQTTLPTHVPPFSTSLVTPSTGTVIT PTHAQMATSASIHSTPTGTIPPPTTL KATGSTHTAPPMTPTTSGTSQAHSS FSTAKTSTSLHSHTSSTHHPEVTPTS TTTITPNPTSTGTSTPVAHTTSATSS RLPTPFTTHSPPTGS	(129)
MUC7	Salivary	sec	23	4q13-q21	TTAAPPTPSATTPAPPSSSAPPG	(130)
MUC8[c]	Tracheal	?	13-41	12q24.3	TSCPRPLQEGTRV TSCPRPLQEGTPGSRAAHALSRRG HRVHELPTSSPGGDTGF	(131)
MUC9[c]	oviduct	?	15	1p13	GAMTMTSVGHQSMTP	(132)
MUC11[c]	Colon	?	28	7q22	SGLSEESTTSHSSPGSTHTTLSPASTTT	(45)
MUC12[c]	Colon	mem	28	7q22	SGLSQESTTFHSSPGSTETTLSPASTTT	(45)

[a]mem = membrane-bound; sec, secreted.
[b](), imperfectly conserved.
[c]putative mucins based on partial sequence data.

56

operon encoding enzymes in the L-Fuc metabolic pathway with expression of another locus that regulates production of fucosylated glycans in intestinal enterocytes. This presumably allows the bacteria to coordinate its nutritional and microenvironmental requirements with a host-derived energy source from mucosal cells.

3. MUCINS IN THE GASTROINTESTINAL TRACT

3.1. Molecular Biology of Mucin Glycoproteins

Biochemical analysis and characterization of mucin proteins has been limited because of their large size and abundant glycosylation. The structure of mucins has been deduced from molecular sequence data derived from the cloning of several human and animal mucins. These data have demonstrated that all mucins share certain structural features. For example, mucin proteins contain regions with a high proportion of threonine and/or serine glycosylation sites that are repeated in tandem along the length of the molecule and, thus, are called tandem repeats. However, the specific amino acid sequences, the lengths of these repeats, and the nonrepetitive domains of these molecules are quite variable (Table 1) (27–29).

3.1.1. Membrane Mucins

Two distinct families of mucins have been defined based on structural characteristics. The first family consists of membrane-bound glycoproteins including MUC1. MUC1 is synthesized by most, if not all, epithelial tissues and is highly expressed in breast and other adenocarcinomas (30–32). Two thirds of this protein consists of 20-amino acid (aa) tandem repeats, which contain 25% serine or threonine glycosylation sites, followed by a 31-aa transmembrane sequence and a 69-aa cytoplasmic tail. The mature protein exists on the cell surface as a heterodimer composed of subunits derived from cleavage of the full-length mucin precursor (33). This protein is targeted to the apical membrane of epithelial cells, with the tandem-repeat domain extending approx 150 nm above the cell surface. This structure is thought to physically shield epithelial surface antigens or receptors from luminal agents. Secreted forms of MUC1 have also been described, which lack the transmembrane domain due to a cleavage of the full-length mucin protein. High levels of this secreted form of MUC1 have been found in vivo in human breast milk and bile and as well as in vitro from cultured cells (34–37).

Descriptions of the human MUC3 and mouse Muc3 carboxyl terminal structures have recently been published (Fig. 1). Gum et al describe the presence of a single cysteine-rich region with homology to a three-lobed epidermal growth factor (EGF)-like tertiary structure within the MUC3 carboxyl terminus (38). Splice variants of this region have been found that contain 366 aa with two EGF domains and a transmembrane domain in the carboxyl terminus (39). The region of MUC3 located upstream of the tandem repeat region encodes another large serine and threonine-rich domain with an imperfect repeat structure of 375 aa. Expression cloning techniques using a mouse cecal cDNA library have identified a mouse Muc3 (mMuc3) mucin that contains two EGF-like domains and a transmembrane domain in its 379-aa carboxyl terminus (40). The tandem repeat domain of mMuc3 is 3000–4000 aa, with an 104-aa amino terminus. These structural data suggests that the MUC3 mucins exist as large membrane-bound and/or soluble glycoproteins, which may participate in ligand–receptor or protein–protein interactions with pathogens, intestinal mucosal surfaces, or other components of mucin or the mucous gel.

A cell surface mucin-like molecule has been isolated from 13,762 rat mammary adenocarcinoma cells, called asialoglycoprotein (ASGP) (41,42). This is a sialomucin which is synthesized as a large precursor that is cleaved in the endoplasmic reticulum to form a sialomucin with tandem repeats of 124 aa (ASGP-1) and a membrane-associated glycoprotein (ASGP-2). The

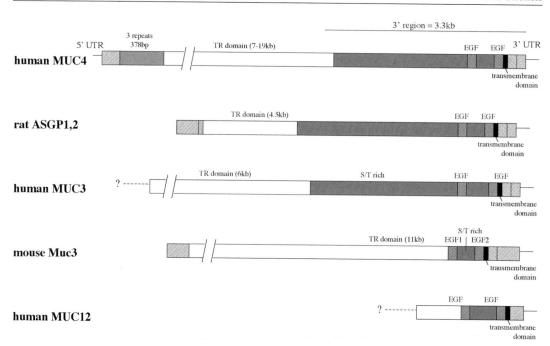

Fig. 1. Comparison of cDNA structures of membrane-bound mucins.

deduced sequence of ASGP-2 consists of a large extracellular domain of 684 aa, a 25-aa transmembrane domain and a 20-aa cytoplasmic tail. The extracellular domain has two EGF-like repeats and is able to bind a tyrosine kinase type receptor. The entire ASGP1/2 protein consists of approx an 80-aa amino terminus, a 1500-aa tandem repeat domain, and a 1339-aa carboxyl terminus. Sequence data for the 5' region and the 3' region of human MUC4 has recently been described. The 5' untranslated region of human MUC4 contains an 82-bp signal peptide with a high degree of similarity with ASGP-1 *(43)*. Additional sequence data regarding the 3' sequence of MUC4 indicates that it contains 1099 aa with two EGF-like domains and a transmembrane sequence *(44)*. Based on sequence similarity between the human MUC4 and ASGP1 and -2 nonrepetitive regions, ASGP represents the rat homologue of MUC4 (ASGP/ rMuc4). The 5' coding region of MUC4 is unique and only one cysteine residue is encoded by this 42-aa region. In the tandem repeat region the human MUC4 gene exhibits a large variation in the number of repeats (7–19 kb).

Partial mucin-like sequences have been isolated by comparison of the differential display of mRNA species in normal colon and colon cancer *(45)*. Two clones were isolated that were highly expressed in normal colon and poorly expressed in colon cancer. One clone encoded a degenerate 28-aa mucin-like tandem repeat and was labeled MUC11. The other clone was labeled MUC12 and encoded a different 28 aa tandem repeat and a carboxyl terminus with two cysteine-rich EGF-like domains and a putative transmembrane domain, similar to the structural organization of MUC3 and MUC4 (Fig. 1). Each clone was mapped to chromosome 7q22, which is the location of the MUC3 mucin gene, and appeared to have different tissue-specific patterns of expression. The structural homology between MUC12 and MUC3 and the similar chromosomal localization suggest that a cluster of related membrane-type mucin genes may exist at this locus.

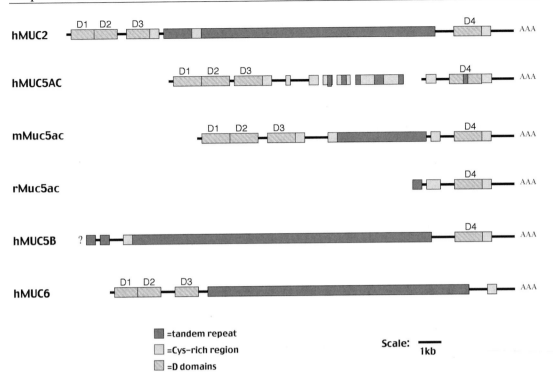

Fig. 2. Comparison of cDNAs structures for secretory mucin genes mapped to 11p15.5.

The specific functional roles of membrane-bound mucins in the intestinal tract have yet to be determined. The presence of both membrane-bound and secretory forms suggests a bifunctional role or tissue-specific differences in function. In the rat colon, Rossi et al. have shown that ASGP/rMuc4 is present primarily as a secretory protein located in goblet cell vacuoles *(42)*. MUC3 has been shown to be expressed by both columnar and goblet cells in the colon, implying a possible bifunctional role. Thus, the contribution of secretory forms of MUC1, MUC3, and MUC4 to the extracellular mucous gel in the intestine and colon may be significant. The presence of EGF-like domains also may suggest a role in growth modulation. EGF-like domains are found in growth factors and extracellular proteins involved in cell adhesion, chemotaxis, wound healing, and matrix interactions. No ligands for MUC3 have been identified, but preliminary data suggest that ASGP-2 may interact with the c-erbB-2 growth factor receptor *(46)*.

3.1.2. Secretory Mucins.

The second family of mucins consists of the secretory mucins. Electron microscopic studies by Carlstedt and Sheehan, working with human cervical mucin, have demonstrated that secreted mucins form long polymers, with molecules linked end-to-end *(47)*. Mucin monomers are thought to be linked together by terminal disulfide bonds via cysteine residues in the terminal nonrepetitive domains, since reduction of disulfide bonds results in the loss of viscosity in mucous gels. To date, five human secretory mucin cDNAs have been cloned and sequenced (Table 1 and Fig. 2).

Investigating the MUC2 intestinal mucin, Gum and coworkers have shown that the MUC2 carboxyl terminal domain contains 984 residues and can be divided into mucin-like (139 residues) and cysteine-rich (845 residues) subdomains *(48)*. The amino terminal segment upstream of the tandem repeats contains a repetitive mucin-like subdomain and a second cysteine-rich region. Both cysteine-rich regions have sequence similarity with the von Willebrand factor (vWF) D domains and most likely function to form disulfide-linked polymers as has been observed for the D domains in vWF. This polymerization is responsible for the viscoelasticity of mucin oligomers. vWF D domains have also been found in a number of other secretory mucins sequenced to date (Fig. 2). These include human, rat, and mouse MUC5AC, the human MUC5B mucin, porcine submaxillary mucin, bovine submaxillary mucin-like protein, and frog integumentary mucin B.1 *(40,49–51)* . The human MUC6 mucin has D domains in the 5' region and a cysteine-rich region (a cysteine-knot [CK] domain) in the 3' terminal domain *(52)*. These structural similarities suggest that these proteins share the ability to form disulfide-linked oligomers or are secretory mucins of the gel-forming type. Their common location on chromosome 11p15 suggests a common derivation from a single ancestral gene.

Direct evidence for the participation of D domain sequences in mucin processing comes from transfection studies of plasmids encoding normal and mutated D domains of porcine submaxillary mucin *(53,54)*. These studies indicate that CGLCG motifs in the D1 and D3 domains in the amino terminus play a critical role. The three D1, D2, and D3 domains must be contiguously located to avoid multimerization in the non acidic endoplasmic reticulum and the *cis-* and *medial*-Golgi compartments. Furthermore, normal multimerization at low pH in the acidic *trans*-Golgi compartments requires an intact CGLCG motif in the D1 domain.

The secretory mucins are typically quite large. The tandem repeat arrays are encoded by a single large exon. The MUC2 exonic repeat region is typically 8700 bp, which compares with the tandem repeat exon of MUC1, which varies from 3500–6200 bp, depending on the number of repeats. The entire MUC2 mucin encodes a protein of about 5200 aa. The MUC5B mucin has the largest central repeat exon reported to date, which is 10,713 bp and encodes a polypeptide with 3570 aa and a calculated apparent molecular weight (Mr) of 370,000 *(49)*; the total mucin protein encodes 5662 aa. The central exons of these secretory mucions are considerably larger than one of the largest coding regions described in vertebrates previously, the 7572 bp exon of lipoporotein ApoB.

The MUC7 is a relatively small molecular weight protein (120–150 kDa) of 377 aa that exists as a monomer and appears to be free of disulfide bonds. MUC7 is expressed in salivary glands and is absent in stomach, tonsils, uterus, placenta, and ovaries.

3.2. Mucin Biochemistry

The protective properties of mucin proteins are derived, in part, from their high molecular weight and the ability, of some types, to form oligomers, thus becoming highly viscous in solution. They have extensive and heterogeneous oligosaccharide side chains, which protect the core peptide from hydrolysis and likely contribute to binding of microbes. Biochemical studies demonstrate that mucins have an average molecular weight of 2×10^6 dal. They are characterized by their exclusion on Sepharose® CL-4B column chromatography and by minimal entry into polyacrylamide gels during electrophoresis. The majority of the mature mucin molecule consists of carbohydrate side chains, which can comprise up to 80–85% of the molecule by weight. Colon mucins contain less carbohydrate than small intestine mucins. Mucin carbohydrates consist primarily of Fuc, galactose (GAL), N-acetylgalactosamine (GalNAc), N-acetylglucosamine (GlcNAc), and sialic acid (SA), with no glucose and trace mannose. The core peptide composition is characteristically rich in serine, threonine, and proline residues, and it is to the hydroxyl amino acids that the carbohyrate chains attach via an O-glycosidic bond.

Goblet cells in both the human and rat colon have been shown to produce a heterogeneous collection of mucin glycoproteins, which can be distinguished by histochemical stains, lectin binding, immunohistochemistry, and ion exchange chromatography *(1,28,55)* . Goblet cells within colon crypts predominantly have sulfomucins and more GlcNAc, whereas the mature goblet cells on the surface contain neutral mucins, less GlcNAc, and more terminal Fuc. These differences in glycoprotein characteristics may be related to differences in core mucin peptide structures, but the precise relationship between different mucin proteins and glycosylation is incompletely known.

Biosynthesis of mucins MUC2–6 in gastrointestinal tissues was performed using metabolic labeling and immunoprecipitation *(56)*. Each of the MUC2 (Mr 600,000), MUC3 (Mr 550,000), MUC4 (Mr > 900,000), MUC5AC (Mr 500,000), and MUC6 (Mr 400,000) precursors could be distinguished electrophoretically in specific regions of the gastrointestinal (GI) tract. MUC2 proteins displayed differences in mobility from samples of small and large intestine, indicating differences in glycosylation. Some individuals displayed double bands for MUC2 and MUC3 precursors, suggesting allelic variation with the respective genes.

The biosynthesis of MUC2-type mucins have been determined in mucin-producing cell cultures and by expression of plasmids encoding specific mucin domains in cell culture *(54,57,58)*. The initial apomucin core protein are formed in the rough endoplasmic reticulum, where they begin to form dimers through the carboxyl terminal CK domains before any O-glycosylation takes place. N-glycosylation of the nascent protein is necessary to insure the correct folding and dimerization and transfer to the Golgi apparatus *(57)*. The tandem repeat domains of the MUC2 mucin monomers and dimers become heavily O-glycosylated in the Golgi apparatus of mucin-producing cells, which confers proteolytic resistance to the protein. When the glycosylated dimers reach the trans Golgi compartments they are assembled into disulfide-bonded multimers through the carboxyl terminal D domains. Insoluble forms of MUC2 are also formed early in biosynthesis, but after initial O-glycosylation *(59,60)*. This insoluble mucin is form by non reducible intermolecular bonds, the nature of which is unknown, but may represent cross-links between linear MUC2 oligomers. The cysteine-rich N-terminal and C-terminal ends of the rat Muc2 protein are very readily cleaved, even in the presence of multiple proteinase inhibitors *(61)*. This suggests that degradation of secreted Muc2 mucin begins in the terminal ends, and conditions that further increase this degradation may increase mucous solubility and decrease the protective barrier. The large glycosylated domains of rat intestinal mucin have been isolated and demonstrate variable glycosylation between rat strains and the small and large intestine *(62)*. The oligosaccharides characterized by gas chromatography mass spectrometry were identical in the large intestine in two different rat strains, but the oligosaccharide pattern from the small intestines differed. Large intestine Muc2 were enriched in sulfated oligosaccharides, and the small intestine contained higher amounts of sialylated species. The identification of at least three different glycoforms of the rat Muc2 mucin is presumably related to the differential regulation of glycosyltransferases, implying a highly flexible system that is able to respond to changing stimuli in the intestinal lumen.

3.3. Localization of Mucin Gene Expression

Studies using mucin-specific cDNA probes and antibodies indicate that expression of mucin genes is organ and cell-type specific (see Table 2). Studies to date indicate that the tissue distribution of the MUC2 and MUC3 mucins are largely restricted to the intestinal tract. MUC2 mRNA and protein are localized to goblet cells of normal jejunum, ileum, and colon. While its expression is normally rare in respiratory tissue, MUC2 expression can be induced there by

Table 2
Expression of Secretory Mucin Genes *(80,131,133–136)*

	MUC2	MUC3	MUC4	MUC5AC	MUC5B	MUC6	MUC7	MUC8
Trachea	+	–	++	++	+	–		++
Salivary	–	–		–	+	–	+++	
Esophagus	–	–	–	–	++	–		
Stomach	–	–	–	+++ surface mucous	–	+++ neck, antral glands		–
Duodenum	++ goblet cells	++ columnar cells	–	–	–	+ brunner glands		
Small intestine	++	++	–	–	–	+		
Colon	++	++	++	–	–	–		
Gallbladder	–	++	–	++	+++	++		
Pancreas	–	±	–	–	–	++		
Endocervix	–	–	+	++	+++	+		

disease. MUC3 mRNA and protein are highly expressed in columnar and goblet cells of normal jejunum, ileum, colon, and gallbladder. Sparse MUC3 expression has been observed in some pancreatic-biliary duct cells. Conversely, MUC1, MUC4, MUC5AC, MUC5B, and MUC6 mRNA and protein have a wider organ distribution. MUC1 is expressed ubiquitously in virtually all epithelial tissues. MUC4 mRNA and protein have been found in isolated goblet cells of the rat and human colon, otherwise this mucin in present primarily in ocular, respiratory, and reproductive tract tissues. Sparse amounts of MUC5B have been shown to be present in human colon goblet cells at the crypt base, co-localizing with MUC2-containing goblet cells *(63)*. MUC5AC and MUC6 are the primary mucin proteins in the stomach. Goblet cells found in the conjunctiva, middle ear, and pulmonary repiratory tissue largely express the MUC5AC mucin. Little data exists comparing expression patterns of MUC7 and 8. The functional importance of different mucin gene products found in different organs is unknown.

Ultrastructural localization of MUC1, MUC2, and MUC4 apomucins in human colon biopsies was performed using immunoelectron microscopy with monoclonal antibodies against tandem repeat peptide sequences *(64)*. MUC1 mucin was present in both columnar and goblet cells, where it was present in secretory vesicles, microvilli, and in cytoplasmic remnants in goblet cell theca. MUC2 expression was restricted to goblet cells of both the upper and lower crypts. MUC4 expression was seen in both columnar and goblet cells, primarily at the crypt base. Within the upper crypt areas, MUC4 was primarily in goblet cells.

4. REGULATION OF MUCIN GENE EXPRESSION

To further understand the regulation of the mucin genes, investigators have recently begun to examine the regulatory elements found in the promoters of several of the mucin genes. Analysis of *MUC1* genomic fragments suggests that tissue-specific regulatory elements are found in the proximal core promoter sequence as well as in upstream sequences (at –150 to –60 from the transcription start site). DNA binding assays and mutation analysis identified an

Sp1 site at –99 to –90 and an E box at –84 to –72 in the *MUC1* promoter *(65)*. Abe and Kufe identified a novel *MUC1* transcription factor in MCF-7 breast cancer cells that recognizes sequences between positiions –505 and –485 *(66)*. Gum et al. have identified two regions in the *MUC2* promoter that are necessary for high level transcription, located –1308 to –641 and –91 to –73 relative to the cap site *(67)*. Recently the promoter region of rat *Muc4* was characterized in rat mammary epithelial cells and a human colon cancer cell line *(68)*. Within 2.4 kb of the *Muc4* promoter lie elements controlling epithelial-specific expression with positive regulatory elements found in both the proximal and distal promoter region and negative regulatory elements lying within the intermediate and far distal regions of the promoter.

Exposure of *Pseudomonas aeruginosa* to cultured cells has been shown to activate a c-Src-Ras-MEK1/2-MAPK-pp90rsk signaling pathway which leads to activation of nuclear factor (NF)-κB *(69)*. This in turn binds to a site in the 5' flanking region of the *MUC2* gene and activates *MUC2* mucin transcription. The role of this pathway in controlling *MUC2* gene expression in bacterial–epithelial interactions in the colon remains to be determined.

Recent data indicates that inflammatory mediators and cytokines may alter mucin gene expression. Temann et al. demonstrated that expression of *Muc5AC* but not *Muc2* is up-regulated in the presence of interleukin (IL)-4 overexpression in transgenic mice *(70)*. Tumor necrosis factor (TNF)α has been shown to increase mucin secretion and steady state MUC2 expression in cultured human tracheal epithelial cells *(71)*. This action was inhibited by agents that block PKC and tyrosine kinase phosphorylation. TNFα has also been shown to stimulate mucin secretion and gene expression in tracheal epithelial cells of the guinea pig *(72)*. In these experiments TNFα was also shown to induce nitric oxide (NO) production, which may also stimulate mucin secretion. These data suggest that TNFα alters mucin expression through a PKC-dependent pathway. Stimulation of PKC results in activation of transcription factors, such as activator protein (AP)1 and NF-κB. A PKC-independent path may also be involved. Interaction of IL-4, TNFα, and intestinal epithelial cells is of considerable interest due to the recent findings that mucosal IL-4 levels are decreased in Crohn's disease *(73)* and that TNFα production is increased in T cells from ulcerative colitis biopsies *(74)*. IL-13-induced mucin gene expression in airway epithelium has recently been shown to involve signaling through the EGF receptor *(75)*. Within the mouse intestine, the parasitic infection by the nemotode *Trichinella spiralis* induces goblet cell hyperplasia and increased Muc2 and Muc 3 mucins *(76)*. This appears to be independent of the cytokines interferon γ, TNF, and IL-4; but the role of other cytokines has not been determined *(76)*.

5. TREFOIL FACTORS AND OTHER GOBLET CELL SECRETORY PRODUCTS

In addition to several distinct mucin glycoproteins discussed above, the mucous gel contains other components that contribute to its cytoprotective properties. Small proteins called TFF have been identified, which play an essential role in strengthening the mucous layer and promoting epithelial cell restitution after injury *(77)*. These peptides share a distinctive motif of six cysteine residues forming a "P domain" and are synthesized by mucin-synthesizing cells of the GI tract. They include pS2/TFF1, spasmolytic polypeptide SP/TFF2, and intestinal trefoil factor(ITF)/TFF3. One P domain is present in TFF1 and TFF3, whereas two P domains are present in TFF2. TFF are synthesized by mucin-producing cells in the GI tract. TTF3 is expressed in goblet cells of the intestine with the MUC2 mucin, whereas in the stomach TFF1 and MUC5AC mucin are co-expressed by surface mucous cells, and TFF2 and MUC6 are co-expressed in mucous neck glands and Brunner's glands *(78–81)*.

Mice that are deficient in TFF3 by targeted gene deletion have normal growth and development, but are very sensitive to toxin-induced intestinal injury compared to wild-type mice. Treatment of TFF3-deficient mice with recombinant trefoil peptides reduces their susceptibility to lumenal toxic agents (82). The addition of recombinant trefoil peptides to epithelial monolayers in vitro increases their tolerance of phytohemagglutinin, bile acids, and Clostridium dificile toxin A (83). The addition of trefoil peptides in addition to colonic mucins augments the protective effect. Trefoils have been postulated to increase the viscosity of mucin glycoproteins, however, the specific mechanism of their protective effects are not understood. Tomasetto et al. have used a yeast two-hybrid system to screen stomach and duodenal cDNA expression libraries to identify proteins that interact with murine TFF1 (84). Four positive clones were isolated that correspond to the murine Muc2 and Muc5ac mucin proteins. Mutagenesis experiments showed that TFF1 interacts with these mucins by binding with their vWF factor cysteine-rich domains. These data suggest that TFF may interact with mucin proteins to organize the surface mucous layer. Recently, recombinant rat intestinal trefoil protein has been shown to cause decreased cell adhesion by inducing phosphorylation of E-cadherin–catenin complex and the EGF receptor, resulting in diminished cell–cell adhesion (85). The mechanism or protein–receptor interaction, which mediates these actions of the trefoils on intestinal cells, has not been determined, but it is known that trefoils do not directly bind EGF receptors.

Lipids and phospholipids are found bound noncovalently to mucin and a small amount of fatty acid is bound covalently to mucin proteins in the mucous gel. Removal of bound lipids has been shown to increase mucin susceptibility to oxygen radicals and to increase the diffusion rate of H^+ through gastric mucous. The gastric mucosa is covered by a layer of surfactant-like phospholipids attached to the mucosal surface that has protective qualities against acid and ulcerogens. The surface hydrophobicity of intestinal mucosa increases from the small intestine to the distal colon (86). The surface tension overlying inflamed colonic mucosa is greater than normal colon and, thus has a lower hydrophobicity than normal colon, which may influence the attachment of certain types of bacterial pili (86). Goblet cells also contain a kallikrein protease (87), lactose-binding lectins (88),a vitamin B_{12} binding protein (89), and a serine protease capable of cleaving EGF and cobalamin-binding protein (90).

6. PATHOBIOLOGY OF GOBLET CELLS
6.1. Transgenic Ablation of Goblet Cells

ITF has been shown to be selectively expressed by goblet cells throughout the small and large intestine. The goblet cell-specific transcriptional mechanism was localized to a 6.35-kbp 5' flanking region of the *ITF* gene (91,92). Itoh et al. created transgenic mice that expressed the diphtheria toxin (DT)-A chain protein driven by the *ITF* gene 5'flanking region (93). This resulted in targeted ablation of goblet cells expressing this transgene. Transgenic mice expressing high copy numbers of the *mITF/DT-A* transgene exibited a 60% reduction in goblet cell numbers in the proximal and distal colon, with no change in the numbers of goblet cells in the small intestine. Increased levels of total endogenous ITF and unchanged levels of MUC2 and MUC3 mucins were found in the colons of *mITF/DT-A* transgenic mice compared with normal mice, indicating a compensatory increase in these components from fewer goblet cells in the transgenic mice. Surprisingly, the transgenic mice were less susceptible to colon injury following dextran sodium sulfate (DSS) or acetic acid administration. After oral administration of DSS, 55% of control mice died compared with 5% of *mITF/DT-A* transgenic mice. Similarly, after rectal administration of acetic acid, 30% of control mice died compared with 3% of the transgenic mice. Other studies of experimental colitis have shown that ITF levels increase in the recovery phase of the colitis *(94,95)*. Furthermore, as noted above, *MUC2* and *MUC3* gene expression have been shown to be preserved in the setting of ulcerative colitis or Crohn's disease despite a reduction in goblet cell number, indicating that compensatory increases in goblet cell products occur in colitis *(96,97)*. These studies indicate that goblet cell damage induces a compensatory increase in ITF and mucin glycoproteins, which can result in enhanced mucosal protection.

6.2. Mucin Gene Knock-Out

The role of specific mucin gene products in the protective surface mucous coat of the intestine has not been determined. One method to determine the function of specific mucins in vivo is the use of homologous recombination techniques to create a mouse strain with a targeted deletion of a specific gene. To date, one mucin, Muc1, has been successfully deleted or knocked out in mice. The Muc1 mucin is a transmembrane mucin produced by most simple secretory epithelia. In the small intestine and colon, the Muc1 mucin is produced by both columnar and goblet cells at relatively low levels. Mice lacking the *Muc1* gene have a relatively normal phenotype, indicating that Muc1 by itself is not critical for normal growth and development *(98)*. Cystic fibrosis (CF) is characterized by defects in the CF transmembrane conductance regulator (*CFTR*) gene. Humans with CF have abnormal accumulations of viscous mucus in the lungs and gastrointestinal tract. Homozygous *CFTR* knock-out mice have severe intestinal obstruction, which often leads to death at weaning. *CFTR* knock-out mice have been shown to have lower levels of Muc2, Muc3, and Muc5ac mRNA levels and similar levels of protein compared to control mice *(99)*. In contrast, elevated levels of Muc1 mRNA and protein are present in the colon of CFTR mice compared with control mice. *CFTR* mice were cross-bred with homozygous *Muc1* knock-out mice resulting in *CFTR* mice lacking *Muc1*. These mice demonstrated greatly diminished intestinal mucus obstruction when compared with Muc1-expressing CF mice and improved survival on solid food. These data indicate that Muc1 mucin may play an important role in the extracellular mucus accumulations observed in the GI tract of *CFTR* knock-out mice. This raises the possibility that other mucins with membrane-spanning domains, such as Muc3 and Muc4, may be expressed as a secreted form and significantly contribute to the secreted mucous layer of the colon.

Recently, Velcich et al. have described a mouse strain genetically deficient in *Muc2*. The intestinal crypts of *Muc2*-deficient mice displayed increased cell proliferation, decreased apoptosis, and lacked histologic goblet cells. Over a one-year period, these mice developed adenomas in the small intestine that progressed to invasive adenocarcinoma *(100)*.

6.3. Mucin Alterations in Colonic Neoplasia

Goblet cell morphology and mucin protein and carbohydrate expression become altered in during the development of preneoplastic hyperproliferative and aberrant crypts in the colon and in neoplastic polyps and cancer (see reviews in refs. *101–105*). Various mucin-related carbohydrate antigens, such as sialylated T antigens and sialylated Lewis-related antigens may be useful markers of colon mucosa with increased risk for malignant transformation *(106,107)*.

6.4. Mucin Alterations in Inflammatory Bowel Disease

Defects in the pre-epithelial mucous barrier, thus, may play an important role in the pathogenesis of inflammatory bowel disease. Mucin abnormalities may represent the primary defect or could interact with other putative etiologic factors at different levels in the pathogenesis of the disease. Abnormal mucin protein or carbohydrate structures could result in increased susceptibility to degrading enzymes, increased adherence by toxic bacteria, or decreased interaction with trefoils, lipids, or IgA. Abnormal mucin regulation could result in decreased responsivenes to luminal or cytokine stimulation (108).

Histochemical, lectin studies and immunohistochemical studies have indicated that mucin carbohydrate structures are altered in inflammatory bowel disease (7,109–113). These alterations include the finding of depleted mucins in ulcerative colits, but not in Crohn's disease; increased amounts of sialomucins in colon with both ulcerative colitis and Crohn's disease; and an increase in O-acetylated sialomucins in the ileum of active Crohn's disease. These changes are nonspecific and have also been described in hyperplastic polyps, neoplastic mucosa, and ischemic colitis. These changes, in part, reflect a relative reduction in oligosaccharide chain completion on mucin glycoprotein in these diseases (114,115).

Podolsky and coworkers have studied colonic mucins using anion exchange chromatography that separates mucins based on their ionic properties. They identified a selective reduction in the fourth migrating mucin species (labeled species IV) which appears to be specifically associated with ulcerative colitis (116,117). This alteration was not present in a variety of other inflammatory and infectious conditions. It was also found in the uninvolved mucosa of patients with ulcerative colitis. The reduction in this mucin species appeared to persist during histologic disease remission. More recent studies performed in a blinded fashion indicate the presence of this abnormality in healthy identical twins of patients with ulcerative colitis (118). Similar alterations of this mucin fraction have been found in cotton-top tamarins with spontaneous colitis, irrespective of the amount of colon inflammation (119). These observations indicate that this alteration is not directly related to the inflammatory process but may constitute a genetically determined predisposing factor. The structural basis for this abnormality is unknown. Podolsky has performed detailed structural analysis of the oligosaccharide side chains of the six chromatographically distinguishable mucin species, and this does not appear to be the sole basis for the species differences (120,121). Colonic explants from patients with ulcerative colitis are able to secrete apparently normal mucin species IV, which argues against a major structural apomucin abnormality; however, it is possible that a mutation in this mucin, which resides in the portion that interacts with the molecules responsible for mucin packaging and regulated secretion may be the possible defect (108). In opposition to these data, one study using different methods of ion exchange chromatography of mucins from patients with inflammatory bowel disease did not find a selective subclass defect (122).

Few studies have examined the role of mucin gene expression in inflammatory bowel disease. Tytgat et al. analyzed mucins purified from resection specimens of patients with ulcerative colitis (96). Immunoprecipitation and RNA analysis indicated that the MUC2 mucin was the major mucin in these specimens. Biosynthetic studies indicated that MUC2 biosynthesis was qualitatively unchanged in ulcerative colitis specimens compared with controls. MUC2 and MUC3 mRNA levels have been shown to be preserved in the setting of active inflammatory bowel disease. This may represent a compensatory up-regulation in these gene products due to the reduced numbers of goblet cells that are found in active inflammatory bowel disease. Further studies examining the quantitative and qualitative changes in specific mucin gene products are needed in controls and patients with inflammatory bowel disease. If abnormal mucins in animal models are shown to increase susceptibility to intestinal damage then genetic studies in human populations would be warranted.

REFERENCES

1. Neutra M, Forstner JF. Gastrointestinal mucus: synthesis, secretion, and function. In *Physiology of the Digestive Tract*. Johnson L (ed.), Raven Press, New York, NY, 1987, pp. 975–1009.

2. Cheng H, LeBlond CP. Origin, differentiation and renewal of the four main epithelial cell types of the mouse small intestine. V. Unitarian theory of the origin of the four epithelial cell types. *Am. J. Anat.*, **141** (1974) 537–562.

3. Specian RD, Oliver MG. Functional biology of intestinal goblet cells. *Am. J. Physiol.*, **260** (1991) C183–C193.

4. Lipkin M. Growth and development of gastrointestinal cells. *Annu. Rev. Physiol.*, **47** (1985) 175–197.

5. Akamatsu T, Ota T, Ishii K et al. Histochemical study of the surface mucous gel layer of the human large intestine. In *Cytoprotection and Cytobiology.* Yunoki K (ed.), Excerpta Medica, Amsterdam, 1991, pp. 90–95.

6. Matsuo K, Ota H, Akamatsu T, Sugiyama A, Katsuyama T. Histochemistry of the surface mucous gel layer of the human colon. *Gut*, **40** (1997) 782–789.

7. Pullan RD, Thomas GAO, Rhodes M, et al. Thickness of adherant mucus gel on colonic mucosa in humans and its relevance to colitis. *Gut*, **35** (1994) 353–359.

8. Phillips TE, Wilson J. Morphometric analysis of mucous granule depletion and replenishment in rat colon. *Dig. Dis. Sci.*, **38** (1993) 2299–2304.

9. Phillips T, Wilson J. Signal transduction pathways mediating mucin secretion from intestinal goblet cells. *Dig. Dis. Sci.*, **38** (1993) 1046–1054.

10. Neutra MR, O'Malley LJ, Specian RD. Regulation of intestinal goblet cell secretion. II. A survey of potential secretagogues. *Am. J. Physiol.*, **242** (1982) G380–G387.

11. Castagliuolo I, Leeman S, Bartolak-Suki E, et al. A neurotensin antagonist, SR48692, inhibits colonic responses to immobilization stress in rats. *Proc. Natl. Acad. Sci. USA*, **93** (1996) 12,611–12,615.

12. Bou-Hanna C, Berthon B, Combettes L, Claret M, Laboisse C. Role of calcium in carbachol- and neurotensin-induced mucin exocytosis in a human colonic goblet cell line and cross-talk with the cyclic AMP pathway. *Biochem. J.*, **299** (1994) 579–585.

13. Moore B, Sharkey K, Mantle M. Role of 5-HT in cholera toxin-induced mucin secretion in the rat small intestine. *Am. J. Physiol.*, **270** (1996) G1001–G1009.

14. Rozee KR, Cooper D, Lam K, Costerton JW. Microbial flora of the mouse ileum mucous layer and epithelial surface. *Appl. Environ. Microbiol.*, **43** (1982) 1451–1463.

15. Poulson LK, Lan F, Kristensen CS, Hobolth P, Molin S, Krogfelt KA. Spatial distribution of *E. coli* in the mouse large intestine inferred from rRNA in situ hybridization. *Infect Immun.,* **62** (1994) 5191–5194.

16. Ensgraber M, Genitsariotis R, Storkel S, Loos M. Purification and characterization of a *Salmonella typhimurium* agglutinin from gut mucus secretions. *Microb. Pathog.*, **12** (1992) 255–266.

17. Sajjan SU, Forstner JF. Role of the putative link glycopeptide of intestinal mucin in binding of piliated *Escherichia coli* serotype O157:H7 strain CL–49. *Infect. Immun.*, **58** (1990) 868–873.

18. Chadee K, Petri WA, Innes DJ, Ravdin JI. Rat and human colonic mucins bind to and inhibit adherence lectin of *Entamoeba histolytica*. *J. Clin. Invest.*, **80** (1987) 1245–1254.

19. Smith CJ, Kaper JB, Mack DR. Intestinal mucin inhibits adhesion of human enteropathogenic *E. coli* to HEp-2 cells. *J. Pediatr. Gastroenterol. Nutr.*, **21** (1995) 269–276.

20. Belley A, Keller K, Grove J, Chadee K. Interaction of LS174T human colon cancer cell mucins with *Entamoeba histolytica*: an in vitro model for colonic disease. *Gastroenterology*, **111** (1996) 1484–1492.

21. Sajjan SU, Forstner JF. Characteristics of binding of *Escherichia coli* serotype O157:H7 strain CL-49 to purified intestinal mucin. *Infect. Immunol.*, **58** (1990) 860–867.

22. Yolken RH, Ojeh C, Khatri IA, Sajjan U, Forstner JF. Intestinal mucin inhibits rotavirus infection in an oligosaccharide-dependent manner. *J. Infect. Dis.*, **169** (1994) 1002–1006.

23. Magnusson KE, Stjernstrom I. Mucosal barrier mechanisms. Interplay between secretory IgA (SIgA), IgG and mucins on the surface properties and association of salmonellae with intestine and granulocytes. *Immunology*, **45** (1982) 239–248.

24. Mack DR, Michail S, Wei S, McDougall L, Hollingsworth MA. Probiotics inhibit enteropathogenic *E. coli* adherence in vitro by inducing intestinal mucin gene expression. *Am. J. Physiol.* **276** (1999) G941–G950.

25. Hooper LV, Wong MH, Thelin A, Hansson L, Falk PG, Gordon JI. Molecular analysis of commensal host-microbial relationships in the intestine. *Science*, **291** (2001)881–884.

26. Hooper LV, Xu J, Falk PG, Midtvedt T, Gordon JI. A molecular sensor that allows a gut commensal to control its nutrient foundation in a competitive ecosystem. *Proc. Natl. Acad. Sci. USA*, **96** (1999) 9833–9838.

27. Ho SB, Ewing S, Montgomery CK, et al. Mucin core peptide expression in the colon polyp-carcinoma sequence. *Gastroenterology*, **100** (1991) A370.

28. Strous GJ, Dekker J. Mucin-type glycoproteins. *Crit. Rev. Biochem. Mol. Biol.*, **27** (1992) 57–92.

29. Gendler SJ, Spicer AP. Epithelial mucin genes. *Annu. Rev. Physiol.*, **57** (1995) 607–634.

30. Hilkens J, Buijs F, Ligtenberg M. Complexity of MAM-6, an epithelial sialomucin associated with carcinomas. *Cancer Res.*, **49** (1989) 786–793.

31. Gendler SJ, Lancaster CA, Taylor-Papdimitriou J, et al. Molecular cloning and expression of human tumor-associated polymorphic epithelial mucin. *J. Biol. Chem.*, **265** (1990) 15,286–15,293.

32. Siddiqui J, Abe M, Hayes D, Shani E, Yunis E, Kufe D. Isolation and sequencing of a cDNA coding for the human DF3 breast carcinoma-associated antigen. *Proc. Natl. Acad. Sci. USA*, **85** (1988) 2320–2323.

33. Ligtenberg MJL, Vos HL, Gennissen AMC, Hilkens J. Episialin, a carcinoma-associated mucin, is generated by a polymorphic gene encoding splice variants with alternative amino termini. *J. Biol. Chem.*, **265** (1990) 5573–5578.

34. Baeckstrom D, Karlsson N, Hansson GC. purification and characterization of sialyl-LeA-carrying mucins of human bile. Evidence for the presence of MUC1 and MUC3 apoproteins. *J. Biol. Chem.*, **269** (1994) 14,430–14,437.

35. Patton S, Gendler SJ, Spicer AP. The epithelial mucin MUC1, of milk, mammary gland, and other tissues. *Biochim. Biophys. Acta.*, **1241** (1995) 407–424:

36. Zhang K, Baeckstrom D, Breving H, Hansson GC. Secreted MUC1 mucins lacking their cytoplasmic part and carrying sialyl-Lewis a and x epitopes from a tumor cell line and sera of colon carcinoma patients can inhibit HL-60 leukocyte adhesion to E selectin-expressing endothelial cells. *J. Cell. Biochem.*, **60** (1996) 538–549.

37. Boshell M, Lalani E-N, Pemberton L, Burchell J, Gendler SJ, Taylor-Papadimitriou J. The product of the human MUC1 gene when secreted by mouse cells transfected with the full-length cDNA lacks the cytoplasmic tail. *Biochem. Biophys. Res. Commun.*, **185** (1992) 1–8.

38. Gum JR, Ho JJL, Pratt WS, et al. MUC3 human intestinal mucin. Analysis of gene structure, the carboxyl terminus, and a novel upstream repetitive region. *J. Biol. Chem.*, **272** (1997) 26,678–26,686.

39. Crawley SC, Gum JR, Hicks JW, et al. Genomic organization and structure of the 3' region of human MUC3: alternative splicing predicts membrane-bound and soluble forms of the mucin. *Biochem. Biophys. Res. Commun.*, **263** (1999) 728–736.

40. Shekels LL, Hunninghake DA, Tisdale AS, et al. Cloning and characterization of mouse intestinal MUC3 mucin: 3' sequence contains epidermal-growth-factor-like domains. *Biochem. J.*, **330** (1998) 1301–1308.

41. Sheng Z, Wu K, Carraway K, Fregien N. Molecular cloning of the transmembrane component of the 13762 mammary adenocarcinoma sialomucin complex. *J. Biol. Chem.*, **267** (1992) 16,341–16,346.

42. Rossi EA, McNeer RR, Price-Schiavi S, et al. Sialomucin complex, a heterodimeric glycoprotein complex. *J. Biol. Chem.*, **271** (1996) 33,476–33,485.

43. Nollet S, Moniaux N, Maury J, et al. Human mucin gene MUC4: organization of its 5'-region and polymorphisms of its central tandem repeat array. *Biocehm. J.*, **332** (1998) 739–748.

44. Moniaux N, Nollet S, Porchet N, Degand P, Laine A, Aubert J-P. Complete sequence of the human mucin MUC4: a putative cell membrane-associated mucin. *Biochem. J.*, **338** (1999) 325–333.

45. Williams S, McGuckin M, Gotley D, Eyre H, Sutherland G, Antalis TM. Two novel mucin genes downregulated in colorectal cancer identified by differential display. *Cancer Res.* **59** (1999) 4083–4089.

46. Mcneer RR, Price-Schiavi SA, Komatsu M, Fregien N, Carraway CAC, Carraway KL. Sialomucin complex in tumors and tissues. *Front. Biosci.*, **2** (1998) 449–459.

47. Carlstedt I, Sheehan JK. Structure and macromolecular properties of mucus glycoproteins. *Monogr. Allergy*, **24** (1988) 16–24.

48. Gum JR, Hicks JW, Toribara NW, Rothe E-M, Lagace RE, Kim YS. The human MUC2 intestinal mucin has cysteine-rich subdomains located both upstream and downstream of its central repetitive region. *J. Biol. Chem.*, **267** (1992) 21,375–21,383.

49. Desseyn J-P, Guyonnet-Duperat, V, Porchet N, Aubert J-P, Laine A. Human mucin gene MUC5B, the 10.7-kb large central exon encodes various alternate subdomains resulting in a super-repeat. *J. Biol. Chem.*, **272** (1997) 3168–3178.

50. Desseyn J-L, Aubert J-P, Van Seuningen I, Porchet N, Laine A. Genomic organization of the 3' region of the human mucin gene MUC5B. *J. Biol. Chem.*, **272** (1997) 16,873–16,883.

51. Inatomi T, Tisdale AS, Zhan Q, Spurr-Michaud S, Gipson IK. cloning of rat Muc5AC mucin gene: Comparison of its structure and tissue distribution to that of human and mouse homologues. *Biochem. Biophys. Res. Commun.*, **236** (1997) 789–797.

52. Toribara NW, Ho SB, Gum E, Gum JR, Lau P, Kim YS. The carboxyl-terminal sequence of the human secretory mucin, MUC6: Analysis of the primary amino acid sequence. *J. Biol. Chem.*, **272** (1997) 16,398–16,403.

53. Perez-Vilar J, Hill RL. Identification of the half-cystine residues in porcine submaxillary mucin critical for multimerization through the D-domains. *J. Biol. Chem.*, **273** (1998) 34,527–34,534.

54. Perez-Vilar J, Hill RL. The structure and assembly of secreted mucins. *J. Biol. Chem.*, **274** (1999) 31,751–31,754.

55. Wesley A, Mantle M, Man D, Qureshi R, Forstner G, Forstner J. Neutral and acidic species of human intestinal mucin. Evidence for different core peptides. *J. Biol. Chem.*, **260** (1985) 7955–7959.

56. Van Klinken BJ-W, Dekker J, Buller HA, De Bolos C, Einerhand AWC. Biosynthesis of mucins (MUC2-6) along the longitudinal axis of the human gastrointestinal tract. *Am. J. Physiol.*, **273** (1997) G296–G302.

57. Asker N, Axelsson MAB, Olofsson S-O, Hansson GC. Dimerization of the human MUC2 mucin in the endoplasmic reticulum is followed by a N-glycosylation-dependent transfer of the mono- and dimers to the golgi apparatus. *J. Biol. Chem.*, **273** (1998) 18,857–18,863.

58. Sheehan JK, Thornton DJ, Howard M, Carlstedt I, Corfield AP, Paraskeva C. Biosynthesis of the MUC2 mucin: evidence for a slow assembly of fully glycosylated units. *Biochem. J.*, **315** (1996) 1055–1060.

59. Axelsson MAB, Asker N, Hansson GC. O-glycosylated MUC2 monomer and dmer from LS174T cells are water soluble, whereas larger MUC2 species formed early during biosynthesis are insoluble and contain nonreducible intermolecular bonds. *J. Biol. Chem.*, **273** (1998) 18,864–18,870.

60. Herrmann A, Davies JR, Lindell G, et al. Studies on the "insoluble" glycoprotein complex from human colon. *J. Biol. Chem.*, **274** (1999) 15,828–15,836.

61. Khatri IA, Forstner GG, Forstner JF. Susceptibility of the cysteine-rich N-terminal and C-terminal ends of rat intestinal mucin Muc2 to proteolytic cleavage. *Biochem. J.*, **331** (1998) 323–330.

62. Karlsson NG, Herrmann A, Karlsson H, Johansson MEV, Carlstedt I, Hansson GC. The glycosylation of rat intestinal Muc2 mucin varies between rat strains and the small and large intestine. *J. Biol. Chem.*, **272** (1997) 27,025–27,034.

63. Van Klinken BJ-W, Dekker J, Van Gool SA, Van Marle J, Buller HA, Einerhand AWC. MUC5B is the prominent mucin in human gallbladder and is also expressed in a subset of colonic goblet cells. *Am. J. Physiol.*, **274** (1998) G871–G878.

64. Winterford CM, Walsh MD, Leggett BA, Jass JR. Ultrastructural localization of epithelial mucin core proteins in colorectal tissues. *J. Histochem. Cytochem.*, **47** (1999) 1063–1074.

65. Kovarik A, Peat N, Wilson D, Gendler SJ, Taylor-Papadimitriou J. Analysis of the tissue-specific promoter of the MUC1 gene. *J. Biol. Chem.*, **268** (1993) 9917–9926.

66. Abe M, Kufe D. Characterization of cis-acting elements regulating transcription of the human DF3 breast carcinoma-associated antigen (*MUC1*) gene. *Proc. Natl. Acad. Sci. USA*, **90** (1993) 282–286.

67. Gum JR, Hicks JW, Gillespie A-M, et al. Goblet cell-specific expression mediated by the MUC2 mucin gene promoter in the intestine of transgenic mice. *Am. J. Physiol.*, **276** (1999) G666–G676.

68. Price-Schiavi SA, Perez A, Barco R, Carraway KL. Cloning and characterization of the 5' flanking region of the sialomucin complex/rat *Muc4* gene: promoter activity in cultured cells. *Biochem. J.*, **349** (2000) 641–649.

69. Li J-D, Feng W, Gallup M, et al. Activation of NF-kB via a Src-dependent RasMAPK-pp90rsk pathway is required for *Pseudomonas aeruginosa*-induced mucin overproduction in epithelial cells. *Proc. Natl. Acad. Sci. USA*, **95** (1998) 5718–5723.

70. Temann U-A, Prasad B, Gallup MW, et al. A novel role for murine IL-4 in vivo: Induction of MUC5AC gene expression and mucin hypersecretion. *Am. J. Respir. Cell Mol. Biol.*, **16** (1997) 471–478.

71. Levine SJ, Larivee P, Logun C, Angus CW, Ognibene FP, Shelhamer JH. Tumor necrosis factor-alpha induces mucin hypersecretion and MUC2 gene expression by human airway epithelial cells. *Am. J. Resp. Cell Mol. Biol.* **12** (1995) 196–204.

72. Fischer BM, Krunkosky TM, Wright DT, Dolan-O'Keefe M, Adler KB. Tumor necrosis factor-alpha stimulates mucin secretion and gene expression in airway epithelium in vitro. *Chest*, **107** (1995) 133S–135S.

73. Nielsen OH, Koppen T, Rudiger N, Horn T, Eriksen J, Kirman I. Involvement of interleukin-4 and-10 in inflammatory bowel disease. *Dig. Dis. Sci.*, **41** (1996) 1786–1793.

74. Kusugami K, Haruta J, Ieda M, Shioda M, Ando T, Kuroiwa A. Phenotypic and functional characterization of T-cell lines generated from colonoscopic biopsy specimens in patients with ulcerative colitis. *Dig. Dis. Sci.*, **40** (1995) 198–210.

75. Shim J, Dabbagh K, Ueki I, et al. IL-13 induces mucin production by stimulating epidermal growth factor receptors and by activating neutrophils. *Am. J. Physiol. Lung Cell Mol. Physiol.*, **280** (2001) L134–L140.

76. Shekels LL, Anway RE, Lin J, et al. Coordinated Muc2 and Muc3 mucin gene expression in *Trichinella spiralis* infection in wild-type and cytokine deficient mice. *Dig. Dis. Sci.*, **46** (2001) 1757–1764.

77. Podolsky DK. Mucosal immunity and inflammation V. Innate mechanisms of mucosal defense and repair: the best offense is a good defense. *Am. J. Physiol.*, **277** (1999) G495–G499.

78. Lefebvre O, Wolf C, Kedinger M, et al. The mouse one P-domain (pS2) and two P-domain (mSP) genes exhibit distinct patterns of expression. *J. Cell Biol.*, **122** (1993) 191–198.

79. Suemori S, Lynch-Devaney K, Podolsky DK. Identification and characterization of rat intestinal trefoil factor: tissue- and cell-specific member of the trefoil protein family. *Proc. Natl. Acad. Sci. USA*, **88** (1991) 11,017–11,021.

80. Ho SB, Shekels LL, Toribara NW, et al. Mucin gene expression in normal, preneoplastic, and neoplastic human gastric epithelium. *Cancer Res.* **55** (1995) 2681–2690.

81. Chang S-Y, Dohrman AF, Basbaum CB, et al. Localization of mucin (MUC2 and MUC3) messenger RNA and peptide expression in human normal intestine and colon cancer. *Gastroenterology*, **107** (1994) 28–36.

82. Mashimo H, Wu D-C, Podolsky DK, Fishman MC. Impaired defense of intestinal mucosa in mice lacking intestinal trefoil factor. *Science*, **274** (1996) 262–265.

83. Kindon H, Pothoulakis C, Thim L, Lynch-Devaney K, Podolsky DK. Trefoil peptide protection of intestinal epithelial barrier function: cooperative interaction with mucin glycoprotein. *Gastroenterology*, **109** (1995) 516–523.

84. Tomasetto C, Masson R, Linares J-S, et al. pS2/TFF1 interacts directly with the VWFC cysteine-rich domains of mucins. *Gastroenterology*, **118** (2000) 70–80.

85. Efstathiou JA, Noda M, Rowan A, et al. Intestinal trefoil factor controls the expression of the adenomatous polyposis coli-catenin and the E-cadherin-catenin complexes in human colon carcinoma cells. *Proc. Natl. Acad. Sci. USA*, **95** (1998) 3122–3127.

86. Mack DR, Neumann AW, Policova Z, Sherman PM. Surface hydrophobicity of the intestinal tract. *Am. J. Physiol.*, **262** (1992) G171–G177.

87. Schacter M, Peret MW, Billing AG, Wheeler GD. Immunolocalization of the protease kallikrein in the colon. *J. Histochem. Cytochem.*, **31** (1983) 1255–1260.

88. Beyer EC, Tokuyasu KT, Barondes SA. Localization of an endogenous lectin in chick liver, intestine, and pancreas. *J. Cell. Biol.*, **82** (1979) 565–571.

89. Kudo H, Inada M, Ohshio G, et al. Immunohistochemical localization of vitamin B12 R-binder in the human digestive tract. *Gut*, **28** (1987) 339–345.

90. Nexo E, Poulsen SS, Hansen SN, Kirkegaard P, Olsen PS. Characterization of a novel proteolytic enzyme localized to goblet cells in rat and man. *Gut*, **25** (1984) 656–664.

91. Ogata H, Inoue N, Podolsky DK. Identification of a goblet cell-specific enhancer element in the rat intestinal trefoil factor gene promoter bound by a goblet cell nuclear protein. *J. Biol. Chem.*, **273** (1998) 3060–3067.

92. Itoh H, Inoue N, Podolsky DK. Goblet-cell specific transcription of mouse intestinal trefoil factor gene results from collaboration of distinctive positive and negative regulatory elements. *Biochem. J.* **341** (1999) 461–472.

93. Itoh H, Beck PL, Inoue N, Xavier R, Podolsky DK. A paradoxical reduction in susceptibility to colonic injury upon targeted transgenic ablation of goblet cells. *J. Clin. Invest.*, **104** (1999) 1539–1547.

94. Tomita M, Itoh H, Ishikawa N, et al. Molecular cloning of mouse intestinal trefoil factor and its expression during goblet cell changes. *Biochem. J.*, **311** (1995) 293–297.

95. Itoh H, Tomita M, Uchino H, et al. cDNA cloning of rat pS2 peptide and expression of trefoil peptides in acetic acid-induced colitis. *Biochem. J.* **318** (1996) 939–944.

96. Tytgat KMAJ, Opdam FJM, Einerhand AWC, Buller HA, Dekker J. MUC2 is the prominent colonic mucin expressed in ulcerative colitis. *Gut*, **38** (1996) 554–563.

97. Weiss AA, Babyatsky MW, Ogata S, Chen A, Itzkowitz SH. Expression of MUC2 and MUC3 mRNA in human normal, malignant, and inflammatory intestinal tissues. *J. Histochem. Cytochem.*, **44** (1996) 1161–1166.

98. Spicer AP, Rowse GJ, Lidner TK, Gendler SJ. Delayed mammary tumor progression in Muc1 null mice. *J. Biol. Chem.*, **270** (1995) 30,093–30,101.

99. Parmley RR, Gendler SJ. Cystic fibrosis mice lacking Muc1 have reduced amounts of intestinal mucus. *J. Clin. Invest.*, **102** (1998) 1798–1806.

100. Velcich A, Yang WC, Heyer J, et al. Colorectal cancer in mice genetically deficient in the mucin Muc2. *Sci.*, **295** (2002) 1726–1729.

101. Ho SB, Kim YS. Carbohydrate antigens on cancer-associated mucin-like molecules. *Semin. Cancer Biol.*, **2** (1991) 389–400.

102. Hakomori SI. Aberrant glycosylation in tumors and tumor-associated carbohydrate antigens. *Adv. Cancer Res.*, **52** (1989) 257–331.

103. Bartman AE, Sanderson SJ, Ewing SL, et al. Aberrant expression of *MUC5AC* and *MUC6* gastric mucin genes in colorectal polyps. *Int. J. Cancer*, **80** (1999) 210–218.

104. Devine PL, McKenzie IFC. Mucins: structure, function, and associations with malignancy. *BioEssays*, **14** (1992) 619–625.

105. Jass JR, Roberton AM. Colorectal mucin histochemistry in health and disease:a critical review. *Pathol. Int.*, **44** (1994) 487–504.

106. Ho SB. The use of mucosal biopsy markers to predict colon cancer risk. *Gastroenterol. Clin. N. Am.*, **3** (1993) 623–638.

107. Karlen P, Young E, Brostrom O, et al. Sialyl-Tn antigen as a marker of colon cancer risk in ulcerative colitis: relation to dysplasia and DNA aneuploidy. *Gastroenterology*, **115** (1998) 1395–1404.

108. Podolsky DK. Role of mucins in inflammatory bowel disease. In *Inflammatory Bowel Disease*. MacDermott RP, Stenson WF (eds.), Elsevier, New York, NY, 1992, pp. 311–322.

109. Boland CR, Lance P, Levin B, Riddell RH, Kim YS. Abnormal goblet cell glycoconjugates in rectal biopsies associated with an increased risk for neoplasia in patients with ulcerative colitis. Early results of a prospective study. *Gut*, **25** (1984) 1364–1371.

110. Jacobs LR, Huber PW. Regional distribution and alterations of lectin binding to colorectal mucin in mucosal biopsies from controls and subjects with inflammatory bowel disease. *J. Clin. Invest.* **75** (1985) 112–118.

111. Filipe M. Mucins in the gastrointestinal epithelium. A review. *Invest. Cell Pathol.* **2** (1979) 195–216.

112. Culling CFA, Reid PE, Dunn WL, Clay MG. Histochemical comparison of the epithelial mucins in the ileum in Crohn's disease and in normal controls. *J. Clin. Pathol.*, **30** (1977) 1063–1067.

113. Ehsanullah M, Filipe MI, Gazzard B. Mucin secretion in inflammatory bowel disease: correlation with disease activity and dysplasia. *Gut*, **23** (1982) 485–489.

114. Clamp JR, Fraser G, Read AE. Study of the carbohydrate content of mucus glycoproteins from normal and diseased colons. *Clin. Sci.*, **61** (1981) 229–234.

115. Boland CR, Deshmukh GD. The carbohydrate composition of mucin in colonic cancer. *Gastroenterology*, **98** (1990) 1170–1177.

116. Podolsky D, Isselbacher K. Composition of human colonic mucin. Selective alteration in inflammatory bowel disease. *J. Clin. Invest.* **72** (1983) 142–153.

117. Podolsky DK, Isselbacher KJ. Glycoprotein composition of colonic mucosa. Specific alterations in ulcerative colitis. *Gastroenterology*, **87** (1984) 991–998.

118. Tysk C, Riedesel H, Lindberg E, Panzini B, Podolsky D, Jarnerot G. Colonic glycoproteins in monozygotic twins with inflammatory bowel disease. *Gastroenterology*, **100** (1991) 419–423.

119. Podolsky DK, Madara JL, King N, Sehgal P, Moore R, Winter HS. Colonic mucin composition in primates. *Gastroenterology*, **88** (1985) 20–25.

120. Podolsky D. Oligosaccharide structures of human colonic mucin. *J. Biol. Chem.*, **260** (1985) 8262–8271.

121. Podolsky D. Oligosaccharide structures of isolated human colonic mucin species. *J. Biol. Chem.*, **260** (1985) 15,510–15,515.

122. Raouf A, Parker N, Idden D, et al. Ion exchange chromatography of purified colonic mucus glycoproteins in inflammatory bowel disease: absence of a selective sublcass defect. *Gut*, **32** (1991) 1139–1145.

123. Gendler SJ, Burchell JM, Duhig T, et al. Cloning of partial cDNA encoding differentiation and tumor-associated mucin glycoproteins expressed by human mammary epithelium. *Proc. Natl. Acad. Sci. USA*, **84** (1987) 6060–6064.

124. Gum JR, Byrd JC, Hicks JW, Toribara NW, Lamport DTA, Kim YS. Molecular cloning of human intestinal mucin cDNAs. Sequence analysis and evidence for genetic polymorphism. *J. Biol. Chem.*, **264** (1989) 6480–6487.

125. Gum JR, Hicks JW, Swallow DM, et al. Molecular cloning of cDNAs derived from a novel human intestinal mucin gene. *Biochem. Biophys. Res. Commun.*, **171** (1990) 407–415.

126. Porchet N, Cong NV, Dufosse J, et al. Molecular cloning and chromosomal localization of a novel human tracheo-bronchial mucin cDNA containing tandemly repeated sequences of 48 base pairs. *Biochem. Biophys. Res. Commun.*, **175** (1991) 414–422.

127. Ho SB, Roberton AM, Shekels LL, Lyftogt CT, Niehans GA, Toribara NW. Expression cloning of gastric mucin complementary DNA and localization of mucin gene expression. *Gastroenterology*, **109** (1995) 735–747.

128. Dufosse J, Porchet N, Aubert J-P, et al. Degenerate 87-base-pair tandem repeats create hydrophilic/hydrophobic alternating domains in human mucin peptides mapped to 11p15. *Biochem. J.*, **293** (1993) 329–337.

129. Toribara NW, Roberton AM, Ho SB, et al. Human gastric mucin; identification of a unique species by expression cloning. *J. Biol. Chem.*, **268** (1993) 5879–5885.

130. Bobek LA, Tsai H, Biesbrock AR, Levine MJ. Molecular cloning, sequence, and specificity of expression of the gene encoding the low molecular weight human salivary mucin (MUC7). *J. Biol. Chem.*, **268** (1993) 20,563–20,569.

131. Shankar V, Gilmore MS, Elkins RC, Sachdev GP. A novel human airway mucin cDNA encodes a protein with unique tandem-repeat organization. *Biochem. J.*, **300** (1994) 295–298.

132. Lapensee L, Paquette Y, Bleau G. Allelic polymorphism and chromosomal localization of the human oviductin gene (MUC9). *Fertil. Steril.*, **68** (1997) 702–708.

133. Ho SB, Niehans GA, Lyftogt C, et al. Heterogeneity of mucin gene expression in normal and neoplastic tissues. *Cancer Res.*, **53** (1993) 641–651.

134. Carrato C, Balague C, De Bolos C, et al. Differential apomucin expression in normal and neoplastic human gastrointestinal tissues. *Gastroenterology*, **107** (1994) 160–172.

135. Balague C, Gambus G, Carrato C, et al. Altered expression of *MUC2*, *MUC4*, and *MUC5* mucin genes in pancreas tissues and cancer cell lines. *Gastroenterology*, **106** (1994) 1054–1061.

136. Gipson IK, Ho SB, Spurr-Michaud SJ, et al. Mucin genes expressed by human female reproductive tract epithelia. *Biol. Reprod.*, **56** (1997) 999–1011.

5 Endocrine Cells of the Colon

Sebastian G. de la Fuente, Christopher R. Mantyh, and Theodore N. Pappas

CONTENTS

INTRODUCTION

The histologic features of the large intestine are constant from the ileocecal valve to the anus. From the outer surface inward, the layers that constitute the normal histology of the colon include: serosa, muscularis externa, submucosa and mucosa. The serosa contains small pendulous protuberances of adipose tissue called appendices epiploicae. The muscularis externa is composed of an inner circular muscular layer and an outer longitudinal muscular layer gathered into three thick bands known as teniae coli. The submucosa contains lymph nodes that are especially abundant in the vermiform appendix. The mucosa is flat and presents small holes that correspond to the openings of straight long tubular glands formed by crypts of Lieberkühn. Structurally, the mucosa is formed by a simple columnar epithelium along the lamina propia and a thin muscular layer known as muscularis mucosae. Although the epithelium that covers the luminal surface and the crypts is of the same type, the cytologic distribution has some unique patterns. Mature absorptive cells and globet cells formed the luminal surface epithelium while the epithelium lining the crypts consists of undifferentiated precursor cells, immature absorptive cells, globet cells, and enteroendocrine cells. Enteroendocrine cells are interspersed among other nonendocrine epithelial cells and are generally located in the deepest portions of the crypts.

Colonic enteroendocrine cells share similarities with other enteroendocrine distributed throughout the gastrointestinal tract. Although these cells are numerous in other segments of gut, they are estimated to represent only 0.4% of all colonic epithelial cells in the mice (1). In the colon, enteroendocrine cells predominate in proximal and distal segments and are specially numerous in the rectum (2,3) (Fig. 1).

The morphologic appearance of enteroendocrine cells is characterized by a small round or pyramidal cytoplasm filled with secretory granules located between the round nucleus and the base of the cell. The cytoplasm is in direct contact with the basal lamina and usually has an apical pole extension that reaches the gastrointestinal lumen, thus allowing secretion of the

From: *Colonic Diseases*
Edited by: T. R. Koch © Humana Press Inc., Totowa, NJ

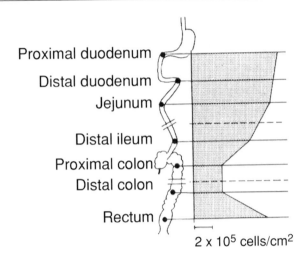

Proximal duodenum
Distal duodenum
Jejunum

Distal ileum
Proximal colon
Distal colon

Rectum

2 x 10⁵ cells/cm²

Fig. 1. Regional distribution of enteroendocrine cells in the intestines. The cell number is expressed per square centimeter mucosal surface. The bar represents 20×10^5 cells/cm² mucosal surface. Adapted with permission from ref. 3.

synthesized peptidergic products. The ultrastructure organelles are typical of other active secreting cells: sparse rough endoplasmic reticulum, abundant Golgi apparatus, and secretory products packed in granules (4). The secretory granules discharge their contents by exocitosis into the bloodstream or luminal surface. Secreted products can cross the basal membrane, and once they reach the bloodstream, exert their modulating effects on distant target organs. This type of secretion is referred to as endocrine secretion in contrast to paracrine secretion, in which the secreted substance effects neighbor cells.

The embryonic origin of enteroendocrine cells has been a controversial issue in the past (5). Proposed sources of enteroendocrine cells include endodermal, mesodermal, and neural crest tissues. Currently, it is accepted that most of these cells are derived from endoderm (6). Immature pre-enteroendocrine cells with small endocrine-like secretory granules give raise to mature cells that will constitute the definitive enteroendocrine cell population of the gut. It has been estimated that approx 7 d are necessary for a pre-enteroendocrine cells to reach the mid crypt and differentiate into a mature enteroendocrine cells. The overall turnover time of enteroendocrine cells was estimated to be 23 d in the descending colon (7).

Although an enteroendocrine cell is capable of synthesizing various peptides, usually only one predominates and is secreted. Once secreted, the peptide affects target cells and can induce an immediate or delayed response. The response is obtained when the peptide binds to a specific protein receptor on the membrane of the target cell. Most of these receptors belong to the guanosine 5'-triphosphate (GTP)-binding proteins (G proteins) family (8,9). The peptide-G protein complex affects the target cell by modifying membrane potentials or by generating second messengers such as inositol triphosphate (IP_3) and cyclic adenosine 5'-monophosphate (AMP). Peptides are then inactivated by tissue peptidases that can either cleave internal bonds (i.e., endopeptidases), the amino terminus (i.e., amino peptidases), or the carboxyl terminus (i.e., carboxyl peptidases).

Staining methods using heavy metal salts were originally utilized to identify entero-endocrine cells. Based on the precipitation properties of their granules, enteroendocrine cells were classified as argentaffin, enterochromaffin, or argyrophyllic cells. Argentaffin cells were named after their attribute of precipitating silver from ammoniacal silver nitrate. Entero-chromaffin cells are stained only by solutions with potassium dichcromate, and argyrophyllic cells have the ability to precipitate silver only in the presence of an external reducing agent. These terms have been used for many years; however, some subpopulations of cells were excluded in this cell categorization, making this classification inaccurate. Modern electron microscopy and inmunohistochemical methods permitted the correlation between cellular morphology and granular content, thus the classification that is currently in use is based on the peptide contained in the cell and not on the staining properties of the granules. To date, 20 different types of enteroendocrine cells have been identified, but only a few of all these cells are present in the colon.

2. SPECIFIC COLONIC ENTEROENDOCRINE CELLS

2.1. D cells or Somatostatin Secreting Cells

2.1.1. PEPTIDE BIOSYNTHESIS

Somatostatin was first isolated from the hypothalamus on the basis of its ability to inhibit growth hormone secretion (10). In the digestive tract, it is produced by D cells, which are widely distributed along the digestive tract mucosa and pancreatic islets, and are present in significant amounts in nerves and nerve plexus (11). Somatostatin is synthesized as a preprohormone and converted into prosomatostatin by microsomal membrane peptidase cleavage (12). The prosomatostatin is first processed as a 28-amino acid peptide and then as a 14-amino acids molecule (13). Both 14- and 28-amino acids forms are biologically active.

2.1.2. BIOLOGIC AND PHYSIOLOGIC ACTIONS

Intestinal D cells are described as "flask-shaped open type" cells with an apical pole reaching the intestinal lumen. Somatostatin is secreted into the lumen and exerts its effects through a family of homologous receptors collectively known as somatostatin receptors (SSTR). To date, five subtypes (SSTR-1, SSTR-2, SSTR-3, SSTR-4, and SSTR-5) have been cloned. The gastrointestinal distribution of these receptors is still under investigation, however it has been demonstrated that SSTR-1 is present in jejunum, stomach, and pancreatic islets, while STTR-2 was found in cerebrum and kidney and in lower concentrations in jejunum, colon, pancreatic islets, and liver (14). Through these receptors, somatostatin has shown to inhibit adenylate cyclase activity, which results in a decrease of intracellular cyclic AMP (cAMP). Additionally, the interaction between somatostatin and SSTR can reduce intracellular Ca^{2+} concentration and increase K^+ conductance. Most of these functions seem to be mediated by GTP-binding proteins (15).

The biological actions of somatostatin include inhibition of several hormones such as acetylcholine, cholecystokinin, enteroglucagon, gastrin, insulin, and glucagon, as well as exocrine pancreatic and gastric acid pepsin secretion. It also has the ability to decrease the cyclic interdigestive motor activity in stomach and small intestine. In the small intestine, the absorption of amino acids is inhibited, and the glucagon-induced jejunal water and electrolyte secretion is blocked by somatostatin. However, somatostatin was ineffective in antagonizing diarrhea caused by small intestine hypersecretion in cholera-infected humans (14). To date, the role of somatostatin in the large intestine is not well known in detail. The fact that somatostatin reduces the proliferation of lymphocytes isolated from Peyer's patches or the immunoglobulin synthesis (15), has attracted the attention of investigators searching for answers to explain the mechanisms involved in inflammatory conditions, such as inflammatory bowel disease (IBD).

Cells / cm

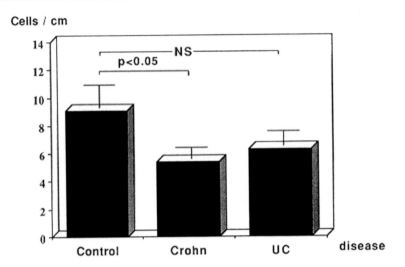

Fig. 2. Somatostatin-containing cells in IBD. Adapted with permission from ref. *16*.

2.1.3. CLINICAL RELEVANCE

SSTR have been observed not only in normal tissues, but also expressed in several pathologic conditions of the gastrointestinal tract, including cancer *(16)*. The importance of somatostatin and its receptor have been extensively studied in inflammatory colonic conditions, such as IBD *(17–20)*. Affected sections of the colon in patients with IBD were found to have lower somatostatin concentration levels in the mucosa and submucosa layers *(17,19)* (Fig. 2). Conversely, the density of SSTR is significantly augmented in the intestinal wall veins of florid IBD cases *(20)*. Moreover, unaffected segments of colon in Crohn's disease cases seem to be excluded in the increment of SSTR. These observations, which appear to be controversial, motivated Reubi et al. *(20)* to hypothesize that the lack of somatostatin concentrations in mucosal layers may trigger the up-regulation of SSTR in the vessels.

The role of somatostatin-producing cells was also investigated in patients with familial amyloidosis with polyneuropathy *(21,22)*, an autosomal dominant form of systemic amyloidosis geographically limited to Portugal, Sweden, and Japan. Rectal somatostatin cells were reported to be decreased in these patients *(21)*; however, a recently published investigation demonstrated opposite results *(22)*. The authors attributed these discrepancies between studies to the different duration of the disease, genetic and environmental factors, major gastrointestinal symptoms, and especially to the colonic segment studied.

Duodenal endocrine cells were reported to be augmented in patients with myotonic dystrophy (MD) *(23)* and diarrhea, including serotonin (5-hydroxytryptamine [5-HT])-, gastrin/cholecyxtokinin (CCK)-, secretin-, gastric inhibitory peptide (GIP)-, and somatostatin-reactive cells. However, this increment was not seen in the colon. Although the rectal total endocrine area was increased in MD patients in comparison to control, the analysis of individual cell populations showed no significant differences.

2.2. Enterochromaffin Cells or 5-HT-Secreting Cells

2.2.1. PEPTIDE BIOSYNTHESIS

5-HT is a potent smooth muscle stimulant and vasoconstrictor synthesized from 5-hydroxy-*L*-tryptophan. The enzyme responsible for catalyzing this reaction is the tryptophan hydroxylase. The tryptophan hydroxylase belongs to the family of aromatic L-amino acid hydroxylases and is the rate-limiting enzyme in the biosynthesis of 5-HT (24). It is generally accepted that the synthesis of 5-HT occurs in the enterochromaffin cells interspersed among the mucosal epithelium and in serotoninergic neurons of the nerve plexus. However, it has recently been documented that tryptophan hydroxylase is also present in normal enterocytes of the small intestine (24). Although this is an interesting and novel finding, the fact that these cells failed to react with anti-5-HT antibodies proves that it is unlikely that enterocytes synthesized significant amounts of 5-HT.

Enterochromaffin cells represent the largest enteroendocrine cell population in the human intestine (3). The prevalence of enterochromaffin cells is more significant in the rectum than in proximal colon. It has been proposed that 5-HT-producing cells co-synthesized other peptides, such as substance P (25). Although this may be true in other segments of the digestive, it does not appear to be the case in the colon. Immunocytochemical methods demonstrated that less than 5% of the serotoninergic cells contained substance P in the distal colon (26).

2.2.2. Biologic and Physiologic Actions

The physiological role of 5-HT has been subject to extensive investigations, and several agonists and antagonists are under development for treatment of motility disorders. 5-HT is known to stimulate motility in the small intestine and the proximal and distal colon (27). In small intestine, the contraction rate is augmented, and mixing motor patterns are converted to propulsive contractions (28). It also accelerates ileocolonic junction transit in animal models (29). A high energy meal stimulates colonic propulsion presumably by activation of 5-HT3 receptor (30). Furthermore, mucosal stimulation produces release of 5-HT that initiates the peristaltic reflex, however, the mechanisms implicated are believed to be through stimulation of 5-HT4/5-HT1$_p$ receptors on sensory calcitonin gene-related peptide (CGRP) containing neurons (31).

5-HT inhibits NA^+Cl^- absorption and stimulates active anion secretion in the intestinal tract (32). Sidhu and Cooke (33) reported that stroking of distal colonic lining mucosa evokes chloride secretion by activating neural reflex pathways via serotoninergic receptors. 5-HT is most likely to be released from enterochromaffin cells, mast cells or neurons in the mucosa–submucosa and stimulate 5-HT2 receptor on the epithelial cell. The stimulation of 5-HT2 receptors produces an increase in the intracellular Ca^+ with subsequent inhibition of NA^+Cl^- absorption and Cl^- and bicarbonate secretion. Certainly, tachykinins and cholinergic containing neurons are also implicated in this mechanism (34).

2.2.3. Clinical Relevance

The regulatory role of 5-HT on intestinal motility has been extensively studied in motility disorders. Results are inconsistent when measuring immunoreactive 5-HT cells. Patients with slow-transit constipation have a lower number of 5-HT secreting cells (35). However, a recently published study showed that the number of 5-HT containing cells is augmented in the mucosa of patients with colonic inertia (36). According to these later results, it is unclear if the increment of 5-HT in pathologies with motility disorders is the initial step in the pathogenesis of the disease or a defensive mechanism to correct the abnormal colonic transit.

5-HT immunoreactive nerve fibers and enteroendocrine cells were also studied in Hirschprung's disease patients (37,38). The frequency of serotoninergic fibers in the aglanglonic segments of Hirschprung's patient(s) gut is decreased (39), however, the enteroendocrine cell population is maintained despite derangements in the nerve supply (40).

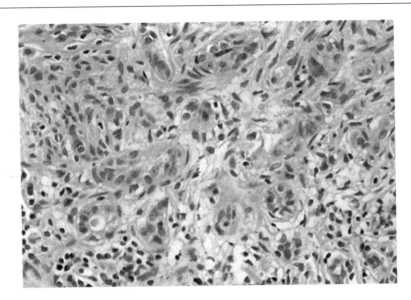

Fig. 3. Appendicular carcinoid tumor. Adapted with permission from ref. *46*.

The number of somatostatin and 5-HT immunoreactive cells/mm^3 and the secretory index is significantly reduced in patients with colon carcinoma *(41)*. Colonic 5-HT is also abnormal in other entitles such MO *(23)*, and familial amyloidotic polyneuropathy *(42)*, and IBD *(43)*.

Carcinoid tumors are the most common endocrine tumors of the intestine, detected in up to 1% of autopsies *(44)* with an incidence of 1.5/100,000 in the general population *(45)*. Eighty-five percent of these tumors arise from the gut, but they can also occur in other localizations, such as pancreas, biliary tract, or thymus. The most common localization in the gut is the appendix (Fig. 3) *(46)*, followed by jejunum–ileum and rectum (Fig. 4) *(46)*. Carcinoid tumors arise from enterochromaffin cells and produce a wide variety of products, including amines, tachykinins (substance P, neurokinin A), 5-HT, histamin, gastrin, etc. Histologically, carcinoid tumors can be classified as nodular, trabecular, tubular (Fig. 5A) *(46)*, rosette-like (Fig. 5B) *(46)*, or mixed tumors. Although the histology of large intestine carcinoid tumors resembles small intestine tumors, the atypia and higher mitotic rate exhibit in colonic tumors predispose them to behave more aggressively. The symptoms related with these neoplasms include rectal bleeding, pain, and diarrhea, which is usually a consequence of the passage of stools over the tumor surface. The carcinoid syndrome, characterized by vasomotor, cardiopulmonary, and gastrointestinal symptoms, is uncommon, even in patients with liver metastases. Patients with functioning carcinoid tumors usually have increases in the urinary excretion of 5-hydroxyindolacetic acid (5-HIAA), a product of the 5-HT metabolism. However, the metabolism of 5-HT varies in relation to the tissue origin of the tumor. Carcinoid tumors should be treated by surgical resection regardless of the presence of metastasis.

2.3. L Cells or Enteroglucagon and Glucagon-Like Peptides-Secreting Cells

2.3.1. PEPTIDE BIOSYNTHESIS

L cells are present throughout the entire gut mucosa with the highest density in the distal ileum and rectum *(3)*. These cells are responsible for producing enteroglucagon and other peptides, all synthesized from preproglucagon. The amino terminal region of preproglucagon

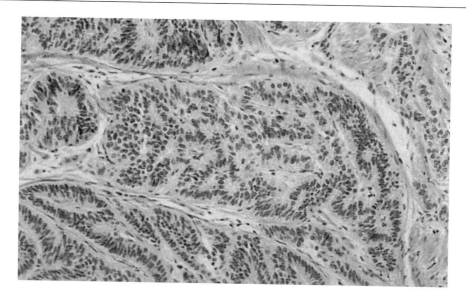

Fig. 4. Carcinoid tumor of the rectum. Adapted with permission from ref. *46*.

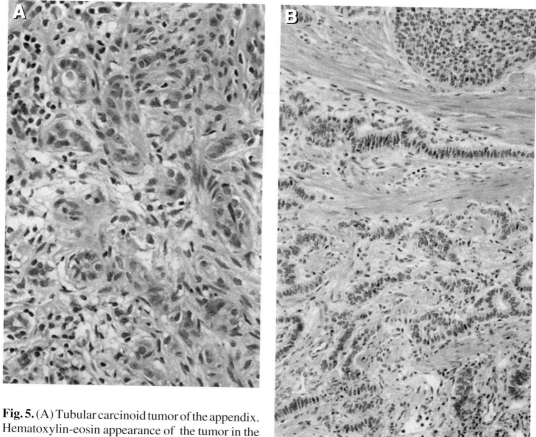

Fig. 5. (A) Tubular carcinoid tumor of the appendix. Hematoxylin-eosin appearance of the tumor in the submucosa and muscularis mucosae.
(B) Rectal carcinoid tumor. Ribbons of cells infiltrating the mucosa. Adapted with permission from ref. *46*.

gives rise to glicentin, and oxyntomodulin while the carboxyl terminal portion produces biologically active glucagon-like peptides (GLP-1 and GLP-2). Although GLP-2 biological actions are currently under investigation, GLP-1 is known to be a potent stimulator for insulin release *(47)*.

Secretion of enteroglucagons is closely regulated by the presence of alimentary products in the digestive tract. An ordinary meal is a potent stimulus in humans for secretion of glicentin–oxyntomodulin and GLP-1 and GLP-2 *(48)*. The load of glucose infused into the jejunum produce a proportional increase in the enteroglucagon release (49). The gastric emptying rate is also a determinant factor in enteroglucagons secretion (50).

2.3.2. Biologic and Physiologic Actions

GLP-1 seems to be the most active glucagon gene product synthesized in the intestines. Its functions include stimulation of insulin release with an effect that is dependant on blood glucose level *(47,51)*, inhibition of gastric emptying *(52)* and gastric acid secretion *(53)*, and inhibition of glucagon release. GLP-2 has been shown to regulate intestinal mucosal growth in small intestine by increasing the crypt cell proliferation rate and reducing apoptosis *(54,55)*, however the effects of GLPs in the colon is currently unknown. Although glicentin and oxyntomodulin are co-synthesized with GLP-1 and GLP-2 from the gut, little is currently known about their biological actions. Glicentin stimulates intestinal growth in rodents *(54)*, and oxyntomodulin regulates gastric acid secretion.

2.3.3. Clinical Relevance

Conditions in which excessive amounts of nutrients are derived to the distal small intestine and proximal colon have associated with increase levels of enteroglucagon. Excessive plasma enteroglucagon values have been measured in patients with dumping syndrome *(56)*, jejunoileal bypass *(57)*, and Billroth II gastrectomy *(58)*.

2.4. Peptide YY-Secreting Cells

2.4.1. Peptide Biosynthesis

Peptide YY (PYY) is a member of the pancreatic polypeptide (PP) family named after its tyrosine amino and carboxyl terminal amio acid residues. Although PYY-producing cells are uncommon in stomach and duodenum, numerous cells are observed in the distal small intestine, colon, and rectum of different species *(59,60)*. Immunohistochemical studies have previously established the co-localization of PYY and enteroglucagon-secreting cells in the colonic mucosa *(61,62)*.

2.4.2. Biologic and Physiologic Actions

The most potent stimulant for PYY secretion is the presence of fat in the intestinal lumen *(63,64)*. PYY plasma concentrations rise progressively in humans after ingestion *(65)* and can remain augmented for 6 h following a meal in the dog *(64)*. Infusion of PYY in dogs induces a reduction in basal and meal-stimulated pancreatic secretion *(64)*. Gastric acid secretions are also inhibited by PYY infusion, probably responding to a neurally mediated mechanism *(66)*. PYY also inhibits propagation of interdigestive myoelectric complex from the duodenum to the jejunum, and large doses also inhibit colonic motility *(67)*.

PYY and neuropeptide Y (NPY) interact with three common receptors known as Y1, Y2, and Y3. Although both peptides act through all three receptors, Y3 has a higher affinity for NPY. PYY/NPY receptors have been identified in a variety of tissues, including small and large intestine, spleen, and brain.

2.4.3. CLINICAL RELEVANCE

The potent effect that PYY has on canine *(63)* and human gastric emptying *(68)* makes it the perfect candidate responsible for the "ileal brake". The term ileal brake refers to the mechanism whereby perfusion of ileum and colon with fat slows intestinal transit and delays gastric emptying *(59)*. This phenomenon is especially important in diseases associated with malabsorption of foods.

2.5. Guanylin

2.5.1. PEPTIDE BIOSYNTHESIS

Guanylin is a 15-amino acid peptide that was first isolated from the rat jejunum in an effort to find an endogenous ligand of the intestinal guanylate cyclase, which is the target of the heat-stable enterotoxin of *Escherichia coli (69)*. The intraluminal cleavage of proguanylin gives rise to biologically active guanylin, which acts on intestinal guanylate cyclase receptors promoting Cl^- and HCO_3^- secretion *(70)*.

Guanylin is present in very low concentrations in the proximal small bowel, increasing its concentration in the distal small bowel and throughout the colon *(71)*. The exact cellular origin of guanylin is still under debate, because the immunoreactive products have been localized in different cells, including enterocytes *(72)*, globet cells *(73,74)*, and enterochromaffin cells *(75,76)*.

2.5.2. BIOLOGIC AND PHYSIOLOGIC ACTIONS

Activation of guanylate cyclase produces an intracellular increment of cyclic guanosine 5'-monophosphate (cGMP). Intracellular cGMP influences Cl^- and HCO_3^- secretion by interacting with the enzymatic activities of either cGMP-dependant protein kinase II *(77)* or cAMP-dependant protein kinase II *(70)*. This provokes the physiological driving forces for inhibition of NA^+ absorption and secretion of water into the intestine, causing diarrhea.

2.5.3. CLINICAL RELEVANCE

The *E. coli* heat-stable enterotoxin causes watery diarrhea, acting in a similar manner to uroguanylin (found in urine and small intestine) and/or guanylin. Other diarrheal diseases that have been associated with guanylin include diarrhea from zinc deficiency syndrome and carcinoid syndrome diarrhea *(70)*.

Guanylin mRNA expression has been found to be reduced in colon polyps and colorectal adenocarcinomas *(78,79)*. Further studies are needed to determine if the loss of endogenous guanylin expression contributes in the development of colonic malignancy.

REFERENCES

1. Karam S. Linage commitment and maturation of epithelial cells in the gut. *Front Biosci.*, **4** (1999) d286–d298.
2. Buffa R, Capella C, Fontana P, et al. Types of endocrine cells in the human colon and rectum. *Cell Tissue Res.*, **192** (1978) 227–240.
3. Sjolund K, Sanden G, Hakanson R, et al. Endocrine cells in the human intestine: an immunocytochemical study. *Gastroenterology*, **86** (1983) 1120–1130.
4. Lewin KJ. The endocrine cells of the gastrointestinal tract. The normal endocrine cells and their hyperplasias. *Pathol. Annu.*, **21** (1986) 1–27.
5. Andrew A, Kramer B, Rawdon BB. The origin of gut and pancreatic neuroendocrine (APUD) cells-the last word? *J. Pathol.*, **186** (1998) 117–118.
6. Andrew A, Kramer B, Rawdon BB. The embryonic origin of endocrine cells of the gastrointestinal tract. *Gen. Comp. Endocrinol.*, **47** (1982) 149–265.

7. Tsubouchi S, Leblond CP. Migration and turnover of entero-endocrine and caveolated cells in the epithelium of the descending colon, as shown by radioautography after continuous infusion of 3H-thymidine into mice. *Am. J. Anat.*, **156** (1979) 431–451.

8. Savarece TM, Fraser CM. In vitro mutagenesis and the search for structure-function relationship among G protein-coupled receptors. *Biochem. J.*, **283** (1992) 1.

9. Conklin BR, Bourne. Structural elements of Ga subunits that interact with Gbg, receptors and effectors. *Cell*, **73** (1993) 631–641.

10. Brazeu P, Vale W, Burgus R, et al. Hypothalamic polypeptide that inhibits the secretion of immunoreactive pituitary growth hormone. *Science*, **179** (1973) 77–79.

11. Costa M, Patel Y, Furness JB, et al. Evidence that some intrinsic neurons of the intestine contain somatostatin. *Neurosci. Lett.*, **6** (1977) 215–222.

12. Goodman R, Aron D, Roos B. Rat pre-prosomatostatin. *J. Biol. Chem.*, **258** (1983) 5570–5573.

13. Patel Y, Oneil W. Peptides derived from cleavage of prosomatostatin at carboxyl- and amino-terminal segments. *J. Biol. Chem.*, **263** (1988) 745–751.

14. Walsh J. Gastrointestinal hormones. In *Physiology of the gastrointestinal tract*. 3rd ed., Johnson L, Alpers DH, Christensen J, Jacobson ED, and Walsh JH (eds.), Raven Press, New York, NY, 1994.

15. Stanisz AM, Befus D, Bienenstock J. Differential effects of vasoactive intestinal polypeptide, substance P, and somatostatin on immunoglobulin synthesis and proliferation by lymphocytes from Peyer's patches, mesenteric lymph nodes, and spleen. *J. Immunol.*, **136** (1986) 152–156.

16. Reubi JC, Laissue J, Waser B, et al. Expression of somatostatin receptors in normal, inflamed, and neoplasic human gastrointestinal tract. *Ann. NY Acad. Sci.*, **733** (1994) 122–137.

17. Watanabe T, Kubota Y, Sawada T, Muto T. Distribution and quantification of somatostatin in inflammatory bowel disease. *Dis. Colon Rectum*, **35** (1992) 488–494.

18. Payer J, Huorka M, Duris I, et al. Plasma somatostatin levels in ulcerative colitis. *Hepatogastroenterology*, **4** (1994) 552–553.

19. Koch T. Carney JA, Morris V, et al. Somatostatin in the idiopathic inflammatory bowel diseases. *Dis. Colon Rectum*, **31** (1988) 198–203.

20. Reubi JC, Mazzucchelli L, Laissue J. Intestinal vessel express a high density of somatostatin receptors in human inflammatory bowel disease. *Gastroenterology*, **106** (1994) 951–959.

21. El-Salhy M, Suhr O. Endocrine cells in rectal biopsy specimens from patients with familial amyloidotic polyneuropathy. *Scand. J. Gastroenterol.*, **31** (1996) 68–73.

22. Anan I, El-Salhy M, Ando Y, et al. Colonic endocrine cells in patients with familial amyloidotic polyneuropathy. *J. Intern. Med.*, **245** (1999) 469–473.

23. Ronnblom A, Danielsson A, El-Salhy M. Intestinal endocrine cells in myotonic dystrophy: an Immunocytochemical and computed image analytical study. *J. Intern. Med.*, **245** (1999) 91–97.

24. Meyer T, Brinck U. Differential distribution of serotonin and tryptophan hydroxylase in the human gastrointestinal tract. *Digestion*, **60** (1999) 63–68.

25. Heitz PH, Polak J, Timson C, et al. Enterochromaffin cells as the endocrine source of gastrointestinal substance P. *Histochemistry*, **49** (1976) 343–347.

26. Roth K, Gordon J. Spatial differentiation of the intestinal epithelium: analysis of enteroendocrine cells containing immunoreactive serotonin, secretin and substance P in normal and transgenic mice. *Proc. Natl. Acad. Sci. USA*, **87** (1990) 6408–6412.

27. Jacoby H, Bonfilio A, Raffa R. Central and peripheral administration of serotonin produces opposite effects on mouse colonic propulsive motility. *Neur. Sci Lett.*, **122** (1991) 122–126.

28. Brand SJ, Schmidt WE. Gastrointestinal hormones. In *Textbook of Gastroenterology*. 2nd ed., Yamada T, Alpers DH, and Laine L (eds.), J.B Lippincort, Philadelphia, PA 1995, pp. 25–71.

29. Oosterboch L, von der Ohe M, Valdovinos MA, et al. Effects of serotonin on rat ileocolonic transit and fluid transfer in vivo: possible mechanisms of action. *Gut*, **34** (1993) 794–798.

30. von der Ohe M, Hanson RB, Camilleri M. Serotoninergic mediation of postprandial colonic tonic and phasic responses in humans. *Gut*, **35** (1994) 536–541.

31. Grider JR, Kuemmerle JF, Jin J. 5-HT released by mucosal stimuli initiates peristalsis by activating 5-HT$_4$/ 5-HT$_{1p}$ receptors on sensory CGRP neurons. *Am. J. Physiol.*, **270** (1996) G778–G782.

32. Brown DR. Mucosal protection through active intestinal secretion: neural and paracrine modulation by 5-hdroxytryptamine. *Behav. Brain Res.*, **73** (1996) 193–197.

33. Sidhu M, Cooke H. Role for 5-HT and ACh in submucosal reflexes mediating colonic secretion. *Am. J. Physiol.*, **269** 1995: G346–G351.

34. Cooke H, Sidhu M, Wang Y. 5-HT activates neural reflexes regulating secretion in the guinea pig colon. *Neurogastroenterol. Motil.*, **9** (1997) 181–186.

35. El-Salhy M, Norrgard O, Spinnel S. Abnormal colonic endocrine cells in patients with chronic idiopathic slow-transit constipation. *Scand. J. Gastroenterol.*, **34** (1999) 1007–1011.
36. Zhao R, Fhurrum Baig M, Wexner S, et al. Enterochromaffin and serotonin cells are abnormal for patients with colonic inertia. *Dis. Colon Rectum*, **43** (2000) 858–863.
37. Toyhara T, Nada O, Nagasaki A, et al. An immunohistochemical study of serotoninergic nerves in the colon and rectum of children with Hirschprung's disease. *Acta Neuropathol.*, **68** (1985) 306–310.
38. Lolova I, Davidoff M, Itzev D, et al. Histochemical, Immunocytochemical and ultrastrucural data on the inervation of the smooth muscle of the large intestine in Hirschprung's disease. *Acta Physiol. Pharmacol. Bulg.*, **12** (1986) 55–62.
39. Lolova I, Davidoff M, Itzev D, et al. Distribution of substance P-, methionine-enkephalin-, somatostatin- and serotonin- immunoreactive nerve elements of the bowel bowl in Hirschprung's disease. *Zentralbl. Allg. Pathol.*, **132** (1986) 25–32.
40. Larsson LT, Sundler F, Ekman R. Intestinal endocrine cells in Hirschprung's disease. No reduction in density in aganglionic compared with ganglionic segment. *Int. J. Colorectal Dis.*, **5** (1990) 155–160.
41. El-Salhy M, Mahdavi J, Norrgard O. Colonic endocrine cells in patients with carcinoma of the colon. *Eur. J. Gastroenterol. Hepatol.*, **10** (1998) 517–522.
42. El-Salhy M, Suhr O. Endocrine cells in rectal biopsy specimens from patients with Familial Amyloidotic Polyneuropathy. *Scand. J. Gastroenterol.*, **31** (1996) 68–73.
43. El-Salhy M, Dannielson A, Stenling R., et al. Colonic endocrine cells in inflammatory bowel disease. *J. Intern. Med.*, **242** (1997) 413–419.
44. Berge T, Linell F. Carcinoids tumors: Frequency in a defined population during a 12-year period. *Acta Pathol. Microbiol. Scand. [A]*, **84** (1976) 322–330.
45. Buchanan KD, Johnston CF, O'Hare MM, et al. Neuroendocrine tumors. A European view. *Am. J. Med.*, **81** (1986) 14–22.
46. Fenoglio-Preiser C, Lantz P, Listrom M, Noffsinger A, Rilke A. (eds.) In *Gastrointestinal Pathology: An Atlas and Text.* 2nd ed., Lippincott-Raven, Philadelphia, PA, 1999.
47. Thompson DG. GLP-1 and the gut. *Gut*, **46** (2000) 591–594.
48. Kreymann B, Williams G, Ghatei MA, et al. Glucagon-like peptide-1 7–36: a physiological incretin in man. *Lancet*, **2** (1987) 1300–1304.
49. Petersen B, Christiansen J, Holst JJ. A glucose-dependant mechanism in jejunum inhibits gastric acid secretion: a response mediated through enteroglucagon? *Scand. J. Gastroenterol.*, **20** (1985) 193–197.
50. Lauritsen KB, Frederiksen HJ, Uhrenholdt A, et al. The correlation between gastric emptying time and the response of GIP and enteroglucagon to oral glucose in duodenal ulcer patients. *Scan. J. Gastroenterol.*, **17** (1982) 513–516.
51. Nathan DM, Fogel H, Mojsov S, Habener JF. Insulinotropic action of glucagonlike peptide-I, (7-37 [GLP-I (7-37)] *Diabetes*, **39** (1990) 142A.
52. Schirra J, Houck P, Wank U, et al. Effects of glucagon-like peptide-1 (7-36) amide on antro-pyloro duodenal motility in the interdigestive state and duodenal lipid perfusion in humans. *Gut*, **46** (2000) 622–631.
53. Imeryuz N, Yegen BC, Bozkurt A, et al. Glucagon-like peptide-1 inhibits gastric emptying via vagal afferent-mediated central mechanisms. *Am. J. Physiol.*, **273** (1997) G920–G927.
54. Drucker DJ, Erlich P, Asa SL, et al. Induction of intestinal epithelial proliferation by glucagon-like peptide 2. *Proc. Natl. Acad. Sci. USA*, **93** (1996) 7911–7916.
55. Drucker DJ. Glucagon peptide 2. *Trends Endocrinol. Metab.*, **10** (1999) 153–156.
56. Lawaetz O, Blackburn AM, Bloom SR, et al. Gut hormone profile and gastric emptying in the dumping syndrome. A hypothesis concerning the pathogenesis. *Scand. J. Gastroenterol.*, **18** (1983) 73–80.
57. Holst JJ, Sorensen TI, Andersen AN, Stadil F, Andersen B. Lauritsen KB. Klein HC. Plasma enteroglucagon after jejunoileal bypass with 3:1 or 1:3 jejunoileal ratio. *Scand. J. Gastroenterol.*, **14** (1979) 205–207.
58. Tamburrano G, Mauceri M, Lala A, et al. Plasma levels of glucagon-like polypeptides in gastrectomized patients transformed from Billroth II into Billroth I. *Horm. Metab. Res.*, **14** (1982) 642–645.
59. Tailor I. Pancreatic polypeptide family, pancreatic polypeptide, neuropeptide Y and peptide YY. In *Handbook of Physiology. The Gastrointestinal System.* Vol II, Rauner BB (ed.), American Physiological Society, Bethesda, MD, 1989.
60. El-Salhy M, Grimelius L, Wilander E, et al. Immunocytochemical identification of polypeptide YY (PYY) cells in the human gastrointestinal tract. *Histochemistry*, **77** (1983) 15–23.
61. Fiocca R, Capella C, Buffa R, et al. Glucagon-, glicentin-, and pancreatic polypeptide- like immunoreactivities in rectal carcinoids and related colorectal cells. *Am. J. Pathol.*, **100** (1980) 81–92.
62. Holst J. Gut glucagon, enteroglucagon, gut glucagonlike immunoreactivity, glicentin–current status. *Gastroenterology*, **84** (1983) 1602–1613.

63. Pappas TN, Debas HT, Chang AM, et al. Peptide YY release by fatty acids is sufficient to inhibit gastric emptying in dogs. *Gastroenterology*, **91** (1986) 1386–1389.

64. Pappas TN, Debas HT, Goto Y, et al. Peptide YY inhibits meal-stimulated pancreatic and gastric secretion. *Am. J. Physiol.*, **248** (1985) G118–G123.

65. Adrian TE, Savage AP, Sagor GR, et al. Effect of peptide YY on gastric, pancreatic, and biliary function in humans. *Gastroenterology*, **89** (1985) 494–499.

66. Pappas TN, Debas HT, Taylor IL. Enterogastrone-like effect of peptide YY is vagally mediated in the dog. *J. Clin. Invest.*, **77** (1986) 49–53.

67. Lunberg JM, Tatemoto K, Terenius L, et al. Localization of peptide YY (PYY) in gastrointestinal endocrine cells and effects on intestinal blood flow and motility. *Proc. Natl. Acad. Sci. USA*, **79** (1982) 4471–4475.

68. Allen JM, Fitzpatrick ML, Yeats JC, et al. Effects of peptide YY and neuropeptide Y on gastric emptying in man. *Digestion*, **30** (1984) 255–262.

69. Currie M, Fok K, Kato J, et al. Guanylin: An endogenous activator of intestinal guanylate cyclase. *Proc. Natl. Acad. Sci. USA*, **89** (1992) 947–951.

70. Forte LR. Guanylin regulatory peptides: structures, biological activities mediated by cyclic GMP and pathobiology. *Regul. Pept.*, **81** (1999) 25–39.

71. Qian X, Prabhakar S, Nandi A, et al. Expression of GC-C, a receptor-guanylate cyclase, and its endogenous ligands uroguanylin and guanylin along the rostracaudal axis of the intestine. *Endocrinol.*, **141** (2000) 3210–3224.

72. Lewis G, Witte D, Laney W, et al. Guanylin mRNA is expressed in villous enterocytes of the rat small intestinal and superficial epithelia of the rat colon. *Biochem. Biophys. Res. Commun.*, **196** (1993) 553–560.

73. Li Z, Taylor-Blake B, Light A, et al. Guanylin, an endogenous ligand for C-type guanylate cyclase, is produced by globet cells in the rat intestine. *Gastroenterology*, (1995) **109** 1863–1875.

74. Cohen M, Witte D, Hawkins JA, et al. Immunohistochemical localization of guanylin in the rat small intestine and colon. *Biochem. Biophys. Res. Commun.*, **209** (1995) 803–807.

75. Cetin Y, Kuhn M, Kulaksiz H, et al. Enterochromaffin cells of the digestive system: cellular source of guanylin, a guanylate cyclase-activating peptide. *Proc. Natl. Acad. Sci. USA*, **91** (1994) 2935–2939.

76. Perkins A, Goy M, Li Z. Uroguanylin is expressed by enterochromaffin cells in the rat gastrointestinal tract. *Gastroenterology*, **113** (1997) 1007–1014.

77. Vaandrager A, Bot A, Ruth P, et al. Differential role of cyclic GMP-dependant protein kinase II in ion transport in murine small intestine and colon. *Gastroenterology*, **118** (2000) 108–114.

78. Shailubhai K, Yu H, Karunanandaa K, et al. Uroguanylin treatment suppresses polyp formation in the Apc$^{Min/+}$ mouse and induce apoptosis in human colon adenocarcinoma cells via cyclic GMP. *Cancer Res.*, **60** (2000) 5151–5157.

79. Cohen MB, Hawkins JA, Witte DP. Guanylin mRNA expression in human intestine and colorectal adenocarcinoma. *Lab. Invest.*, **78** (1998) 101–108.

6 Micronutrients

Emmanuel C. Opara

CONTENTS

1. INTRODUCTION

1.1. Classes of Micronutrients

Micronutrients are essential dietary factors, which cannot be synthesized in the human body and other vertebrate animals. They are required only in small quantities for the enhancement of a diverse array of metabolic processes in the body. They include vitamins and trace elements, and a significant deficiency of these essential micronutrients in the body results in disease *(1)*. The abundance or deficiency of any given essential micronutrient in the body is determined by dietary sources, and by their utilization for different biological processes. It is, therefore, difficult to have a complete directory of trace elements, as there is significant diversity in the types of diets consumed by different individuals. In this chapter, we will limit the discussion to antioxidant vitamins and certain trace elements, which are involved in biological processes that have pathophysiological implications for the colon.

There are two distinct classes of micronutrients, as shown in Table 1 (vitamins) and Table 2 (trace elements). Vitamins are further subdivided into two groups, the fat-soluble vitamins (vitamins A, D, E, K) and the water-soluble vitamins as shown in Table 1. One class of micronutrients acts as cofactors for some enzymatic processes in metabolism, and the other is recognized as antioxidants involved in the destruction of toxic free radicals produced in the body as a normal consequence of the metabolic processes *(2)*. Among these antioxidant micronutrients, while the vitamins act as donors and acceptors of reactive oxygen species (ROS), including free radicals, the trace elements regulate the activity of certain antioxidant enzymes shown in Table 3.

2. MICRONUTRIENT INTERACTIONS AND SUPPLEMENTATION

In the last decade, we have seen a tremendous increase in consumer use of antioxidant micronutrient supplements for disease prevention and treatment *(3,4)*. There is, therefore,

From: *Colonic Diseases*
Edited by: T. R. Koch © Humana Press Inc., Totowa, NJ

a growing need for research devoted to understanding the bioavailability, tissue uptake, metabolism, micronutrient interactions, and their biological activities. A pertinent segment of research with an urgent need for public health nutrition guidelines is the use of antioxidant micronutrients in the prevention of age-associated diseases, including cancer (3,5,6). The prime targets of free radical reactions are unsaturated bonds in membrane phospholipids. The consequence of these reactions, termed lipid peroxidation, is the loss of membrane fluidity, receptor alignment, and potential cellular lysis (7). Also, free radical damage to sulfur-containing enzymes and other proteins results in inactivation, cross-linking, and denaturation. In addition, nucleic acids can be attacked and subsequent damage to the DNA can cause mutations that may be carcinogenic (6–8). All these cellular and molecular perturbations induced by free radical reactions have been associated with the process of aging and the development of chronic disabling diseases (5–10). The relationship between oxidative stress (increased ROS levels) and the process of aging is currently not clear. While some investigators propose that oxidative stress is the result of aging, others argue that it is the cause of aging and disease (9–12). However, there is consensus that a strong association exists between oxidative stress, aging, and chronic diseases of aging, such as colorectal cancer, leading to the proposal that nutrition-based antioxidative strategies, including antioxidant micronutrient supplementation, should be adopted in the prevention and treatment of age-associated diseases (3,5,6,11–18).

Based on this rationale, it has become common practice to use high doses of single antioxidant supplements. Biochemically, this is not a safe approach, because micronutrient antioxidants interact with each other in a biochemical chain of defense against free radicals, and the use of high doses of a single antioxidant poses potential risks, since it could perturb the antioxidant–prooxidant balance (7,19). It has, therefore, been recommended that high doses of micronutrient antioxidant vitamins should be administered in combination rather than as single supplements (2). There is a growing number of preparations containing mixtures of antioxidant vitamins and/or trace elements. It has been reported that supplementation with a multivitamin–mineral formulated appropriately at the level of the daily recommended dietary allowance (RDA) caused a decrease in the prevalence of suboptimal vitamin status in older adults and improved their micronutrient status to levels associated with reduced risk for several chronic diseases (18). Table 4 shows the RDA levels, also referred to as the dietary reference intake (DRI), for the various micronutrients in popular use as supplements for disease prevention and treatment (20). It is possible that, while appropriate combination of micronutrients formulated with these RDA levels may be useful for disease prevention (18), higher levels may be required for treatment (21). A recent study has shown that supplementation with a cocktail of folic acid (650 µg), vitamin B_{12} (400 µg), and the antioxidants, vitamins, vitamin E (150 IU), vitamin C (150 mg), and β-carotene (12,500 IU) twice a day for 15 d, resulted in the reduction of serum levels of homocysteine and in vitro low density lipoprotein (LDL) oxidation in patients with coronary artery disease (22). In specific cases, micronutrient supplementation may augment tissue levels better than dietary sources. For instance, it has been reported that folic acid supplements are more effective in raising serum folate levels than dietary intake (23). However, it should be noted that the absorption of micronutrients in the gastrointestinal tract is a saturable process that operates with the economic principle of diminishing returns. For example, it has been shown that at low doses <180 mg/d, vitamin C is nearly completely absorbed, but absorption falls to 50% with a dose of 1.5 g/d, and to 16% with a dose of 12 g/d (3). Also, at RDA levels, approx 20–40% of vitamin E is absorbed, and the percentage of absorption decreases as the dose increases (3). An unresolved issue with these observations is whether the pharmacokinetics of micronutrient absorption is altered in disease.

Table 1
Dietary Vitamins and their Roles as Coenzyme Precursors

Water-soluble vitamin	Coenzyme	Fat-soluble vitamins
Thiamine (vitamin B_1)	Thiamine pyrophosphate (TPP)	Vitamin A (retinol)
Riboflavin (vitamin B_2)	Flavin adenine dinucleotide (FAD)	Vitamin D
Niacin (nicotinic acid)	Nicotinamide adenine dinucleotide (NAD)	Vitamin E (tocopherol)
Folate	Tetrahydrofolate	Vitamin K (quinone)
Biotin	Pyruvate carboxylase	
Pantothenic acid	Coenzyme A (CoA)	
Pyridoxine (vitamin B_6)	Pyridoxal phosphate	
Vitamin B_{12}	5'-Deoxyadenosyl-cobalamine	
Vitamin C (ascorbate)		

Table 2
Trace Elements as Cofactors for Antioxidant Enzymes

Element	Enzymes
Copper	Cytochrome oxidases
	Cytosolic superoxide dismutase
Zinc	Cytosolic superoxide dismutase
Manganese	Mitochondrial superoxide dismutase
Selenium	GPX
Iron	Catalase

Table 3
Micronutrients as Components of the Antioxidant Network

Trace elements	Role as antioxidant enzyme cofactor	Antioxidant vitamins
Selenium	GPX	Vitamin A (retinol)
Iron	Catalase	β-Carotene (previtamin A)
Zinc	Cytosolic superoxide dismutase	Vitamin C (ascorbic acid)
Copper	Cytosolic superoxide dismutase and ceruloplasmin	Vitamin E (tocopherol)
Manganese	Mitochondrial superoxide dismutase	Vitamin K (quinones)

The role of trace elements as micronutrient antioxidants has not received the same attention as vitamins, and this may probably be due to the relatively narrow range of safety between deficiency and toxicity. By virtue of their abilities to donate or accept electrons, all transition metals have potential antioxidant properties. Three key trace elements whose antioxidant activities are gradually gaining attention are zinc, selenium, and iron. In the last two decades, a substantial body of evidence has been accumulated to support the role of zinc as a cellular antioxidant (24). Although zinc does not react directly with ROS, a number of indirect mechanisms have been described (24,25). One of the ways by which zinc acts as an antioxidant is through the induction of the metallothioneins, a group of low-molecular-weight amino acid residues, the production of which is induced by zinc in many tissues including the liver, gut, and kidney. The metallothioneins have been shown to scavenge free

Table 4
RDA for Selected Micronutrients

Compound	RDA (DRI)
Vitamin E	1500 IU[a]
βCarotene (previtamin A)	800–1000 IU
Vitamin C (L-ascorbic acid)	2000 mg[a]
Vitamin B$_6$	1.6–2 mg
Vitamin B$_{12}$	2 µg
Thiamine	1.2 mg
Riboflavin	1.2 mg
Niacin	8–12 mg
Folate	200 µg
Biotin	30–100 µg
Pantothenic acid	None
Calcium	800–1200 mg
Phosphorus	1000–1500 mg
Iodine	150 µg
Magnesium	280–300 mg
Zinc	12–15 mg
Selenium	400 µg[a]
Iron	14–22 µg
Copper	1.5–3 mg
Manganese	2.0–5 mg

[a]On April 12, 2000, the National Academy of Sciences report on dietary reference intakes for antioxidants recommended these new values as the upper intake levels for these micronutrients.

radicals and bind some oxidants in a relatively inert state and have been shown to act in this manner under a variety of conditions, including radiation exposure, drug toxicities, ethanol toxicity, and mutagenesis (24–28). Zinc status has also been shown to regulate the levels of the extracellular form of superoxide dismutase (SOD), which is an enzyme that destroys the superoxide radical (7) and may also protect against nitric oxide-mediated free radical formation (29). Zinc may also protect sulfyhydryl group, and reduce the formation of the highly toxic hydroxyradical (OH$^-$) from H_2O_2 produced through the antagonism of redox-active transition metals, such as iron and copper (24). There is considerable evidence to show that mild zinc deficiency is common in elderly subjects and that this deficiency may contribute to the high prevalence of chronic disease in this population (30,31). The potential adverse effects of zinc supplementation are mild and include a reduction in serum copper levels (32) and dyslipidemia at high very doses of zinc.

Selenium is a trace element that is known to be essential for the activation of glutathione peroxidase (GPx), which is a key enzyme in the defense against oxidative stress (7). In a study of selenium supplementation (in combination with vitamins C and E) in elderly subjects > 65 yr of age, it was found that a dose of 100 µg selenium increased GPx activity and improved red blood cell antioxidant defense after 2 yr (16). In another study, Galan et al. supplemented hospitalized elderly subjects for 1 y with 100 µg selenium, along with 20 mg zinc, and found an increase in GPx levels (33). Other investigators have also studied the effect of supplementation with 200 µg selenium and have described a decrease in the incidence and mortality ascribed to certain types of cancer (34) and an increase in immune function (35). An interesting aspect of selenium supplementation is the observation that, while either vitamin E or selenium alone was ineffective in preventing chemically induced mammary cancer, the combined supplementation of both micronutrients resulted in the prevention of tumor development (36). Selenium toxicity ascribable to supplementation appears to be rare. However, it has been suggested that selenium toxicity, which primarily affects the immune system, may be limited to inorganic rather than the organic forms of this trace element (37).

Most people use iron supplementation to prevent or treat anemia. It is rarely recognized that iron supplementation has any implications for antioxidant defense. Catalase, the enzyme that catalyzes the decomposition of hydrogen peroxide, is a hemeprotein, and it is, therefore, difficult to take iron supplements without an impact on the body's antioxidant status. Iron supplementation, for whatever purpose, should be done with great caution, because electron transfer from transition metals, such as iron, to oxygen-containing molecules can initiate free radical reactions (7). It is particularly important to avoid iron supplementation with vitamin C, since it has been shown that ascorbate can provoke the formation of free radicals in the presence of transition metals (7).

As with trace elements, an important issue to consider in vitamin supplementation is the potential toxicity of a given dose of a single vitamin or compound formula. Vitamin E has been extensively evaluated as an antioxidant micronutrient (3,6,8,13,38–43). It has also been proposed as an anti-aging micronutrient (13,40,41). As a fat-soluble vitamin, once absorbed, vitamin E is located in cell membranes, where it is thought to be active in preventing lipid peroxidation (1,5). Although most adults appear to tolerate doses of vitamin E alone up to 800 mg/d without gross signs or biochemical evidence of toxicity (40–43), as previously noted, under these circumstances, the antioxidant–prooxidant balance may be altered particularly during prolonged use. Also, β-carotene (previtamin A analogue), which participates in the chain of antioxidant reactions, has been proposed as an antioxidant that may be useful for the prevention of chronic diseases associated with aging (6,16). When ingested in very high doses either acutely or chronically, vitamin A may cause toxic manifestations, including headache, vomiting, diplopia, alopecia, dryness of the mucous membrane, bone abnormalities, and liver damage. However, signs of toxicity usually appear only with sustained daily intakes, including both foods and supplements, exceeding 15,000 IU (20). These toxicity signs have not been observed during supplementation with β-carotene, the previtamin A analogue. Although vitamin C, another antioxidant involved in the chain of antioxidant reactions, appears to be useful when used in combination with vitamin E (7), questions have been raised about the potential risk of very large doses (20).

Besides vitamin E, another fat-soluble vitamin capable of acting as an antioxidant is vitamin K. Vitamin K is the name given to a group of compounds, all of which contain the 2-methyl-1,4-naphthoquinone moiety, and these compounds are essential for the formation of prothrombin and at least five other factors (factors VII, IX, and X, and proteins C and S) involved in the regulation of blood clotting (1,20). Under normal conditions, vitamin K is moderately (40–70%) well absorbed from the jejunum and ileum, but very poorly absorbed in the colon (44). As with the other lipid-soluble vitamins, the absorption of vitamin K depends on the normal flow of bile and pancreatic juice and is enhanced by dietary fat. Absorbed vitamin K is transported primarily in chylomicrons through the lymphatic fluid to the liver, from which it is distributed widely among body tissues. Once inside the cell, it is mainly associated with membranes (1,20). In humans, the total body pool of vitamin K is small, and its turnover is rapid. However, most of the daily requirements for this vitamin is provided through its biosynthesis by the intestinal flora *(20)*. Except when there is the need to assess the adequacy of plasma prothrombin levels, vitamin K supplementation is not usually desirable, even though toxicity ascribable to high doses of vitamin is K very rare *(20)*.

3. MICRONUTRIENT DISTURBANCE AND COLONIC DISEASE

Studies on the role of antioxidants in the maintenance of the integrity and function of the gut received tremendous impetus from the observation that glutathione (GSH) deficiency induced by buthionine sulfoximine (BSO) administration in the mouse resulted in severe degeneration of epithelial cells of the jejunum and colon *(45)*. GSH is a simple tripeptide (glutamate-cysteine-glycine) that acts as a cellular antioxidant and is necessary for the maintenance of multiple metabolic processes *(46)*. The rate-limiting enzyme in the biosynthesis of GSH is γ-glutamylcysteine synthetase, which is inhibited by BSO *(45)*. Considerable evidence has since accumulated to support the initial observation of the deleterious effect of GSH depletion on the colon. For example, it has been shown that the regions of the bowel that are more susceptible to malignancy, such as the colon and rectum, have low levels of GSH in the cells lining the mucosa *(46)*. Also, it has consistently been shown that tissue GSH levels are depleted in Crohn's disease *(47–49)* and acquired megacolon *(50)*. GSH metabolism is linked to antioxidant micronutrient reactions in a biochemical chain that results in the destruction of free radicals *(7)*. It is, therefore, not surprising that various disturbances of micronutrient antioxidant homeostasis have been described in colonic diseases *(5)*.

It has been shown that reduced levels of different trace elements involved in the enzymatic arm of antioxidant defense are present in colonic disease. In one study, it was found that a diminished activity of copper–zinc-containing SOD (CuZn-SOD) occurred simultaneously with decreased levels of zinc and copper in uninflammed mucosal samples obtained from patients with inflammatory bowel disaease (IBD) *(51)*. In another study, the zinc deficiency was linked to a functional defect of zinc transport in patients with Crohn's disease *(52)*. It has also been shown that patients with moderately active ulcerative colitis had significantly lower levels of iron, selenium and GPx than patients in remission and those without the disease *(53)*. It has been reported that multiple vitamin and trace element deficiencies may be present in 20–50% of patients with IBD, and that these deficiencies are primarily due to malabsorption, which is sometimes exacerbated by some drugs, such as sulfasalazine, which is used for treatment *(21)*. Some investigators have examined prediagnostic serum levels of several antioxidant vitamins in cohorts of patients, some of whom were subsequently afflicted with colorectal cancer. In a retrospective study, which compared serum vitamin E levels with the risk of developing colorectal carcinoma, it was found that a modest reduction in risk was associated with higher levels of vitamin E *(54)*. In another study involving 36,265 Finnish subjects, it was reported that a modest, but statistically significant, reduction in prediagnostic serum vitamin A levels was observed in those patients who went on to develop colorectal malignancy over a 9-yr period *(55)*. However, in a study with a follow-up period of 12 y, it was suggested that low initial serum β-carotene (previtamin A) level was a significant risk factor for the development of stomach cancer, but not colon cancer *(56)*. It has been difficult to perform studies of prediagnostic vitamin C levels largely because of the need to store the serum in acid solution *(5)*.

4. INTERVENTIONAL STUDIES WITH MICRONUTRIENTS IN COLONIC DISEASE

A good number of studies have examined the potential use of micronutrient antioxidant supplementation for both prevention and treatment of colonic disease. While some studies have examined the preventive and therapeutic effects of supplementation with these micronutrients on colorectal neoplasia and cancer, others have been devoted to the micronutrient effects in IBD. In studies that have employed both single and combinations of micronutrients for prevention or treatment of colonic adenoma or carcinoma, the results have been conflicting. It does appear that differences in the doses of micronutrients used, as well as short periods of follow-up, have contributed to the mixed results observed in these studies (5). For these same reasons and other deficiencies in experimental design, micronutrient supplementation in patients with IBD have also provided conflicting results. In one study, supplementation with vitamin A alone at the dose of 50,000 U twice daily for over 1 yr was not shown to be of any benefit to patients with Crohn's disease who were in remission (57). An unresolved question from this study is the effect of appropriate micronutrient supplementation in patients with active disease. It is of interest that in a phase II trial with Cu/Zn-SOD in 26 patients with severe Crohn's disease, more than 80% of these patients derived long-term benefit in the management of symptoms (58).

In conclusion, the role of micronutrient antioxidant supplementation in the control and management of colonic disease remains to be completely elucidated. What is needed in further studies in this area of research is the use of appropriate combinations and doses of relevant micronutrients in properly controlled experimental designs. Research opportunities in this area include the need for studies to determine the relative contribution of individual micronutrients to antioxidant status in health and disease. There is also a need for studies to delineate what would constitute appropriate supplementation regimens based on biochemically defined interactions between the different antioxidant micronutrients. Considering the theoretical benefits, the high therapeutic index, and the lack of long-term side effects of optimal doses of micronutrient antioxidants, there is a great chance that interventional studies with these micronutrients may prove to be beneficial as a preventive strategy and as an adjunct therapy in colonic disease.

REFERENCES

1. Lehninger AL, Nelson DL, Cox MM (eds.). In *Principles of Biochemistry*. 2nd ed., Worth Publishers, New York, NY, 1993.
2. Opara EC. Oxidative stress, micronutrients, diabetes and its complications. *J. R. Soc. Health*, **122** (2002) 28–34.
3. Rock CL, Jacob RA, Bowen PE. Update on biological characteristics of the antioxidant micronutrients: vitamin C, vitamin E, and the carotenoids. *J. Am. Diet Assoc.*, **96** (1996) 693–702.
4. Eisenberg DM, Davis RB, Ettner SL, et al. Trends in alternative medicine use in the United States, 1990–1997. Results of a follow-up national survey. *JAMA*, **280** (1998) 1569–1575.
5. Thomson A, Hemphill D, Jeejeebhoy KN. Oxidative stress and antioxidants in intestinal disease. *Dig. Dis.*, **16** (1998) 152–168.
6. Ames BN, Shigenaga MK. Oxidants, antioxidants, and the degenerative diseases of aging. *Proc. Natl. Acad. Sci. USA*, **90** (1993) 7915–7922.
7. Machlin LJ, Bendich A. Free radical tissue damage: protective role of antioxidant nutrients. *FASEB J.*, **1** (1987) 441–445.
8. Cross CE, Halliwell B, Borish ET, et al. Oxygen radicals and human disease. *Ann. Intern. Med.*, **107** (1987) 526–545.
9. Emerit I, Chance B (eds.), In *Free Radicals and Aging*, Birkhauser Verlag, Basel, 1992.
10. Yu, BY (ed.), In *Free Radicals in Aging*, CRC Press, Boca Raton, FL, 1993.
11. Julius M, Lang CA, Gleiberman L, Harburg E, DiFranceisco W, Schork A. Glutathione and morbidity in a community-based sample of elderly. *J. Clin. Epidemiol.*, **47** (1994) 1021–1026.
12. Rikans LE, Hornbrook KR. Lipid peroxidation, antioxidant protection and aging. *Biochim. Biophy. Acta.*, **1362** (1997) 116–127.
13. Traber MG. Vitamin E, oxidative stress and healthy aging. *Eur. J. Clin. Invest.*, **27** (1997) 822–824.

14. Otamiri T, Sjodahl R. Oxygen radicals: their role in selected gastrointestinal disorders. *Dig. Dis.*, **9** (1991) 133–141.
15. Garewal HS, Diplock AT. How safe are antioxidant vitamins? *Drug Safety*, **13** (1995) 8–14.
16. Girodon F, Blanche D, Monget AL, et al. Effect of a two-year supplementation with low doses of antioxidant vitamins and/or minerals in elderly subjects on levels of nutrients and antioxidant defense parameters. *J. Am. Coll. Nutr.*, **16** (1997) 357–365.
17. Ward JA. Should antioxidant vitamins be routinely recommended for older people? *Drugs Aging*,**12** (1998) 169–175.
18. McKay DL, Perrone G, Rasmussen H, et al. The effects of a multivitamin/mineral supplement on micronu-trient status, antioxidant capacity and cytokine production in healthy older adults consuming a fortified diet. *J. Am. Coll. Nutr.*, **19** (2000) 613–621.
19. Halliwell B. The antioxidant paradox. *Lancet*, **355** (2000) 1179–1180.
20. National Research Council. *Recommended Dietary Allowances,* 10th ed., National Academy Press, Washing-ton, DC, 1989.
21. Keshavarzian A, Mobarhan S. Inflammatory bowel disease in the elderly. In *Digestive diseases and the elderly.* Vellas BJ, Russel R, Dyard F, Garry PJ, Albarede JL (eds.), Springer, New York, NY, 1996, pp. 35–52.
22. Bunout D, Garrido A, Suazo M, et al. Effects of supplementation with folic acid and antioxidant vitamins on homocysteine levels and LDL oxidation in coronary patients. *Nutrition*, **16** (2000) 107–110.
23. Elkin AC, Higham J. Folic acid supplements are more effective than increased dietary folate intake in elevating serum folate levels. *Br. J. Obstetr. Gynalcol.*, **107** (2000) 285–289.
24. Powell SR. The antioxidant properties of zinc. *J. Nutr.*, **130** (2000) 1447S– 1454S.
25. DiSilvestro RA. Zinc in relation to diabetes and oxidative stress. *J. Nutr.*, **130** (2000) 1509S–1511S.
26. Rossman TG, Goncharova EI. Spontaneous mutagenesis in mammalian cells is caused mainly by oxidative events and can be blocked by antioxidants and metal-lothionein. *Mutat. Res.*, **402** (1998) 103–111.
27. Sato M, Brenner I. Oxygen free radicals and metallothionein. *Free Radic. Biol. Med.*, **14** (1993) 325–342.
28. DiSilvestro RA, Cousind RJ. Mediation of endotoxin-induced changes in zinc metabolism in rats. *Am. J. Physiol.*, **247** (1984) E436–E441.
29. Oury TD, Day BJ, Crapo JD. Extracellular superdioxide dismutase: a regulator of nitric oxide availability. *Lab. Invest.*, **75** (1996) 617–636.
30. Craig GM, Evans SJ, Brayshaw BJ, Raina SK. A study of serum zinc, albumin, alpha-2-macroglobulin and tranferrin levels in acute and long-stay elderly hospital patients. *Postgrad. Med. J.*, **66** (1990) 205–209.
31. Prasad AS, Fitsgerald JT, Hess JW, et al. Zinc deficiency in elderly patients. *Nutrition*, **9** (1993) 218–224.
32. Sanstead HH. Zinc interference with copper metabolism. *JAMA*, **240** (1978) 188–189.
33. Galan P, Preziosi P, Monget AL, et al. Effects of trace element and/or vitamin supplementation on vitamin and mineral status, free-radical metabolism, and immunological markers in elderly long-term-hospitalized subjects. Geriatric Network MIN.VIT.AOX *Int. J. Vitam. Nutr. Res.*, **67** (1997) 450–460.
34. Clark L, Combs GF, Turnbull BW, et al. Effects of selenium supplementation for cancer prevention in patients with carcinoma of the skin. *JAMA*, **276** (1996) 1957–1963.
35. Kiremidjian-Schumacher L, Glickman R, Schneider K, et al. Selenium and immunocompetence in patients with head and neck cancer. *Biol. Trace Elem. Res.*, **73** (2000) 97–111.
36. Horvath PM, Ip C. Synergistic effect of vitamin E and selenium on the chemoprevention of mammary carcinogenesis in rats. *Cancer Res.*, **43** (1983) 693–792.
37. Johnson VJ, Tsunoda M, Sharma RP. Increased production of proinflammatory cytokines by murine mac-rophages following oral exposure to sodium selenite but not to seleno-L-methionine. *Arch. Environ. Contam. Toxicol.*, **39** (2000) 243–250.
38. Rice-Evans CA, Diplock AT. Current status of antioxidant therapy. *Free Rad. Biol. Med.*, **15** (1993) 77–96.
39. Halliwell B. Free radicals, antioxidants, and human disease: curiosity, cause or consequence? *Lancet*, **344** (1994) 721–724.
40. Meydani SN, Meydani M, Blumberg JB, et al. Assessment of safety of supplementation with different amounts of vitamin E in healthy older adults. *Am. J. Clin. Nutr.*, **68** (1998) 311–318.
41. Meydani M. Dietary antioxidants modulation of aging and immune-endothelial cell interaction. *Mech. Ageing Dev.*, **111** (1999) 123–132.
42. Bendich A, Machlin LJ. Safety of oral intake of vitamin E. *Am. J. Clin. Nutr.*, **48** (1988) 612–619.
43. Farrell PM, Bieri JG. Megavitamin E supplementation in man. *Am. J. Clin. Nutr.*, **28** (1975) 1381–1386.
44. Shearer MJ, McBurney A, Barkhan P. Studies on the absorption and metabolism of phylloquine (vitamin K) in man. *Vitam. Horm.*, **32** (1974) 513–514.
45. Martensson J, Jain A, Meister A. Glutathione is required for intestinal function. *Proc. Natl. Acad. Sci. USA*, **87** (1990) 1715–1719.

46. White AC, Thannickal VJ, Fanburg BL. Glutathione deficiency in human disease. *J. Nutr. Biochem.*, **5** (1994) 218–226.

47. Ruan EA, Rao S, Burdick JS, et al. Glutathione levels in chronic inflammatory disorders of the human colon. *Nutr. Res.* **17** (1997) 463–473.

48. Miralles-Barrachina O, Savoye G, Belmonte-Zalar L, et al. Low levels of glutathione in endoscopic biopsies of patients with Crohns colitis: role of malnutrition. *Clin. Nutr.* **18** (1999) 313–317.

49. Iantomasi T, Marraccini P, Favilli F, Vincenzini MT, Ferretti P, Tonelli F. Glutathione metabolism in Crohns disease. *Biochem. Med. Metabol. Biol.*, **53** (1994) 87–91.

50. Koch TR, Schulte-Bockholt A, Otterson MF, et. Decreased vasoactive intestinal peptide levels and glutathione depletion in acquired megacolon. *Dig. Dis. Sci.*, **41** (1996) 1409–1416.

51. Lih-Brody L, Powell SR, Collier KP, et al. Increased oxidative stress and decreased antioxidant defenses in mucosa of inflammatory bowel disease. *Dig. Dis. Sci.*, **41** (1996) 2078–2086.

52. Stoll R, Schmidt H, Stern H, Ruppin H, Domschke W. Functional defect of zinc transport in patients with Crohns disease. *Hepatogastroenterology*, **34** (1987) 178–181.

53. Sturniolo GC, Mestriner C, Lecis PE, et al. Altered plasma and mucosal concentrations of trace elements and antioxidants in active ulcerative colitis. *Scand. J. Gastroenterol.*, **33** (1998) 644–649.

54. Longnecker M, Martin-Moreno J-M, Knekt P, et al. Serum alpha tocopherol concentration in relation to subsequent colorectal cancer: Pooled data from five cohorts. *J. Natl. Cancer. Inst.*, **84** (1992) 430–435.

55. Knekt P, Aromaa A, Maatela J, et al. Serum vitamin A, and subsequent risk of cancer: cancer incidence follow-up of the Mobile Clinic Health Examination Survey. *Am. J. Epidemiol.*, **132** (1990) 857–870.

56. Stahelin H, Gey F, Eicholzer M, Ludin E. Beta carotene and cancer prevention: the Basel Study. *Am. J. Clin. Nutr.*, **53(Suppl)** (1991) 265–269.

57. Wright JP, Mee AS, Parfitt A, et al. Vitamin A therapy in patients with Crohn's Disease. *Gastroenterology*, **88** (1985) 512–514.

58. Emerit J, Pelletier S, Tosoni-Verlignue D, Mollet M. Phase II trial of copper zinc superoxide dismutase (CuZnSOD) in treatment of Crohns disease. *Free Rad. Biol. Med.*, **7** (1989) 145–149.

7 Aging

Emmanuel C. Opara and Timothy R. Koch

Contents

1. INTRODUCTION

Definition of Aging

Aging has been defined by some authorities as an accumulation of changes responsible for sequential alterations that accompany advancing age and progressively increase the chance of disease and death *(1)*. The presence of the process of aging involving the colon would be expected to have a major impact on colonic diseases. By 1985, the number of Americans aged 65 and older increased to 28 million, and it is estimated that this population of elderly individuals will reach 64 million by the year 2020 *(2)*. An estimated $8 billion of $22 billion spent yearly for care of institutionalized elderly is required for patients who have disorders of defecation *(3)*.

Whether there is a true aging process involving the colon, e.g. separate from a concomitant disease process, environmental exposure, or somatic gene mutation, is therefore a major scientific and health issue. This chapter will examine major proposed theories of aging and experimental evidence that an aging process alters colonic function. This area of scientific work provides an important bridge between basic science and clinical research and management of clinical disorders of the colon.

2. THEORIES OF AGING

Several specific processes related to aging can not be generalized to all mammals *(4)*. Two interesting processes that have been examined in specific species include a defined genetic

From: *Colonic Diseases*
Edited by: T. R. Koch © Humana Press Inc., Totowa, NJ

etiology and the occurrence of chronic degeneration. The former model is illustrated by the Pacific salmon model. In this species, during mating, adrenal glucocorticoid secretion increases, and death will occur after a few days. The latter model is illustrated by dormancy, which has been termed stopping the aging clock. This process may be illustrated by diapause in worker bees and hibernation in Turkish hamsters.

Dozens of specific theories have been proposed to explain the aging process (5,6). Many of the major theories are summarized in Table 1. In 1908, Rubner proposed a modern scientific theory when he presented evidence linking metabolic rate and aging. The Rate of Living Theory, proposed by Pearl in 1928, was based on the concept that the duration of life varies inversely with the rate of energy expenditure.

Dr. Leo Szilard, who had aided in the development of the atomic bomb, proposed the Somatic Mutation Theory in 1959. This theory implied that genetic mutations of DNA accumulate with time resulting in miscopying and functional failure. The Somatic Mutation Theory has been extensively investigated by many researchers, but there is little confirmatory evidence.

In 1963, Dr. Leslie Orgel proposed a related theory termed the Error Catastrophe Theory. It was suggested that if an error were made in molecular copying processes (either transcription or translation) resulting in the synthesis of an altered protein, the mutated protein could initiate a chain of flawed events resulting in a cascade of altered biochemical processes. This theory postulated that an error could occur in information transfer at a site other than at the level of DNA. Unfortunately, experimental support for this theory is not consistent.

Dr. Johan Bjorksen proposed the Cross-Linkage Theory in 1968. It was suggested that an alteration occurred in structural proteins that induced inter- and intramolecular cross-linkage with other proteins. Bjorksen hypothesized that a process of progressive cross-linking in the body was responsible for age-related changes. He believed that two potential approaches to preventing cross-linking of proteins were physical exercise and chelation therapy with ethylene diamine tetra acetic acid (EDTA).

Dr. A. Cerami has proposed the Glycation Theory of Aging. He suggested that nonenzymatic reactions of glucose and other reducing sugars with amino groups of proteins and nucleic acids result in a series of events that alter protein and nucleic acid structure and function. This process is similar to the caramelization of sugar.

Professor Vladimir Dilman of the Petrov Institute in St. Petersburg, Russia, proposed the Neuroendocrine Theory in 1983. He hypothesized that the aging process is due to the loss of receptor sensitivity to feedback inhibition during aging, resulting in a progressive shifting of homeostasis and alterations of hormone levels and their effect with time.

Telomeres are short noncoding nucleoprotein structures at the ends of eukaryotic chromosomes. The telomere hypothesis of cell aging suggests that this structure is involved in a component of cellular aging due to a lower critical limit in telomere length. Telomeres appear involved in the accurate transcription of DNA during cell division. Telomere shortening occurs during each cell division during replication, and so it is hypothesized that telomeres eventually become too short to permit cell division (7). In examination of human tissues (leukocytes, skin, and synovial tissue), there does appear to be an inverse relationship between patient age and telomere fragment length (8).

Mitochondrial oxidative phosphorylation is involved in the synthesis of ATP in cells. The Mitochondrial Theory of Aging suggests that an accumulation of somatic mutations involving mitochondrial DNA induces a decline in mitochondrial function (9). This aging hypothesis includes the notion that mitochondrial DNA mutations and deletions will accumulate in tissues during the aging process and are, therefore, responsible for aging.

Table 1
Theories of Aging

Year	Proponent	Chief Element of Theory
1908	Rubner	Metabolic rate influences aging.
1928	Pearl	Duration of life varies with energy expenditure.
1959	Szilard	Somatic mutation of DNA theory.
1963	Orgel	Error (transcription or translation) catastrophe.
1968	Bjorksen	Alteration of structural protein cross-linkage.
	Cerami	Glycation of reducing sugars with amino groups.
1983	Dilman	Neuroendocrine loss of receptor sensitivity.
1995		Telomere shortening hypothesis of cell aging.
1989		Mitochondrial theory of aging.
1956	Harman	Free radical theory of aging.

The Free Radical Theory of Aging was proposed by Dr. Denham Harman. He hypothesized that aging results from an accumulation of changes caused by reactions in the body initiated by highly reactive free radicals. Changes induced by free radicals are believed to be a major cause for aging, disease development, or death. Free radicals and their precursors can be produced endogenously (within the body) through normal metabolic processes, as well as exogenously (outside the body), from sources such as cigarette smoking. This has been a popular and widely tested theory.

3. FREE RADICAL THEORY OF AGING

Defense mechanisms against exogenous and endogenous free radicals are reducing agents termed antioxidants. When the levels of available antioxidants are insufficient to interact with free radicals, these very reactive molecules easily react with vital molecules in the body, such as DNA, causing mutations in the sequence of genetic material. An accumulation of induced changes is thought to lead to the process of aging.

The free radical theory of aging, which hypothesizes that aging is due to damage to DNA and molecular membranes, induced by highly reactive molecules or free radicals, is very appealing. There are a number of reasons why this theory has remained popular and withstood the test of time. First, it provides a unifying mechanism for different theories. The free radical theory is the only theory that encompasses concepts from many other theories of aging (an exception being the Neuroendocrine Theory). Second, it may be experimentally verified. There is a growing number of studies that implicate free radical reactions in the development of many chronic age-related diseases. Third, it suggests a number of parameters that can be evaluated to determine the progress of aging and the success of anti-aging therapies. In addition, it proposes a mechanism that could be altered by appropriate antioxidant therapies or supplements.

The free radical theory integrates theories that pertain to metabolism and energy expenditure with theories dealing with molecular changes (or mutations) at the DNA level. It is possible to propose mechanisms by which increasing the metabolic rate in a mammal would generate an increase in free radicals or reactive oxygen species. The reactive oxygen species would, in turn, react with DNA to cause mutations that could lead to aging. This sequence could provide an explanation for the potential benefit of lowering the metabolic rate of a mammal with regards to increasing its length of survival.

Free radicals are derived from two major sources: (i) endogenous and (ii) exogenous. Endogenous free radicals are produced in the body by four different mechanisms. The first includes the normal metabolism of oxygen-requiring nutrients. Mitochondria, which produce the universal energy molecule, adenosine triphosphate (ATP), normally consume oxygen in this process and convert it to water. Unwanted byproducts such as the superoxide anion, hydrogen peroxide, and the hydroxyl radical are produced because of incomplete reduction of the oxygen molecule. It has been estimated that more than 20 billion molecules of oxidants per day are produced by each cell during normal metabolism. Inefficient cell metabolism could further increase this free radical production during the aging process.

Second, white blood cells destroy parasites, bacteria, and viruses by producing oxidants, including nitric oxide, superoxide, and hydrogen peroxide. Chronic infection could prolong phagocytic activity and increase exposure of organs in the body to oxidants. Certainly the presence of large numbers of bacteria in the lumen of the colon warrants investigation.

A third potential mechanism is the production of hydrogen peroxide by peroxisomes as a byproduct of the degradation of fatty acids and other molecules. While mitochondria oxidize fatty acids to produce ATP and water, peroxisomes oxidize fatty acids to produce heat and hydrogen peroxide. Hydrogen peroxide is then degraded by the enzymatic antioxidant, catalase. Under certain conditions, hydrogen peroxide could escape to damage other compartments in the cell.

As a fourth mechanism, cytochrome P450 is a cellular enzyme that is one of the body's primary defenses against toxic chemicals that are ingested with food. The induction of these enzymes in order to prevent damage by toxic foreign chemicals, such as drugs and pesticides, can result in the production of oxidant byproducts. This could also be important in the process of aging.

Exogenous sources of free radicals include air pollution, which includes industrial waste and cigarette smoke. Cigarette smoke itself contains oxidants. Radiation and trace metals, notably lead, mercury, iron, and copper, are also major sources of free radical generation. Normal diets containing plant foods with large quantities of compounds such as phenols and caffeine could contribute to the exogenous supply of oxidants in the colon.

The combination of oxidative damage by exogenously and endogenously produced free radicals could have ominous consequences for body tissues. Oxidants may induce alterations in the structures of tissues and in their functions, which could then manifest as aging or chronic diseases, including cancer.

The relationship between oxidative damage and aging is a double-edged sword. On one hand, oxidative damage to DNA, lipids, proteins, and other macromolecules could be a major contributing factor to aging, while at the same time, oxidative damage accumulates with aging, despite attempts by an individual's cellular machinery to repair it. The colon is equipped with antioxidant defense systems to detoxify these dangerous agents. This suggests that if the colon's defense system becomes less effective as we get older, this could lead to the accumulation of oxidative damage and the development of chronic colonic diseases. There are only preliminary studies of age-associated changes in colonic antioxidants. In a small study of 16 patients with nonobstructing neoplasia, there was no apparent age-associated change in total antioxidant capacity of the human colon (10). In a second small study of 10 patients with nonobstructing neoplasia, there was a strong trend toward age-associated reduction in colonic levels of the nonenzymatic cellular antioxidant, glutathione, in human colon (11). Certainly, an age-related decrease in colonic antioxidants would support this mechanism as a potential explanation for altered colonic function in aging.

4. COLONIC CANCER AND AGING

Colorectal cancer is the second most common cause of cancer deaths for both males and females in the United States. Oxidative damage may play a significant role in the development of this cancer. Oxidants are produced as a result of normal digestive metabolism. The slower the transit time of stool in the colon, the greater the concentration of potential cancer-causing free radicals. It has been proposed that tissue damage could increase as bowel habits become less regular, and the cancer-susceptible mucous membranes of the colon could be exposed to progressively more active cancer-causing oxidative agents for longer periods of time.

This hypothesis is supported by the increased incidence of cancer as digestive products pass through the colon toward the rectum. If this hypothesis is true, it would suggest that the a way to reduce the risk of colon cancer would be to maintain rapid colonic transit time.

Since colon cancer is associated with oxidative stress and is a leading cause of death in most developed countries, cancer therapy with antioxidants has been extensively researched. Investigators have examined the benefits of various antioxidants in high risk individuals and in individuals with colon cancer. Antioxidants that have been examined in chemoprevention of colorectal cancer include N-acetylcysteine and vitamins A, C, and E. The choice of antioxidants and the examined doses depended upon the desired goals of the study. For disease prevention, moderate dosages of a combination of antioxidants have generally been examined, since antioxidants work best when combined. For adjuvant therapies in disease, high doses of antioxidants have been examined for beneficial effect. Antioxidant supplements appear to be extremely safe, even when used at high doses for adjuvant therapy in disease.

In a different approach, chitosan and other forms of soluble and insoluble fibers, such as apple pectin, guar gum, and oat bran fiber, may be effective in decreasing colonic transit time and may influence the incidence of colon cancer.

5. EPIDEMIOLOGIC EVIDENCE SUPPORTING AGING OF COLON

Epidemiologic studies have defined the prevalence of gastrointestinal (GI) symptoms in young, old, hospitalized, and nonhospitalized patients. These studies of age-associated constipation have demonstrated that this disorder is one of the most common chronic digestive disorders in the United States, affecting one out of every 50 people (an estimated 4.5 million Americans) (12,13). Chronic constipation is the cause for an estimated 2.5 million physician visits yearly in the United States. Although prevalence is high, mortality is rare, leading to a chronic disorder. For these reasons, age-related defecatory disorders produce major symptomatic and financial impacts on public health. The occurrence of constipation increases with advancing age, showing an exponential increase in prevalence after the age of 65. Constipation occurs in an estimated 4.5% of individuals age 65–74 and 10.2% of those age 75 yr and older. Overall, constipation is three times more common in females than males (see Table 2). We have proposed that age-related constipation may reduce the risk of development of fecal incontinence in elderly individuals.

Diverticular disease of the colon is quite common in Western countries. The prevalence of colonic diverticular disease has been correlated with age (14). Epidemiologic studies have suggested that an origin of colonic diverticulosis may involve the use of a low fiber diet in Western countries. This suggests that colonic diverticulosis may be induced by an environmental exposure rather than being related to a process of aging.

Studies of fecal incontinence have shown that it is more common in women than in men and that there is an age-related increase in the prevalence of fecal incontinence. Fecal incontinence has been reported by approx 1.2% of individuals age 65 yr and older (15).

Table 2
Evidence Supporting Aging of Colon

Technique	Major findings	Reference
Epidemiology	Increased occurrence of constipation.	12,13
	Increased prevalence of diverticulosis.	14
	Increased prevalence of fecal incontinence.	
Morphology	Decreased numbers of neurons in colonic myenteric plexus.	17–19
	Increased connective tissue in internal anal sphincter.	20
Immunochemistry	Decreased staining of peptide-containing enteric nerves.	21
	Decreased tissue levels of intestinal neuropeptides.	22,23
In vivo physiology	Colonic contractile activity unchanged.	
	Slow colonic transit of solid markers	25–27
	Declines in resting anal canal pressure and maximal squeeze pressure.	29,30
In vitro physiology	Decline in amplitude of inhibitory junction potentials.	24
	Decline in calcium channel current.	32

In surveys of patients with consistent symptoms, it has been reported that 11% of individuals 60 yr and older have irritable colon (16). Due to the high prevalence of this disorder, there is presently no evidence for an age-related increase in this disorder.

6. MORPHOLOGIC EVIDENCE SUPPORTING AGING OF COLON

There has been considerable scientific interest in the potential for an age-associated alteration of colonic enteric nerves. The density of enteric nerves in young and old individuals has been studied in man and in animal models. In the rat model, a 60% decrease in the number of neurons in colonic myenteric plexus has been reported, when 24-mo-old rats were compared to 6-mo-old rats (17). Previous morphologic studies demonstrated age-related declines in the numbers of neurons in human myenteric plexus (18,19). In examination of nerve cells in the myenteric plexus of human colon, subjects over 65 yr old had 37% fewer neurons that individuals less than age 35 yr (19).

It has also been suggested that there is increased sclerosis or connective tissue in the internal anal sphincter in elderly patients (20).

7. ENTERIC NEUROTRANSMITTERS AND AGING OF COLON

There have been some studies that showed an age-associated alteration in colonic inhibitory neurochemicals. In a rat model, elderly animals have decreased density of vasoactive intestinal peptide (VIP)-containing, substance P-containing, and somatostatin-containing intestinal nerve fibers (21). A study of rat small intestine showed that VIP tissue levels were significantly decreased in 28 mo-old animals compared to 3 mo-old animals (22). In rectal biopsies from young and elderly humans, declines in VIP, substance P, and neurokinin A levels have been reported (23). In studies of surgical tissues obtained from nonobstructing colonic neoplasia, there were no age-associated changes in levels of the inhibitory neuropeptides VIP, peptide histidine–methionine, neuropeptide Y, somatostatin, or methionine–enkephalin identified in the mucosal–submucosal layer or in the muscularis externa layer (24).

8. IN VIVO PHYSIOLOGICAL EVIDENCE FOR AGING OF COLON

In studies of colonic contractile patterns using endoscopically placed perfused manometry catheters, there have been no age-associated changes identified in either colonic segmental contractions or mass movements (termed giant migrating contractions).

In vivo studies involving young and elderly individuals have also utilized radiopaque markers. The transit of solid markers through the colon and rectum has been examined. Older individuals have been shown to have slower mean colonic transit time than younger individuals (25). Other studies have demonstrated that constipated elderly individuals have slow transit of solid markers through the sigmoid colon and rectum (26,27). In a rat model, similar to clinical studies, transit through the colon is slowed in senescent rats compared to young rats (28).

Using a continuously perfused catheter to perform anal–rectal manometry, age-related declines in resting anal canal pressure and maximal squeeze pressure have been reported (29). Consistent with epidemiologic evidence, the decline observed in women in this study preceded that observed in men. Other studies have supported the notion that resting pressure of the internal anal sphincter and voluntary contractile pressure of the external anal sphincter are decreased with age and are lower in women compared to men (30). These findings suggest a mechanism that could explain the epidemiologic evidence for fecal incontinence in elderly women.

9. IN VITRO PHYSIOLOGICAL EVIDENCE FOR AGING OF COLON

Using strips of human colonic smooth muscle, electrical field stimulation evokes release of inhibitory neurotransmitters, which induce hyperpolarization of the smooth muscle membrane by increasing potassium conductance. This hyperpolarization is termed an inhibitory junction potential (IJP). Consistent with this ion transport, high amplitude electrical field stimulation in human colonic circular smooth muscle evokes IJPs that approach the calculated K^+ equilibrium potential (E_k) of –80 mV. The nerve-mediated origin of IJPs is supported by their blockade by the sodiumchannel blocker, tetrodotoxin (31).

Intracellular impalements of human colonic circular muscle in the presence of cholinergic and α- and {b}-adrenergic receptor blocking agents demonstrate that prolonged electrical field stimulation evokes both an immediate IJP and a summed IJP of lower amplitude (24). These two types of IJPs could be produced by release of one or more inhibitory neurotransmitters. The magnitude of smooth muscle relaxation is directly related to the amplitude of IJPs (24).

Using surgical specimens of human colon from patients with nonobstructing colonic neoplasia, in vitro studies of inhibitory nerve input to human colonic circular muscle have been performed (24). Using grossly and histologically normal descending colon, IJPs evoked by electrical field stimulation were recorded and characterized (Fig. 1). Mean IJP amplitudes declined in older patients. Consistent with epidemiologic studies of constipation and patient age in the United States, the decline shown in women preceded that in men. Resting membrane potentials were similar at different ages, and this was evidence against an age-related myopathy.

This study was consistent with a study of cell membrane currents using single smooth muscle cells isolated from human colon (32). In this latter study, there was no identified age-associated change in potassium current, which would be consistent with the absence of an age-associated change in resting membrane potentials. There appeared however to be an age-associated decline in calcium channel current, which physiologically could be expected to influence excitation and contraction of human colonic smooth muscle (32).

To summarize these studies, electrophysiologic methods provide quantitative data during studies of intrinsic nerve input to colonic circular muscle. Decreased IJPs would be expected to be associated with diminished circular smooth muscle relaxation. An age-associated

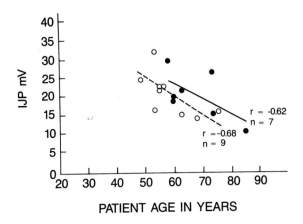

Fig. 1. Inverse relationship between patient age and the mean amplitude of membrane hyperpolarization evoked by activating intrinsic inhibitory nerves in circular smooth muscle from human colon. Note that the decline in women (open circles) preceded the decline in men (solid circles). The magnitude of smooth muscle relaxation can be directly related to the amplitude of membrane hyperpolarization. Reprinted with permission from ref. *24*.

decline in calcium channel current could effect excitation and contraction of human colonic smooth muscle. The results support two mechanisms, one neurogenic and one myogenic, that could be tested to explain slowed colonic transit associated with aging human colon.

In addition, there has been an in vitro physiologic study of the human internal anal sphincter (*33*). This study supported absence of intramural α-adrenergic excitatory nerve input to the internal anal sphincter in patients with idiopathic fecal incontinence. This finding could provide a potential mechanism to explain an age-related loss in resting pressure of the internal anal sphincter.

10. FUTURE DIRECTIONS

Questions remain on an appropriate strategy for proceeding in studies of the aging colon. We would suggest four potential approaches to future studies. Additional epidemiologic studies of colonic diseases and patient age in countries with differing dietary intake should provide important information about the potential influence of this environmental factor on the development of colonic diseases.

A second approach could be based upon studies of whole organ physiology. Available studies suggest that pathophysiological changes in colonic function during senescence need to be better defined. Interstudy variability supports the real concern that age-associated changes in colon function could be induced by either an underlying disease process or environmental influences, which may be difficult to delineate from an ongoing aging process.

As a third approach, if markers for altered colonic function could be validated, this area of research could then progress more reliably into studies of cellular and molecular mechanisms designed to understand abnormal colonic function. Improving our understanding of these potential underlying mechanisms could permit examination of specific aging theories, for example the free radical theory, to determine whether the specific theory would be capable of inducing the proposed mechanism. This approach would be different from common strategies in which a new theory is proposed, and then multiple species or organs are examined to look for evidence of an abnormality that could be explained by the new aging theory.

In a fourth approach, the free radical theory of aging could be indirectly tested by studying the physiologic effects of supplementing subjects with antioxidant nutrients, including vitamins A, C, and E, with minerals such as selenium, and with nutritional antioxidant cofactors, including lipoic acid. As an allied approach, one could test chelating substances, such as EDTA, in order to remove free radical promoting toxic heavy metals. If the free radical theory of aging proves to be correct, antioxidants could offer tremendous potential benefit to individuals during the aging process.

REFERENCES

1. Ashok BT, Ali R. The aging paradox: free radical theory of aging. *Exp. Gerontol.*, **34** (1999) 293–303.
2. Anderson MS, Gilchrist A, Mondeika T, et al. and the American Medical Association Council on Scientific Affairs. American Medical Association white paper on elderly health: report of the Council on Scientific Affairs. *Arch. Intern. Med.*, **150** (1990) 2459–2472.
3. Szurszewski JH, Holt PR, Schuster M. Proceedings of a workshop entitled "Neuromuscular function and dysfunction of the gastrointestinal tract in aging". *Dig. Dis. Sci.*, **34** (1989) 1135–1146.
4. Sapolsky RM, Finch CE. On growing old: not every creature ages, but most do. The question is why. *Sciences*, **31** (1991) 30–38.
5. Carlson JC, Riley JCM. A consideration of some notable aging theories. *Exp. Gerontol.*, **33** (1998) 127–134.
6. McClearn GE. Biogerontologic theories. *Exp. Gerontol.*, **32** (1997) 3–10.
7. Allsopp RC. Models of initiation of replicative senescence by loss of telomeric DNA. *Exp. Gerontol.*, **31** (1996) 235–243.
8. Friedrich U, Griese E–U, Schwab M, Fritz P, Thon K-P, Klotz U. Telomere length in different tissues of elderly patients. *Mech. Ageing and Dev.*, **119** (2000) 89–99.
9. Gadaleta MN, Cormio A, Pesce V, Lezza AMS, Cantatore P. Aging and mitochondria. *Biochimie*, **80** (1998) 863–870.
10. Koch TR, Yuan L-X, Stryker SJ, Ratliff P, Telford GL, Opara EC. Total antioxidant capacity of colon in patients with chronic ulcerative colitis. *Dig. Dis. Sci.*, **45** (2000) 1814–1819.
11. Koch TR, Schulte-Bockholt A, Otterson MF, et al. Decreased vasoactive intestinal peptide levels and glutathione depletion in acquired megacolon. *Dig. Dis. Sci.*, **41** (1996) 1409–1416.
12. Sonnenberg A, Koch TR. Physician visits in the United States for constipation: 1958 to 1986. *Dig. Dis. Sci.*, **34** (1989) 606–611.
13. Sonnenberg A, Koch TR. Epidemiology of constipation in the United States. *Dis. Colon Rectum*, **32** (1989) 1–8.
14. Parks TG. Natural history of diverticular disease of the colon. *Clin. Gastroenterol.*, **4** (1973) 53–60.
15. Madoff RD, Williams JG, Caushaj PF. Fecal incontinence. *N. Engl. J. Med.*, **326** (1992) 1002–1007.
16. Talley NJ, Zinsmeister AR, Van Dyke C, Melton LJ III. Epidemiology of colonic symptoms and the irritable bowel syndrome. *Gastroenterology*, **101** (1991) 927–934.
17. Santer RM, Baker DM. Enteric neuron numbers and sizes in Auerbach's plexus in the small and large intestine of adult and aged rats. *J. Auton. Nerv. Syst.*, **25** (1988) 59–67.
18. Koberle F. Quantitative pathologie des vegetativen nervensystems. *Wiener klin Wochenschrift*, **74** (1962) 144–151.
19. Gomes OA, de Souza RR, Liberti EA. A preliminary investigation of the effects of aging on the nerve cell number in the myenteric ganglia of the human colon. *Gerontology*, **43** (1997) 210–217.
20. Klosterhalfen B, Offner F, Topf, N, Vogel P, Mittermayer C. Sclerosis of the internal anal sphincter-A process of aging. *Dis. Colon Rectum*, **33** (1990) 606–609.
21. Feher E, Penzes L. Density of substance P, vasoactive intestinal polypeptide and somatostatin-containing nerve fibers in the ageing small intestine of the rats. *Gerontology*, **33** (1987) 341–348.
22. Ferrante F, Geppetti P, Amenta F. Age-related changes in substance P and vasoactive intestinal polypeptide immunoreactivity in the rat stomach and small intestine. *Arch. Gerontol. Geriatr.*, **13** (1991) 81–87.
23. Donckier J, McGregor GP, Impallomeni M, Calam J, Bloom SR. Age-related changes in regulatory peptides in rectal mucosa. *Acta. Gastroenter. Belg.*, **50** (1987) 405–410.
24. Koch TR, Carney JA, Go VLW, and Szurszewski JH. Inhibitory neuropeptides and intrinsic inhibitory innervation of descending human colon. *Dig. Dis. Sci.*, **36** (1991) 712–718.
25. Madsen JL. Effects of gender, age, and body mass index on gastrointestinal transit times. *Dig. Dis. Sci.*, **37** (1992) 1548–1553.

26. Melkersson M, Andersson H, Bosaeus I, Falkheden T. Intestinal transit time in constipated and non-consti-
    pated geriatric patients. *Scand. J. Gastroentol.*, **18** (1983) 593–597.
27. Varma JS, Bradnock J, Smith RG, Smith AN. Constipation in the elderly: a physiologic study. *Dis. Colon
    Rectum*, **31** (1988) 111–115.
28. McDougal JN, Miller MS, Burks TF, Kreulen DL. Age-related changes in colonic function in rats. *Am. J.
    Physiol.*, **247** (1984) G542–G546.
29. McHugh SM, Diamant NE. Effect of age, gender and parity on anal canal pressures: contribution of impaired
    anal sphincter function to fecal incontinence. *Dig. Dis. Sci.*, **32** (1987) 726–736.
30. Enck P, Kuhlbusch R, Lubke H, Frieling T, Erckenbrecht JF. Age and sex and anorectal manometry in
    incontinence. *Dis. Colon Rectum*, **32** (1989) 1026–1030.
31. Koch TR, Carney JA, Go VLW, Szurszewski JH. Altered inhibitory innervation of circular smooth muscle
    in Crohn's colitis: association with decreased vasoactive intestinal peptide levels. *Gastroenterology*, **98**
    (1990) 1437–1444.
32. Xiong Z, Sperelakis N, Noffsinger A, Fenoglio-Preiser C. Ca^{2+} currents in human colonic smooth muscle
    cells. *Am. J. Physiol.*, **269** (1995) 269 G378–G385.
33. Speakman CTM, Hoyle CHV, Kamm MM, Henry MM, Nicholls RJ, Burnstock G. Abnormalities of inner-
    vation of internal anal sphincter in fecal incontinence. *Dig. Dis. Sci.*, **38** (1993) 1961–1969.

Immunology
of the Gastrointestinal Tract

Jonathan R. Fulton, Cynthia A. Cunningham,
and Christopher F. Cuff

CONTENTS

INTRODUCTION
INNATE IMMUNITY
ADAPTIVE IMMUNITY
ORAL TOLERANCE
CONCLUSIONS
ACKNOWLEDGMENTS
REFERENCES

1. INTRODUCTION

The gastrointestinal system is essentially a long muscular tube, the functional surface of which is a thin, mucus-coated layer approx 1 mm thick, that is joined at both ends with the external integument and, thus, is a contact surface with the external environment *(1)*. The surface area of the adult human intestine is estimated to be approx 300 M^2 *(2)*. This surface is constantly exposed to antigens, which, proximally, is mostly of dietary origin and, distally, tends to be bacterial products derived from colonic flora. Providing a protective barrier at this external surface is complicated by the need to selectively absorb nutrients. To prevent the colonization and/or invasion of the intestinal mucosa by foreign organisms, the intestine makes use of a number of innate and adaptive defense factors. This chapter provides a broad overview of immune responses in the intestine.

2. INNATE IMMUNITY

A palisade of columnar intestinal epithelial cells (IEC) with interspersed mucus-secreting goblet cells maintains the first line of innate mucosal defense. Mucus sheaths the mucosal epithelium and, together with the glycoproteins of the IEC glycocalyx, forms a size-restrictive permeability barrier against lumenal antigens *(3)*. Tight junctions between adjacent IEC serve to prevent intercellular passage of antigens and organisms into the intestinal tissues. Thus, under ideal conditions, the majority of lumenal contents that gain access to the intestinal tissues are small nutrient molecules transported transcellularly across the IEC.

From: *Colonic Diseases*
Edited by: T. R. Koch © Humana Press Inc., Totowa, NJ

The integrity of the IEC barrier in the villi and crypts is maintained by constant proliferation of epithelial stem cells located approx halfway down the villi, the progeny of which migrate either downward into the crypt or upward to the tips of the villi. Progeny cells initially have the ability to differentiate into a number of epithelial cell types, such as absorptive IEC, Paneth cells, and goblet cells, undergoing progressive differentiation during migration. These cell types have specialized functions in protection of the mucosa. For instance, Paneth cells, which are located at the bases of the crypts, produce a number of exocrine antimicrobial factors, such as the anion-binding pore-forming α-defensins (cryptins) (4), peptidoglycan hydrolyzing lysozyme (5), and phospholipase A2 (6), that contest microbial colonization of the crypt epithelium. In addition to secreting the mucus barrier (7), goblet cells also produce trefoil proteins (8), factors that enhance IEC migration toward sites of injury and are thus believed to play a role in maintaining the integrity of the epithelial barrier (9).

3. ADAPTIVE IMMUNITY

3.1. Organization and Location of Intestinal Lymphocytes

While passive and active innate factors of the intestinal epithelium provide a basic outermost layer of defense against a broad assortment of environmental antigens and organisms, a diverse array of cells of hematopoietic origin are dispersed throughout the underlying lamina propria, clustered in highly organized secondary lymphoid tissues, and intercalated within the IEC palisade. These bone marrow-derived cells include CD4+ T cells, which support and direct many of the effector functions of other cells, CD8+ T cells, and natural killer (NK) cells, which mediate cytotoxicity against infected, transformed, or physiologically stressed self cells. Other cells involved include B lymphocytes, which produce antigen-specific immunoglobulin (Ig) of primarily the IgA isotype and lesser quantities of IgM and IgG (2), macrophages, dendritic cells, and tissue granulocytes, such as mast cells and eosinophils.

Lymphoid tissues of the intestine are typically categorized into two types: (i) inductive tissues, wherein naïve T and B cells as well as antigen-experienced memory cells are primed by gut lumenal antigens and then induced to proliferate; and (ii) effector tissues, the sites to which primed lymphocytes migrate and mediate protective immune function (10). Inductive tissues include the Peyer's patches (PP), the mesenteric lymph nodes (MLN), the appendix, isolated lymphoid follicles (LF), and potentially such structures as the lymphocyte-filled villi (11). Inductive LF, which are aggregates of B and T cells, interdigitating dendritic cells, and macrophages separated from the lumenal contents by specialized follicle-associated epithelium (FAE), are distributed along the length of the intestine from the duodenum to the anorectal junction (11). While usually located in the lamina propria (LP) of the antimesenteric gut wall, human follicles may be distributed randomly around the circumference of the gut. Although generally not macroscopically visible, histological examination reveals that they can be extensive and may be either entirely contained within the LP or may have long extensions under the muscularis mucosa, creating structures previously identified as submucosal lymphoid aggregates (11). Effector tissues include the intestinal LP underlying the villus and crypt absorptive epithelium, and the T lymphocyte-dominated intraepithelial lymphocyte (IEL) compartment (1). Collectively, all these tissues are referred to as the gut-associated lymphoid tissue (GALT).

The largest aggregates of inductive lymphoid tissue in the GALT, the PP are considered the premier priming tissue of intestinal immunity (12). Defined as collections of 5 or more LF, PP are roughly analogous to peripheral lymph nodes. Histologically and functionally, the LF and appendix are very similar to the PP, although some question still remains as to whether the appendix may also serve as a primary B cell organ in the human perinatal gut (13). The quantity of follicular lymphoid tissue in the gut is considerable; with an estimated 11,000–14,000 scattered LF in the large intestine alone *(14)*.

The lumenal face of the PP, as with all gut follicular tissues, is covered with a specialized dome of epithelial cells, known as the FAE *(15)*. Among the conventional columnar epithelial cells of the FAE are interspersed thin flat microfold (M) cells that lack the long organized apical microvilli, glycocalyx, and mucus coating that characterize the villus absorptive epithelium. The lack of these covering structures, which form a size-selective permeability barrier to prevent access of large antigenic molecules and organisms from the absorptive epithelium, make M cells natural portals of ingress for lumenal antigens and organisms into the PP *(16)*. In animal studies, intestinal pathogens such as *Salmonella typhi (17)*, *Shigella flexneri (18)*, *Yersinia enterocolitica (19)*, reovirus *(20)*, poliovirus type 1 *(21)*, and *Cryptosporidium (22)* are believed to bind to glycoproteins on the M cell surface, thus facilitating their ingress. M cells also have been shown to express Fcα receptors (FcαR), which selectively allow the binding and uptake of lumenal antigens bound by secreted IgA, the Ig most associated with mucosal humoral immunity *(23)*. Additionally, particulate and soluble antigen may be nonspecifically internalized and transcytosed by M cells.

Although M cells have been demonstrated to contain lysosomal vesicles, they express major histocompatibility class I, and, in the small intestine but not the large intestine, class II molecules *(24)*, and are in intimate contact with a population of T and B lymphocytes *(25)*. It remains uncertain whether they play a role as antigen-presenting cells (APC). However, M cells transcellularly translocate lumenal antigens and organisms into the subepithelial dome region of the PP *(10)*. This area is rich in APC such as macrophages and immature dendritic cells that can internalize, process, and present peptide antigen epitopes in association with immature dentritic MHC class I and class II molecules to antigen-specific T cells *(10)*. Maturing antigen-bearing dendritic cells and macrophages subsequently migrate from the subepithelial dome region deeper into the T cell-enriched parafollicular regions, where they join with networks of interdigitated dendritic cells that serve to prime CD4$^+$ T cells and cytolytic CD8$^+$ T cells *(26)*.

3.2. Cellular Immunity

3.2.1. T-Helper Cells

Adaptive immune responses can be broadly divided into two arms: (i) the cellular response, mediated primarily by CD4$^+$ and CD8$^+$ T cells, and the myeloid cells they influence, and (ii) the humoral response, consisting of B cells and the specific antibodies that they produce under the influence primarily of CD4$^+$ T cells. Central to both arms of adaptive immunity is the priming of antigen-specific naive T lymphocytes by antigen-presenting dendritic cells. Interaction of T cells bearing T cell receptors (TCR) specific for antigenic epitopes expressed in association with MHC class I or II molecules on the surface of dendritic cells results in mutual stimulation and activation of the T cell and dendritic cell. Binding of dendritic cell CD40 to T cell CD40 ligand (CD40L) induces the dendritic cells to up-regulate expression of T cell co-stimulatory molecules B7.1 and B7.2, which, in turn, interact with T cell surface molecule CD28 to augment the stimulatory signaling of the TCR-CD3 complex with its epitope *(27)*. These multiple interactions required to initiate a T cell-mediated immune response are important controls in preventing the development of aberrant immune responses (Fig. 1).

CD4$^+$ T cells recognizing antigen through the TCR and receiving co-stimulation through B7-CD28 ligation, up-regulate both T cell growth factor interleukin (IL)-2 production *(28)*, and expression of the high affinity IL-2 receptor α-subunit (TAC; CD25) *(29)*, allowing for autocrine induction of proliferation. Activated progeny CD4$^+$ T cells may then either differ-

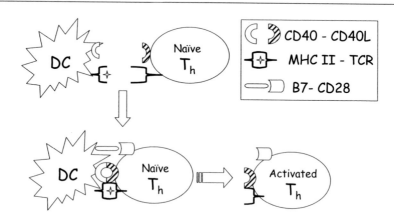

Fig. 1. Initial interactions between a naïve Th cell and a dendritic APC occur through CD40–CD40L and class II MHC-TCR. As a result of this interaction, B7 expression on dendritic cells is increased, and co-stimulatory signals are sent through interactions of B7 with CD28. The activated T cell is now ready to proliferate and differentiate.

entiate into effector cells or migrate from the PP via efferent microlymphatic vessels to complete differentiation and mediate effector function in distant tissues (*30*).

Generally, effector CD4+ T cells are classified as either T-helper type 1 (Th1) or T-helper type 2 (Th2) and are defined by the cytokines that they produce. Th1 cells produce IL-2, interferon (IFN)-γ, and tumor necrosis factor (TNF)-α. IFN-γ activates macrophages, up-regulates MHC class II expression of APC (*31*), induces activated B cells to undergo Ig heavy chain isotype switching to IgG2, and inhibits the establishment of Th2 responses (*31*). Th1 cytokines, in particular IFN-γ and IL-2, can also augment CD8+ cytotoxic T cell responses (*32*). Th2 effector T cells produce predominately IL-4, IL-5, IL-6, and IL-10 (*33*). These cytokines act on humoral responses; IL-4 induces isotype class switching to IgE and IgG1 (*34*), whereas IL-5, IL-6, and IL-10 support proliferation of activated B cells, and their differentiation into antibody-secreting plasma cells (*35*). It has also been suggested that the intestine supports the development of a third population of Th cells referred to as Th3, which preferentially produces transforming growth factor β (TGF-β). TGF-β promotes IgA class switching in β-cells and suppresses systemic immune responses (*36*). This phenomenon is described as "oral tolerance" and is considered in more detail in Subheading 4. Selection of Th1 vs Th2 responses is thought to be influenced by the local cytokine milieu, concurrent immune responses, the nature of the antigen, the APC, and individual genetic predisposition (*33,37–39*). It is thought that Th cells are the most important lymphocyte population in immunopathological inflammatory bowel diseases. This hypothesis and its ramifications are described in detail in Chapters 28 and 29.

3.2.2. Cytotoxic T Lymphocyte Responses

CD8+ T cells are responsible for killing cells infected with intracellular pathogens by effector mechanisms such as membrane pore-forming perforin and granzyme-mediated cytotoxicity, as well as by inducing apoptosis of target cell by Fas–FasL interactions. CD8+ cells can also kill intracellular bacteria, such as mycobacteria, by means of the antimicrobial protein granulysin. Naïve CD8+ T cells are activated by antigen expressed in association with MHC class I molecules by dendritic cells in the parafollicular T cell area of the PP. Effector CD8+ T cells produce cytokines, such as IFN-γ, IL-4, and small amounts of IL-2, which can influence other aspects of immune system. In addition, evidence exists in animal and human models that $CD8^+$ T cells can suppress immune responses.

3.2.3. Effector T cells in the Intestine

T lymphocytes in the intestinal lamina propria and intraepithelial lymphocyte compartment are numerous, and are phenotypically, functionally, and developmentally diverse. In general terms, LP and some IEL T cells can be considered as conventional antigen experienced, chronically activated immigrant lymphocytes from GALT and peripheral immune compartments. Four general functions can be ascribed to both LP and IEL T cells: (i) Th cell support of B cell secretory IgA and IgM production; (ii) protection of the mucosa against invasive organisms; (iii) regulation and attenuation of inflammatory responses; and (iv) repair and maintenance of the integrity of the epithelial barrier. These functions are mediated by secreted cytokines and direct cell contact-dependent ligation of signal-transducing cell surface molecules. As cytokine profiles, cell surface receptor expression and activation requirements of mucosal effector T cells are often quite different. It is likely that the above mentioned functions are mediated, with varying amounts of overlap, by distinct T cell subsets.

3.2.3.1. LP T Cells. Lamina propria T lymphocytes are approx 55% $CD4^+$, 24% $CD8^+$, similar to percentages found in the peripheral blood *(40)*. Most $CD3^+$ T cells (95%) use the $\alpha\beta$ form of the TCR *(41)*, again similar to the peripheral blood. Although LP $\gamma\delta$ TCR^+ cells account for <5% of T cells, they are slightly enriched in the LP as compared to the systemic periphery. The LP also contains a minor T cell population that expresses both CD4 and CD8 (14%) of unknown function *(42)*. These so-called "double positive" cells are rarely found in the peripheral blood. LP T cells bear surface marker phenotypes associated with previous antigen-experience, such as CD45RO (96%), cellular adhesion molecules CD2 *(40)*, $\alpha_4\beta_7$ (70%) *(43)*, $\alpha_E\beta_7$ (52%), and basement membrane binding CD44 (>80%) *(44)*. LP T cells proliferate at relatively low levels, and are refractory to TCR-specific antigen-mediated proliferative responses, although proliferation can be induced by ligation of alternative T cell stimulation molecules such as CD2 and CD28 *(45)*, and epithelial goblet cell-derived cytokine IL-7 *(46)*. Nevertheless, many LP T cells are constitutively activated as evidenced by the expression among roughly 15% of $CD4^+$ and $CD8^+$ cells of CD25 *(47)*. and the apoptosis-inducing FasL *(48)*. Furthermore, LP T cells were shown to spontaneously produce IFN-γ and IL-4 ex vivo. Additionally, high levels of both Th1 cytokines, such as IFN-γ, IL-2, and TNF-α, and Th2 cytokines, such as IL-4, IL-5, and IL-10, can be induced by ligation of CD2 *(49–53)*. Together, the available data suggest that these cells are antigen-experienced, but somewhat refractory to reactivation. This physiologic state of T cells in normal LP probably also contributes to the state of immunologic tolerance of the intestinal immune system.

Perhaps the most important function of LP T cells is the support of B cell proliferation and differentiation. Differentiation of antigen-experienced B cells into pIgA secreting plasma cells is promoted by T cell cytokines TGF-β, IL-5, and IL-10, whereas IL-6 supports IgA, IgM, and IgG3 production *(54)*. Compelling evidence exists that LP T cells are constitutively activated to support B cell function, as LP T cells co-cultured with lipopolysaccharide (LPS)-stimulated LP B cells provided Th cell support for secretion of IgA and IgM, whereas autologous peripheral blood T cells did not support IgA and IgM production *(55)*. Interestingly, TGF-β, IL-6, and IL-15 produced by IEC are thought to augment LP IgA production in vivo *(56,57)*, suggesting a complex array of factors collectively involved in mucosal immunoregulation.

3.2.3.2. IEL. In terms of phenotype, effector mechanisms, priming, and ontogeny, LP T cells are similar to other peripheral antigen-experienced T cells, yet contrast dramatically with IEL. IEL are a dispersed effector lymphocyte population intercalated within the IEC palisade just above the IEC basement membrane and, thus, are in intimate contact with the columnar epithelium. The IEL compartment consists of T lymphocyte-like cells, with diverse and often unconventional phenotypes and developmental backgrounds. Most IEL bear the CD45RO$^+$ phenotype of antigen-experienced cells and the integrin $\alpha_E\beta_7$ (58), which binds to E-cadherin expressed on IEC (59). IEL also express human leukocyte antigen (HLA)-DR and decreased levels of TCR/CD3 as compared to peripheral blood lymphocytes, possibly indicating recent activation (60). Up to 90% of IEL bear the CD8 phenotype. Most CD8$^+$ IEL express the conventional heterodimeric form of CD8 referred to as CD8$\alpha\beta$. About 10% of IEL express CD4, some of which also co-express CD8 in the unconventional homodimeric form of CD8 referred to as CD8$\alpha\alpha$. CD4$^+$ IEL are found throughout the length of the intestine and may respond to antigen presented on HLA-DR by IEC (61). Additionally, small populations of CD4$^-$CD8$^-$ cells are found in the IEL compartment predominantly in the large intestine. Most IEL are $\alpha\beta$ TCR$^+$, with a significant fraction of $\gamma\delta$ TCR$^+$ cells that variably increases in quantity from 2%–10% in the duodenum up to approx 40% in the large intestine (41,62). While $\alpha\beta$ TCR$^+$ IEL can express any of the CD8 and CD4 phenotypes, the most prevalent population is the seemingly conventional CD8$\alpha\beta^+$ $\alpha\beta$ TCR$^+$ IEL. Of $\gamma\delta$ TCR$^+$ IEL, about 58% express the homodimeric CD8$^+$, with the remainder being CD4$^-$CD8$^-$ (63).

The distinct phenotypes of IEL may correlate with ontogeny. Numerous studies undertaken in animals have suggested that CD8$\alpha\alpha^+$ $\alpha\beta$ TCR$^+$ and $\gamma\delta$ TCR$^+$ IEL may be derived from extrathymic maturation pathways. This is less clear in humans. Nevertheless, these distinct phenotypes do correlate with function and specificity. It is well established that IEL with the conventional CD8$\alpha\beta^+$ $\alpha\beta$ TCR$^+$ phenotype contain conventional antigen-specific cytotoxic T cell populations (64,65) and that these CTL are derived from CD8$^+$ T cells primed in PP (66) and other secondary lymphoid tissues (67) and assume effector function upon TCR-mediated recognition of antigen. Analysis of the TCR β-chain sequences have demonstrated that while CD8$\alpha\beta^+$ and CD8$\alpha\alpha^+$ T cells are not derived from the same precursor T cells, they are the clonal progeny of very restricted group of progenitors as compared to peripheral blood CD8$^+$ T cells (68). This restricted clonality is thought to derive from chronic expansion of a few IEL by enteric microfloral or dietary antigens. However, CD8$\alpha\beta^+$ $\alpha\beta$ TCR$^+$ IEL bearing identical TCR β-chain sequences may be simultaneously broadly distributed throughout the length of the intestine and locally enriched (69) and also found within the thoracic duct and LP (70), indicating that clonal populations of IEL may proliferate locally, and that progeny cells may migrate out of the epithelium and recirculate to distant sections of the intestine (70).

While CD8$\alpha\beta^+$ $\alpha\beta$ TCR$^+$ IEL are responsive to TCR-mediated recognition of antigen, CD8$\alpha\alpha^+$ $\alpha\beta$ TCR$^+$ and $\gamma\delta$ TCR$^+$ IEL are much less responsive to TCR-mediated activation (71). However, IEL are stimulated to proliferate and assume effector function by alternative pathways, such as ligation of IEL CD2 (72), and, thus, may be activated in vivo by contact with the IEC surface integrin leukocyte function-associated antigen (LFA)-1, which is a ligand for CD2 (73). Additionally, IEC express surface glycoprotein 180, which can stimulate IEL proliferation through direct binding of CD8 (74). Furthermore, IEL proliferation can be induced by goblet cell secreted IL-7, which is augmented by LP CD4$^+$ T cell TNF-α and IL-2 (75), and by direct contact with LP myofibroblasts underlying the IEC basement membrane (76). CD8 $\alpha\beta^+$ $\alpha\beta$ TCR$^+$ IEL are MHC class I restricted, mediate effector function by perforin and FasL-mediated cytotoxicity (77), and produce cytokines such as IFN-γ, IL-8, and TNF-α and chemokines, such as macrophage inflammatory protein (MIP)-1β (78–80). CD8 $\alpha\alpha^+$ $\alpha\beta$ TCR$^+$ IEL and $\gamma\delta$ TCR$^+$ IEL also have the ability to mediate cytotoxicity and secrete IFN-γ. Both subsets have been shown to recognize alternative nonclassical MHC molecules on IEC, such as CD1d (81,82). Indeed, $\gamma\delta$ TCR$^+$ IEL that express TCR Vγ respond to MHC class I-like

(MICA) molecules MICA-A and MICA-B, which are polymorphic molecules up-regulated on stressed or damaged epithelium (83–85). Additionally, some murine αβ TCR+ and γδ TCR+ IEL have been shown to proliferate and secrete IL-3, myeloid cell growth factor granulocyte-macrophage colony-stimulating factor (GM-CSF), and IFN-γ in response to soluble 65-kDa mycobacterial heat-shock protein (HSP) (86), which has been thought to be a cross-reactive antigen with mammalian HSP. In murine studies, CD8 αα+ αβ TCR+ IEL and γδ TCR+ IEL mediate spontaneous NK cell-like killing, possibly through surface NK cell markers (87). In humans, NK cell marker CD56 and NKG2D have been found on γδ TCR+ IEL, although human IEL do not appear to mediate much spontaneous ex vivo cytotoxicity except in the presence of IL-2, IL-7, or IL-15, which induce so-called lymphokine activated killer (LAK) function (83,88,89). Thus, CD8αα+ αβ TCR+ IEL and γδ TCR+ IEL appear to remain cytolytically inactive until stimulated by a battery of IEC and LP cytokines and epithelial stress markers, thereby fine tuning an otherwise nonspecific response specifically against stressed or infected epithelial cells, possibly an ancient immune function predating the evolution of antigen-specific adaptive immunity (90).

In addition to cytolysis of infected and possibly stressed epithelial cells (91), IEL influence epithelial barrier integrity. IEL have been shown to produce epithelial cell mitogen keratinocyte growth factor (KGF), which can repair damaged epithelium at the resolution of an inflammatory immune response. Mice lacking γδ TCR+ IEL show a reduction in epithelial cell turnover and resolution of mucosal inflammation, with the subsequent restoration of the epithelium greatly impaired (92,93). IEL are reciprocally influenced by IEC-derived cytokines, such as IL-15 and IL-7, which can induce IEL proliferation and LAK function, and TGF (89) and nitric oxide (94), which have been shown to prevent IEL activation (89,95). Thus, as the immediate front line of the immune system in the intestine, different IEL subpopulations function to: (i) maintain normal epithelium growth homeostasis; (ii) non-specifically prevent infection of the epithelium; (iii) specifically resolve infection and guard against re-infection; and (iv) resolve inflammation and repair epithelial damage, all while under the dynamic reciprocal control of numerous in situ factors of immune, epithelial, and stromal cell origin.

3.3. Humoral Immunity

3.3.1. B CELL ACTIVATION

The primary follicles, located within the PP, appendix, or as dispersed isolated lymphoid aggregates, are the sites of initiation of humoral immune responses and appear as spherical lymphocyte aggregates containing predominately naive B cells that express several surface markers including CD19+, CD20+, surface IgD (sIgD+) and IgM (sIgM+) (96). In addition, the follicles contain follicular dendritic cells (FDC) and occasional CD4+ Th cells. Primary follicles initially occur in the developing fetal intestine, but the development of secondary follicles that contain germinal centers (GC) do not occur until after birth, concomitant with the establishment of gut microflora. Naïve antigen-specific B cells initially contact antigen percolating through the parafollicular T cell area by means of their antigen-binding surface IgD and IgM, and subsequently internalize, process, and present epitopes to antigen-specific CD4+ T cells, which themselves have been previously activated by the interdigitating dendritic cells in the parafollicular T cell area. In a manner that is analogous to the interaction between dendritic APC and T cells, CD4+ T cell CD40L interaction with B cell surface CD40 induces up-regulation of co-stimulatory B7 molecules on the B cell, which binds T cell surface CD28 and induces effector cytokine production and B cell proliferation in the subsequently induced GC. GC reactions occurring within extant primary follicles produce a characteristic appearance of the secondary follicle, with a darkly staining zone of rapidly proliferating centroblasts

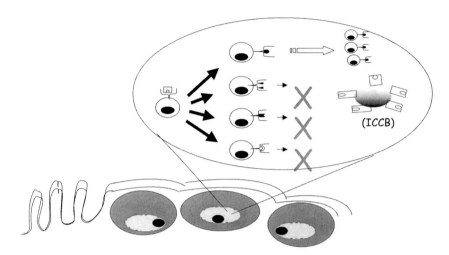

Fig. 2. GC reactions occurring within extant primary follicles produce a characteristic appearance of the secondary follicle, with a dark zone of rapidly proliferating centroblasts, which undergo isotype switching predominately to the IgA1 and IgA2 subclasses, and somatic hypermutation of antigen-binding Ig heavy chains, and a light zone of centrocytes. During a GC reaction, FDC are induced to shed these immune complexes on membrane vesicles known as immune complex-coated bodies (ICCB). Centrocytes with hypermutated heavy chains are competitively positively selected by their ability to bind and internalize these immune complexes and, subsequently, to present epitopes to follicle-infiltrating CD4+ Th cells, thereby avoiding apoptosis. This competitive selection for B cells expressing mutated surface Ig best able to bind limiting amounts of antigen is the basis of the phenomenon of affinity maturation and allows for progressively more effective fine-tuning of humoral immunity.

that undergo isotype switching and hypermutation of Ig heavy chains. The GC also contains a lightly staining zone of centrocytes. Early in the GC reaction, low affinity antigen-specific antibody forms insoluble antigen–antibody immune complexes on the membranes of FDC within the follicle. FDC then shed these immune complexes on membrane vesicles known as immune complex-coated bodies *(97)* (Fig. 2). Centrocytes with hypermutated heavy chains are competitively positively selected by their ability to bind and internalize these immune complexes and, subsequently, to present epitopes to follicle-infiltrating CD4+ T cells. The competitive selection for B cells expressing mutated surface Ig best able to bind limiting amounts of antigen is the basis of the phenomenon of affinity maturation and allows for progressively more effective fine-tuning of humoral immunity.

Following proliferation of activated antigen -specific B cells, somatic hypermutation, and possibly isotype class switching, the resulting centrocytes do not usually immediately terminally differentiate to antibody-secreting plasma cells. Typically, they migrate from the lymphoid tissue via the efferent lymphatics to traffic to effector tissues. Alternatively, they enter the marginal zone around the periphery of the follicular mantle zones to become a quiescent reserve pool of antigen-experienced "memory" cells *(98)*. These cells await subsequent reexposure to antigen, whereupon they can provide a secondary "recall" response, which is more rapid and of greater magnitude than the primary response.

3.3.2. Intestinal Effector B Cells

The intestinal LP, which contains approx 10^{10} Ig-producing B cells and plasma cells per meter, totaling roughly 80% of the body total, is far and away the largest B cell organ of the body*(99)*. In the human gut, IgA+ B cells, expressing either the IgA1 or IgA2 subclasses, predominate over all other isotypes, accounting for about 80% of B cells in the LP of the proximal jejunum (77% IgA1, 23% IgA2), increasing to 84% in the ileum (60% IgA1, 40% IgA2), and 90% in the large intestine (36% IgA1, 64% IgA2) *(100)*. The relative predominance of IgA2$^+$ B cells in the large intestine may be due to the abundance of bacterial products such as LPS, which tend to induce isotype class switching to IgA2 *(100)*. IgM$^+$ cells show a substantial though decreasing representation from 18% of B cells in the jejunum to 6% in the large intestine *(100)*. IgG$^+$ cells represent about 4% of all B cells throughout the intestine, with a subclass distribution of >60% IgG1, 20% IgG2, and <10% IgG3 and IgG4 *(101)*. IgE$^+$ and IgD$^+$ LP B cells are infrequent *(102)*. Commitment to the IgA isotype, which contrasts with the peripheral lymph node isotype class switch preference for IgG, appears to be due to intrinsic factors of the mucosal priming site microenvironment *(103)*. It is now known that the intestinal CD4$^+$ T cell-derived cytokine TGF-β and possibly dendritic cell CD40L interaction with CD40 on the surface of activated B cells, induces the IgA isotype class switching within the intestinal secondary follicles. The exact mechanisms for induction of IgA class switching and its regulation are still being elucidated.

Nearly all LP IgA$^+$ and IgM$^+$ B cells, and >80% of IgG$^+$ B cells also express the 15-kDa joining (J) chain *(104)*, which aggregates intracellular IgA monomers into predominantly dimeric IgA, and occasional larger polymeric masses, and aggregates intracellular IgM into predominantly pentameric forms, and occasional hexameric forms collectively called polymeric IgA (pIgA) and pIgM, respectively *(105)*. Monomeric IgG, by contrast, does not aggregate into polymers, and J chain expression by IgG$^+$ cells is believed to be a by-product of mucosal priming of these cells *(105)*. J chain-dependent pIgA and pIgM secreted by LP plasma cells are bound by the polymeric Ig receptor (pIgR) on IEC, translocated, and released in association with the secretory component (SC) following cleavage of the pIgR on the lumenal face of the IEC *(105)* (Fig. 3). Large amounts of IgG are also secreted into the intestinal lumen, most likely by passive diffusion through paracellular junctions *(106)*, although some evidence exists that an FcγR expressed in the small intestine serves as a bidirectional transporter and can transport LP IgG onto the mucosal surface *(107)*. However, most IgG is probably derived from serum protein filtrate in the LP. These findings suggest a not inconsequential role for IgG in addition to pIgA and pIgM in normal intestinal immunity.

3.3.3. Intestinal Humoral Immunity

Intestinal immunity, mounted under constant challenge by commensal and pathogenic organisms, is further complicated by the requirement to tolerate a massive load of normal floral and dietary-derived antigens. Despite the vast antigenic challenge, and the apparent chronic activation of the GALT, it is striking that not only is the intestinal mucosa not chronically massively inflamed, but with only rare exceptions immune responses to most innocuous antigens are apparently inhibited. Perhaps the most important mechanism of preventing damaging immune responses to normal floral and dietary antigens is prevention of their contact with intestinal lymphocytes. This function is partially mediated by the epithelial cell and mucus barriers and also by secreted antibody. Coating of lumenal organisms and antigens by secretory IgA prevents epithelial invasion by pathogens and commensal opportunists, as well as attenuating uptake of lumenal antigens, a process collectively known as "immune exclusion". It is also believed that during IgA translocation, pIgA may bind to antigen or organisms previously internalized by the IEC and "carry" it back to the lumen. By contrast, although FAE lacks pIgR *(2)* and, therefore, does not transport pIgA into the gut lumen, M cell FcαR binds antigen-bound secretory IgA in the lumen, translocating it and any associated antigen into the PP for subsequent immune priming *(23)* (Fig. 4). Nevertheless, normal human GALT does not

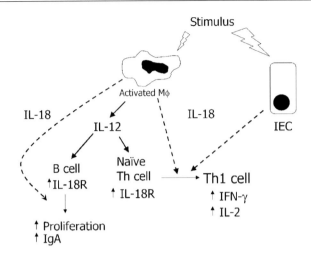

Fig. 3. pIgA produced in the LP is bound by the pIgR on the basolateral surface of the IEC. Receptor bound pIgA is subsequently translocated to the lumenal apical IEC surface and is there released by proteolytic cleavage of the pIgR. In the lumen, pIgA prevents antigen and organism contact with the IEC. It is also believed that, during the translocation event, pIgA may bind to antigen or organisms previously internalized by the IEC and carry it back to the lumen.

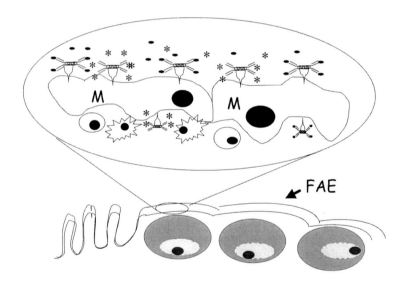

Fig. 4. M cells within the FAE overlying lymphoid follicles express the FcaR, which binds antigen-bound secretory pIgA in the lumen. FcaR-bound pIgA, and any associated antigen, is translocated into the PP for subsequent uptake and expression by dendritic cells. Particulate antigen and organisms are also nonspecifically endocytosed and translocated across M cells, independent of lumenal Ig.

prime humoral responses to dietary antigen, as little or no IgA or IgE is produced against food antigens except in cases of chronic intestinal inflammatory diseases *(108)* or food allergy. Thus, intestinal IgA responses seem predominantly restricted to commensal and pathogenic organisms and their structural constituents and secreted products. This is perhaps most clearly illustrated in studies using germ-free mice, wherein GC reactions are absent until colonization of the mucosa with gut microflora. Interestingly, while PP and appendix-derived B cells have been demonstrated to provide IgA and IgM lymphocytes throughout the gut LP, studies in mice suggest that up to half of all gut LP IgA$^+$ cells are the progeny of an unconventional population of CD5$^+$ B cells derived from the peritoneal cavity that are referred to as B1 B cells *(109)*. B1 B cells tend to produce IgM of low affinity to nonprotein bacterial structural components, such as phosphatidylcholine and lipopolysaccharide, generally considered to be Th cell indepen- dent antigens. Nevertheless, under the influence of Th cell cytokines possibly from peritoneal cavity CD4$^+$ T cell, or LP T cells, or even possibly such novel factors as enteric nervous system neuropeptide vasoactive intestinal peptide *(110)*, activated B1 cells can undergo isotype class switching to IgA. It is thought that B1 B cells represent ancient innate "natural antibody" B cell immunity that forms an initial nonspecific high volume low affinity component of immune exclusion. By contrast, conventional bone marrow-derived B cells (B2 B cells) form a highly selective high affinity response to commensal and pathogenic organisms that manage to pen- etrate the B1 B cell pIgA line of defense *(111)*. Interestingly, low affinity Ig from B1 B cells against some bacterial constituents, such as phosphatidylcholine-coated surface glycopro- teins, can cross react with tissue self antigens. This response potentially precipitates antibody- mediated autoimmunity and is a phenomenon that is currently under investigation *(109)*.

3.4. Migration of Intestinal Lymphocytes

Initiation of immune responses in the PP results in production of antigen-specific antibody and the appearance of activated T cells at effector sites, in the intestine and other mucosal sites such as the respiratory tract, the mammary gland, and perhaps the genitourinary tract. This phenomenon has led investigators to describe a common mucosal immune system (CMIS). The cellular basis for this CMIS has been understood for almost 30 yr. Immune cells activated in the PP preferentially migrate back to the intestine, but a fraction distribute to other mucosal compartments. The phenomenon of shared memory lymphocytes among anatomically distinct mucosal compartments is the rationale behind mucosal vaccine strategies aimed at providing protective immunity at targeted mucosal tissues by antigen application at physically more accessible and convenient locations. The molecular basis for this preferential recirculation has been more clearly elucidated only in the last decade. Most cells leaving the intestine and entering the mesenteric lymphatic vessels are believed to migrate to the MLN. Proliferating T and B cells from the GALT can produce large numbers of progeny in the MLN, which, along with quiescent recirculating naïve and memory cells, can reenter the efferent lymphatics, going on to the thoracic duct and then the systemic venous circulation. Antigen-experienced T and B cells can then migrate to mucosal effector sites or to other secondary lymphoid tissues.

Memory T and B cells exiting the gut express a heterodimeric protein receptor referred to as $\alpha_4\beta_7$ integrin, which allows for the preferential trafficking of gut-primed lymphocytes to the intestinal LP and back to the intestinal priming tissues, such as PP and MLN. The phenomenon of recirculation of antigen-experienced cells back to the gut tissues is mediated by $\alpha_4\beta_7$ ligation of the mucosal addresin cell adhesion molecule 1 (MadCAM-1) constitu- tively expressed on the intravascular surfaces of the flat endothelial cells of the postcapillary venules of the gut LP and also on the specialized cuboidal high endothelial vessels (HEV) cells, which serve as the points of egress of naïve and memory T and B cells from the venous circulation into the organized intestinal priming lymphoid tissues. Differential glycosylation of the MadCAM molecule within the endothelial cells at these locations allow for specific interactions with distinct lymphocyte ligands expressed on naïve or activated lymphocytes. Thus, naïve cells are excluded from effector compartments, which preferentially recruit antigen-experienced $\alpha_4\beta_7$ cells.

Expression of $\alpha_4\beta_7$ is not confined solely to intestinally primed lymphocytes nor even more generally to mucosally primed lymphocytes. Nevertheless, cells primed in distinct mucosal immune compartments show a definite preference for returning to their compartment of priming. This is likely mediated by differential levels of expression of other integrins and chemokine receptors that contribute to lymphocyte homing. However, a detailed discussion of these interactions is beyond the scope of this chapter.

4. ORAL TOLERANCE

Secretory IgA and, to a lesser extent, IgM-mediated immune exclusion and epithelial barrier function to exclude lumenal antigen from the intestinal tissues are important mechanisms by which the intestine prevents uncontrolled immune activation and inflammation. Intestinal T cell responses and, by extension, systemic T cell responses are tightly controlled by mechanisms ranging from outright elimination of antigen-activated T cells known as "clonal deletion", inhibition of proliferation and effector function, known as "anergy", and generation cytokine-secreting effector T cells that attenuate other T and B cell responses by "active suppression". Collectively, these three mechanisms contribute to a phenomenon of antigen-specific hyporesponsiveness, known as oral tolerance. Oral T cell tolerance is generated to protein antigens and therefore requires T cell interaction with APC and antigen. It appears likely that large quantities of antigen and low levels of co-stimulatory molecule expression on APC preferentially induce clonal deletion of anergy (112–114). In the absence of sufficient APC activation by CD40L-CD40 interaction or local inflammatory cytokines such as IL-12, the APC will express B7 at levels insufficient for naïve T cell co-stimulation, rendering responder T cells anergic (113,115,116). Antigen-experienced T cells express cytolytic lymphocyte-associated antigen (CTLA)-4, which also binds to B7 on APC. Binding of B7 by CTLA-4 induces apoptosis (117). Where exceptionally high local concentration of antigen are present, the APC might provide high numbers of MHC antigen complexes, which induce responder T cells to undergo apoptosis, thereby leading to tolerance by clonal deletion (118).

By contrast, active suppression is more complicated, involving CD4[+], CD8[+], or $\gamma\delta$ TCR[+] T cells, and is dependent on CD40L–CD40 interaction and APC activation (119). In general, active suppression is mediated by antigen-specific T cells that produce the pleiotropic cytokine TGF-β, and/or IL-10 (120). TGF-β strongly attenuates T cell responses (121). Thus, TGF-β serves to prevent damaging immunity directly and by augmenting IgA-mediated immune exclusion (122). IL-10 down-regulates antigen processing and presentation and blocks Th1 responses. IL-10 also contributes to the IgA response by promoting IgA[+] B cell differentiation to IgA secreting plasma cells. GALT CD8[+] T cells also mediate active suppressive tolerance by TGF-β production, often in concert with TGF-β producing CD4[+] T cells. Animal studies have also shown a pivotal role for $\gamma\delta$ TCR[+] T cells in oral tolerance induction and maintenance, as oral tolerance to ovalbumin protein could not be established in mice depleted of $\gamma\delta$ TCR[+] T cells (123,124). Furthermore, previously established oral tolerance to ovalbumin could be abrogated by in vivo depletion of $\gamma\delta$ TCR[+] T cells (123). Conversely, adoptive transfer of murine $\gamma\delta$ TCR[+] T cells has been shown to abrogate previously established oral tolerance (125). The complex role of $\gamma\delta$ TCR[+] T cells in oral tolerance induction and maintenance are subject to ongoing investigation. Although the mechanisms of tolerance are not completely understood, numerous clinical studies have been initiated attempting to ameliorate intestinal and systemic immunopathology by inducing tolerogenic intestinal immune responses, thus exploiting a natural protective phenomenon for broad therapeutic benefit.

5. CONCLUSIONS

Mucosal immunologists strive to understand the molecular and cellular mechanisms that result in induction, expression, and regulation of intestinal immunity. Understanding these mechanisms improves our ability to manipulate the immune response, with the goals of increasing resistance to intestinal infection and providing relief from the debilitating effects of inflammatory bowel diseases.

ACKNOWLEDGMENTS

The work in our laboratory is supported by National Institutes of Health grant RO1 AI34544.

REFERENCES

1. MacDonald TT, Bajaj-Elliot M, Pender SLF. T cells orchestrate intestinal mucosal shape and integrity. *Immunol. Today*, **20** (1999) 505–510.
2. Brandtzaeg P, Bjerke K. Human Peyer's patches: lympho-epithelial relationships and characteristics of Ig-producing cells. *Immunol. Invest.*, **18** (1989) 29–45.
3. Pitman RS, Blumberg RS. First line of defense: the role of the intestinal epithelium as an active component of the mucosal immune system. *Gastroenterology*, **35** (2000) 805–814.
4. Jones DE, Bevin CL. Paneth cells of the human small intestine express an antimicrobial peptide gene. *J. Biol. Chem.*, **267** (1992) 23,216–23,225.
5. Valnes K, Brandtzaeg P, Elgio K, Stave R. Specific and nonspecific humoral defense factors in the epithelium of normal and inflamed gastric mucosal. Immunohistochemical localization of Igs, secretory component, lysozyme, and lactoferrin. *Gastroenterology*, **86** (1984) 402–412.
6. Kiyohara H, Egami H, Shibata Y, Murata K, Ohshima S, Ogawa M. Light microscopic immunohistochemical analysis of the distribution of groups II phospholipase A2 in human digestive organs. *J. Histochem. Cytochem.*, **40** (1992) 1659–1664.
7. Jabbal I, Kells DI, Forstner G, Forstner J. Human intestinal goblet cell mucin. *Can. J. Biochem.*, **54** (1979) 707–716.
8. Podolsky DK, Lynch-Devaney K, Stow JL, et al. Identification of human intestinal trefoil factor. Goblet cell-specific expression of a peptide targeted for apical secretion. *J. Biol. Chem.*, **268** (1993) 6694–6702.
9. Modlin IM, Poulsom R. Trefoil peptides: mitogens, motogens, or mirages? *J. Clin. Gastroenterol.*, **1** (1997) S94–S100.
10. Mowat AM, Viney JL. The anatomical basis of intestinal immunity. *Immunol. Rev.*, **156** (1997) 145–166.
11. Moghaddami M, Cummins A, Mayerhofr G. Lymphocyte-filled villi: comparisons with other lymphoid aggregations in the mucosal of the human small intestine. *Gastroenterology*, **115** (1998) 1414–1425.
12. Kelsall BL, Strober W. The role of dendritic cells in antigen processing in the Peyer's patch. *Ann. NY Acad. Sci.*, **778** (1996) 47–54.
13. Dasso JF, Obiakor H, Bach H, Anderson AO, Mage RG. A morphological and immunohistological study of the human and rabbit appendix for comparison with the avian bursa. *Dev. Comp. Immunol.*, **24** (2000) 797–814.
14. Gebbers JO, Kennel I, Laissue JA. Lymphoid follicles of the human large bowel mucosal: structure and function. *Verh. Dtsch. Ges. Pathol.*, **76** (1992) 126–130.
15. Jacob E, Baker SJ, Swaminathan SP. 'M' cells in the follicle-associated epithelium of the human colon. *Histopathology*, **11** (1987) 941–952.
16. Neutra MR, Pringault E, Kraehenbuhl JP. Antigen sampling across epithelial barriers and induction of mucosal immune responses. *Annu. Rev. Immunol.*, **14** (1996) 275–300.
17. Kohbata S, Yokoyama H, Yabuuchi E. Cytopathogenic effect of *Salmonella typhi* GIFU 10007 on M cells of murine Peyer's patches in ligated ileal loops: an ultrastructural study. *Microbiol. Immunol.*, **30** (1986) 1225–1237.
18. Wassef JS, Keren DF, Mailloux JL. Role of M cells in initial antigen uptake and in ulcer formation in the rabbit intestinal loop model of shigellosis. *Infect. Immun.*, **57** (1989) 858–863.
19. Grutzkau A, Hanski C, Hahn H, Riecken EO. Involvement of M cells in the bacterial invasion of Peyer's patches: a common mechanism shared by *Yersinia entercolitica* and other enteroinvasive bacteria. *Gut*, **31** (1990) 1011–1015.

20. Wolfe JL, Rubin DH, Finberg R, et al. Intestinal M cells: a pathway for entry of reovirus into the host. *Scienc* **212** (1983) 471–472.
21. Sicinski P, Rowinski J, Warchol JB, et al. Poliovirus type 1 enters the human host through intestinal M cell *Gastroenterology*, **98** (1990) 56–58.
22. Marcial MA, Madara JL. Cryptosporidium: cellular localization, structural analysis of absorptive cell parasi membrane-membrane interactions in guinea pigs, and suggestion of protozoan transport by M cells. *Gastr enterology*, **90** (1986) 583–594.
23. Neutra MR. M cells in antigen sampling in mucosal tissues. *Curr. Top. Microbiol. Immunol.*, **236** (1999) 17–3
24. Bjerke K, Brandtzaeg P. T cells and epithelial expression of HLA class II determinants in relation putative M cells of follicle-associated epithelium in human Peyer's patches. *Adv. Exp. Med. Biol.*, **2** (1988) 695–698.
25. Farstad IN, Halstensen TS, Fausa O, Brandtzaeg P. Heterogeneity of M-cell-associated B and T cells in huma Peyer's patches. *Immunology*, **83** (1994) 457–464.
26. Steinman RM, Pack M, Inaba K. Dendritic cells in the T cell areas of lymphoid organs. *Immunol. Rev.*, **1** (1997) 25–37.
27. McLellan AD, Sorg RV, Williams LA, Hart DN. Human dendritic cells activate T lymphocytes via a CD4 CD40 ligand-dependent pathway. *Eur. J. Immunol.*, **26** (1996) 1204–1210.
28. Petro TM, Chen SS, Panther RB. Effect of CD80 and CD86 on T cell cytokine production. *Immunol. Inves* **4** (1995) 965–976.
29. Kremer IB, Cooper KD, Teunissen MB, Stevens SR. Low expression of CD40 and B7 on macrophages inf trating UV-exposed human skin; role in IL-2Ralpha-T cell activation. *Eur. J. Immunol.*, **28** (1998) 2936–294
30. Dunkley ML, Husband AJ. Distribution and functional characteristics of antigen-specific helper T cel arising after Peyer's patch immunization. *Immunology*, **61** (1987) 475–482.
31. Farrar MA, Schreiber RD. The molecular cell biology of interferon-gamma and its receptor. *Annu. Re Immunol.*, **11** (1993) 571–611.
32. Biron CA. Cytokines in the generation of the immune responses to, and resolution of, virus infection. *Cur Opin. Immunol.*, **6** (1994) 530–538.
33. McHugh S, Deighton J, Rifkin I, Ewan P. Kinetics and functional implication of Th1 and Th2 cytoki production following activation of peripheral blood mononuclear cells in primary culture. *Eur. J. Immuno* **26** (1996) 1260–1265.
34. Rousset F, Garcia E, Banchereau J. Cytokine-induced proliferation and immunoglobulin production of h man B lymphocytes triggered through their CD40 antigen. *J. Exp. Med.*, **173** (1991) 705–710.
35. Burdin N, Van Kooten C, Galibert L, et al. Endogenous IL-6 and IL-10 contribute to the differentiation CD40-activated human B lymphocytes. *J. Immunol.*, **154** (1995) 2533–2544.
36. Faria AM, Weiner HL. Oral tolerance: mechanisms and therapeutic applications. *Adv. Immunol.*, **73** (199 153–264.
37. Shibuya K, Robinson D, Zonin F, et al. IL-1 alpha and TNF-alpha are required for IL-12-induced developme of Th1 cells producing high levels of IFN-gamma in BALB/C but not C57BL/6 mice. *J. Immunol.*, **160** (199 1708–1716.
38. McHugh SM, Rifkin I, Deighton J, et al. The immunosuppressive drug thalidomide induces T helper cell ty 2 (Th2) and concomitantly inhibits Th1 cytokine production in mitogen- and antigen-stimulated huma peripheral blood mononuclear cell cultures. *Clin. Exp. Immunol.*, **99** (1995) 160–167.
39. Schmitz J, Assenmacher M, Radbruch A. Regulation of T helper cell cytokine expression: function dichotomy of antigen-presenting cells. *Eur. J. Immunol.*, **23** (1993) 191–199.
40. Schieferdecker HL, Ullrich R, Hirseland H, Zeitz M. T cell differentiation antigens on lymphocytes in t human intestinal lamina propria. *J. Immunol.*, **149** (1992) 2816–2822.
41. Ullrich R, Schieferdecker HL, Ziegler K, Riecken EO, Zeitz M. gamma delta T cells in the human intesti express surface markers of activation and are preferentially located in the epithelium. *Cell. Immunol.*, **1** (1990) 619–627.
42. Abuzakouk M, Carton J, Feighery C, O'Donoghue DP, Weir DG, O'Farrelly C. CD4⁺ CD8⁺ a CD8alpha⁺beta- T lymphocytes in human small intestinal lamina propria. *Eur. J. Gastroenterol. Hepatol.*, **1** (1998) 325–329.
43. Farstad IN, Halstensen TS, Lien B, Kilshaw PJ, Lazarovitz AI. Distribution of β7 integrins in the huma intestinal mucosal and organized gut-associated lymphoid tissue. *Immunology*, **89** (1996) 227–237.
44. Ebert EC, Roberts AI. Costimulation of the CD3 pathway by CD28 ligation in the human intestinal lymph cytes. *Cell. Immunol.*, **171** (1996) 211–216.
45. De Maria R, Fais S, Silvestri M, et al. Continuous in vivo activation and transient hyporesponsiveness to Tc CD3 triggering of human gut lamina propria lymphocytes. *Eur. J. Immunol.*, **23** (1993) 3104–3108.

46. Watanabe M, Ueno Y, Yajima T, et al. Interleukin 7 is produced by human intestinal epithelial cells and regulates the proliferation of intestinal mucosal lymphocytes. *J. Clin. Invest.*, **95** (1995) 2945–2953.

47. Zeitz M, Greene WC, Peffer NJ, James SP. Lymphocytes isolated from the intestinal lamina propria of normal nonhuman primates have increased expression of genes associated with T cell activation. *Gastroenterology*, **94** (1988) 647–655.

48. De Maria R, Boirivant M, Cifone MG, et al. Functional expression of Fas and Fas ligand on human gut lamina propria T lymphocytes. A potential role for the acidic sphingomyelinase pathway in normal immunoregulation. *J. Clin. Invest.*, **97** (1996) 316–322.

49. Gonsky R, Deem RL, Bream JH, Lee DH, Young HA, Targan SR. Mucosa-specific targets for regulation of IFN-gamma expression: lamina propria T cells use different cis-elements than peripheral blood T cells to regulate transactivation of IFN-gamma expression. *J. Immunol.*, **1164** (2000) 1399–1407.

50. Gonsky R, Deem RL, Hughes CC, Targan SR. Activation of the CD2 pathway in lamina propria T cells up-regulates functionally active AP-1 binding to the IL-2 promoter, resulting in messenger RNA transcription and IL-2 secretion. *J. Immunol.*, **160** (1998) 4914–4922.

51. Targan SR, Deem RL, Liu M, Wang S, Nel A. Definition of a lamina propria T cell responsive state. Enhanced cytokine responsiveness of T cells stimulated through the CD2 pathway. *J. Immunol.*, **154** (1995) 664–675.

52. Boirivant M, Fuss I, Fiocchi C, Klein JS, Strong SA, Strober W. Hypoproliferative human lamina propria T cells retain the capacity to secrete lymphokines when stimulated via CD2/CD28 pathways. *Proc. Assoc. Am. Physicians.*, **108** (1996) 55–67.

53. Braunstein J, Qiao L, Autschbach F, Schurmann G, Meuer S. T cells of the human intestinal lamina propria are high producers of interleukin-10. *Gut*, **41** (1997) 215–220.

54. Riordan SM, McIver CJ, Wakefield D, Thomas MC, Duncombe VM, Bolin TD. Interleukin-6 and small intestinal lumenal immunoglobulins. *Dig. Dis. Sci.*, **43** (1998) 442–445.

55. Danis VA, Heatly RV. Evidence for regulation of human colonic mucosal immunoglobulin secretion by intestinal lymphoid cells. *J. Clin. Lab. Immunol.*, **22** (1987) 7–11.

56. Goodrich ME, McGee DW. Regulation of mucosal B cell immunoglobulin secretion by intestinal epithelial cell-derived cytokines. *Cytokine*, **10** (1998) 948–955.

57. Hiroi T, Yanagita M, Ohta N, Sakaue G, Kiyono H. IL-15 and IL-15 receptor selectively regulate differentiation of common mucosal immune system-independent B-1 cells for IgA responses. *J. Immunol.*, **165** (2000) 4329–4337.

58. Jarry A, Cerf-Bensussan N, Brousse N, Selz F, Guy-Grand D. Subsets of CD3+ (T cell receptor alpha/beta or gamma/delta) and CD3- lymphocytes isolated from normal human gut epithelium display phenotypical features different from their counterparts in peripheral blood. *Eur. J. Immunol.*, **20** (1990) 1097–1103.

59. Higgins JM, Mandlebrot DA, Shaw SK, et al. Direct and regulated interaction of integrin alphaEbeta7 with E-cadherin. *J. Cell. Biol.*, **140** (1998) 197–210.

60. Abuzakouk M, Kelleher D, Feighery C, O'Farrelly C. Increased HLA-DR and decreased CD3 on human intestinal intraepithelial lymphocytes; evidence of activation. *Gut*, **39** (1996) 396–400.

61. Hoang P, Crotty B, Dalton HR, Jewell DP. Epithelial cells bearing class II molecules stimulate allogeneic human colonic intraepithelial lymphocytes. *Gut*, **33** (1992) 1089–1093.

62. Trejdosiewicz LK, Smart CJ, Oakes DJ, et al. Expression of T cell receptors TcR1 (gamma/delta) and TcR2 (alpha/beta) in the human intestinal mucosa. *Immunology*, **68** (1989) 7–12.

63. Deusch K, Pfeffer K, Reich K, et al. Phenotypic and functional characterization of human TCR gamma delta+ intestinal intraepithelial lymphocytes. *Curr. Top. Microbiol. Immunol.*, **173** (1991) 279–283.

64. Chardes T, Buzoni-Gatel D, Lepage A, Bernard F, Bout D. *Toxoplasma gondii* oral infection induces specific cytotoxic CD8 alpha/beta+ Thy-1+ gut intraepithelial lymphocytes, lytic for parasite-infected enterocytes. *J. Immunol.*, **153** (1994) 4596–4603.

65. Chen D, Lee F, Cebra JJ, Rubin DH. Predominant T cell receptor Vbeta usage of intraepithelial lymphocytes during the immune response to enteric reovirus infection. *J. Virol.*, **71** (1997) 3431–3436.

66. Cuff CF, Cebra CK, Rubin DH, Cebra JJ. Developmental relationship between cytotoxic alpha/beta T cell receptor-positive intraepithelial lymphocytes and Peyer's patch lymphocytes. *Eur. J. Immunol.*, **23** (1993) 1333–1339.

67. Sydora BC, Jamieson BD, Ahmed R, Kronenberg M. Intestinal intraepithelial lymphocytes respond to systemic lymphocytic choriomeningitis virus infection. *Cell. Immunol.*, **167** (1996) 161–169.

68. Pluschke G, Taube H, Krawinkel U, et al. Oligoclonality and skewed T cell receptor V beta gene segment expression in in vivo activated human intestinal intraepithelial T lymphocytes. *Immunobiology*, **192** (1994) 77–93.

69. Regnault A, Kourilsky P, Cumano A. The TCR-beta chain repertoire of gut-derived T lymphocytes. *Semin. Immunol.*, **7** (1995) 307–319.

70. Arstila T, Arstila TP, Calbo S, et al. Identical T cell clones are located in the mouse gut epithelium and lamina propria and circulate in the thoracic duct lymph. *J. Exp. Med.*, **191** (2000) 823–834.

71. Barrett TA, Gajewski TF, Danielpour D, Chang EB, Beagley KW, Bluestone JA. Differential function of intestinal intraepithelial lymphocyte subsets. *J. Immunol.*, **149** (1992) 1124–1130.

72. Van Houten N, Mixter PF, Wolfe J, Budd, RC. CD2 expression on murine intestinal intraepithelial lymphocytes is bimodal and defines proliferative capacity. *Int. Immunol.*, **5** (1993) 665–672.

73. Kvale D, Krajci P, Brandtzaeg P. Expression and regulation of adhesion molecules ICAM-1 (CD54) and LFA-3 (CD58) in human intestinal epithelial cell lines. *Scand. J. Immunol.*, **35** (1992) 669–676.

74. Li Y, Yio XY, Mayer L. Human intestinal epithelial cell induced CD8+ T cell activation is mediated through CD8 and the activation of CD8-associated p56lck. *J. Exp. Med.*, **182** (1995) 1079–1088.

75. Ebert EC. Tumor necrosis factor-alpha enhances intraepithelial lymphocyte proliferation and migration. *Gut*, **42** (1998) 650–655.

76. Roberts AI, Nadler SC, Ebert EC. Mesenchymal cells stimulate human intestinal intraepithelial lymphocytes. *Gastroenterology*, **113** (1997) 144–150.

77. Corazza N, Muller S, Brunner T, Kagi D, Mueller C. Differential contribution of Fas- and perforin-mediated mechanisms to the cell-mediated cytotoxic activity of naïve and in vivo primed intestinal intraepithelial lymphocytes. *J. Immunol.*, **164** (2000) 398–403.

78. Fan JY, Boyce CS, Cuff CF. T-helper 1 and T-helper 2 cytokine responses in gut-associated lymphoid tissue following enteric reovirus infection. *Cell. Immunol.*, **188** (1998) 55–63.

79. Lundqvist C, Melgar S, Yeung MM, Hammarstrom S, Hammarstrom ML. Intraepithelial lymphocytes in human gut have lytic potential and a cytokine profile that suggests T helper 1 and cytotoxic functions. *J. Immunol.*, **157** (1996) 1926–1934.

80. Mattapallil JJ, Smit-McBride Z, McChesney M, Dandekar S. Intestinal intraepithelial lymphocytes are primed for gamma interferon and MIP-1beta expression and display antiviral cytotoxic activity despite severe CD4(+) T cell depletion in primary simian immunodeficiency virus infection. *J. Virol.*, **72** (1998) 6421–6429.

81. Panja A, Blumberg RS, Balk SP, Mayer L. CD1d is involved in T cell-intestinal epithelial cell interactions. *J. Exp. Med.*, **178** (1993) 1115–1119.

82. Sydora BC, Brossay L, Hagenbaugh A, Kronenberg M, Cheroutre H. TAP-independent selection of CD8+ intestinal intraepithelial lymphocytes. *J. Immunol.*, **56** (1996) 4209–4216.

83. Deusch K, Luling F, Reich K, Classes M, Wagner H, Pfeffer K. A major fraction of human intraepithelial lymphocytes simultaneously expresses the gamma/delta T cell receptor, the CD8 accessory molecule and preferentially uses the V delta 1 gene segment. *Eur. J. Immunol.*, **21** (1991) 1053–1059.

84. Groh V, Steinle A, Bauer S, Spies T. Recognition of stress-induced MHC molecules by intestinal epithelial gamma delta T cells. *Science*, **279** (1998) 1737–1740.

85. Griffith E, Ramsburg E, Hayday A. Recognition of human gut gamma-delta cells of stress-inducible major histocompatibility molecules on enterocytes. *Gut*, **43** (1998) 166–167.

86. Beagley KW, Fujihashi K, Black CA, et al. The *Mycobacterium tuberculosis* 71-kDa heat-shock protein induces proliferation and cytokine secretion by murine gut intraepithelial lymphocytes. *Eur. J. Immunol.*, **23** (1993) 2049–2052.

87. Guy-Grand D, Cuenod-Jabri B, Malassis-Seris M, Selz F, Vassalli P. Complexity of the mouse gut T cell immune system: identification of two distinct natural killer T cell intraepithelial lineages. *Eur. J. Immunol.*, **26** (1996) 2248–2256.

88. Bauer S, Groh V, Wu J, et al. Activation of NK cells and T cells by NKG2D, a receptor for stress-inducible MICA. *Science*, **285** (1999) 727–729.

89. Ebert EC. Inhibitory effects of transforming growth factor-beta (TGF-beta) on certain functions of intraepithelial lymphocytes. *Clin. Exp. Immunol.*, **115** (1999) 415–420.

90. Hayday AC. [Gamma][delta] cells: a right time and a right place for a conserved third way of protection. *Annu. Rev. Immunol.*, **18** (2000) 975–1026.

91. Suzuki Y, Mori K, Iwanaga T. Intraepithelial gamma delta T cells are closely associated with apoptotic enterocytes in the bovine intestine. *Arch. Histol. Cytol.*, **60** (1997) 319–328.

92. Komano H, Fujiura Y, Kawaguchi M, et al. Homeostatic regulation of intestinal epithelia by intraepithelial gamma delta T cells. *Proc. Natl. Acad. Sci. USA*, **92** (1995) 6147–6151.

93. Roberts SJ, Smith AJ, West AB, et al. T cell alpha beta+ and gamma delta+ deficient mice display abnormal but distinct phenotypes toward a natural, widespread infection of the intestinal epithelium. *Proc. Natl. Acad. Sci. USA*, **93** (1996) 11,774–11,779.

94. Yoshikai Y. The interaction of intestinal epithelial cells and intraepithelial lymphocytes in host defense. *Immunol. Res.*, **20** (1999) 219–235.

95. Chung CS, Song GY, Wang W, Chaudry IH, Ayala A. Septic mucosal intraepithelial lymphoid immune suppression: role for nitric oxide not Interleukin-10 or transforming growth factor-beta. *J. Trauma* **48** (2000) 807–812.

96. Farstad IN, Carlsen H, Morton HC, Brandtzaeg P. Immunoglobulin A cell distribution in the human small intestine: phenotypic and functional characteristics. *Immunology*, **101** (2000) 354–363.

97. Ahmed R, Gray D. Immunological memory and protective immunity: understanding their relation. *Science*, **272** (1996) 54–60.

98. Dunn-Walters DK, Isaacson PG, Spencer J. Sequence analysis of rearranged IgVH genes from microdissected human Peyer's patch marginal zone B cells. *Immunology*, **88** (1996) 618–624.

99. Brandtzaeg P, Baekkevold ES, Farstad IN, et al. Regional specialization in the mucosal immune system: what happens in the microcompartments? *Immunol. Today*, **20** (1999) 141–151.

100. Kett K, Brandtzaeg P, Radl J, Haaijman JJ. Different subclass distribution of IgA-producing cells in human lymphoid organs and various secretory tissues. *J. Immunol.*, **136** (1986) 3631–3635.

101. Bjerke K, Brandtzaeg P. Terminally differentiated human intestinal B cells. J chain expression of IgA and IgG subclass-producing immunocytes in the distal ileum compared with mesenteric and peripheral lymph nodes. *Clin. Exp. Immunol.*, **82** (1990) 411–415.

102. Brandtzaeg P, Bjerke K, Kett K, et al. Production and secretion of immunoglobulins in the gastrointestinal tract. *Ann. Allergy*, **59** (1987) 21–39.

103. Weinstein PD, Cebra JJ. The preference for switching to IgA expression by Peyer's patch germinal center B cells is likely due to the intrinsic influence of their microenvironment. *J. Immunol.*, **147** (1991) 4126–4135.

104. Bjerke K, Brandtzaeg P. Terminally differentiated human intestinal B cells. IgA and IgG subclass-producing immunocytes in the distal ileum, including Peyer's patches, compared with lymph nodes and palatine tonsils. *Scand. J. Immunol.*, **32** (1990) 61–67.

105. Brandtzaeg P, Farstad IN, Haraldsen G. Regional specialization in the mucosal immune system: primed cells do not always home along the same track. *Immunol. Today*, **20** (1999) 267–277.

106. Prigent-Delecourt L, Coffin B, Colombel JF, Dehinnin JP, Vaerman JP, Raumbaud JC. Secretion of immunoglobulins and plasma proteins from the colonic mucosal: an in vivo study in man. *Clin. Exp. Immunol.*, **99** (1995) 221–225.

107. Dickinson BL, Badizadegan K, Wu Z, et al. Bidirectional FcRn-dependent IgG transport in a polarized human intestinal epithelial cell line. *J. Clin. Invest.*, **104** (1999) 903–911.

108. O'Malony S, Arranz E, Barton JR, Ferguson A. Dissociation between systemic and mucosal humoral immune responses in celiac disease. *Gut*, **32** (1991) 29–35.

109. Murakami M, Honjo T. The involvement of B-1 cells in mucosal immunity and autoimmunity. *Immunol. Today*, **16** (1995) 534–539.

110. Boirivant M, Fais S, Annibale B, Agostini D, Delle Fave G, Pallone F. Vasoactive intestinal polypeptide modulates the in vitro immunoglobulin A production by intestinal lamina propria lymphocytes. *Gastroenterology*, **106** (1994) 576–582.

111. Bos NA, Cebra JJ, Kroese FGM. B-1 cells and the intestinal microflora. *Curr. Top. Microbiol. Immunol.*, **252** (2000) 211–220.

112. Friedman A, Weiner HL. Induction of anergy or active suppression following oral tolerance is determined by antigen dosage. *Proc. Natl. Acad. Sci. USA*, **91** (1994) 6688–6692.

113. Van Gool SW, Vermeiren J, Rafiq K, Lorr K, de Boer M, Ceuppens JL. Blocking of CD40-CD154 and CD80/CD86-CD28 interactions during primary allogeneic stimulation results in T cell anergy and high IL-10 production. *Eur. J. Immunol.*, **29** (1999) 2367–2375.

114. Koenen HJ, Joosten I. Blockade of CD86 and CD40 induces alloantigen-specific immunoregulatory T cells that remain anergic even after reversal of hyporesponsiveness. *Blood*, **95** (2000) 3153–3161.

115. Villegas EN, Elloso MM, Reichmann G, Peach R, Hunter CA. Role of CD28 in the generation of effector and memory responses required for resistance to *Toxoplasma gondii. J. Immunol.*, **163** (1999) 3344–3353.

116. Frauwirth KA, Alegre ML, Thompson CB. Induction of T cell anergy in the absence of CTLA-4/B7 interaction. *J. Immunol.*, **164** (2000) 2987–2993.

117. Perez VL, Van Parijs L, Biuckians A, Zheng XX, Strom TB, Abbas AK. Induction of peripheral T cell tolerance in vivo requires CTLA-4 engagement. *Immunity*, **4** (1997) 411–417.

118. Chen Y, Inobe J, Weiner HL. Inductive events in oral tolerance in the TCR transgenic adoptive transfer model. *Cell. Immunol.*, **178** (1997) 62–68.

119. Kweon MN, Fujihashi K, Wakatsuki Y, et al. Mucosally induced systemic T cell unresponsiveness to ovalbumin requires CD40 ligand — CD40 interactions. *J. Immunol.*, **162** (1999) 1904–1909.

120. Kitani A, Chua K, Nakamura K, Strober W. Activated self-MHC-reactive T cells have the cytokine phenotype of the Th3/T regulatory cell 1 T cells. *J. Immunol.*, **165** (2000) 691–702.

121. Levings MK, Roncarolo MG. T-regulatory 1 cells: a novel subset of CD4 T cells with immunoregulatory properties. *J. Allergy Clin. Immunol.*, **106** (2000) S109–S112.

122. Van Vlasselaer P, Punnonen J, de Vries JE. Transforming growth factor-beta directs IgA switching in human B cells. *J. Immunol.*, **148** (1992) 2062–2067.

123. Mengel J, Cardillo F, Aroeira LS, Williams O, Russo M, Vaz, NM. Anti-gamma delta T cell antibody blocks the induction and maintenance of oral tolerance to ovalbumin in mice. *Immunol. Lett.*, **48** (1995) 97–102.

124. Ke Y, Pearce K, Lake JP, Ziegler HK, Kapp JA. Gamma delta T lymphocytes regulate the induction and maintenance of oral tolerance. *J. Immunol.*, **158** (1997) 3610–3618.

125. Fujihashi K, Taguchi T, Aicher WK,et al. Immunoregulatory functions for murine intraepithelial lymphocytes: gamma/delta T cell receptor-positive (TCR+) T cells abrogate oral tolerance, while alpha/beta TCR+ T cells provide B cell help. *J. Exp. Med.*, **175** (1992) 695–707.

9 Colonic Lymphatics

Stacey A. Weiland and Yang K. Chen

1. INTRODUCTION

Mesenteric lymphatics have been studied since the 16th century. One of the earliest published observations was mady by Asellius (1581–1625), Professor of Anatomy and Surgery in Milan, who, in 1622, documented the presence of a white vessel system, *"venae albae et lacteae"* in a postprandial canine mesentery *(1)*.

Since then, the macroscopic and microscopic anatomy, as well as the physiology and immunology, of mesenteric lymphatics have been extensively evaluated. Multiple disease states related to congenital and acquired disorders of mesenteric lymphatics have also been described. This chapter discusses the normal physiology and anatomy, as well as pathologic states, of the mesenteric lymphatic system, with particular emphasis on the colonic lymphatic system.

2. COLONIC LYMPHATIC ANATOMY

2.1 The Colon Lymphatic Vascular Tree

The well-characterized lacteal of the small intestine, which has a primary role in nutrient absorption, is closely associated with subepithelial capillaries within the lamina propria of the intestinal villus *(2)*. The colonic lymphatic microanatomy, in contrast, was once thought to only reach the muscularis mucosa at the bases of crypts *(3)*. More recent data, however demonstrates that the lymph vessels of the colon penetrate into the mucosa, as well.

Three-dimensional microstructural analysis of the colon has revealed the presence of microscopic lymph vessels surrounding the crypts in the lamina propria mucosa (Fig. 1). In an elegant set of experiments, Hirai et al. *(4)* have demonstrated that superficial colonic lymphatics form both shallow and deep hexagonal reticular layers, which are connected to one another by other vertical lymph vessels. The shallow layer is found just below the

From: *Colonic Diseases*
Edited by: T. R. Koch © Humana Press Inc., Totowa, NJ

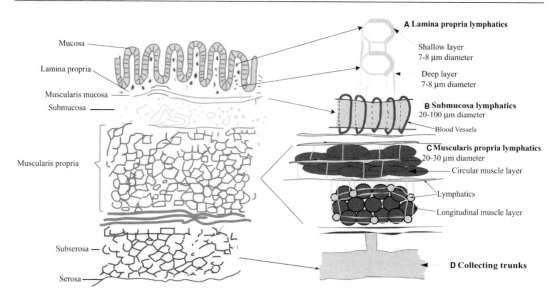

Fig. 1. (A) Lamina propria lymphatics are comprised of shallow and deep hexagonal layers, connected by vertical lymph vessels. (B) Submucosal lymphatics from a denser meshwork and are encircled by vascular capillaries. (C) Muscularis proprialymph vessels course along muscle fibers and are connected by branches between the circular and longitudinal muscle layers. (D) Collecting truck lymphatics collect lymph from the submucosa, muscularis propria, and subserosa.

mucosal surface, while the deep layer lies just above the muscularis mucosae. These vessels are 7 to 8 µm in diameter and are located beneath the blood capillary networks.

Lymphatic vessels in the submucosa form a denser meshwork and send branches into the circular muscle layer. These vessels range in size from 20–100 µm and are encircled by blood capillaries.

In the muscularis propria, lymph vessels course along muscle fibers and send out branches which connect the circular and longitudinal muscle layers. These lymph vessels form an even coarser density than that found in the submucosa, but are of a smaller diameter, at only 20–30 µm.

The density and size of the lymphatics progressing from the muscularis propria into the subserosa remain constant. These vessels run parallel to the intestinal axis.

Lymph vessels in the submucosa, muscularis propria and subserosa then merge into the thicker collecting trunks, which pass through the intestinal wall *(4)*.

From the external surface of the bowel wall, circumferential lymphatic vessels coarse along the vascular arcade toward the mesentery *(5)*. An extramural network of lymphatic vessels and nodes then parallels the vascular system. The colonic lymph node regions include: (i) the epicolic nodes, which rest on the colonic surface; (ii) the paracolic nodes, which lie along the marginal artery and the mesenteric vascular arcade; (iii) the intermediate nodes, which lie in proximity to the main colonic arteries; (iv) and the main (principal) nodes, which rest on the major mesenteric vessels, and are named according the vessels with which they are associated *(6)*.

Cecal and appendiceal lymph drains into the ileocolic lymph nodes, which are located along the superior mesenteric artery, and also into the celiac nodes *(7)*. Lymphatics from the ascending and transverse colon drain into the superior mesenteric group, while the lymphatics from the descending and sigmoid colon drain into the inferior mesenteric group. Lymphatics from the splenic flexure may drain toward either the superior or inferior mesenteric groups *(8)*.

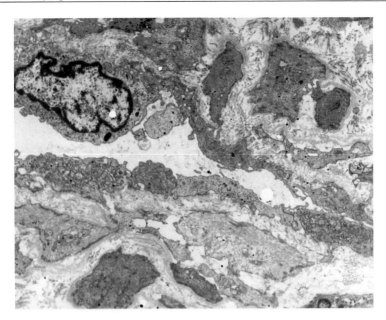

Fig. 2. Submucosal lymphatic in benign colonic adenomatous polyp (electromicrograph, original magnification, 11,500X). Note lack of defined basement membrane and absence of pericytes and adventitial cells. Courtesy of Janet K. Stephens, MD, PhD.

Lymphatics located in the rectum above the middle valve of Houston drain into the superior rectal lymph nodes, eventually progressing to the inferior mesenteric group and the left lumbar para-aortic group. Lymphatics below the middle valve of Houston and above the mucocutaneous junction drain into the middle rectal lymph nodes, progressing to the internal iliac nodes. Lymphatics below the mucocutaneous junction drain into the inferior rectal nodes, progressing to the internal pudendal, posterior sacral, common iliac, internal iliac, and superficial inguinal nodes *(9)*.

From the preaortic nodes, drainage is first into the cysterna chyli, located anterior to the second lumbar veterbra, and then into the thoracic duct, which drains into the venous system at the junction of the left subclavian and internal jugular veins *(10)*. Intestinal and hepatic lymph comprise 50–90% of all thoracic duct lymph *(11)*.

2.2. The Colonic Lymphatic Endothelium

The microstructure of colonic lymphatic capillaries, like those found in other organs, has an irregular endothelial lining, composed only of endothelial cells. Pericytes and adventitial cells are absent, and the isolated endothelial cells are protected only by fibrils of collagen and reticulin. Endothelial cells meet both end-to-end and overlap. There is an incomplete basal lamina and no junctional complexes. This flimsy microanatomy enables the tiny lymphatic capillaries to allow passive transport of various molecules including water, electrolytes, proteins, and macromolecules, as well as cell fragments, inflammatory cells, and even tumor cells (Fig. 2).

The lymphatic collecting vessel wall is also composed of a thin endothelial lining with reticular fibrils, but is additionally surrounded by an incomplete layer of smooth muscle cells, as well as an adventitial layer of connective tissue. Also unlike the lymphatic capillaries, the lymphatic collecting vessels contain multiple valves, pointing toward the direction of lymph flow. The function of the lymphatic collecting system is primarily that of lymph propulsion which is controlled via neural, humoral, and endothelial-derived factors.

The thoracic duct wall is composed of the three complete layers of the tunica intima, media and adventitia *(12–16)*.

3. COLONIC LYMPHATIC EMBRYOLOGY

The gut-associated lymphoepithelial organs (GALT) are characterized by a close morphological and functional correlation between the lymphatic tissue of mesenchymal origin and the endodermal epithelium of the digestive tract. Beginning in the 14th wk of gestation, a system of epithelial crypts grows down into the mesenchyme.

Primitive lymph sacs are thought to bud from the major vessels of the venous system including the anterior cardinal, mesonephric,and Wolffian body associated veins *(17)*. These sacs go through various stages of growth, fusion, and outward branching toward the peripheral aspects of the embryo *(18–20)*.

A possible lymphangiogenesis factor has recently been defined, vascular endothelial growth factor C (VEGF-C) *(21)*, as well as its probable binding site, VEGF receptor-3 or fms-like tyrosine kinase 4 (FLT4) *(22)*. Overexpression of dermal and pancreatic VEGF-C in transgenic murine models has been shown to produce lymphatic vessel proliferation *(23)*. Inactivation of the FLT4 gene results in cardiovascular failure and death in mouse embryos *(24)*. FLT4 mRNA has been demonstrated on adult mesenteric lymphatic sinuses and afferent and efferent lymphatic vessels, high endothelial venule (HEV) cells, lymphangiomas, as well as in lymph nodes containing adenoarcinoma metastases. Interestingly, the lymphatic endothelium of metastatic lymph nodes gives an enhanced signal *(22)*. Other lymphangiogenesis factors, including Prox 1 *(25)*, are being studied.

The gut-associated immune system also begins formation early in gestation.

The divergent T cell populations of the epithelium and lamina propria form within the first 19 wk of gestation. As seen in the adult intestine, the predominant intraepithelial T-lymphocyte population are composed of $CD3^+$, $CD8^+$ cells, and also include $\gamma/\delta+$ T cell receptor (TCR) T cells, or antigen-independent cells. In contrast, the majority of T cells in the lamina propria are $CD4^+$, and all are α/β TCR^+ *(26)*.

The beginnings of the Peyer's patches are shown to develop with the formation of aggregates of $CD4^+$ and $CD3^+$ cells in the lamina propria by 14–16 wk gestation. By 19 wk, distinct B cell follicles form, which are surrounded by T cells in interfollicular zones. All follicles are immunologically naive or primary follicles. Secondary follicles form with the advent of antigenic stimulation as occurs after birth *(26–29)*.

Maternal nutrition and immune status has a large impact on the development of the neonatal immune system both before and after birth *(27)*. Because there is no prior bacterial antigen exposure, the newborn intestine lacks IgA (unless supplied by maternal milk) in the first months of life. It takes several years before IgA levels approach those of adults *(30)*. In the presence of a poor nutritional state, secretory IgA production is low *(31–34)*. An inadequate IgA defense system allows lumenal bacterial invasion and also increases the absorption of proteins, antigens, immune complexes, and cellular breakdown products from the intestinal lumen. Increased absorption of these compounds increases the probability of the formation of immune complexes with dietary antigens *(35–37)*. This may be partially responsible for the increased incidence of relapsing enteritis, infectious celiac disease, cow's milk allergy, and protein intolerance in malnourished children in developing countries *(38,39)*.

4. LYMPHATIC PHYSIOLOGY

The lymphatic vessels play a major role in the prevention of mucosal edema formation in all tissues. Fluid filtered from blood capillaries into the interstitial space is in large part removed by the lymphatic system. Lymph flow must adjust for any variance in the capillary filtration rate, to allow for adequate fluid removal. If lymph flow does not increase directly with increases in the capillary filtration rate, for example, capillary filtrate will accumulate within the tissue and edema will develop (40).

In no organ is the removal of tissue fluid more relevant than in the human colon, where 1.5 L of fluid is absorbed every day (41,42).

4.1. Colon Lymphatic Fluid Removal

The descending colon has been shown to produce a suction tension approaching 4 to 5 atm, or 400–500 kPa, resulting in a water content of less than 70% of the total fecal weight (43–46). This suction tension is in large part thought to be produced by the hypertonic absorption of NaCl by crypts.

A high concentration of hypertonic NaCl in the pericryptal space produces an osmotic pressure gradient across the crypt wall resulting net fluid outflow from the crypt (47). While the distal colon Na^+ conductance channels are aldosterone-sensitive, and inhibited by amiloride (45–50), the proximal colon achieves electroneutral NaCl absorption via a dual Na^+/H^+ and Cl^-/bicarbonate exchange (49,51–53). These differences are thought to contribute to a functional difference between crypts in the distal and proximal colon. The distal colon, in contrast to the proximal colon, has been shown to absorb fluid against a high hydraulic resistance in the lumen(54).

Several mechanical processes are also thought to contribute to colonic suction. The NaCl gradient-generated crypt osmotic pressure is transduced into hydrostatic pressure at the mucosal surface of the crypt lumen. Crypt lumen size varies with colonic transport. Activation of colonic transport raises luminal tension, resulting in a decrease in crypt luminal volume. This effect is countered by crypt epithelial cells, which slow the collapse of the luminal diameter, producing a large hydraulic suction tension at the crypt entrance. When colonic transport is inhibited, the crypt lumen size expands (55).

A physical barrier to Na^+ transport also exists between the pericryptal space, the submucosa and pericryptal capillaries (56–59).

The lymphatic vessel walls and valves themselves contribute to lymph suction and propagation. Directionality of lymph transport is produced by the inflow and outflow valves. In addition, independent contraction cycles have been shown to be produced in the segment between individual valves, creating a functional pumping unit, termed the lymphangion (60).

4.2. The Lymphangion

The contraction cycles of the lymphangion have been compared with that of the heart and are composed of three phases of systole and three phases of diastole with periods of isovolumetric contraction and relaxation (60,61). The magnitude of lymphangion contractile activity is closely linked to the drainage requirements of the particular interstitial compartment with which it is associated (60).

The lymphangion also exhibits a degree of regulatory autonomy, with contractile activity varying with changing systemic conditions even in the absence of lymph input (62–65). With hypovolemia (64,65) or cerebral ischemia (63) as the stimulus, for example, flow through sheep mesenteric lymphatics will still increase even if separated from lymph input, as long as contact with nerve and blood supplies remain intact. Evidence suggests that this may be sympathetic nervous system-mediated effect (63).

Li et al (60) have demonstrated that the pressure–volume characteristics of sheep mesenteri lymphatic vessels, including the ejection fraction, stroke volume, pulse pressure, contractio frequency, and output per minute are affected by increases in transmural pressure as well a by decreases in transmural pressure, as occurs with hemorrhage.

A transmural pressure increase produces a bimodal pattern in the lymphatic vessel pres sure–volume characteristics which varies as the pressure increases. A mild increase in trans mural pressure (from 2–4 cm H_2O) produces an initial increase in ejection fraction, strok volume, contraction frequency, and output per minute. However, as the transmural pressur is increased further, up to 12 cm H_2O, there is a decrease in all parameters. This lymphc dynamic change may reflect a compensatory mechanism to prevent the formation of sever edema. In an inflammatory model developed by Benoit et al (66), increasing lymph produc tion via the activation of an inflammatory response was matched by a rise in lymphati pumping and stroke volume.

A decrease in transmural pressure, as occurs in the case of hemorrhage, produces an increas in postbleed ejection fraction and stroke volume, a decrease in contraction frequency, and n significant change in output per minute. This enhanced contractile state, in large part attrib utable to an up to 40% increase in ejection fraction, most likely contributes to a restitution o plasma protein and volume.

The molecular mechanism by which lymphangion pumping occurs within the lymphati vessel endothelium, as well as the surrounding smooth muscle, has been extensively evaluatec

4.3. The Lymphatic Smooth Muscle

Smooth muscle cells surrounding individual lymphatics have been shown to produce indi vidual action potentials (67–69). These electrical properties are mediated, at least in part, b both calcium and potassium channels (70–77).

Inhibition of L-type calcium channels with caffeine, ryanodine, and cyclopiazonic aci decrease lymphatic pumping ability. This effect is magnified by increases in transmural pres sure, suggesting a relationship between vessel wall stretch and intracellular calcium stores i lymph propulsion (74,75).

Adenosine triphosphate (ATP)-sensitive K^+ channels (K_{ATP}) and inward rectifier K channels contribute to lymphatic smooth muscle resting membrane potential (RMP) an spontaneous activity of lymph microvessels (70–72). Nitric oxide and acetylcholine induc K_{ATP} channel opening and lymphatic smooth muscle hyperpolarization by increasing pro duction of both cyclic guanosine 5'-monophosphate (GMP) and β-adrenoceptor agonis induced production of cyclic adenosine 5'-monophosphate (AMP), thus leading to activatio of protein kinase A (71).

Presynaptic and postjunctional α- and β-adrenoceptors have been identified on lymphati vessels, and have been shown to provide adrenergic regulation of spontaneous lymphati vessel activity. β1- and β2-adrenoceptors induce a negative chronotropic effect, while α1- an α2-adrenoceptors induce stimulation (78–82).

Lymphatic smooth muscle activity has also been demonstrated to be significantly affecte by various inflammatory mediators, including histamine, leukotriene C_4 and D_4, and platele activating factor (PAF). Histamine increases vessel diameter and contractility, leukotriene increase contraction frequency, and PAF induces smooth muscle relaxation, vasodilation, an decreased contraction frequency. These changes may contribute to the pathogenesis of edem formation in inflammatory states (83).

4.4. Lymph Formation

The major function of the mesenteric lymphatic system is to transport water, plasma proteins, fat, and chylomicrons *(84)*.

4.4.1. WATER TRANSPORT

The transport of water from the bowel into lymphatics may occur by both a paracellular route through tight junctions *(42,85)*, as well as by a transcellular route via aquaporin (AQP) receptors *(86)*. Several different AQPs have been described, with differential expression in various areas of the gastrointestinal (GI) tract, as well as in many other non-GI organs. Koyama et al *(86)* have demonstrated that AQP1 and AQP3 are expressed throughout the GI tract with particular prominence in the small and large bowel. In contrast, AQP4 is selectively expressed in the stomach and small intestine, and AQP8 is selectively expressed in the jejunum and colon.

4.4.2. PROTEIN TRANSPORT

Lymph formation has been postulated to occur via one of two mechanisms: hydraulic vs osmotic. The osmotic theory proposes that an osmotic pressure gradient is generated by a protein-concentrating mechanism within the initial lymphatic created by cycles of compression and relaxation *(87–94)*. In the hydraulic theory, one-way valves in the initial lymphatic wall and between lymphangions cause formation of lymph via a balance of hydraulic forces across the initial lymphatic *(95–106)*. A protein concentration differential has been shown to exist as lymph progresses from initial mesenteric lymphatics toward the collecting lymphatic system, with protein concentrations ranging from 2.0–2.5 g/dL *(107)*.

4.4.3. FAT AND CHOLESTEROL TRANSPORT

The absorption of fatty acids, triglycerides, phospholipid, cholesterol, and chylomicrons occurs predominantly in small intestinal lymphatics, the composition of which is highly diet-dependent *(108)*.

5. PATHOPHYSIOLOGY

Perturbations of the bowel lymphatic system at both the macroscopic and microscopic level have been shown to result in various pathophysiologic conditions. Mesenteric lymph and lymph nodes normally act as the safeguard for the body, preventing intraluminal toxins, acids, digestive enzymes, bacteria, and bacterial endo- and exotoxins from contaminating the sterile internal environment of the human body. However, they may also act as the conduit through which potentially lethal sepsis and tumor dissemination occur.

5.1. The Role of Lymphatics in Colorectal Cancer Dissemination

The best known adverse prognosticator in colorectal cancer is morphologic tumor spread manifested by invasion at the primary tumor site (Fig. 3A,3B) and metastases to regional lymph nodes and distant organs *(109–115)*. The 5-y mortality for Dukes Stages A and B, which lack lymph node spread, has been estimated at 5–15% and 30–40%, respectively. These percentages climb to 50–70% in Dukes Stage C, which is defined by the presence of tumor in regional lymph nodes, irrespective of primary site invasion. Postoperative survival has also been shown to be reduced in Dukes C, compared with lower stage tumors *(110,115–117)*.

In primary diffusely infiltrative adenocarcinoma of the colon and rectum, the severity of lymphangiosis (diffuse lymphatic permeation of tumor cells), classified as absent–mild vs moderate–severe is also an independent predictor of patient outcome. Tang et al *(118)* dem-

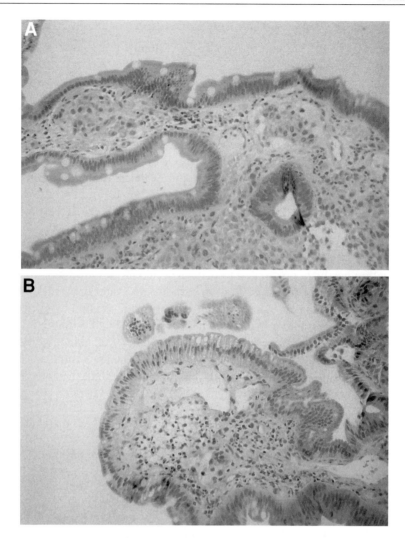

Fig. 3. Invasion of intestinal lymphovascular structures by metastatic melanoma (A) with associated dilatation of uninvolved lymphatic and vascular channels (B). Courtesy of Daniel Merrek, MD.

onstrated that there is an increased mortality odds ratio to 2.4 when comparing tumors with moderate–severe vs an absent–mild degree of lymphangiosis *(118)*.

Why some tumors migrate to lymph nodes while others do not is a subject of intense investigation. Differential expression of various extra and intracellular proteins, including plasminogen activators and gelatinase *(119)*, particular glycoproteins *(120)*, gastrin releasing peptide (GRP) *(121)*, and glycosaminoglycan hyaluronic acid (HA) *(122–126)* have all been studied.

Tumor cells have been shown to stimulate the production of glycosaminoglycan HA by local fibroblasts. Glycosaminoglycan HA then travels into lymph, the extracellular matrix, and connective tissues *(125)*.

5.2. The Role of Lymphatics in Local and Systemic Infection

The lymphatic system has been shown to be a conduit for developing severe sepsis by multiple mechanisms, including mechanical damage (i.e., bowel perforation), micro- and macroscopic lymphatic occlusion, as well as in the absence of a discernible lesion *(127)*. This occurs through a process called "bacterial translocation" *(128,129)*.

Bacterial translocation has been demonstrated in multiple clinical scenarios, including hemorrhagic shock *(128,129,131)*, endotoxemia *(132)*, antibiotic-induced microflora changes *(133)*, long-term parenteral feeding *(134)*, intestinal obstruction *(135)*, abdominal irradiation *(136)*, hematological malignant neoplasms *(137)*, experimentally induced intra-abdominal abscesses *(138)*, and thermal trauma *(127,128,130,140)*, which can cause subsequent systemic infections and the adult respiratory distress syndrome (ARDS).

In bacterial translocation, viable bacteria are recovered from mesenteric lymph nodes (MLNs). Conditions where bacterial translocation into MLNs spreads into a systemic infection include endotoxemia *(132)*, hemorrhagic shock *(130,131)*, disruption of the normal intestinal flora with immunosuppression *(141)*, prolonged intestinal obstruction *(142)*, and burn injury *(127,139,143,144)*. The source of translocation appears to be spread from MLNs to mesenteric lymph.

Burn injury is associated with increased bacterial translocation, most likely by a multitude of mechanisms, including reduced mesenteric arterial flow, altered gut microflora, and increased intestinal permeability *(144–147)*.

In the presence of severe illness and shock, MLN's may be inundated with cell debris and protein fragments, overwhelming the capacity of antigen-presenting macrophages *(148)*.

"Infected" mesenteric lymph then creates havoc in all the major organ systems. In the lungs, it increases lung permeability, promotes pulmonary neutrophil sequestration, and induces alveolar apoptosis, leading to the formation of ARDS *(130,131,139)*

Division of mesenteric lymphatics prior to experimentally induced thermal injury in mice results in a 50% reduction of pulmonary permeability, with subsequent reduced progression to ARDS *(139)*. Diversion of mesenteric lymph *(139)* and even removal of mesenteric lymph nodes *(127)* in acute burn injury has been demonstrated to reduce or prevent the systemic infection of multiple tissues, including the spleen, liver, kidney, and lung.

Microscopic lymphatic occlusion is also thought to have a major role in the development of necrotizing enterocolitis (NEC) and pneumatosis intestinalis. Sibbons et al. *(149)*, demonstrated that isolated ligation of mesenteric lymphatics in neonatal piglets resulted in a prepneumatosis pathology with distended lymphatic vessels in the submocosa. Arterial ligation alone induced NEC-like lesions without pneumatosis. Lymphatic ligation alone produced gross lymphatic engorgement in a prepneumatosis pattern. Arterial plus lymphatic ligation induced lesions showing the complete histopathological spectrum of NEC with mucosal stripping, hemorrhage, submucosal disruption and destruction, full-thickness necrosis, inflammatory infiltration, and pneumatosis intestinalis *(149)*.

The authors concluded that NEC and pneumatosis intestinalis are caused by a cascade of events, beginning with diminished arterial flow resulting in mucosal ischemia. The ischemic tissue is more susceptible to bacterial growth and spread into draining lymphatics. Overwhelming bacterial invasion then overloads the lymph node capacity causing proximal lymphatic distension and a prepneumatosis state. In the absence of lymphatic flow, the lymph components provide an excellent media for the growth of gas-producing facultative anaerobes, leading to a full blown pneumatosis intestinalis *(149)*.

5.3. Gut Immunology and Systemic Disease

Alterations of the gut immune system have been seen in various disease states. Lymphoglandular complexes (LCGs), which are known sites of antigen processing, are diffusely increased in carcinoma and Crohn's colitis *(150)*. In ileocecal tuberculosis, lymphoglandular complexes and Peyer's patches increase at sites of mucosal ulceration, and transmural lymphoid aggregates proliferate in close proximity to lymphatic and blood vessels *(151)*. Aggregating LGCs, Peyer's patches, and lymphoid aggregates are most likely the substrates for granuloma formation in ileocecal tuberculosis, Crohn's disease, and yersinial appendicitis *(143,151)*.

5.4. Lymphatic Cysts

Lymphatic cysts, also known as lymphangiomas, are one of the rarest submucosal colon masses, with fewer than 150 cases reported in the literature *(152–155)*. Demographics indicate a clustering of cases between the fifth and seventh decades, with a male predominance in Japan and a female predominence in western countries *(156–158)*.

The cysts may be found in any part of the colon, and their developmental etiology is uncertain *(157)*. Reported signs and symptoms include abdominal pain, melena, and diarrhea *(156–159)*. However, as these cysts are usually encountered incidentally, symptoms are most likely attributable to coexisting lesions *(158)*. There is a rare association with colon intussusception and protein-losing enteropathy *(160–166)*. In addition, there is a 22% reported incidence of malignant degeneration to lymphangioendothelioma, predominantly in mesenteric rather than luminal cysts *(167)*.

The mucosa overlying a lymphatic cyst is histologically normal, as the cysts are found within the submucosa. They may be either unilocular or multilocular, with fibrous connective tissue separating cysts. They are lined by flattened endothelial cells and contain lymph *(152,156,157)*.

The cysts are smooth, transparent, and compressible at endoscopy, with normal overlying mucosa, and are of varying color, including yellowish gray, blue, white, and red *(156,157,168, 169)*. Their size ranges from 0.1–15 cm in diameter *(157)*.

They produce oval to round radiolucent defects with sharply defined borders on radiographic exam, suggestive of an intramural lesion *(170)*. They are anechoic on endoscopic ultrasound and high density nonenhancing lesions on contrast-enhancing computed tomography *(171)*.

Cysts smaller than 2 cm may be approached via endoscopic mucosal resection, but standard treatment for larger lesions involves radical, segmental, or wedge resection *(157)*.

5.5. Chylous Ascites

Chylous ascites (Fig. 4) or the accumulation of lymph fluid within the peritoneal space may occur secondary to a gross disruption of mesenteric lymphatics, i.e., after an operation, abdominal trauma, pelvic irradiation, and peritoneal dialysis. It has also been documented in the presence of malignant neoplasms, spontaneous bacterial peritonitis, cirrhosis, abdominal tuberculosis, and congenital defects in lacteal formation *(172–186)*.

Blalock et al. *(187)* demonstrated that thoracic duct occlusion alone is insufficient to cause chylous ascites. Rather, a predisposing lack of collateral and anastomotic lymphatic channels, in addition to an acute obstruction or division of lymphatic channels, are required for the creation of persistent chylous effusions and ascites.

Multiple treatment regimens for chylous ascites have been proposed, including salt restriction and diuretics, surgical management with reoperation and ligation or peritoneovenous shunting, as well as dietary manipulation using low-fat diets with medium-chain triglycerides, elemental diets, and total parental nutrition *(188)*.

5.6. Intestinal Lymphangiectasia

Intestinal lymphangiectasia (InL) (Fig. 5) is another rare disease of the mesenteric lymphatic system. Occluded intestinal lymphatics induce lymphatic vessel dilation and leakage of

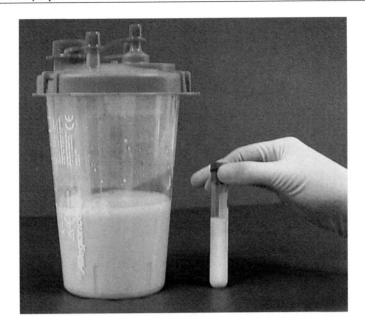

Fig. 4. Chylous ascites.

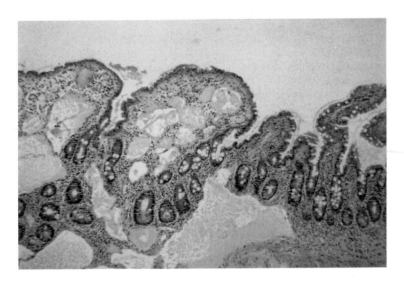

Fig. 5. Intestinal lymphagiectasia with enlargement of intestinal villi. Courtesy of Daniel Merrek, MD.

lymph fluid into the GI tract. This leads to hypoproteinemia, hypogammaglobulinemia, and lymphocytopenia, with a selective loss of $CD4^+/CD45RA^+$ T cells, resulting in skin anergy and impaired allograft rejection (189–191).

InL may be either congenital or acquired and may be associated with abnormal peripheral lymphatic development as well (192–200).

REFERENCES

1. Asellius G. *De Lactibus sive lacteis venis Quarto Vasorum Mesaraicorum Genere Novo Invento*. Apud J Baptistam Bidelliu, Mediolani, Italy, 1627.
2. Barrowman JA. *Physiology of the Gastro-Intestinal Lymphatic System*. Books on Demand, 1978.
3. Cecilia M, Fenoglio MD, Kaye GI, Lane N. Distribution of Human Colonic Lymphatics in Normal, Hype plastic, and Adenomatous Tissue. Its relationship to metastasis from small carcinomas in pedunculate adenomas, with two case reports. *Gastroenterology*, **64** (1973) 51–66.
4. Hirai R, Nimura Y, Sakai H. The three-dimensional microstructure of intramural lymphatics in the canin large intestine. *Gastroenterol. Jpn.*, **25** (1990) 169–74.
5. Sterns EE, Vaughan GER. The Lymphatics of the dog colon: A study of the lymph drainage patterns b indirect lymphography in the dog under normal and abnormal conditions. *Cancer*, **26** (1970) 218–231.
6. Jameson JK, Dobson JF. The lymphatics of the colon. *Proc. R. Soc. Med.*, **2** (1909) 149.
7. Schumpelick V, Dreuw B, Ophoff K, Prescher A. Appendix and cecum: Embryology, anatomy, and surgic applications. *Surg. Clin. N. Am.*, **80** (2000) 295–318.
8. Siddharth P, Ravo B. Colorectal neurovasculature and anal sphincter. *Surg. Clin. N. Am.*, **68** (1988) 118⁵
9. Godlewski G, Prudhomme M. Embryology and anatomy of the anorectum. *Surg. Clin. N. Am.*, **80** (200(319–343.
10. Ablan CJ, Littooy FN, Freeark RJ. Postoperative chyous ascites: diagnosis and treatment A series report ar literature review. *Arch. Surg.*, **125** (1990) 270–273.
11. Lesser GT, Bruno MS, Enselberg K. Chylous ascites. Newer insights and many remaining enigmas. *Arc Intern. Med.*, **125** (1970) 1073–1074.
12. Carmeliet P, Collen D. Vascular development and disorders: molecular analysis and pathogenic insight *Kidney Int.*, **53** (1998) 1519–1549.
13. Kubik S, Manestar M. *Anatomy of the Lymph Capillaries and Pre-Collectors of the Skin*. Stuttgart,Thieme, 198.
14. Rhodin JAG. *The Lymphatic System*. Oxford University Press, New York, NY, 1974.
15. Aukland K, Reed RK. Interstitial-lymphatic mechanisms in the control of extracellular volume. *Physiol. Re\ **73** (1993) 1–78.
16. Ferguson MK, DeFilippi VJ, Reeder LB. Characterization of contractile properties of porcine mesenteric an tracheobronchial lymphatic smooth muscle. *Lymphology*, **27** (1994) 71–81.
17. Sabin FR. The lymphatic system in human embryos, with a consideration of the morphology of the syste as a whole. *Am. J. Anat.*, **9** (1909) 43–91.
18. Hobson B, Denekamp J. Endothelial proliferation in tumours and normal tissues: Continuous labelling stud ies. *Br. J. Cancer*, **49** (1984) 405–413.
19. Van Der Putte SC. The development of the lymphatic system in man. *Adv. Anat. Embryol. Cell. Biol.*, **5** (1975) 3–60.
20. Yoffey JM, Courtic FC. *Lymphatics, Lymph, and the Lymphomyeloid complex*. Academic Press, New Yor NY, 1970.
21. Kukk E, Lymboussaki A, Taira S et al. VEGF-C receptor binding and pattern of expression with VEGFR- suggests a role in lymphatic vascular development. *Development*, **122** (1996) 3829–3837.
22. Kaipainen A, Korhonen J, Mustonen T et al. Expression of the fms-like tyrosine kinase 4 gene becom restricted to lymphatic endothelium during development. *Proc. Natl. Acad. Sci. USA*, **92** (1995) 3566–357(
23. Jeltsch M, Kaipainen A, Joukov V et al. Hyperplasia of lymphatic vessels in VEGF-C transgenic mic *Science*, **276** (1997) 1423–1425.
24. Dumont DJ, Jussila L, Taipale J, et al. Cardiovascular failure in mouse embrys deficient in VEGF recepto 3. *Science*, **282** (1998) 946–949.
25. Wigle JT, Oliver G. Prox1 function is required for the development of the murine lymphatic system. *Cell*, **9** (1999) 769–778.
26. MacDonald TT, Spencer J. Ontogeny of the gut-associated lymphoid system in man. Acta *Paediatr. Supp* **395** (1994) 3–5.
27. Prinhdull G, Ahmad M. The ontogeny of the gut mucosal immune system and the susceptibility to infection in infants of developing countries. *Eur. J. Pediatr.*, **152** (1993) 786–792.
28. Von Gaudecker B, Muller-Hermelink HK. The development of the human tonsilla palatina. *Cell Tissue Re\ **224** (1982) 579–600.
29. Kyriazis AA, Esterly JR. Fetal and neonatal development of lymphoid tissues. *Arch. Pathol.*, **91** (197 444–451.
30. Perkki M, Savilahti E. Time of appearance of immunoglobulin-containing cells in the mucosa of the neonat intestine. *Pediatr. Res.*, **14** (1980) 953–955.

31. Chandra RK. Serum complement and immunoconglutin in malnutrition. *Arch. Dis. Child.*, **50** (1975) 225–229.
32. Chandra RK. Nutritional deficiency and susceptibility to infection. *Bul. World Health Organ.*, **57** (1979) 167–177.
33. McMurray DN, Rey H, Casazza LJ, Watson RR. Effect of moderate malnutrition on concentrations of immunoglobulins and enzymes in tears and saliva of young Colombian children. *Am. J. Clin. Nutr.*, **30** (1977) 1944–1948.
34. Sirisinha S, Suskind R, Edelmann R, Asvapaka C, Olson RE. Secretory and serum IgA in children with protein-calorie malnutrition. *Pediatrics*, **55** (1975) 166–170.
35. Lim PL, Rowley D. The effect of antibody on the intestinal absorption of macromolecules and on intestinal permeability in adult mice. *Int. Arch. Allergy Appl. Immunol.*, **68** (1982) 41–6.
36. Swarbrick ET, Stokes CR, Soothill JF. Absorption of antigens after oral immunization and the simultaneous induction of specific systemic tolerance. *Gut*, **20** (1979) 121–125.
37. Walker WA, Isselbacher KJ. Uptake and transport of macromolecules by the intestine: Possible role in clinical disorders. *Gastroenterology*, **67** (1974) 531–550.
38. MacDonald TT. The role of activated T lymphocytes in gastrointestinal disease. *Clin. Exp. Allergy*, **20** (1990) 247–252.
39. Selby WS, Janossy G, Bofill M, Jewell DP. Intestinal lymphocyte subpopulations in inflammatory bowel disease: an analysis by immunohistological and cell isolation techniques. *Gut*, **25** (1984) 32–40.
40. Drake RE, Teague RA, Gabel JC. Lymphatic drainage reduces intestinal edema and fluid loss. *Lymphology*, **31** (1998) 68–73.
41. Phillips SF. Diarrhea: a current view of the pathophysiology. *Gastroenterology*, **63** (1972) 495–518.
42. Powell DW. Intestinal water and electrolyte transport. *Physiol. Gastrointest. Tract*, **2** (1987) 1267–1305.
43. Van Weerden EJ. The osmotic pressure and concentration of some solutes of the intestinal contents and faeces of the cow, in relation to the absorption of the minerals. *J. Agricul. Sci.*, **56** (1961) 317–324.
44. McKie AT, Goecke IA, Naftalin RJ. Comparison of fluid absorption by bovine and ovine descending colon in vitro. *Am. J. Physiol.*, **261** (1991) G433–G442.
45. McKie AT, Powrie W, Naftalin RJ. Mechanical aspects of rabbit fecal dehydration. *Am. J. Physiol.*, **258** (1990) G391–G394.
46. Pedley KC, Naftalin RJ. Evidence from fluorescence microscopy and comparative studies that rat, ovine, and bovine colonic crypts are absorptive. *J. Physiol.*, **460** (1993) 525–547.
47. Zammit PS, Mendizabal M, Naftalin RJ. Effects on fluid and Na$^+$ flux of varying luminal hydraulic resistance in rat colon in vivo. *J. Physiol.*, **477** (1994) 539–548.
48. Edmonds CJ, Marriott JC. The effect of aldosterone and adrenalectomy on the electrical potential difference of rat colon and on the transport of sodium, potassium, chloride and bicarbonate. *J. Endocrinol.*, **39** (1967) 517–531.
49. Clauss W. Segmental action of aldosterone on water and electrolyte transport across rabbit colon in vivo. *Comp. Biochem. Physiol. A.*, **81** (1985) 873–877.
50. Sellin JH, Oyarzabal H, Cragoe EJ. Electrogenic sodium absorption in rabbit cecum in vivo. *J. Clin. Invest.*, **81** (1988) 1275–1283.
51. Sellin JH, DeSoignie R. Rabbit proximal colon— a distinct transport epithelium. *Am. J. Physiol.*, **246** (1984) G603–G610.
52. Fromm M, Hegel U. Net ion fluxes and zero flux limiting concentrations in rat upper colon and rectum during anesthesia-induced aldosterone liberation. *Pflugers Arch.*, **408** (1987) 185–193.
53. Turnamian SG, Binder HJ. Aldosterone and glucocorticoid receptor-specific agonists regulate ion-transport in rat proximal colon. *Am. J. Physiol.*, **258** (1990) G492–G498.
54. Naftalin RJ, Zammit PS, Pedley KC. Regional differences in rat large intestinal crypt function in relation to dehydrating capacity in vivo. *J. Physiol.*, **514** (1999) 201–210.
55. Bleakman D, Naftalin RJ. Hypertonic fluid absorption from rat descending colon in vitro. *Am. J. Physiol.*, **258** (1990) G377–G390.
56. Naftalin RJ, Pedley KC. Regional crypt function in rat large intestine in relation to fluid absorption and growth of the pericryptal sheath. *J. Physiol.*, **514** (1999) 211–227.
57. Singh SK, Binder HJ, Boron WF, Geibel JP. Fluid absorption in isolated perfused colonic crypts. *J. Clin. Invest.*, **96** (1995) 2373–2379.
58. Skinner SA, O'Brien PE. The microvascular structure of the normal colon in rats and humans. *J. Surg. Res.*, **61** (1996) 482–490.
59. Araki K, Furuya Y, Kobayashi M, Matsuura K, Ogata T, Isozaki H. Comparison of mucosal microvasculature between the proximal and distal human colon. *J. Elec. Microsc.*, **45** (1996) 202–206.

60. Li B, Silver I, Szalai JP, Johnston MG. Pressure-volume relationships in sheep mesenteric lymphatic vessels in situ: response to hypovolemia. *Microvasc. Res.*, **56** (1998) 127–138.
61. Benoit JN, Zawieja DC, Goodman AH, Granger HJ. Characterization of intact mesenteric lymphatic pump and its responsiveness to acute edemagenic stress. *Am. J. Physiol.*, **257** (1989) H2059–H2069.
62. Hayashi A, Johnston MG, Nelson W, Hamilton S, McHale NG. Increased intrinsic pumping activity of intestinal lymphatics following hemorrhage in anesthetized sheep. *Circ. Res.*, **60** (1987) 265–272.
63. McHale NG, Adair TH. Reflex modulation of lymphatic pumping in sheep. *Circ. Res.*, **64** (1989) 1165–1171.
64. Elias R, Johnston MG. Modulation of lymphatic pumping by lymph-borne factors after endotoxin administration in sheep. *J. Appl. Physiol.*, **68** (1990) 199–208.
65. Boulanger BR, Lloyd SJ, Walker M, Johnston MG. Intrinsic pumping of mesenteric lymphatics is increased after hemorrhage in awake sheep. *Circ. Shock*, **43** (1994) 95–101.
66. Benoit JN, Zawieja DC. Effects of f-Met-Leu-Phe-induced inflammation on intestinal lymph flow and lymphatic pump behavior. *Am. J. Physiol.*, **262** (1992) G199–G202.
67. Kirkpatrick CT, McHale NG. Electrical and mechanical activity of isolated lymphatic vessels. *J. Physiol.*, **272** (1977) 33P–34P.
68. Allen JM, McHale NG, Rooney BM. Effect of norepinephrine on contractility of isolated mesenteric lymphatics. *Am. J. Physiol.*, **244** (1983) H479–H486.
69. Van Helden DF. Pacemaker potentials in lymphatic smooth muscle of the guinea-pig mesentery. *J. Physiol.*, **471** (1993) 465–479.
70. Der Weid PY, Van Helden DF. Functional electrical properties of the endothelium in lymphatic vessels of the guinea-pig mesentery. *Am. J. Physiol.*, **504** (1997) 439–451.
71. Der Weid PY. ATP-sensitive K^+ channels in smooth muscle cells of guinea-pig mesenteric lymphatics: role in nitric oxide and b-adrenoceptor agonist-induced hyperpolarizations. *Br. J. Pharmacol.*, **125** (1998) 17–22.
72. Mizuno R, Ono N, Ohhashi T. Involvement of ATP-sensitive K^+ channels in spontaneous activity of isolated lymph microvessels in rats. *Am. J. Physiol.*, **277** (1999) H1453–H1456.
73. Cotton KD, Hollywood MA, McHale NG, Thronbury KD. Outward currents in smooth muscle cells isolated from sheep mesenteric lymphatics. *J. Physiol.*, **503** (1997) 1–11.
74. Atchison DJ, Rodela H, Johnston MG. Intracellular calcium stores modulation in lymph vfessels depends on wall stretch. *Can. J. Physiol. Pharmacol.*, **76** (1998) 367–372.
75. Atchison DJ, Johnston MG. Role of extra- and intracellular Ca^{2+} in the lymphatic myogenic response. *Am. J. Physiol.*, **272** (1997) R326–R333.
76. Mizuno RA, Dornyei G, Koller A, Kaley G. Myogenic responses of isolated lymphatics: modulation by endothelium. *Microcirculation*, **4** (1997) 413–420.
77. Azuma T, Ohhashi T, Roddie IC. Bradykinin-induced contractions of bovine mesenteric lymphatics. *J. Physiol.*, **342** (1983) 217–227.
78. Mahe L, Chapelain B, Neliat G, Gargouil YM. The role of α- and β-adrenoceptors in the response to noradrenaline of lymphatic vessels isolated from the bovine mesentery. *Eur. J. Pharmacol.*, **167** (1989) 31–39.
79. Watanabe N, Kawai Y, Ohhashi T. Demonstration of both β1- and β2-adrenoceptors mediating negative chronotropic effects on spontaneous activity in isolated bovine mesenteric lymphatics. *Microvasc. Res.*, **39** (1990) 50–59.
80. Mahe L, Chapelain B, Gargouil YM, Neliat G. Characterization of β-Adrenoceptor subtypes and indications for two cell populations in isolated bovine mesenteric lymphatic vessels. *Eur. J. Pharmacol.*, **199** (1991) 19–25.
81. Ikomi F, Kawai Y, Ohhashi T. Beta-1 and beta-2 adrenoceptors mediate smooth muscle relaxation in bovine isolated mesenteric lymphatics. *J. Pharmacol. Exp. Ther.*, **259** (1991) 365–370.
82. Allen JM, McCarron JG, McHale NG, Thornbury KD. β-Adrenoceptor-mediated facilitation of [3H]-noradrenaline release from the intramural nerves of bovine mesenteric lymphatic vessels. *Br. J. Pharmacol.*, **96** (1989) 45–50.
83. Ferguson MK, Shahinian HK, Michelassi F. Lymphatic smooth muscle responses to leukotrienes, histamine, and platelet activating factor. *J. Surg. Res.*, **44** (1988) 172–177.
84. Bohlen HG, Lash JM. Intestinal lymphatic vessels release endothelial-dependent vasodilators. *Am. J. Physiol.*, **262** (1992) H813–H818.
85. Powell DW. Barrier function of epithelia. *Am. J. Physiol.*, **241** (1981) G275–G288.
86. Koyama Y, Yamamoto T, Tani T et al. Expression and localization of aquaporins in rat gastrointestinal tract. *Am. J. Physiol.*, **276** (1999) C621–C627.
87. Brace RA, Taylor AE, Guyton AC. Time course of lymph protein concentration in the dog. *Microvasc. Res.*, **14** (1977) 243–249.
88. Casley-Smith JR. Protein concentrations in regions with fenestrated and continuous blood capilaries and in initial and collecting lymphatics. *Anthol. Med. Santoriana*, **12** (1972) 245–257.

89. Casley-Smit JR. The functioning and interrelationships of blood capillaries and lymphatics. *Experentia*, **32** (1976) 1–12.

90. Casley-Smith JR. The concentrating of proteins in the initial lymphatics and their rediluting in the collecting lymphatics. *Anthol. Med. Santoriana*, **25** (1977) 81–99.

91. Casley-Smith JR. A fine structural study of variations in protein concentration in lacteals during compression and relaxation. *Lymphology*, **12** (1978) 59–65.

92. Hargens AR, Tucher BJ, Blantz RC. Renal lymph protein in the rat. *Am. J. Physiol.*, **233** (1977) F269–F273.

93. Rusznyak I, Foldi M, Szabo G. In *Lymphatics and Lymph Circulation; Physiology and Pathology*. Youlten L (ed.), Oxford, New York, NY, 1967, pp. 220–225.

94. Vriem CE, Snashall PD, Demling RH, Staub NC. Lung lymph and free interstitial fluid protein composition in sheep with edema. *Am. J. Physiol.*, **230** (1976) 1650–1653.

95. Allen L. Volume and pressure changes in terminal lymphatics. *Am. J. Physiol.*, **123** (1938) 3–4.

96. Allen L, Vogt E. A mechanism of lymphatic absorption from serous cavities. *Am. J. Physiol.*, **119** (1937) 776–782.

97. Casley-Smith JR. The function of the lymphatic system under normal and pathological conditions: its dependence on the fine structure and permeability of the vessels. In *Progress in Lymphology. Proceedings of the International Symposium on Lymphology*. xvi, 425, Ruttimann A (ed.), Stuttgart, Thieme, 1967, pp. 348–359.

98. Clough G, Smaje LH. Simultaneous measurement of pressure in the intertittium and the terminal lymphatics of the cat mesentery. *J. Physiol. (Lond)*, **283** (1978) 457–468.

99. Hogan RD. The initial lymphatics and interstitial fluid pressure. In *Tissue Fluid Pressure and Composition*, Williams and Wilkens, Baltimore, MD, 1981, pp. 155–163.

100. Leak LV, Burke JF. Ultrastructural studies on the lymphatic and the anchoring filaments. *J. Cell Biol.*, **36** (1968) 129–249.

101. McMaster PD. The relative pressures within cutaneous lymphatic capillaries and the tissues. *J. Exp. Med.*, **86** (1947) 293–308.

102. Nicolaysen G, Staub NC. Time course of albumin equilibration in interstitium and lymph of normal mouse lyngs. *Microvasc. Res.*, **9** (1975) 29–37.

103. Nicoll PA, Hogan RD. Pressures associated with lymphatic capillary contraction. *Microvasc. Res.*, **15** (1978) 257–258.

104. Rutili G, Arfors KE. Protein concentration in interstitial and lymphatic fluids from the subcutaneous tissue. *Acta Physiol. Scand.*, **99** (1977) 1–8.

105. Taylor AE, Gibson WH, Granger HJ, Guyton AC. The interaction between intrecapillary and tissue forces in the overall regulation of interstitial fluid volume. *Lymphology*, **6** (1972) 192–208.

106. Wiederhielm CA, Weston BV. Microvascular, lymphatic, and tissue pressures in the unanesthetized mammal. *Am. J. Physiol.*, **225** (1973) 992–996.

107. Zawieja DC, Barber BJ. Lymph protein concentration in initial and collecting lymphatics of the rat. *Am. J. Physiol.*, **252** (1987) G602–G606.

108. Bernard A, Echinard B, Carlier H. Differential intestinal absorption of two fatty acid isomers: elaidic and oleic acids. *Am. J. Physiol.*, **253** (1987) G751–G759.

109. Astler VB, Coller F. The prognostic significance of direct extension of carcinoma of the colon and rectum. *Ann. Surg.*, **139** (1954) 846–851.

110. Dukes CE, Bussey HJ. The spread of rectal cancer and its effect on prognosis. *Br. J. Surg.*, **12** (1958) 309–320.

111. Spiessl B, Hermanek P, Scheibe O, Wagner G (eds.). *TNM Atlas: Illustrated Guide to the TNM/pTNM-Classification of Malignant Tumours*. 2nd ed., xiii, Springer-Verlag, Berlin, New York, NY, 1985.

112. Chapuis PH, Dent OF, Fisher R. A multivariate analysis of clinical and pathological variables in prognosis after resection of large bowel cancer. *Br. J. Surg.*, **72** (1985) 698–702.

113. Jass JR, Atkin WS, Cuzick J. The grading of rectal cancer: historical perspectives and a multivariate analysis of 447 cases. *Histopathology*, **10** (1986) 437–459.

114. American Joint Committee on Cancer. *Manual of Staging of Cancer*. Lippincott-Raven, Philadelphia, PA, 1992.

115. Lindmark G, Gerdin B, Pahlman L, Bergstrom R, Glimelius B. Prognostic predictors in colorectal cancer. *Dis. Colon Rectum*, **37** (1994) 1219–1227.

116. Cohen AM, Tremiterra S, Candela F, Thaler HT, Sigurdson ER. Prognosis of node–positive colon cancer. *Cancer*, **67** (1991) 1859–1861.

117. Brodsky JT, Richard GK, Cohen AM, Minsky BD. Variables correlated with the risk of lymph node metastasis in early rectal cancer. *Cancer*, **69** (1992) 322–326.

118. Tang R, Wang JY, Tsao KC, Ho YS. Lymphangiosis as a predictor of outcome in patients with primary diffusely infiltrative adenocarcinoma of the colon and rectum. *Arch. Surg.*, **134** (1999) 157–160.

119. Shah V, Kumar S, Zirvi KA. Metastasis of human colon tumor cells in vivo: correlation with the overexperssion of plasminogen activators and 72 kDa gelatinase. *In Vivo*, **8** (1994) 321–326.
120. Laferte S, Prokopishyn NL, Moyana T, Bird RP. Monoclonal antibody recognizing a determinant on type 2 chain blood group A and B oligosaccharides detects oncodevelopmental changes in azoxymethane-induced rat colon tumors and hyman colon cancer cell lines. *J. Cell. Biochem.*, **57** (1995) 101–119.
121. Saurin JC, Rouault JP, Abello J, Berger F, Remy L, Chayvialle JA. High gastrin releasing peptide receptor mRNA level is related to tumour dedifferentiation and lymphatic vessel invasion in human colon cancer. *Eur. J. Canc.*, **35** (1999) 125–132.
122. Kubens BS, Zanker KS. Differences in the migration capacity of primary human colon carcinoma cells (SW480) and their lymph node metastatic derivatives (SW620). *Cancer Lett.*, **131** (1998) 55–64.
123. Bertrand P, Girard N, Delpech B, Duval C, d'Anjou J, Dauce JP. Hyaluronan (hyaluronic acid) and hyaluronectin in the extracellular matrix of hyman breast carcinomas: comparison between invasive and non-invasive areas. *Int. J. Cancer*, **52** (1992) 1–6.
124. de la Torre M, Wells AF, Bergh J, Lindgren A. Localization of hyaluronan in normal breast tissue, radial scar, and tubular breast carcinoma. *Hum. Pathol.*, **24** (1993) 1294–1297.
125. Knudson W, Biswas C, Toole BP. Interactions between human tumor cells and fibroblasts stimulate hyaluronic acid synthesis. *Proc. Natl. Acad. Sci. USA*, **81** (1984) 6767–6771.
126. Pauli BU, Knudson W. Tumor invasion: a consequence of destructive and compositional matrix alterations. *Hum. Pathol.*, **19** (1988) 628–639.
127. Tokyay R, Zeigler ST, Loick HM, et al. Mesenteric lymphadenectomy prevents postburn systemic spread of translocated bacteria. *Arch. Surg.*, **127** (1992) 384–388.
128. Sori AJ, Rush BF, Lysz TW, Smith S, Machiedo GW. The gut as source of sepsis after hemorrhagic shock. *Am. J. Surg.*, **155** (1988) 187–192.
129. Maejima K, Deitch EA, Berg RD. Bacterial translocation from the gastrointestinal tracts of rats receiveing thermal injury. *Infect. Immun.*, **43** (1984) 6–10.
130. Magnotti LJ, Upperman JS, Xu DZ, Lu Q, Deitch EA. Gut-derived mesenteric lymph but not portal blood increases endothelial cell permeability and promotes lung injury after hemorrhagic shock. *Ann. Surg.*, **228** (1998) 518–527.
131. Upperman JS, Deitch EA, Guo W, Lu Q, Xu DZ. Post-hemorrhagic shock mesenteric lymph is cytotoxic to endothelial cells and activates neutrophils. *Shock*, **10** (1998) 407–414.
132. Deitch EA, Berg RD. Endotoxin but not malnutrition promotes bacterial translocation of the gut flora in burned mice. *J. Trauma.*, **27** (1987) 161–166.
133. Deitch EA, Maejima K, Berg R. Effect of oral antibiotics and bacterial overgrowth on the translocation of the GI tract microflora in burned rats. *J. Trauma*, **25** (1985) 385–392.
134. Alverdy JC, Aoys E, Moss GS. Total parenteral nutrition promotes bacterial translocation from the gut. *Surgery*, **104** (1988) 185–190.
135. Deitch EA. Simple intestinal obstruction causes bacterial translocation in man. *Arch. Surg.*, **124** (1989) 699–701.
136. Guzman-Stein G, Bonsack M, Liberty J, Delaney JP. Abdominal radiation causes bacterial translocation. *J. Surg. Res.*, **46** (1989) 104–107.
137. Tancrede CH, Andremont AO. Bacterial translocation and gram-negative bacteremia in patients with hematological malignancies. *J. Infect. Dis.*, **152** (1985) 99–103.
138. Wells CL, Rotstein OD, Pruett TL, Simmons RL. Intestinal bacteria translocate into experimental intraabdominal abscesses. *Arch. Surg.*, **121** (1986) 102–107.
139. Magnotti LJ, Xu DZ, Lu Q, Deitch EA. Gut-derived mesenteric lymph: a link between burn and lung injury. *Arch. Surg.*, **134** (1999) 1333–1341.
140. Deitch EA, Winterton J, Berg R. Thermal injury promotes bacterial translocation from the gastrointestinal tract in mice with impaired T-cell-mediated immunity. *Arch. Surg.*, **121** (1986) 97–101.
141. Tomono K. Etiology of sepsis occurring in the immunocompromised host and its prevention,1: analysis fo the bacterial portal of entrance in experimental mice with vacteremia. *Kansenshogaku Zasshi*, **63** (1991) 479–488.
142. Deitch EA, Bridges WM, Ma JW, Ma L, Berg RD, Specian RD. Obstructed intestine as a reservoir for systemic infection. *Am. J. Surg.*, **211** (1990) 399–405.
143. Jones W, Minei JP, Barber AE. Bacterial translocation and intestinal atrophy after thermal injury and burn wound sepsis. *Ann. Surg.*, **211** (1990) 399–405.
144. Morris SE, Navaratnam N, Herndon DN. A comparison of effects of thermal injury and smoke inhalation on bacterial translocation. *J. Trauma*, **30** (1990) 639–643.
145. Maejima K, Deitch E, Berg R. Promotion by burn stress of the translocation of bacteria from the gastrointestin tracts of mice. *Arch. Surg.*, **119** (1984) 166–172.

146. Carter EA, Tomkins RG, Yarmush ML, Walker WA, Burke JF. Redistribution of blood flow after thermal injury and hemorrhagic shock. *J. Appl. Physiol.*, **65** (1988) 1782–1788.

147. Ziegler TR, Smith RJ, O'Dwyer ST, Demling RH, Wilmore DW. Increased intestinal permeability associated wtih infection in burn patients. *Arch. Surg.*, **123** (1988) 1313–1319.

148. Faist E, Storck M, Ertel W, and Meves A. *Shock, Sepsis, and Organ Failure First Wiggers Bernard Conference.* Springer-Verlag, New York, NY, 1990, pp. 307–328.

149. Sibbons P, Spitz L, van Valzen D. The role of lymphatics in the pathogenesis of pneumatosis in experimental bowel ischemia. *J. Pediatr. Surg.*, **27** (1992) 339–343.

150. O'Leary AD, Sweeney EC. Lymphoglandular complexes of the colon: structure and distribution. *Histopathology*, **10** (1986) 267–283.

151. Haggitt RC. Granulomatous diseases of the gastrointestinal tract. In *Pathology of Granulomas.* Ioachim HL (ed.), Raven Press, New York, NY, 1983, pp. 257–305.

152. Fleming MP, Carlson HC. Submucosal lymphatic cysts of the gastrointestinal tract: a rare cause of a submucosal mass lesion. *Am. J. Roentgenol.*, **110** (1970) 842–845.

153. Geboes K, Wolf-Peeters C, Rutgeerts P, Vantrappen G, Desmet V. Submucosal tumors of the colon: experience with twenty-five cases. *Dis. Col. Rectum.*, **21** (1978) 420–425.

154. Okamoto J, Sasaki T, Staake Y. Non-epithelial tumors of the large intestine. *Gastrointest. Endosc.*, **31** (1989) 866–871.

155. Hara K, Kanazawa K, Yamashiro M. Non-epithelial benign tumors of the colon. *J. Jpn. Soc. Coloproctol.*, **30** (1977) 498–504.

156. Stuart M, Bursle G. Lymphatic cyst of the descending colon: a report of a case. *Aust. N. Z. J. Surg.*, **50** (1980) 186–189.

157. Kuramoto S, Sakai S, Tsuda K. Lymphangioma of the large intestine: report of a case. *Dis. Col. Rectum*, **31** (1989) 900–905.

158. Matsumoto T, Matsumoto F, Hashimoto N. A case of lymphangioma coexistent with tubular adenoma in the descending colon and a review of the literature. *Dig. Endosc.*, **5** (1993) 277–284.

159. Girdwood TG, Phillips LD. Lymphatic cysts of the colon. *Gut*, **12** (1971) 933–935.

160. Matsui A, Okajimi K, Ishii M. Lymphangioma of the cecum with intussusception—a case report and review of the literature. *Nippon Rinsho Geka Igakkai Zasshi*, **47** (1985) 234–239.

161. Fujumoto S, Imaoka T, Suou T. Cystic lymphangioma of the cecum—a report of a case and a review of the literature. *Yonago Acta Med.*, **25** (1981) 28–33.

162. Nagle R. Lymphangiomatous hamartoma with intussusception of the caput caeci. *Br. J. Surg.*, **55** (1968) 879–880.

163. Lam A, Ternberg JL. Cystic lymphangioma of the cecum with ileal intussusception—case report. *Am. Surg.*, **41** (1975) 648–649.

164. Corman ML, Haggitt RC. Lymphangioma of the rectum: report of a case. *Dis. Col. Rectum*, **16** (1973) 524–529.

165. Zilko PJ, Lawerance BH, Sheiner H, Pollard J. Cystic lymphangiomyoma of the colon causing a protein-losing enteropathy. *Dig. Dis.*, **20** (1975) 1076–1080.

166. Kato S, Asakura H, Miura S. A case of localized colonic lymphangiectasia associated with a protein depletion syndrome. *Jpn. J. Gastroenterol.*, **82** (1985) 765–770.

167. Beahrs OH, Judd ES, Dockerty MB. Chylous cysts of the abdomen. *Surg. Clin. N. Am.*, **30** (1950) 1081–1097.

168. Yamamoto J, Matsumoto K, Furuya T. Lymphangioma of the ascending colon. *J. Clin. Gastroenterol.*, **11** (1989) 598–599.

169. Poulos JE, Presti ME, Phillips N, Longo WE. Presentation and management of lymphatic cyst of the colon. Report of a case. *Dis. Colon Rectum*, **40** (1997) 366–369.

170. Arnett NL, Friedman PS. Lymphangioma of the colon: roentgen aspects: a case report. *Radiology*, **67** (1956) 882–885.

171. Fujimura Y, Nishishita C, Lida M, Jajihara Y. Lymphangioma of the colon diagnosed with an endoscopic ultrasound probe and dynamic CT. *Gastrointest. Endosc.*, **41** (1995) 252–254.

172. Meinke AH, Estes NC, Ernst CB. Chylous ascites following abdominal aortic aneurysmectomy: Management with total parenteral hyperalimentation. *Ann. Surg.*, **190** (1979) 631–633.

173. Savlov ED. Chylous ascites following retroperitoneal lymph node dissection successfully treated with peritoneovenous shunting. *J. Surg. Oncol.*, **36** (1987) 228–229.

174. Fleisher HL, Oren JW, Sumner DS. Chylous ascites after abdominal aortic aneurysmectomy: successful management with a peritoneovenous shunt. *J. Vasc. Surg.*, **6** (1987) 403–407.

175. Leport J, Devars D, Mayne JF, Hay JM, Cerf M. Chylous ascites and encapsulating peritonitis: unusual complications of spontaneous bacterial peritonitis. *Am. J. Gastroenterol.*, **82** (1987) 463–466.

176. Segal R, Waron M, Reif R, Zecler E. Chylous ascites and chylothorax as presenting manifestations of stomach carcinoma. *Isr. J. Med. Sci.*, **22** (1986) 897–899.

177. Allen W, Parrott TS, Saripkin L, Allan C. Chylous ascites following retroperitoneal lymphadenectomy for granulosa cell tumor of the testis. *J. Urol.*, **135** (1986) 797–798.
178. Sarazin WG, Sauter KE. Chylous ascites following resection of a ruptured abdominal aneurysm: treatment with a peritoneovenous shunt. *Arch. Surg.*, **121** (1986) 246–247.
179. Sipes SL, Newton M, Lurain JR. Chylous ascites: a sequel of pelvic radiation therapy. *Obstet. Gynecol.*, **66** (1985) 832–835.
180. Savrin RA, High R. Chylous ascites after abdominal aortic surgery. *Surgery*, **98** (1985) 866–869.
181. Ferrigni RG, Novicki DE. Chylous ascites complicating genitourinary oncological surgery. *J. Urol.*, **134** (1985) 774–746.
182. Varma JS. Acute chylous ascites with carcinoid of the pancreas. *Scott. Med. J.*, **30** (1985) 111.
183. Humayun HM, Daugirdas JT, Ing TS, Leehey DJ, Gandhi VC, Popli S. Chylous ascites in a patient treated with intermittent peritoneal dialysis. *Artif. Organs*, **8** (1984) 358–360.
184. Rector WG. Spontaneous chylous ascites of cirrhosis. *J. Clin. Gastroenterol.*, **6** (1984) 369–372.
185. Jansen TT, Debruyne FM, Delaere KP, de Vries JD. Chylous ascites after retroperitoneal lymph node dissection. *Urology*, **23** (1984) 565–567.
186. Selli C, Carini M, Mottola A, Barbagli G. Chylous ascites after retroperitoneal lymphadenectomy: successful management with peritoneovenous shunting. *Urol. Int.*, **39** (1984) 58–60.
187. Blalock A, Robinson CS, Cunningham RS. Experimental studies on lymphatic blockage. *Arch. Surg.*, **34** (1937) 1049–1071.
188. Press OW, Press NO, Kaufman SD. Evaluation and management of chylous ascites. *Ann. Intern. Med.*, **96** (1982) 358–364.
189. Fuss IJ, Strober W, Cuccherini BA et al. Intestinal lymphangiectasia, a disease characterized by selective loss of naive CD45RA[+] lymphocytes into the gastrointestinal tract. *Eur. J. Immunol.*, **28** (1998) 4275–4285.
190. Waldmann TA. Protein-losing enteropathy. *Gastroenterology*, **50** (1966) 422–443.
191. Strober W, Wochner RD, Carbone PP, Waldmann TA. Intestinal lymphangiectasia: a protein-losing enteropathy with hypogammaglobulinemia, lymphocytopenia and impaired homograft rejection. *J. Clin. Invest.*, **46** (1967) 1643–1656.
192. Kinmonth JB, Cox SJ. Protein-losing enteropathy in primary lymphoedema: mesenteric lymphography and gut resection. *Br. J. Surg.*, **61** (1974) 589–593.
193. Levine C. Primary disorders of lymphatic vessels—a unified concept. *J. Pediatr. Surg.*, **24** (1989) 233–240.
194. Hennekam RC, Geerdink RA, Hamel BC et al. Autosomal recessive intestinal lymphangiectasia and lymphedema with facial anomalies and mental retardation. *Am. J. Med. Genet.*, **34** (1989) 593–600.
195. Mucke J, Hoepffner W, Scheerschmidt G, Gornig H, Beyreiss K. Early onset lymphedema, recessive form— a new form of genetic lymphoedema syndrome. *Eur. J. Pediatr.*, **145** (1986) 195–198.
196. Wilkinson P, Pinto B, Senior JR. Reversible protein-losing enteropathy with intestinal lymphangiectasia secondary to chronic constrictive pericarditis. *N. Engl. J. Med.*, **273** (1965) 1178–1181.
197. Broder S, Callihan TR, Jaffe ES et al. Resolution of longstanding protein-losing enteropathy in a patient with intestinal lymphangiectasia after treatment for malignant lymphoma. *Gastroenterology*, **80** (1981) 166–168.
198. Takagi S, Oshimi K, Sumiya M, Gonda N, Kano S, Takaku F. Protein-losing enteropathy in systemic lupus erythematosus. *Am. J. Gastroenterol.*, **3** (1983) 152–154.
199. Warshaw AL, Waldmann TA, Laster L. Protein-losing enteropathy and malabsorption in regional enteritis: cure by limited ileal resection. *Ann. Surg.*, **178** (1973) 578–580.
200. Weiden PL, Blaese RM, Strober W, Block JB, Waldman TA. Impaired lymphocyte transformation in intestinal lymphangiectasia: evidence for at least two functionally distinct lymphocyte populations in man. *J. Clin. Invest.*, **51** (1972) 1319–1325.

10 Probiotics and the Colon
Therapeutic and Prophylactic Uses

Thomas J. Borody and Patricia L. Conway

CONTENTS

1. INTRODUCTION

In the past, probiotic use has been shrouded by scepticism because of a lack of scientifically valid evidence of efficacy and with the science behind the concept lost to the culinary world of yogurt production. A new generation of probiotics is emerging in the new millennium as the potential savior of colonic disturbances that plague up to 30% of the general public. It is now recognized that with stringent probiotic strain selection criteria and demonstration of measurable parameters of functionality, probiotics can effectively prevent, reduce, or even eliminate many colonic disorders. Some of the targeted disorders have only recently been linked to the indigenous bowel flora, and as yet, no specific pathogens have been identified. Probiotics can be used either directly or indirectly to affect these putative causal agents, even if they have not yet been unmasked, and to restore the balance of beneficial microbes, thereby improving symptoms. While these new probiotic preparations can be included in foods, clinical evidence of efficacy will lead to the development of effective pharmaceutical probiotic products for colonic applications.

Probiotics of the future will probably allow the realization of American humorist, Josh Billing's belief in the importance of bowel health. He stated that: "I have finally come to the conclusion that a good reliable set of bowels is worth more to a man than any quantity of brains" *(1)*.

1.1. Definition of Probiotics

The definition of Fuller, in 1992, is commonly used and refers to probiotics as live microbial supplements that improve the health of the host by beneficially influencing the indigenous

From: *Colonic Diseases*
Edited by: T. R. Koch © Humana Press Inc., Totowa, NJ

microbes *(2)*. More recently, this definition was modified somewhat and generally probiotics are now referred to as living microorganisms that, upon ingestion in certain numbers, exert health benefits beyond inherent basic nutrition *(3)*.

1.2. Historical Perspective

The term "probiotics" was coined by Parker as the opposite of antibiotic, i.e., "for life" *(4)*. However, the concept dates back to the time when the Russian scientist Metchnikoff in 1908 proposed that one could reduce intestinal putrefaction and improve longevity by consumption of fermented milk products *(5)*. Subsequently, there was considerable interest in using yogurt bacteria such as lactobacilli, for improving intestinal health in man *(6)*. Research into the use of lactobacilli for improving health virtually stopped with the discovery of antibiotics, since effective disease control could be achieved with antibiotics. It was not until the excessive use of antibiotics in animal production became the focus of public attention in some countries in the mid-1980s and the emergence of antibiotic resistance in hospitals, that alternative methods of disease control were needed. Consequently, interest in the use of lactobacilli was rekindled. An evaluation of the efficacy of lactobacilli identified that some strains of lactobacilli can effectively reduce disease in animals, however, the particular strain used and the viability and stability of the strain needed to be examined *(7)*. Unfortunately, a veil of controversy still surrounds probiotics, since over the years, there have been many anecdotal or contradictory reports and inconclusive studies and the papers entitled "Probiotics—snake oil for the new millennium" *(8)* and "Probiotics, prebiotics or conbiotics" *(9)* address these issues.

Since 1996, there have been several collaborative projects within the European Union addressing function and efficacy of probiotics, the most recent of which was called the PROBDEMO project *(10)*. From this work, it was concluded that with the application of a scientific basis to the selection of probiotic strains, it is possible to develop safe and efficacious probiotic products with demonstrable benefit to the health of consumers. Successful clinical trials are being achieved with the new generation of probiotic strains, and consequently, probiotics are being evaluated for a number of colonic disorders.

1.3. Development of the Science of Probiotics

Many of the probiotic products of bygone years were ineffective. It is agreed that in some cases, the viability of the preparation was very poor, and often, the particular strain used was not specified *(7,11–13)*. It is now recognized that not all strains of the same species have comparable probiotic properties and that one can not extrapolate from data obtained from taxonomically related strains. The designation of the strain used must be specified. While this often occurs for the species that are not commonly used in fermented foods, it is often neglected when *Lactobacillus acidophilus* is used. This lack of strain designation contributes to the conflicting findings that have been reported for *L. acidophilus*.

It is agreed that stringent selection criteria should be used, since the selected strains must be biologically active against the identified target, have the capacity to colonize, be metabolically active in the host, and must be evaluated under strict scientifically controlled conditions. Adhesion is considered a prerequisite for successful colonization of the tract by the probiotic and there has been an identified need to develop appropriate in vitro adhesion assays for preliminary evaluation of the adhesive nature of the strains *(14)*. Furthermore the desirable properties of the strains must be stable during production, storage, and usage. It is envisaged that there will be particular probiotic strains for specific applications and that, ideally, the strains should originate from the host for which it is developed.

The list of probiotic applications for improving human health is long, and one can appreciate the views of the sceptics in questioning the application of a single microbe for so many different conditions. It is conceivable that one strain can influence a number of conditions if they are linked to an alteration in the composition or metabolic activity of the indigenous microbes of the colon. In such cases, the introduction of the probiotic shifts the balance of the microbes in favor of the more desirable ones. At present, research groups focus on a limited number of probiotic strains and then trial them for a huge range of applications. It is presumed that the introduction of the single strain will lead to the development of the desirable complex beneficial profile as seen in the developing indigenous microbial flora of the infant (15). It is well recognized that the breast-fed infant has high numbers of *Bifidobacterium*, and after the introduction of other foods, a more complex and stable microbial community gradually develops. Pure cultures of *Bifidobacterium* or *Lactobacillus* are commonly used for oral administration to improve health. Combinations of *Lactobacillus* and *Bifidobacterium* strains are also used rather extensively. More complex mixtures of lactic acid bacteria and even mixtures including additional genera may facilitate a more rapid restoration of the healthy profile of microbes in the colon rather than allowing the succession of development that occurs with single strains and simple mixtures.

The application of strict scientific principles for evaluation of probiotic preparations is crucial. There is an absolute requirement for scientifically valid clinical trials, including randomized double-blind placebo-controlled human studies, in which defined products are tested in defined study groups of individuals. There should be confirmation of the findings and documentation of the strain in independent centers with publication of the findings in peer-review journals.

2. PROBIOTIC PREPARATIONS

2.1. Types of Preparations

Both single strains and mixtures of microbes are used as probiotics. Traditionally probiotics were pure strains of lactobacilli. Today, lactic acid bacteria, especially lactobacilli, bifidobacteria, and enterococci are used either alone or in combination (16–18). There is also considerable usage of the yeast *Saccharomyces boulardii (19,20)*. The most common lactobacilli are the *L. acidophilus* strains and *L. bulgaricus*, because traditionally, these were the ones first used in fermented milk products and believed to be beneficial. Today, a number of *L. acidophilus* strains are used and, in some instances, are combined with *L. bulgaricus* strains and with *Streptococcus thermophilus*, which is also frequently included in fermented milk products. With the renewed interest in probiotics in the late 1980s and early 1990s, it was agreed that strains originating from the gastrointestinal tract that were more resistant to stomach and bile acids may have a better capacity to colonize and be more metabolically active *in situ*. In addition, the capacity of the strains to inhibit pathogens was considered an important criterion (11,13). This approach has led to the emergence of a new generation of probiotics as listed in Table 1. A range of *Lactobacillus* species is now considered for use as probiotics and these include *L. johnsonii, L. rhamnosus, L. casei, L. gasseri, L. reuteri, L. fermentum, L. plantarum,* and *L. salivarus. Bifidobacterium* strains used as probiotics include *B. lactis, B. animalis, B. longum,* and *B. infantis*. In addition, *Lactococcus lactis,* originating from a traditional fermented milk product from northern Sweden, and *Enterococcus faecium* are available as powdered commercial products, but are not found in foods.

Nonlactic acid bacteria available commercially as probiotics for human usage include *Escherichia coli, Clostridium butyricum,* and *Saccharomyces boulardii*. While most of the

Table 1
Strains Currently Used as Probiotics Either as Single Cultures or in Combination

L. acidophilus NCFB1748	*B. adolescentis*
L. acidophilus NFCM	*B. animalis*
L. acidophilus La-5	*B. bifidum*
L. bulgaricus	*B. infantis*
L. casei strain Shirota	*B. lactis* Bd 12
L. casei	*B. longum* B536
L. fermentum KLD	*B. breve*
L. gasseri	
L. johnsonii LA1(LC1 or LJ1)	*S. boulardii*
L. planatarum 299V	*S. cerevisiae*
L. reuteri	
L. rhamnosus GG	
L. rhamnosus	
L. salivarius	
L. lactis	*E. coli*
C. butyricum	
S. salivarius ssp. *thermophilu*	

lactic acid bacteria sold as probiotics are marketed as functional foods, the nonlactic acid bacteria are not used in foods. Two different strains of *E. coli* have been used in commercial preparations, namely strain A0 34/86 serotype 083 and strain Nissle 1917 (DSM 6601). These strains belong to the human intestinal *E. coli* type strains according to biochemical properties. The Nissle 1917 strain exhibits antagonistic activity against pathogenic enterobacteria. *E. coli* cultures have been tested in the newborn to prevent establishment of less desirable *E. coli* and to prevent nosocomial infections *(21)* possibly by triggering a protective immune response. *C. butyricum* is used as a commercial probiotic preparation in Japan and has been shown to have health benefits *(22,23)*. In addition, complex mixes of microbes have been evaluated in humans. While there are no complex mixtures widely available as commercial products for humans, most of the commercial probiotic preparations for the chicken industry are complex mixtures of about 30 different microbes *(24)*.

2.2. Mode of Function of Probiotics

In unraveling the mysteries associated with probiotics, it is desirable to understand how they function, as this may shed light on why they may fail to be efficacious in some situations. It is now accepted that probiotic microbes need to be live and metabolically active within the digestive tract in order to induce demonstrable beneficial effects on the host *(25)*. Furthermore, some probiotic strains will be effective for some applications but not all. For example, those which function well as immunomodulators may not have any capacity to reduce the growth of pathogens. There is now considerable focus on ensuring that the probiotic microbes maintain viability in the food product and during passage through the digestive tract to the site where they will be active. Traditionally, lactic acid bacteria used for producing cultured dairy products were used as probiotics, however it is now established that there are differences between strains of lactic acid bacteria and that some are more effective as probiotics than others. Stringent strain selection criteria have been developed for isolation of effective probiotics. We are seeing the emergence now of a new generation of specifically selected probiotic strains with demonstrated modes of action and efficacy *(26,27)*.

The indigenous microbes contribute to the health of the host in a number of ways including protecting the host from invasion of pathogens (28,29), contributing to digestion, and by producing valuable metabolites, such as vitamins and short chain fatty acids. While many ingested microbes may be desirable, potential pathogens can enter the tract and colonize. The stability and composition of these indigenous microbes is affected by stress to the host, medications, and dietary changes, and thus, may allow the increase in the undesirable microbes, which may be present in low numbers. Probiotics can ensure the establishment or reestablishment of a healthy microbial population that prevents the growth of pathogens (30). This can occur by competitive exclusion, whereby the desirable microbes out-compete the pathogens for either nutrients or colonization sites (31) or by the production of metabolites, which are inhibitory to the growth or adhesion of the pathogen (32), thus preventing their establishment in the gut. The metabolites can include short chain fatty acids, which are either inhibitory to the growth of many pathogens or of lower *in situ* pH, such that the pathogens grow poorly (33). In addition, some probiotic microbes produce bacteriocins that inhibit the growth of the pathogen (34), while others have immunomodulating properties (35). It is proposed that the respiratory nature of the yeast strains, mostly *Saccharomyces*, may be beneficial, because as the yeast respires, it consumes traces of oxygen, thus allowing the more anaerobic bacteria to develop (36). Some probiotics may also interfere with toxicity by preventing toxins from binding to receptors on the mucosal surface (19).

2.3. Monitoring the Probiotic Effect

Well-conducted clinical trials are required for monitoring the probiotic effect, and these should ideally be double-blind placebo-controlled randomized trials. This involves multidisciplinary research teams and is preferable as a multicenter study. The important features of such studies are the parameters monitored, the methodology used, the size of the research groups, and the statistical evaluation of the data generated. These aspects are linked, since the size of the research group is influenced by the parameters monitored and the methodology used. When symptoms of a disease are monitored, considerable benefit of a probiotic can be demonstrated (37). For example, *L. salivarius* UCC118 has been shown to reduce the severity of inflammatory bowel disease (IBD) symptoms, even though the etiological agent has not been identified. The uniformity of a condition and the severity also influence the outcome. For example, the most promising clinical trials using probiotics have involved rotavirus diarrhea in children (see Subheading 4.1.). These studies involve a single causative agent that has severe implications for the health of the child.

Boosting resistance to infection requires larger numbers of subjects and is dependent on the development of a condition or the increased levels of a pathogen, for example antibiotic-associated diarrhea (AAD) and the increase in numbers of *C. difficile*. With larger numbers of subjects in a study, the parameters being monitored need to be manageable. For example, a requirement to enumerate pathogen levels will be labor-intensive. Quantifying changes in the colonic microbes using culture techniques has limitations, both in terms of the microbes that can be cultured, the number of samples that can be analysed and the need to have fresh samples. To address these difficulties, the concept of monitoring microflora-associated characteristics (MACs) has been developed and used successfully to study the colonic microbes of the infant (38). The MACs refer to changes in biochemical parameters as a result of microbial growth, and hence, can be carried out on frozen samples, thus alleviating the need for culturing of fresh fecal material. The rapidly developing molecular techniques also hold promise as a way of characterizing changes in colonic microbes and, thus, allow the processing of larger numbers of samples, which can be stored frozen prior to analysis (39).

Monitoring the probiotic effect that addresses disease prevention such as colon cancer has inherent problems. It is not surprising that this is the area with the least proof of efficacy of probiotics. For colon cancer, inference of a probiotic effect is obtained from animal models and indicators of risk are assessed in humans, as discussed in Subheading 6.3. Reliance is also placed on epidemiological studies correlating incidence with a particular parameter in a population.

2.4. Industrial Development of Probiotic Preparations

An important consideration in the development of efficacious probiotic preparations is the production of the commercial product and the regulatory requirements relating to statements of health claims. At present, dairy products are the most common form used for probiotics, and attention has been directed to the technological aspects of such (40). It is recognized that the impact of the probiotic strain on the food needs to be assessed and may involve considerable product development. While the organoleptic characteristics can not be overlooked, the survival of the probiotic microbes in the product is of paramount importance. Failure to demonstrate efficacy of a particular probiotic may be attributable to the fact that low numbers of viable organisms are consumed. With the emergence of novel probiotic strains of intestinal origin, difficulties are encountered in the production of the cultures. Tailor-made growth medium can be required as noted for L. salivarius (40) and L. johnsonii LA1 (41). Stability of characteristics during production and in the final product are important, especially for those linked to a probiotic effect, such as adhesion. It is recognized that some adhesive strains lose the potential to adhere on subculturing and storage (12).

With the emerging evidence of efficacy of probiotics, the question of therapeutic claims arises. At present, food products carry very simple descriptions of the health benefits with statements, such as "helps every day your body to be stronger". It is anticipated that as the mechanisms of function of probiotics are better understood, it will be easier to monitor specific host responses, and then more specific claims could be developed.

2.5. Safety Considerations of Probiotic Preparations

Conventional toxicology and safety evaluation methodology has limitations when applied to probiotics. Parameters for assessing the safety of probiotics are being developed (42–45). Safety is generally discussed in terms of metabolic activity including the production of potentially harmful enzymes and toxins, the risk of systemic infection, excessive immunostimulation, and the potential for transfer of genetic material, especially antibiotic resistance. The lactic acid bacteria are generally regarded as safe and have been used extensively in humans for many years. Consequently, the potential risks associated with lactic acid bacteria are considered to be low (46), except for the Enterococcus genus. The safety of Enterococcus-based probiotics requires more attention than that of probiotic products containing lactobacilli and bifidobacteria, because the enterococci have a greater capacity for transfer of genetic material, including antibiotic resistance. The safety of nonlactic acid bacteria probiotics needs close scrutiny using the same parameters being developed for lactic acid bacteria. Such strains need to be assessed for the absence of genes or gene products of virulence factors, or undesirable metabolites, such as enzymes and toxins.

Lactobacilli have been isolated from the blood of endocarditis patients in a very limited number of cases, however there has been no link implicating the isolated strain in the disease. As a consequence however, an in vitro adhesion assay assessing the capacity of the probiotic strains to agglutinate blood platelets has been developed (47). Adhesion is a criterion considered desirable for probiotic strains, since the capacity to adhere can increase the potential of the strain to colonize the digestive tract (14). It is highly likely that desirable adhesive strains will also agglutinate platelets. One needs to question the value of the platelet assay since the relevance of this assay for in vivo induction of endocarditis has not been demonstrated. Furthermore, in a 4- to 6-mo study in Southern Finland, no cases of bacteraemia due to *Lactobacillus* species could be linked to probiotic cultures used extensively in dairy products in the area *(48,49)*. There have been rare cases of infection associated with lactic acid bacteria used in foods. There was a case of endocarditis due to *L. rhamnosus* in a patient who chewed a probiotic capsule containing probiotic lactobacilli after dental surgery *(50)*. A liver abscess contained a *L. rhamnosus* similar to the commercial strain *L. rhamnosus* GG that the patient had ingested *(51)*. There have been a number of cases of fungaemia due to usage of *S. boulardii (52–54)* and also in patients with a central catheter while hospitalized in intensive care units *(55)*. There are a number of known risk factors, which include the presence of catheters and serious underlying diseases that predispose the patient to infection. It is recognized that zero risk does not exist and that probiotics can potentially have side effects. Nonetheless, the safety of existing products based on lactic acid bacteria is excellent *(45)*. It is important to assess the safety of new probiotics in terms of the intrinsic properties of the strain, the interactions of the strain with the host, and the pharmocokinetics of the strain *(44,45)*.

3. THE COLONIC ECOSYSTEM

The digestive tract of humans is sterile at birth, and within the first few days of life, it becomes colonized by microbes, which in breast-fed infants are predominantly bifidobacteria *(15)*. With the introduction of other foods, a unique and diverse microbial population develops in the gastrointestinal tract. While the upper regions of the tract are sparsely populated with microbes, a large microbial community resides in the large bowel *(56)*. This population comprises predominantly strict anaerobic bacteria, such as *Bacteroides, Fusobacterium, Bifidobacterium, Lactobacillus*, and *Eubacterium*, with lower levels of coliforms. These microbes play an important role in the health of the host *(25)* in terms of producing short chain fatty acids for colonocyte nutrition and essential vitamins, assisting with degradation of complex nutrients, and protecting the host from invasion by pathogens. In addition, it has been proposed that the microbes in the bowel are involved in immunomodulation. Some undesirable effects such as diarrhea, constipation, liver damage, flatulence, IBD, and bowel cancer have been linked to enteric microbes. These unfavorable situations can occur if there is a shift in either the composition or perhaps metabolism of the indigenous microbes of the healthy individual. It is established that some microbes such as the *Lactobacillus* and *Bifidobacterium* are more beneficial than others.

The microbial community of the bowel is a part of a complex ecosystem that is regulated by the diet of the host, microbial interactions, and host factors, such as gut motility and intestinal secretions *(25,57)*. External factors, such as stress, dietary changes, and medications, can affect the microbial community in the bowel and may induce an alteration in the diversity of the microbes or in the metabolism of the microbes. This can be detrimental to the host, however it can also be utilized for the benefit of the host. In addition to maintaining a healthy microbial population by dietary means, one can also supplement the indigenous microbes with foods containing beneficial microbes such as the *Lactobacillus* and *Bifidobacterium*. It is envisaged that one can ensure a healthy body if one can maintain a stable population of beneficial microbes.

4. THERAPEUTIC APPLICATIONS OF PROBIOTICS: COLONIC DISEASES

Probiotics have been tested for efficacy against a range of conditions with 37% of studies representing general gastrointestinal tract effect, 26% relating to cholesterol lowering activities,

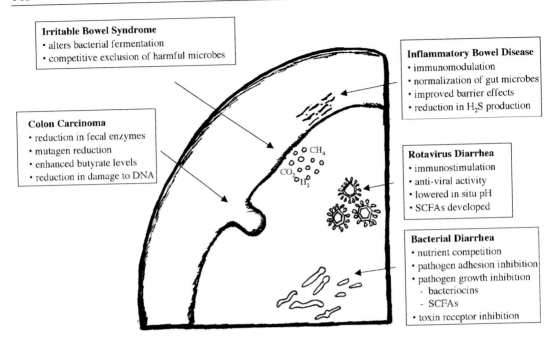

Irritable Bowel Syndrome
• alters bacterial fermentation
• competitive exclusion of harmful microbes

Inflammatory Bowel Disease
• immunomodulation
• normalization of gut microbes
• improved barrier effects
• reduction in H_2S production

Colon Carcinoma
• reduction in fecal enzymes
• mutagen reduction
• enhanced butyrate levels
• reduction in damage to DNA

Rotavirus Diarrhea
• immunostimulation
• anti-viral activity
• lowered in situ pH
• SCFAs developed

Bacterial Diarrhea
• nutrient competition
• pathogen adhesion inhibition
• pathogen growth inhibition
  - bacteriocins
  - SCFAs
• toxin receptor inhibition

Fig. 1. Proposed mechanisms of function of probiotics in the colon.

and 23% investigating the immunostimulatory activities (3,25,37,58). Of the various studies, it is apparent that among others, probiotics can clinically influence the following: (i) reduce infantile rotavirus-induced diarrhea; (ii) reduce adult diarrhea from a range of infectious agents; (iii) reduce AAD; (iv) stimulate the immune system by activating macrophages and stimulating cytokine production as well as induce a specific immune response to an introduced antigen; (v) reduce harmful intestinal bacterial enzymes; (vi) decrease fecal mutagenicity; and (vii) treat constipation and IBD.

Some proposed mechanisms by which probiotics can induce these benefits are illustrated in Fig. 1.

4.1. Diarrheal Disease

The therapeutic use of probiotics for amelioration of infectious diarrhea holds promise. Since infantile diarrhea can be severe and even life threatening, there has been considerable interest in this application. Some studies have addressed the reduction in the occurrence of rotavirus diarrhea, and these are discussed as prophylactic applications (Subheading 6.2.). Probiotics have been successfully used to reduce the symptoms or severity of infantile diarrhea. For example, *E. faecium* has been shown to reduce the duration of acute diarrhea in children with an unidentified causative agent (59,60). Feeding *E. faecium* SF68 to adults suffering *E. coli* and *Vibrio*-associated diarrhea failed to exert any effect on the subjects (61). The administration of *Lactobacillus* GG has promoted recovery of children suffering from rotavirus induced diarrhea in two separate studies. Isolauri et al. showed a significant reduction ($p < 0.05$) in the number of motions per day from 3.4 in the placebo group to 2.1 in the test group using a double-blind placebo-controlled study with 71 children suffering diarrhea (62). Of these cases of diarrhea, 82% were attributable to rotavirus. Subsequently, these workers showed a significant ($p < 0.05$) reduction in the duration of rotavirus diarrhea from 2.3 d to 1.5 d with children receiving the *Lactobacillus* GG (n = 42 children) *(63)*. The administration of *L. reuteri* to young children suffering acute diarrhea reduced its duration from 2.9 d to 1.7 d (n = 40) *(64)*. *S. boulardii* administration has improved the outcome in human immunodeficiency virus (HIV)-associated acute diarrhea with 56% of patients receiving the *S. boulardii* having their symptoms resolved, while only 6% of the placebo group showed improvement *(65)*. These workers showed a reduction in bowel movements from 9.0 to 2.1/d in these subjects (n = 17). When the *S. boulardii* was administered together with an oral rehydration therapy to children, an improved outcome was obtained *(66)*. The effect of probiotic administration on *C. difficile*-induced diarrhea has also been examined. There are a number of scientifically controlled studies showing an improvement in *C. difficile*-induced diarrhea with administration of *S. boulardii (67,68)* and two studies showing a reduction in relapsing diarrhea with dosage of *Lactobacillus* GG in a small number of subjects *(69,70)*.

4.2. Constipation

Constipation is generally regarded as an idiopathic condition in which fiber deficiency has been implicated. While fiber has long been used to treat constipation, it is not a cure, and in many patients, constipation persists in spite of adequate fiber supplementation, which suggests an alternate etiology. There are indications that the indigenous microbes of the bowel may play a contributory or even an etiological role, since the symptoms have been reversed in a chronically constipated subject in whom the bowel flora was restored using fecal enema infusions *(71)*. Subsequently, it was shown that antibiotic administration can markedly alleviate symptoms and, in fact, in one patient, completely reverse the condition *(72)*. These workers showed that vancomycin treatment altered transit times and improved bowel symptoms. In the light of such findings, one could postulate that constipation is mediated by abnormal or pathogenic bacterial components that can modify gut motility and/or water absorption, and consequently, probiotics could act to affect such luminal microbes such that the symptoms of constipation would be reduced.

In a double-blind placebo-controlled randomized crossover study, 134 chronically constipated subjects, who had suffered constipation for an average of 18.8 yr and whose condition was resistant to the action of dietary fiber, were dosed with *E. coli* (Nissle 1917) strain, for 28 d *(73)*. Transit times and daily bowel symptoms were monitored. The patients who received the *E. coli* preparation had a significantly higher stool frequency than the placebo treated controls ($p < 0.001$). Following crossover of the therapy the results were similar in both groups and it was concluded that the use of this *E. coli* strain is successful in the treatment of chronic constipation. The effect of lactic acid bacteria has also been studied in constipation in several controlled trials. Using *B. animalis* fermented milk in a double-blind trial, transit time (pellet technique) was studied in 72 healthy volunteers. After an 11-d treatment, the fermented milk significantly reduced total colonic transit by approx 22% from initial value and also when compared with the placebo group, which received milk containing heat-denatured bifidobacteria *(74)*. In a separate trial using yogurt containing *B. animalis*, a marker technique was used to measure orocecal transit time *(75)*. In a total of 350 subjects using a parallel design, it was shown that using increasing doses of the yogurt servings (125, 250 and 375g/d) taken for 2 wk accelerated transit time significantly in a dose-dependent fashion by 22, 40, and 47%, respectively, when compared with initial values. The effect continued from 2–6 wk after the end of the consumption of the product, suggesting that the bacteria persist within the bowel. In a further double-blind crossover, trial using 500 mL of yogurt containing *B. longum* together with lactulose *(76)*, the mouth-to-cecum time accelerated during the period of ingestion of yogurt-enriched *B. longum* plus lactose from initial values when compared with conventional yogurt. In this instance however, one cannot ignore the fact that the addition of lactulose may have contributed to the increased transit speed.

It is, therefore, proposed that the use of probiotics may be successful in the treatment of constipation whose etiology may indeed, in part, be of microbial origin.

4.3. Pouchitis

Pouchitis is a nonspecific inflammation of the ileal reservoir remaining after an ileoanal anastomosis carried out usually for severe ulcerative colitis. Although some patients respond promptly to metronidazole or other antibiotic treatment, 5–10% of patients may develop refractory or relapsing symptoms called "chronic pouchitis".

Just as patients with chronic ulcerative colitis respond to probiotic therapy, a new therapy has been trialed for restoring luminal microbial balance and controlling inflammation in chronic pouchitis. Gionchetti et al. (77), in a double-blind placebo-controlled trial in 40 patients, used oral bacteriotherapy with a mixture of probiotics (VSL#3) including 3 strains of bifidobacteria, 1 strain of *Streptococcus salivarius* ssp. *thermophilus*, and 4 strains of *Lactobacillus* at a dose of 6 g/d or placebo for 9 mo. Only 3 patients (15%) relapsed in the VSL#3 group within the 9-mo period, compared to all 20 patients (100%) in the placebo group ($p < 0.001$). These results suggest that oral administration of a mixture of probiotics can be effective in preventing flare-ups of chronic pouchitis. A separate study by Freedman and George (78), using *Lactobacillus* GG and fructooligosaccharide for 1 mo, reported induction of remission in 10 patients with chronic pouchitis. These findings suggest that multiple and even single probiotics with high efficacy can be beneficial in reducing inflammation in pouchitis. Restoring a microbial balance by combining antibiotics, probiotics, and prebiotics may offer the most physiological and nontoxic approach to treating chronic pouchitis.

4.4. Irritable Bowel Syndrome

Irritable bowel syndrome (IBS) is considered to be a disorder of gut motility with symptoms that can include altered bowel habit, abdominal pain, flatulence, and bloating, among others. Data are accumulating that there may be a close relationship between the intestinal flora and motility. Indeed, there is direct evidence that luminal bacteria can stimulate the migratory motor complex and that transit is slower in germ-free animals (79). If abnormal luminal bacteria could result in aberrant motility, then it would not be unreasonable to suggest that such pathogenic microbes might be implicated in the etiology of IBS. Clinically, chronic gastrointestinal symptoms caused by specific microbial pathogens such as *C. difficile* or *Giardia lamblia* can mimic IBS, further implicating microbial involvement in the condition. Recently, antibiotic therapy in nonspecific bacterial overgrowth has been shown to improve IBS symptoms (80). Consequently, given that probiotics possess antimicrobial properties and can effectively compete with and displace enteric pathogens, it is reasonable to anticipate that probiotic administration to IBS patients will improve intestinal dysmotility. Evidence to support this hypothesis is accumulating. Da-Rong et al. effectively used *C. butyricum* strain MIYARI 588 to treat diarrhea-predominant IBS, although the dose used was not specified (81). The subjects were randomized, but the data was analyzed in terms of the symptoms of the patients who were grouped into three groups, namely (i) abdominal pain type (n = 7); (ii) diarrheic type (n = 14); and (iii) the postprandial abdominal pain type (n = 9). They reported a >80% global clinical response and restoration of bowel flora when the *C. butyricum* was dosed to the diarrheic-type patients. This included increases in lactobacilli and bifidobacteria and decreases in clostridia. Other workers administered 2×10^{10} colony-farming units/d of *L. plantarum* DSM 9843 for 4 wk to 60 IBS patients suffering abdominal bloating and pain in a randomized study. A rapid decrease in pain and flatulence was seen, and it was concluded that the treatment held promise for alleviation of symptoms of IBS *(82)*. In contrast, O'Sullivan and O'Morain *(83)* failed to significantly improve symptoms in a subgroup of patients with IBS using *L. rhamnosus* GG dosed at a level of 10^{10} cfu/d, though a trend was noted in the reduction of unformed stools. These workers proposed that while no significantly measurable improvement in symptoms was noted, the diarrhea-predominant subgroup may warrant further investigation. While it is completely plausible that the various subgroups of IBS may have differ microbial components contributing to the condition, and thus some, but not all, subgroups may be improved by various probiotics, one must also consider that not all strains of *Lactobacillus* will perform similarly. It is possible that the DSM strain 9843 is more efficacious than the GG strain. This could only be proven in a comparative study of similar subgroups of patients. Studies to date suggest that, with further development of probiotics, these products are likely to have a direct application in the treatment of all subgroups of IBS.

4.5. Inflammatory Bowel Disease

Chronic IBD is a group of "idiopathic" disorders, yet they can at times resemble clinically, colonoscopically, and histologically specific infectious disorders, e.g., *C. difficile* colitis, *Shigella* dysentery, or *Mycobacterium tuberculosis* enteritis. Such examples have long pointed to IBD having an infective etiology. Our inability to find a microbial cause of idiopathic IBD has caused physicians to conclude that these IBDs are not infectious diseases. However, given the complexity of intestinal flora, it is quite possible that one or more infectious agents exist for IBD, but are yet to be detected *(84)*. From animal models, we can confidently state that in the absence of luminal bacteria, together with a genetic predisposition, colitis will not develop *(85)*. Hence, the luminal bacteria seem to be a crucial factor in the development of IBD.

Since probiotics have been effective in managing bacterial infective diseases, e.g., *Lactobacillus* GG in *C. difficile* colitis, it seemed reasonable to trial probiotics in IBD on the premise that, although specific pathogens have not yet been detected, probiotics may be capable of detecting them and so modify the clinical outcome. In addition, probiotics might play a direct role in immunomodulation promoting host defences and down-regulating hypersensitivity reactions in inflammatory responses *(86)*.

Several controlled trials have now demonstrated the ability of probiotics to influence the course of IBD, and it was recently concluded that there is considerable promise with the use of probiotics in controlling IBD *(37)*. In two trials, patients with ulcerative colitis (UC) were given either capsules of *E. coli* (Nissle 1917) or mesalazine *(87,88)*. No significant difference in relapse rates was observed between the two treatments. Venturi et al. used VSL#3 twice daily for 12 mo *(89)*. Fifteen of twenty (75%) treated patients remained in remission during this study.

In studying postoperative recurrence of Crohn's disease, Rizzello et al. compared mesalazine vs VSL#3 *(90)*. At 12 mo, only 20% of patients on VSL#3 suffered a relapse vs 40% of patients on mesalazine when assessed at only 4 mo.

S. boulardii has also been used in combination with mesalazine *(91)* to reduce Crohn's disease relapse. Some 37% of patients sustained a recurrence of Crohn's disease on mesalazine alone vs only 6% on mesalazine plus *S. boulardii*.

Hence, in chronic IBD, anti-inflammatory therapy may well find a useful complementary, if not "stand-alone" treatment in probiotics *(92)*. Furthermore, probiotic effectiveness augurs well for an ultimate discovery of a microbial cause of IBD.

5. FECAL INFUSIONS AS PROBIOTICS FOR COLONIC DISEASES

Persky and Brandt *(93)* have published the latest of a series of sporadic reports over the last 40 or so years, on the use of fecal flora to treat chronic colonic infections. Their report demonstrated how preparations of normal human bacterial flora were capable of permanently eradicating *C. difficile* from the bowel. This type of therapy is, at this stage, considered a treatment of last resort, generally, because it is unconventional, distasteful, and because the physiological role of the human flora remains poorly understood. Nonetheless, because it is a probiotic colonic therapy, and often dramatically curative, it will be briefly reviewed here.

Fecal bacteriotherapy has been most commonly reported in the treatment of *C. difficile*-associated diarrhea and pseudomembranous colitis (PMC). In this setting, it has been very effective, and indeed, its results have been described as "dramatic" *(94)*. In 9 reports *(93–101)*, the overall cure rate was 61 in 68 treated patients, and most of those patients who failed to be cured had, in fact, been treated too late and died from overwhelming PMC *(94)*. Clinical improvement usually occurred within 1–4 d and has been reported to be curative without recurrence. There are few medical therapies that reverse severe illness so dramatically. This fact should lead us to question the mechanism of this treatment and ponder possible therapies for other bowel infections. Tvede and Rask-Madsen demonstrated in vitro how some but not other bacteria can profoundly inhibit growth of pathogenic strains *(97)*. A less powerful phenomenon has been described for *Lactobacillus* GG *(102)*. It would seem that inhibitory substances, perhaps bacteriocins and other antimicrobial peptides *(103)* elaborated by bacteria, possess antimicrobial properties. Unlike available antibiotics, it is possible that these substances have the power to eliminate bacterial spores. In addition, the incoming mix of bacteria implants missing flora components, such as *Bacteroides* species, thus restoring fecal physiology *(101,104)* and deficient composition *(97,105)*, which may have initially permitted implantation of the pathogen, e.g., *C. difficile*. Hence, colonic infusion of enteric flora may serve both as an antimicrobial and replacement therapy.

The human fecal flora is a complex mix of organisms and is arguably the largest organ of the body containing in a compact mass of living bacterial cells almost nine times more living cells than does the entire body *(106)*. Given the bactericidal nature of fecal flora, as judged by the approx 90% cure of *C. difficile*, it is instructive to realize that *C. difficile* may be but one of many established infective agents mediating chronic gastrointestinal (GI) disease. As *Helicobacter pylori* was found to be the infective cause of ulcer disease, so chronic clostridial (or other) infections may cause a portion of chronic GI disorders, such as constipation, IBS, or IBD, as illustrated above. Indeed, constipation responds to vancomycin *(72,107)* and to fecal flora therapy *(71,108)* as does IBS *(96,109)*. Ulcerative colitis (UC) has also been reported to undergo prolonged remission following fecal flora infusion *(110)*. We have confirmed this finding in our own prospective series of 12 patients with severe UC, five of whom remain in clinical remission without other therapy 1–11 yr after treatment *(109)*. Similarly when Eiseman et al. *(95)* treated his four PMC cases in 1957, *C. difficile* had not been discovered, yet the therapy was successful. This very finding teaches us that we can use probiotic (fecal or other) bacteriotherapy to treat enteric infections without necessarily identifying the pathogen. Fecal bacteria appear to eradicate or suppress the pathogen, possibly because of their broad-spectrum activity. Hence, when the bacterial species is unknown, fecal bacteria act upon the pathogen without our need to detect and diagnose the infection. Although scientifically, it is satisfying to recognize the pathogen, strictly speaking fecal bacteriotherapy can get around this problem. As alluded to in preceding sections, it is possible that progress in the discovery of the etiology of IBS/IBD could spring from a successful probiotic therapy rather than from pathogen identification.

When planning to use this fecal bacteriotherapy, some practical issues need to be considered which include: (i) the method of treatment, and (ii) selection of donor. It appears that a successful result can be achieved regardless of method of delivery of the fecal slurry into the bowel. Success has been achieved when given by an enema suspended in saline *(94–96,98–100,109)* or milk for acute infections (never reported for chronic *C. difficile*) *(101,104)*, by a small bowel infusion via a nasoduodenal tube *(96,98)*, a gastrostomy *(100)*, or through a colonoscope *(93)*. However, there may be advantages to delivering via a colonoscope, to infuse as proximally as possible and to detect any colonic pathology. Selection of the donor is of crucial importance to avoid infecting the recipient with a separate disease. The donor should be tested at least for HIV, hepatitis A, B, and C, cytomegalovirus, Ebstein-Barr virus, syphilis, and any other relevant infective disorders, and have stools negative for any detectable parasites or bacterial pathogens. In our experience, choosing the patient's partner offers a theoretical advantage that any existing transmissible disease would have been transmitted and emerged by now.

In the future, it is conceivable that fecal bacteriotherapy may become more frequently used for recalcitrant enteric infections and perhaps for those GI disorders that we now call "idiopathic," but may well have an infective etiology *(111)*.

6. PROPHYLACTIC APPLICATIONS OF PROBIOTICS

6.1. Prevention of Diarrhea

Because of the severity of infectious diarrhea in infants, a suitable prophylactic treatment is needed. Probiotics have been effectively used to reduce the severity or duration of diarrhea in children. Pedone et al. *(112)* used a mixture of *L. casei*, *S. thermophilus*, and *L. bulgaricus* in a randomized blinded placebo-controlled study involving 287 children in a daycare center who were given the probiotic mixture for 6 mo. These workers noted a significantly ($p < 0.05$) shorter duration of the diarrhea in the children given the probiotic mixture. Similarly, administration of a mixture of *B. bifidum* and *S. thermophilus* to children suffering from rotavirus-induced diarrhea in a double-blind placebo-controlled study and resulted in a reduction rate of rotavirus-associated diarrhea from 8 in 26 cases to 2 in 29 cases and decreased rotavirus shedding in the test group *(113)*. In a large multicenter study in Europe, a reduction in diarrhea in children was noted using *Lactobacillus* GG *(114)*. Use of this strain in Peru also reduced the incidence of diarrhea in children *(115)*. *L. plantarum* 299V was shown to reduce the cases of diarrhea in a daycare center with a high frequency of diarrhea *(116)*.

AAD is a major problem in hospitals, with about 20% being attributable to the opportunistic pathogen, *C. difficile* *(117)*. AAD may develop into colitis, and in extreme cases, even death. Prophylactic probiotic administration has been shown to effectively reduce AAD in a number of studies. A reduction from 14 to 0% was noted with administration of a mixture of *L. acidophilus* and *L. bulgaricus* in one study *(118)*. However, a similar mixture but not necessarily the same strains, only decreased the incidence from 69 to 66% *(119)*. The combination of *L. acidophilus* and *B. longum* has been shown to decrease the incidence from 70 to 20% *(120)* while *B. longum* given alone resulted in a decrease from 60 to 10% in diarrhea incidence in a single-blind placebo-controlled study *(121)*. The administration of *Lactobacillus* GG in a single-blind placebo-controlled study reduced the duration of AAD from 8 to 2 d *(122)*. *S. boulardii*, given together with antibiotics, also decreased AAD in a study involving 124 patients, with significantly fewer (26%) patients in the test group (n = 57) experiencing recurrent diarrhea over 2 mo following the antibiotic treatment *(123)*. With appropriate control of the specific probiotics used and the dosages, effective reductions in AAD can be achieved.

6.2. Prevention of Traveler's Diarrhea

Antibiotics can be used to prevent the establishment of traveler's diarrhea and can reduce the incidence by up to 90% *(124,125)*. This prophylactic antibiotic treatment is not generally recommended, because of problems with increasing drug resistance and potential side effects, including AAD. While bismuth has been effectively used for reducing traveler's diarrhea *(126)*, this treatment is not popular, and an alternative is needed. Probiotics have been investigated with modest success, probably mostly attributable to the complexity of causative agents and the limited number of published studies. In a double-blind placebo-controlled study, a significant reduction ($p < 0.05$) in the incidence of diarrhea was noted in the probiotic-treated group when the incidence was high *(127)*. This group was given a mixture of *L. acidophilus*, *L. bulgaricus*, *B. bifidum*, and *S. thermophilus* and had 43% incidence of diarrhea compared to the 71% level observed in the placebo group. Other workers failed to show an effect of probiotic administration using a mixture of *L. acidophilus* and *L. bulgaricus* in 50 subjects in a double-blind placebo-controlled study over 8 d *(128)*. It must be recognized that the strains of *L. acidophilus* and *L. bulgaricus* were probably different, and no conclusions can be drawn on the role the *B. bifidum* and *S. thermophilus* may have had. *Lactobacillus* GG has been evaluated in Finnish travelers to two different locations, and no overall effect was noted, however, when only one travel destination was considered, a reduction in the incidence of diarrhea was noted *(129)*. The use of *S. boulardii* in another double-blind, placebo-controlled study failed to show an effect on the condition in 3000 subjects *(130)*. Katelaris et al., 1995, showed no effect in a double-blind placebo-controlled study in soldiers (n = 282) given either a *L. fermentum* or *L. acidophilus* when the incidence of diarrhea was low (22%) *(131)*. While the use of probiotics for traveler's diarrhea has potential, the studies to date do not offer proof. There is a trend that a high incidence is required before effective prevention can be demonstrated.

6.3. Colonic Carcinoma

The role of diet and colonic microbes in colon cancer suggests that probiotic administration could be combined with dietary regimes to reduce risks of tumor development. While there are many phases in the development of tumors, probiotic administration has focused largely on the initiation phase rather then being studied as a therapeutic agent. Practical limitations with humans studies has contributed to the fact that probiotic studies have been carried out in animal models and then extrapolated to human studies with reliance on epidemiological human data for support. It is recognized that bacterial fermentation and high protein diets lead to elevated levels of phenols, tryptophane metabolites, ammonia, and amines, while high fat diets yield aromatic polycyclic hydrocarbons. These compounds are known to enhance carcinogenesis. In addition, ingested nitrate can be converted to carcinogenic nitroso compounds. Interest has focused on a number of bacterial enzymes that may be involved in this carcinogenesis. These include azoreductase, nitroreductase, β-glucuronidase and β-gluconase. The immune mechanism may be stimulated or inhibited, and thereby, also play a role in carcinogenesis. It is proposed that probiotics may play a beneficial role in reducing the risk of colon carcinoma development by reducing levels of these harmful enzymes by shifting the profile or metabolism of the indigenous microbes, by binding the carcinogens and mutagens, and thereby, removing them from the system, as well as by increasing levels of metabolites, such as butyrate, which can reduce the frequency of DNA damage leading to tumor formation, and by triggering the immune system *(132)*. Such detoxification of genotoxins in the colon can be measured by the extent of the damage to the DNA in animals exposed to a mutagen for a short period of time or by the development of aberrant crypt focus (ACF) with a slightly extended exposure to the mutagen. Animals exposed to the mutagen for longer periods of time are studied, and the number and size of tumors noted. These parameters can then be used as indicators of the risk for the occurrence of carcinogenesis. Only the bacterial enzymes and levels of carcinogens in human feces can be used for generating data from humans consuming probiotics.

Parodi reviewed the effects of probiotics on the risk of colon cancer and concluded that animal studies show suppression in tumor development and that epidemiological studies show consumption of fermented milk products may help reduce the risk of cancer *(133)*. The particular strains and formulations can alter the results obtained. It has been shown that milk fermented with *L. bulgaricus* and *S. thermophilus* was more effective in deactivating risk factors than cellular components of the *L. bulgaricus* and *S. thermophilus* administered to rats exposed to the mutagen 1,2-dimethylhydrazine (DMH) *(134)*. Rats given an *L. acidophilus* preparation and exposed to DMH had reduced numbers and size of tumors compared to controls *(135)*. Similar results were obtained for rats dosed with *Lactobacillus* GG *(136)*, and this correlated with a reduction in the fecal enzymes in humans dosed with the *Lactobacillus* GG *(137)*. Yamazaki et al. *(138)* showed that *L. casei* strain Shirota inhibited chemically induced colon cancer in rats with significantly less tumors per rats given the mutagen azoxymethane (AOM). These workers also showed a reduction in large ACF (4 or more) in rats dosed with the Shirota strain of *L. casei*. Reddy showed that an oral dosage of *B. longum* resulted in a suppression of colon tumor development and tumor burden *(139)*.

The capacity of probiotics to bind mutagens has also been evaluated in vitro using mutagenic heterocyclic amines formed during cooking of protein-rich food, and all probiotic strains tested bound the mutagens *(140)*. A radioactively labeled heterocylic amine was administered to mice, and the fate of the radioactivity was monitored in mice also dosed with lactic acid bacteria *(141)*. It was shown that oral dosage of the mixture of *L. acidophilus* 1748 and *B. longum* 536 reduced the amount of labeled amine entering the tissues and organs, and it was concluded that the amine most probably bound to the bacteria was removed from the system. At present, there are no indicators that can be measured to determine the role of the immune system in tumor development. From studies to date, there is a promising correlation between the consumption of lactic acid bacteria and the indicators of risk of tumor development.

7. CONCLUSIONS

Live microbial supplements, probiotics, have originally been proposed to improve health. Progress in probiotic development was slowed with the introduction of antibiotics. However, probiotics are once again receiving considerable attention, since there is a concerted effort to decrease antibiotic usage and because of their potential health promoting activities. While there are nonconclusive or contradictory clinical probiotic studies, it is agreed that if one specifically selects appropriate probiotic strains and carries out adequate controlled clinical studies, probiotic-mediated improvements in health are likely to be significant. Currently, probiotic supplements generally include single species and/or mixtures of *Lactobacillus* and *Bifidobacterium*. Probiotics have been shown to reduce the numbers of enteric pathogens and lessen diarrhea, improve AAD, reduce the risk of colon cancer, and induce a protective immune response. Furthermore, beneficial effects on IBD, constipation, IBS and pouchitis have been reported. While emerging data is confirming efficacy of specific probiotics for specific applications, information on the mechanisms of the function of probiotics remains scarce. Foods have been the preferred vehicle for probiotics, but claims on food products do not yet reflect the scientific evidence of therapeutic capacity, since food products do not address disease states. Pharmaceutical probiotic preparations will resolve this situation through clinical findings reflected in defined claims. It is speculated that future probiotic preparations will contain species focused on specific activities and are likely to contain mixtures of probiotics to achieve clinical effects by copying components of perhaps the ideal or original probiotic, the human flora.

REFERENCES

1. Shaw HW. *The Complete Works of Josh Billings.* (With one hundred illustrations by Thomas Nast and others, and a biographical introduction.) Dillingham, New York, NY, 1876.
2. Fuller R. History and development of probiotics. In *Probiotics: The Scientific Basis.* Fuller R (ed.), Chapman & Hall, London, UK, 1992, pp. 1–4.
3. Salminen S, Bouley C, Boutron-Ruault M-C, et al. Functional food science and gastrointestinal physiology and function. *Brit. J. Nutr.,* **80** (1998) 147–171.
4. Parker RB. Probiotics, the other half of the antibiotic story. *Anim. Nutr. Health,* **29** (1974) 4–8.
5. Metchnikoff E. *The Prolongation of Life,* 1st ed., Putnam Sons, New York, NY, 1908.
6. Rettger LF, Chaplin HA. *Treatise on the Transformation of the Intestinal Flora with Special Reference to the Implantation of* Bacillus acidophilus. Yale University Press, New Haven, CT, 1921.
7. Conway PL. Lactobacilli: fact and fiction. In *The Regulatory and Protective Role of the Normal Microflora.* Grubb R, Midtvedt T, Norin E (eds.), The MacMillan Press LDT, London, UK, 1989, pp. 263–282.
8. Altas R. Probiotics—snake oil for the new millennium. *Environ. Microbiol.,* **1** (1999) 377–382.
9. Berg RD. Probiotics, prebiotics or conbiotics. *Trends Microbiol.,* **6** (1998) 89–92.
10. Mattila-Sandholm T. The PROBDEMO project: demonstration of the nutritional functionality of probiotic foods. *Tr. Food Sci. Tech.,* **10** (1999;) 385–386.
11. Havenaar H, Ten Brink B, Huis In't Veld J. Selection of strains for probiotic use. In *Probiotics: The Scientific Basis.* Fuller R (ed.), Chapman & Hall, London, UK, 1992, pp. 209–224.
12. Conway PL, Henriksson A. Strategies for the isolation and characterisation of functional probiotics. In *Human Health: The Contribution of Microorganisms.* Gibson S (ed.), Springer-Verlag, London, UK, 1994 pp. 119–144.
13. Conway PL. Selection criteria for probiotic microorganisms. *Asian Pac. J. Clin. Nutr.,* **5** (1996) 10–14.
14. Blum S, Reniero R, Schiffrin EJ, et al. Adhesion studies for probiotics: need for validation and refinement *Tr. Food Sci. Tech.,* **10** (1999) 405–410.
15. Conway PL: Acquisition and Succession of the gut microflora. In *The Gastrointestinal Microflora.* Vol. 2 Mackie RI, White BA, Isaacson RE (eds.), International Thomson Publishing, New York, NY, 1996, pp. 3–38
16. Salminen S. Human studies on probiotics. Aspects of scientific documentation. *Scand. J. Nutr.,* **45** (2001) 8–12
17. Pathmakanthan SA, Meance S, Edwards CA. Probiotics: A review of human studies to date and methodological approaches. *Microb. Ecol. Health Dis.,* **12** (2000) S10–S30.
18. Sanders ME, Huis in't Veld J. Bringing a probiotic-containing functional food to the market: microbiological product regulatory and labelling issues. *Antonie van Leeuwenhoek,* **76** (1999) 293–315.
19. Elmer GW, Surawicz CM, McFarland LV. Biotherapeutic agents. A neglected modality for the treatment and prevention of selected intestinal and vaginal infections. *JAMA,* **275** (1996) 870–876.
20. McFarland LV. A review of the evidence of health claims for biotherapeutic agents. *Microb. Ecol. Health. Dis.,* **12** (2000) 65–76.
21. Lodinova-Zadnikoa R, Sonnenborn U, Tlaskalova H. Probiotics and *E. coli* infections in man. *Vet. Q.,* **2** (1998) S78–S91.
22. Okamoto T, Sasaki M, Tsujikawa T, Fujiyama Y, Bamba T, Kusunoki M. Preventive efficacy of butyrate enemas and oral administration of *Clostridium butyricum* M588 in dextran sodium sulfate-induced colitis in rats. *J. Gastroenterol.,* **35** (2000) 341–346.
23. Kuroika T, Iwanaga M, Kobari K, Higashionna A, Kinjyo F, Saito A. Preventive effect of *Clostridium butyricum* M588 against the proliferation of *Clostridium difficile* during antimicrobial therapy. *J. Jpn. Assoc. Infect. Dis.,* (1990) 1425–1432.
24. Pascual M, Hugas M, Badiola JI, Monfort JM, Garriga M. *Lactobacillus salivarius* CTC2197 prevent *Salmonella enteritidis* colonisation in chickens. *Appl. Environ. Microbiol.,* **65** (1999) 4981–4986.
25. Conway PL. Probiotics and the gastrointestinal microbiota. In *Germfree Life and Its Ramifications.* Hashimo K, Sakakibara B, Tazume S, Shimizu K (eds.), XII ISG Publishing Committee, Shiozawa, Japan, 199 pp. 97–100.
26. Jacobsen CN, Rosenfeldt-Nielsen V, Hayford AE, et al. Screening of probiotics activities of forty-seve strains of *Lacatobacillus* spp by in vitro techniques and evaluation of the colonisation ability of five selecte strains in humans. *Appl. Environ. Microbiol.,* **65** (1999) 4949–4956.

27. Dunne C, Murphy L, Flynn S, et al. Probiotics: from myth to reality. Demonstration of functionality in animal models of disease and in human clinical trials. *Antonie von Leeuwenhoek*, **76** (1999) 279–292.

28. Barrow PA, Fuller R, Newport MJ. Changes in the microflora and physiology of the anterior intestinal tract of pigs weaned at 2 d, with special reference to the pathogenesis of diarrhea. *Infect. Immun.*, **18** (1977) 586–595.

29. Blomberg L, Conway PL. An in vitro study of colonisation resistance to *Escherichia coli* strain Bd 1107/7508 (K88) in relation to indigenous squamous gastric colonisation in piglets of varying ages. *Microb. Ecol. Health Dis.*, **2** (1989) 285–291.

30. Fuller R. Probiotics in man and animals. *J. Appl. Bacteriol.*, **66** (1989) 365–378.

31. van der Waaij D, Berguis-de Vries JM, Lekkerkerk-v. Colonisation resistance of the digestive tract in conventional and antibiotic-treated mice. *J. Hyg.*, **69** (1971) 405–411.

32. Blomberg L, Henriksson A, Conway PL. Inhibition of *Escherichia coli* K88 to piglet ileal mucus by *Lactobacillus* spp. *Appl. Environ. Microbiol.*, **59** (1993) 34–39.

33. Fox SM. Probiotics: intestinal inoculants for production animals. *Vet. Med.*, **83** (1988) 806–830.

34. Lindgren SE, Dobrogosz WJ. Antagonistic activities of lactic acid bacteria in food and feed fermentations. *FEMS Microbiol. Rev.*, **87** (1990) 149–164.

35. Cunningham-Rundles S, Ahrne S, Bengmark S, et al. Probiotics and immune response. *Am. J. Gastoenterol.*, **95** (2000) S22–S25.

36. Wallace RJ, Newbold CJ. Microbial feed additives for ruminants. In *Old Herborn University Seminar Monographs*. Fuller R, Heidt PJ, Rusch V, Van der Waaij D (eds.), Institute for Microbiology & Biochemistry, Herborn, Germany, 1995, pp. 101–125.

37. Mattila-Sandholm T, Blum S, Collins JK, et al. Probiotics: towards demonstrating efficacy. *Tr. Food Sci. Tech.*, **10** (1999) 393–399.

38. Bottcher MF, Nordin EK, Sandin A, Midtvedt T, Bjorksten B. Microflora-associated characteristics in faeces from allergic and nonallergic infants. *Clin. Exp. Allergy*, **30** (2000) 1590–1596.

39. Vaughan EE, Heilig HGHJ, Zoetendal EG, et al. Molecular approaches to study probiotic bacteria. *Tr. Food Sci. Tech.*, **10** (1999) 400–404.

40. Saxelin M, Grenov B, Svenson U, Fondèn R, Reniero R, Sandholm-Mattila T. The technology of probiotics. *Tr. Food Sci. Tech.*, **10** (1999) 387–392.

41. Elli M, Zink R, Reniero R, Morelli L. Growth requirements of *Lactobacillus johnsonii* in skim and UHT milk. *Int. Dairy J.*, **9** (1999) 507–513.

42. Aguirre M, Collins MD. Lactic acid bacteria and human clinical infection. *J. Appl. Bacteriol.*, **75** (1993) 95–107.

43. Gasser F. Safety of lactic acid bacteria and their occurrence in human clinical infections. *Bull. Inst. Pasteur*, **92** (1994) 45–67.

44. O'Brien JO, Crittenden R, Ouwehand A, Salminen S. Safety evaluation of probiotics. *Tr. Food Sci. Tech.*, **10** (1999) 418–424.

45. Marteau P. Safety aspects of probiotic products. *Scand. J. Nutr.*, **45** (2001) 22–24.

46. Adams MR. Safety of industrial lactic acid bacteria. *J. Biotechnol.*, **68** (1999) 171–178.

47. Harty DWS, Oakey JH, Patrikakis M, Hume EBH, Knox KW. Pathogenic potential of lactobacilli. *Int. J. Food Microbiol.*, **24** (1994) 179–189.

48. Saxelin M, Chuang NH, Chassy B, et al. Lactobacilli and bacteremia in Southern Finland 1989–1999. *Clin. Infect. Dis.*, **22** (1996) 564–566.

49. Saxelin M, Rautelin H, Salminen S, Makela P. The safety of commercial products with viable *Lactobacillus* strains. *Infect. Dis. Clin. Pract.*, **5** (1996) 331–335.

50. MacKay AD, Tylor MB, Kibbler CC, Hamilton-Miller JMT. *Lactobacillus* endocarditis caused by a probiotic organism. *Clin. Microbiol. Infect.*, **5** (1999) 290–292.

51. Rautio M, Jousimies H, Kauma H, et al. Liver abscess due to a *Lactobacillus rhamnosus* indistinguishable from *L. rhamnosus* GG. *Clin. Infect. Dis.*, **28** (1999) 1159–1160.

52. Pletinex M, Legein J, Vanenplas Y. Fungicemia with *Saccharomyces boulardii* in a 1-year-old girl with protracted diarrhea. *J. Pediatr. Gastroenterol. Nutr.*, **21** (1995) 113–115.

53. Niault M, Thomas F, Prost J, Ansari FH, Kalfon P. Fungemia due to *Saccharomyces* species in a patient treated with enteral *Saccharomyces boulardii*. *Clin. Infect. Dis.*, **28** (1999) 930.

54. Perapoch J, Planes AM, Querol A, et al. Fungemia with *Saccharomyces cerevisiae* in two newborns, only one of whom had been treated with Ultra-Levura. *Eur. J. Clin. Microbiol. Infect. Dis.*, **19** (2000) 468–470.

55. Hennequin C, Kauffmann-Lacroix C, Jobert A, et al. Possible role of catheters in *Saccharomyces boulardii* fungemia. *Eur. J. Clin. Microbiol. Infect. Dis.*, **19** (2000) 16–20.

56. Mitsuoka T. *Intestinal Bacteria and Health*. Harcourt Brace Jovanovich, Tokyo, 1978.

57. Tannock GW. Analysis of the intestinal microflora: a renaissance. *Antonie von Leeuwenhoek*, **76** (1999) 265–278.

58. Shortt C. The probiotic century: historical and current perspectives. *Tr. Food Sci. Tech.*, **10** (1999) 411–4

59. Wunderlich PF, Braun L, Fumagalli I, et al. Double-blind report on the efficacy of lactic acid-produci *Enterococcus* SF68 in the prevention of antibiotic-associated diarrhea and in the treatment of acute diarrh *J. Int. Med. Res.*, **17** (1989) 333–338.

60. Bellomo G, Mangiagle A, Nicastro L, Frigerio G. A controlled double-blind study of SF68 strain as a n biological preparation for the treatment of diarrhea in pediatrics. *Curr. Ther. Res.*, **28** (1980) 927–936.

61. Mitra AK, Rabbani GB. A double-blind, controlled trial of Bioflorin (*Streptococcus faecium* SF68) in ad with acute diarrhea due to *Vibrio cholerae* and enterotoxigenic *Escherichia coli*. *Gastroenterology*, **99** (199 1149–1152.

62. Isolauri E, Juntunen M, Rautanen T, Sillanaukee P, Koivula T. A human *Lactobacillus* strain (*Lactobacil casei* sp GG) promotes recovery from acute diarrhea in children. *Pediatrics*, **88** (1991) 90–97.

63. Isolauri E, Aila M, Mykkanen H, Ling WH, Salminen S. Oral bacteriotherapy for viral gastroenteritis. *D Dis. Sci.*, **39** (1994) 2595–2600.

64. Shornikova AV, Casas IA, Mykkanen H, Salo E, Vesikari T. Bacteriotherapy with *Lactobacillus reuteri* rotavirus gastroenteritis. *Pediatr. Infect. Dis. J.*, **16** (1997) 1103–1107.

65. Saint-Marc T, Blehaut H, Touraine JL. AIDS-related diarrhea: a double blind trial of *Saccharomyces boulard Sem. Hop.*, **71** (1995) 735–741.

66. Chapoy P. Traitement des diarrhees aigues infantiles: essai contrôlé de *Saccharomyces boulardii*. *A Pediatr.*, **32** (1985) 561–563.

67. Surawiscz CM, McFarland LV, Elmer GW, Chinn J. Treatment of recurrent *Clostridium difficile* colitis w vancomycin and *Saccharomyces boulardii*. *Am. J. Gastroenterol.*, **84** (1989) 1285–1287.

68. Mcfarland LV, Surawicz CM, Greenberg RN, et al. A randomized placebo-controlled trial of *Saccharomy boulardii* in combination with standard antibiotics for *Clostridium difficile* disease. *JAMA*, **271** (1994) 191 1918.

69. Gorbach SL, Chang TW, Goldin B. Successful treatment of relapsing *Clostridium difficile* colitis with *L tobacillus* GG. *Lancet*, **2** (1987) 1519.

70. Biller JA, Katz AJ, Flores AF, Buie TM, Gorbach SL. Treatment of recurrent *Clostridium difficile* colitis w *Lactobacillus* GG. *J. Pediatr. Gastroenterol. Nutr.*, **21** (1995) 224–226.

71. Andrews PJ, Barnes P, Borody TJ. Chronic constipation reversed by restoration of bowel flora. A case a a hypothesis. *Eur. J. Gastroenterol. Hepatol.*, **4** (1992) 245–247.

72. Celik AF, Tomlin J, Read NW. The effect of oral vancomycin on chronic idiopathic constipation. *Alime Pharmacol. Ther.*, **9** (1995) 63–68.

73. Mollenbrink M, Bruckschen E. Treatment of chronic constipation with physiologic *Escherichia coli* bacter Results of a clinical study of the effectiveness and tolerance of microbiological therapy with the *E. coli* Nis 1917 strain (Mutaflor). *Med. Klin.*, **89** (1994) 587–593.

74. Grimaud JC, Bouvier JG, Bertolini JG, Salducci J, Chiarelli P, Bouley C. Effects du lait fermenté content du Bifidobacterium sur le temps de transit colique. *Gastroenterol. Clin. Biol.*, **17** (1993) A127.

75. Mance S, Turchet P, Raimondi A, Antoine JM. Cayuéla C, Postaire E, Lucas C. Effects of a milk ferment by Bifidobacterium SP. Dn_173010 (BIO™) on the oro-fecal transit time in elderly. *Gut*, **45** (1999) A32

76. Bartram HP, Scheppach W, Gerlach S, Ruckdeschel G, Kelber E, Kasper H. Does yoghurt enriched wi Bifidobacrterium longum affect colonic microbiology and fecal metabolites in healthy subjects? *Am. J. Cl Nutr.*, **59** (1994) 428–432.

77. Gionchetti P, Rizzello F, Venturi A, et al. Oral bacteriotherapy as maintenance treatment in patients w chronic pouchitis: a double-blind, placebo-controlled trial. *Gastroenterology*, **119** (2000) 305–309.

78. Friedman G, George J. Treatment of refractory pouchitis with prebiotic and probiotic therapy. *Gastroent ology*, **118** (2000) A778.

79. Husebye E, Hellstrom PM, Midtvedt T. Intestinal microflora stimulates myoelectric activity of rat sm intestine by promoting cyclic initiation and aboral propagation of migrating myoelectric complex. *Dig. D Sci.*, **39** (1994) 946–956.

80. Pimentel M, Chow EJ, Lin HC. Eradication of small intestinal bacterial overgrowth reduces symptoms irritable bowel syndrome. *Am. J. Gastroenterol.*, **95** (2000) 3503–3506.

81. Da-Rong Z, Xiao-Xv D, Takahashi M, Bao Y. Intestinal microflora changes in patients with irritable bow syndrome after ingestion of *Clostridium butyricum* preparation. *Chin. J. Gastroenterol.*, **3** (1998).

82. Nobaek S, Johansson M-L, Molin G, Ahrne S, Jeppsson B. Alteration of intestinal microflora is associat with reduction in abdominal bloating and pain in patients with irritable bowel syndrome. *Am. J. Gastroentero* **95** (2000) 1222–1238.

83. O'Sullivan MA, O'Morain CA. Bacterial supplementation in the irritable bowel syndrome. A randomis double-blind placebo-controlled crossover study. *Digest. Liver Dis.*, **32** (2000) 294–301.

84. Blaser MJ. Microbial causation of the chronic idiopathic inflammatory bowel diseases. *Inflamm. Bowel Dis.*, **3** (1997) 225–229.

85. Campieri M, Gionchetti P. Bacteria as the cause of ulcerative colitis. *Gut*, **48** (2001) 132–135.

86. Isolauri E. Probiotics and gut inflammation. *Curr. Opin. Gastroenterol.*, **15** (1999) 534–537.

87. Kruis W, Schutz E, Fric P. Double-blind comparison of an oral *Escherichia coli* preparation and mesalazine in maintaining remission of ulcerative colitis. *Aliment. Pharmacol. Ther.*, **11** (1997) 853–859.

88. Rembacken BJ, Snelling AM, Hawkey PM, Chalmers DM, Axon AT. Non-pathogenic *Escherichia coli* versus mesalazine for the treatment of ulcerative colitis: a randomised trial. *Lancet*, **354** (1999) 635–639.

89. Venturi A, Gionchetti F, Rizello F, et al. Impact on the composition of the fecal flora by a new probiotic preparation: preliminary data on maintenance treatment of patients with ulcerative colitis. *Aliment. Pharmacol. Ther.*, **13** (1999) 1103–1108.

90. Rizzello F, Gionchetti P, Venturi A, et al. Prophylaxis of postoperative recurrence of Crohns disease combination of antibiotic and probiotic versus mesalazine. *Digest. Liver Dis.*, **32** (2000) A69.

91. Guslandi M, Mezzi G, Massimo S, Testoni PA. *Saccharomyces boulardii* in maintenance treatment of Crohns disease. *Dig. Dis. Sci.*, **45** (2000) 1462–1464.

92. Schulz M, Sartor RB. Probiotics and inflammatory bowel diseases. *Am. J. Gastroenterol.*, **95** (2000) S19–S21.

93. Persky SE, Brandt LJ. Treatment of recurrent *Clostridium difficile*-associated diarrhea by donated stool directly through a colonoscope. *Am. J. Gastroenterol.*, **95** (200) 3283–3285.

94. Bowden TA, Mansberger AR, Lykins LE. Pseudomembranous enterocolitis: mechanism of restoring floral homeostasis. *Am. Surg.*, **47** (1981) 178–183.

95. Eiseman B, Silen W, Bascom GS, Kauvar AJ. Fecal enema as an adjunct in the treatment of pseudomembranous enterocolitis. *Surgery*, **44** (1958) 854–859.

96. Schwan A, Sjolin S, Trottestam U. Relapsing *Clostridium difficile* enterocolitis cured by rectal infusion of homologous faeces. *Lancet*, **2** (1983) 845.

97. Tvede M, Rask-Madsen J. Bacteriotherapy for chronic relapsing *Clostridium difficile* diarrhea in six patients. *Lancet*, **1** (1989) 1156–1160.

98. Flotterod O, Hopen G. Refractory *Clostridium difficile* infection. Untraditional treatment of antibiotic-induced colitis. *Tidsskr. Nor. Laegeforen.*, **111** (1991) 1364–1365.

99. Paterson DL, Irdell J, Whitby M. Putting back the bugs: bacterial treatment relieves chronic diarrhea. *Med. J. Aust.*, **160** (1994) 232–233.

100. Lund-Tonnesen S, Berstad A, Schreiner A, Midtvedt T. *Clostridium difficile*-associated diarrhea treated with homologous feces. *Tidsskr. Nor. Laegeforen.*, **118** (1998) 1027–1030.

101. Gustafsson A, Lund-Tonnesen S, Berstad A, Midtvedt T, Norin E. Fecal short-chain fatty acids in patients with antibiotic-associated diarrhea before and after fecal enema treatment. *Scand. J. Gastroenterol.*, **33** (1998) 721–727.

102. Gorbach SL. Lactic acid bacteria and human health. *Ann. Med.*, **22** (1990) 37–41.

103. Mahida YR, Rose F, Chan WC. Antimicrobial peptides in the gastrointestinal tract. *Gut*, **40** (1997) 161–163.

104. Gustaffson A, Berstad A, Lund-Tonnesen S, Midtvedt T, Norin E. The effect of fecal enema on five microflora-associated characteristics in patients with antibiotic-associated diarrhea. *Scand. J. Gastroenterol.*, **34** (1999) 580–586.

105. Butt HL, Dunstan RH, McGregor NR, Roberts TK, Zerbes M, Klineberg IJ. Alteration of the bacterial microbial flora in chronic fatigue/pain patients. In *Proceedings of the Clinical and Scientific Basis of Chronic Fatigue Syndrome: From Myth Towards Management*. Sydney, Australia, Feb 1998.

106. Hart CA. Antibiotic resistance: an increasing problem? *BMJ*, **316** (1998) 1255–1256.

107. Borody TJ, Noonan S, Cole P, et al. Oral vancomycin can reverse idiopathic constipation. *Gastroenterology*, **96** (1989) A52.

108. Andrews PJ, Borody TJ. Putting back the bugs: bacterial treatment relieves chronic constipation and symptoms of irritable bowel syndrome. *Med. J. Aust.*, **159** (1993) 633–634.

109. Borody TJ, George L, Andrews PJ, et al. Bowel flora alteration: a potential cure for inflammatory bowel disease and irritable bowel syndrome? *Med. J. Aust.*, **150** (1989) 604.

110. Bennet JD, Brinkman M. Treatment of ulcerative colitis by implantation of normal colonic flora. *Lancet*, **1** (1989) 164.

111. Borody TJ. "Flora Power". Fecal bacteria cure chronic *C. difficile* diarrhea. *Am. J. Gastroenterol.*, **95** (2000) 3028–3029.

112. Pedone C, Bernabeu A, Postaire E, Bouley A, Reinert P. The effect of supplementation with milk fermented by *Lactobacillus casei* (strain DN-114) on acute diarrhea in children attending day care centres. *Int. J. Clin. Pract.*, **53** (1999) 179–184.

113. Saavadra JM, Baumann NA, Oung I, Pernan JA, Yolken RH. Feeding of *Bifidobacterium bifidum* and *Streptococcus thermophilus* to infants in hospital for prevention of diarrhea and shedding of rotavirus. *Lancet*, **344** (1994) 1046–1049.

114. Guandalini S, Pensabene L, Zibri MA, et al. *Lactobacillus* GG administered in oral rehydration solution to children with acute diarrhea: a multicentre European trial. *J. Pediatr. Gastroenterol.*, **30** (2000) 54–60.

115. Oberhelman R, Gilman RH, Sheen P, et al. A placebo controlled trial of *Lactobacillus* GG to prevent diarrhea in undernourished Peruvian children. *J. Paediatr.*, **134** (1999) 15–20.

116. Ribeiro H, Vanderhoof JA. Reduction of diarrheal illness following administration of *Lactobacillus plantarum* 299v in a daycare facility. *J. Pediatr. Gastroenterol. Nutr.*, **26** (1998) 561.

117. McFarland LV, Mulligan ME, Kwok RY, Stamm WE. Nosocomial acquisition of *Clostridium difficile* infection. *N. Engl. J. Med.*, **320** (1989) 204–210.

118. Gotz V, Romankiewicz JA, Moss J, Murray HW. Prophylaxis against ampicillin-associated diarrhea with a *Lactobacillus* preparation. *Am. J. Hosp. Pharm.*, **36** (1979) 754–757.

119. Tankanow RM, Ross MB, Ertel IJ, Dickinson DG, McCormick LS, Garfinkel JF. A double-blind, placebo-controlled study of the efficacy of Lactinex in the prophylaxis of amoxicillin-induced diarrhea. *DICP*, **24** (1990) 382.

120. Orrhage, Brismar B, Nord CE. Effects of supplements of *Bifidobacterium longum* and *Lactobacillus acidophilus* on the intestinal microbiota during administration of clindamycin. *Microb. Ecol. Health Dis.*, **7** (1994) 17–25.

121. Colombel JF, Cortot A, Neut C, Romond C. Yoghurt with *Bifidobacterium longum* reduces erythromycin-induced gastrointestinal effects. *Lancet*, **2** (1987) 43.

122. Siitonen S, Vapaatalo H, Salminen S, et al. Effect of *Lactobacillus* GG yoghurt in prevention of antibiotic associated diarrhea. *Ann. Med.*, **22** (1990) 57–59.

123. McFarland LV, Surawicz CM, Greenburg RN, et al. Prevention of beta lactam associated diarrhea by *Saccharomyces boulardii* compared to placebo. *Am. J. Gastroenterol.*, **90** (1995) 439–448.

124. Freeman LD, Hooper DR, Lathen DF, Nelson, Harrison WO, Anderson DS. Brief prophylaxis with doxycyline for the prevention of traveler's diarrhea. *Gastroenterology*, **4** (1983) 276–280.

125. Wistrom J, Norrby SR, Burman LG, Lundholm R, Jellheden B, Englund G. Norfloxacin versus placebo for prophylaxis against traveler's diarrhea. *J. Antimicrob. Chemother.*, **20** (1987) 563–574.

126. Dupont HL, Sulivan P, Evans DG, et al. Prevention of traveller's diarrhea (emporiatric enteritis): prophylactic administration of subsalicylate bismuth. *JAMA*, **243** (1980) 237–241.

127. Black FT, Andersen PL, Orskov J, Orskov F, Gaarslev K, Laulund S. Prophylactic efficacy of lactobacilli on traveler's diarrhea. In *Travel Medicine. Conference on International Travel Medicine 1.* Steffen R (ed.), Springer, Zurich, 1989, pp. 333–335.

128. Pozo-Olano JD, Warram JH, Gomez RG, Cavazos MG. Effect of a *Lactobacilli* preparation preparation on traveler's diarrhea. *Gastroenterology*, **74** (1978) 829–830.

129. Orksanen PJ, Salminen S, Saxelin M, et al. Prevention of travellers diarrhea by *Lactobacillus* GG. *Ann. Med.*, **22** (1990) 53–56.

130. Kollaritsch H, Holst H, Grobara P, Wiedermann G. Prophylaxe der Reisediarrhee mit *Saccharomyces boulardii*. *Fortschr. Med.*, **111** (1993) 153–156.

131. Katelaris PH. Probiotic control of diarrheal disease. *Asian Pac. J. Clin. Nutr.*, **5** (1995) 39–43.

132. Hirayama K, Rafter J. The role of lactic acid bacteria in colon cancer prevention: mechanistic considerations. *Antonie van Leeuwenhoek*, **76** (1999) 391–394.

133. Parodi PW. The role of intestinal bacteria in the causation and prevention of cancer: modulation by diet and probiotics. *Am. J. Dairy Technol.*, **54** (1999) 103–121.

134. Wollowski I, Rechkemmer G, Pool-Zobel BL. Protective role of probiotics and prebiotics in colon cancer. *Am. J. Clin. Nutr.*, **73** (2001) S451–S455.

135. McIntosh GH, Royle PJ, Playne MJ. A probiotic strain of *L. acidophilus* reduces DMH-induced large intestinal tumors in male Sprague-Dawley rats. *Nutr. Cancer*, **35** (1999) 153–159.

136. Gorbach S. Probiotics and gastrointestinal health. *Am. J. Gastroenterol.*, **95** (2000) S2–S4.

137. Goldin B. The metabolic activity of the intestinal microflora and its role in colon cancer. *Nutr. Today*, **31** (1996) S24–S27.

138. Yamazaki K, Tsunoda A, Sibusawa M, et al. The effect of an oral administration of *Lactobacillus casei* strain Shirota on azoxymethane-induced colonic aberrant crypt foci and colon cancer in the rat. *Oncol. Rep.*, **7** (2000) 977–982.

139. Reddy BS. Possible mechanisms by which pro- and prebiotics influence carcinogenesis and tumor growth. *J. Nutr.*, **129** (1999) S1478–S1482.

140. Orrhage K, Sillerstrom E, Gustafsson JA, Nord CE, Rafter J. Binding of mutagenic heterocyclic amines by intestinal lacttic acid bacteria. *Mutat. Res.*, **311** (1994) 239–248.
141. Orrhage K. Impact of *Bifidobacterium longum* and *Lactobacillus acidophilus* on the intestinal microflora and bioavailability of some food mutagens. PhD Thesis, Karolinska Institute, Stockholm, Sweden 1999.

11 Physiology and Pathophysiology of Colorectal Sensory Processes

Michael D. Crowell and Brian E. Lacy

1. INTRODUCTION

Pain referred to the abdomen is the symptom most commonly reported by patients evaluated in gastroenterology clinics. In many instances, abdominal pain is acute and short-lived, and symptoms resolve without a clear diagnosis being made. In other cases, the underlying cause is identified, treatment is initiated, and the pain is relieved. In some patients, however, abdominal pain becomes a chronic problem and may exist as an episodic or recurrent problem with multiple exacerbations over time, or as an intractable, persistent symptom that can be debilitating. Extensive diagnostic testing often fails to reveal an organic cause for the pain. These patients are often diagnosed with one of the functional gastrointestinal (GI) disorders, which include disorders of colonic afferent processes (e.g., colonic hypersensitivity), characteristic of disorders such as the irritable bowel syndrome (IBS). This chapter will focus on the physiology and pathophysiology of colorectal sensory processes and their relationship to chronic abdominal pain and functional GI pain.

To understand the complex nature of pain originating from the viscera, it is useful to analyze the stimulus, the nervous structures that encode, relay, and modify the stimulus, and finally the central processing that produces the perception of the sensation. The perception of acute pain begins with a specific stimulus. The GI viscera are, however, relatively insensitive to most stimuli, compared to skin and other somatic structures. Early reports consistently showed the abdominal organs to be generally insensitive to light touch, pinching, cutting, and even burning *(1–4)*. The poor correlation between injury and pain in the abdominal viscera led investigators to differentiate noxious from nociceptive stimuli. Cervero suggested that the term noxious

From: *Colonic Diseases*
Edited by: T. R. Koch © Humana Press Inc., Totowa, NJ

should be applied only to stimuli that signal the ". . . relationship between the stimulus and the integrity of the organism", whereas the term nociceptive should define the ". . . relationship between the stimulus and the nervous system of the subject" (5). These criteria infer that a noxious stimulus produces actual damage to the organ or tissue and may or may not be associated with the perception of pain, while a nociceptive stimulus produces affective and/or autonomic reflex responses and results in the perception of pain or discomfort. A single stimulus can be simultaneously noxious and nociceptive. For example, overdistention of hollow visceral organs produces both pain and tissue damage (noxious), but at lower levels, distention produces autonomic reflexes and the perception of pain (nociceptive) without damage to the organ system. Similarly, irradiation can produce severe damage to the visceral organs and tissue (noxious) without producing an immediate perception of pain (nociception). Therefore, visceral nociceptors can be operationally defined as sensory afferents that encode nociceptive stimuli from the periphery and produce autonomic reflexes or pseudoaffective responses and the perception of pain.

2. NEUROANATOMY OF VISCERAL PAIN PATHWAYS

Morphologically, visceral nociceptors consist of afferent fibers that terminate in free nerve endings. These receptors are located between the smooth muscle layers of hollow organs such as the colon, on their serosal surface, in the mesentery, and within the mucosa of the GI tract. The majority of afferent sensory fibers are small, nonmyelinated, and belong to the C-polymodal class (C-PMNs). These fibers are sensitive to mechanical, chemical, and thermal stimulation. A second major group of receptors are fine myelinated Aδ fibers, also called A-mechano-heat (AMH) receptors. These receptors respond predominantly to mechanical and thermal stimuli, although certain chemicals, such as bradykinin and capsaicin, are able to activate them (6). The receptive field of the Aδ fibers lies within the mucosa, while in uninflamed tissue, the receptive field of C-PMNs is located in the muscle layer, serosa, and mesentery. Inflammation in the gastrointestinal tract extends the receptive field of C-fibers to the mucosa (7,8).

Although not directly related to the sensation of pain from the viscera, the enteric nervous system (ENS) deserves mention. The cell bodies are located in the submucosal and myenteric plexuses and are intricately involved in the control of local reflexes, smooth muscle contractile patterns, absorption, and secretion. The ENS serves to integrate motor activity within the GI tract. These neurons do not project to the central nervous system directly, and therefore, do not appear to play a major role in the transmission of sensory information from the colon or the perception of visceral pain. However, the ENS modulates the local environment and may enhance or inhibit the activation of nociceptors through alteration in smooth muscle tone.

2.1. Classic Afferent Pain Pathways

The neuronal pathways that mediate sensation of abdominal pain arising from the colon involve three levels of neurons between the abdominal viscera and the cerebral cortex (Fig. 1). First order neurons travel from the viscera to the spinal cord, second order neurons link the spinal cord and the brain stem, and third order neurons travel from the brain stem to higher levels of the brain. After leaving the viscus they innervate, the first order nerves pass through the adjacent autonomic nerve plexus. In general, the plexus appears as a web of nerve tissue associated with the major artery supplying the organ (e.g., celiac, hepatic, superior mesenteric). These plexuses then coalesce to form ganglia from which the afferent fibers then travel. Fibers run within the regional splanchnic nerve to the associated sympathetic chain parallel to the spinal cord on either side. They then proceed to the spinal nerve

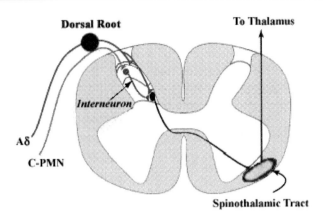

Fig. 1. The primary neuronal pathway that mediates the sensation of pain from the colon involves three levels of neurons between the abdominal viscera and the cerebral cortex. First order neurons travel from the viscera through the dorsal root ganglia to the spinal cord. The postsynaptic (i.e., second order) neurons that mediate abdominal visceral sensory processes begin in the superficial laminae of the dorsal horn, cross the midline to the contralateral side, and then travel cephalad within the ventrolateral quadrant of the spinal cord. These neurons run in several ascending pathways (mainly the spinothalamic and spinoreticular tracts) and synapse within several thalamic and reticular nuclei, including the pons and medulla. Third order neurons travel from the brain stem to higher levels of the brain.

via the white ramus communicans and enter the spinal cord and synapse in the dorsal horn, predominantly in laminae I, II, and V (9–12). The cell bodies of the first order neurons lie in the dorsal root ganglia.

Virtually all nerve fibers that carry visceral nociceptive afferent information travel with the sympathetic nervous system (i.e., thoracolumbar input) (9,10,13–15). Many afferents travel via parasympathetic vagal pathways and are thought to primarily serve regulatory autonomic functions. These enteroceptors consist of mechanoreceptors that respond to light touch, chemoreceptors sensitive to acidity, alkalinity, and nutrients, and osmoreceptors sensitive to changes in the extracellular fluid. Thermoreceptors are also present and, under certain conditions, may contribute to nociception. Vagal fibers, however, are thought to have little direct effect on pain or pressure perception under normal conditions (16,17). This observation is based largely on investigations that have demonstrated that stimulation of the splanchnic nerves produced pain, whereas stimulation of the vagus nerve did not (18). Additionally, inhibition of chronic pain and experimentally induced pain arising from the viscera can be achieved by sectioning the dorsal roots of spinal nerves, while the vagus nerve remains intact (19,20). Recent data, however, have shown that the parasympathetic fibers serve a modulatory role in the transmission of pain from the periphery to the central nervous system (CNS) and from the CNS to the periphery, possibly through gating mechanisms. For example, electrical simulation of the vagus inhibits some, and facilitates other, spinothalamic tract neurons associated with pain (21), while vagotomy at the cervical level attenuates the antinociceptive effects of analgesics (22). These observations suggest that spinal visceral afferents interact with vagal afferents at the level of the brainstem and that complex interactions of these two groups of afferents are likely to occur at this level.

The postsynaptic (i.e., second order) neurons that mediate abdominal visceral sensory processes begin in the superficial laminae of the dorsal horn, cross the midline to the contralateral side, and then travel cephalad within the ventrolateral quadrant of the spinal cord. These neurons run in several ascending pathways (mainly the spinothalamic and spinoreticular tracts) and synapse within several thalamic and reticular formation nuclei of the pons and medulla *(9,11)*. Few data are available regarding the pathways of third order neurons that transmit visceral pain sensation to higher brain centers, but by analogy to somatic pain pathways, they probably travel widely throughout the brain. By this analogy, pain pathway projections from the spinothalamic tract travel primarily to the somatosensory cortex, which seems to subserve the sensory discriminative components of pain perception that are concerned with the quality and localization of the pain. Third order neurons that synapse with spinoreticular tract neurons seem to terminate largely in the limbic system and frontal cortex and are thought to subserve the motivational affective aspects of pain perception, known clinically as the aversive or unpleasant features *(23,24)*.

2.2. Newly Discovered Spinal Pathways

According to the classical model of nociceptive transmission, sensory pathways, either somatic or visceral, along with sensations of temperature and touch, are conducted in the anterolateral spinal cord via the spinothalamic and spinomesencephalic tracts. This view has recently been seriously challenged with the findings that visceral pain may be relayed in the dorsal spinal column. This spinal tract has long been held to subserve only the "finer" qualities of sensation, such as joint position sense and two-point discrimination. This postsynaptic dorsal column pathway may be relatively specific to visceral sensation in that it does not appear to play a significant role in cutaneous pain *(25–26)*. In contrast, both mechanical and chemical irritation of viscera results in stimulation of postsynaptic dorsal column cells as well as cells of the gracile nucleus *(27)*. The gracile nucleus in turn projects to the contralateral ventral posterolateral (VPL) nucleus in the thalamus. Evidence for the functional importance of this pathway comes from studies in patients with intractable pelvic cancer pain in whom a limited midline myelotomy resulted in complete or near-complete relief of pain *(28–30)*.

3. NEUROPHYSIOLOGY OF VISCERAL PAIN
3.1. Nociceptive Encoding

The encoding of nociceptive information from the viscera and the transmission of this information to the CNS has generated considerable controversy. Three theories of peripheral encoding are at the forefront of this debate: (i) the patterning theory; (ii) the intensity theory; and (iii) the specificity theory. The patterning theory suggests that peripheral afferent neurons fire in highly specific temporospatial patterns that can differentiate between various sensory events *(31)*. This theory of peripheral encoding has received little electrophysiologic support, however. The intensity theory of pain transmission suggests that both innocuous and noxious stimuli act on an identical group of nonspecific afferents and that these different sensations can be distinguished simply by the frequency of neuronal firing *(32,33)*. Consequently, the intensity of neuronal stimulation would directly correlate with the intensity of neuronal firing and sophisticated central processes would act to summate and decode incoming signals. Lastly, the specificity theory proposes that specific populations of afferent fibers exist that respond only to noxious stimulation and, thus, represent the recruitment of specific nociceptors *(34)*. Additional theories, including central and peripheral convergence, and peripheral transduction, have been proposed to explain the facilitation or inhibition of sensory information from the viscera to the CNS.

After many years of debate, investigators have begun to make significant progress at integrating these theories into a more comprehensive model of peripheral encoding. Recently three types of afferent mechanoreceptors were identified according to their discharge frequency

(17). These afferents were described functionally as: (i) low-threshold mechanoreceptors that respond to innocuous stimulation; (ii) high-threshold mechanoreceptors that respond only to noxious stimulation; and (iii) wide-dynamic range mechanoreceptors that fire to both innocuous and noxious stimuli. All vagal mechanoreceptors were found to be of the low-threshold type, whereas splanchnic afferents were found to be a mixture of the wide-dynamic range and the high-threshold fibers. Subsequently, these investigators demonstrated that vagal fibers discharged maximally during both peristaltic activity and luminal distention, whereas only a small percentage of splanchnic afferents fired during contractile events, while maximal firing rates occurred during luminal distention. It has been suggested that the wide-dynamic range of the splanchnic mechanoreceptors supports the hypothesis of a homogeneous population of visceral afferents responsible for encoding both regulatory information and innocuous and noxious stimuli within the gut *(16)*. To be effective, this hypothesis requires the progressive recruitment of intensity-encoding afferents and a central mechanism responsible for decoding intensity-summation signals from the periphery.

These electrophysiologic data lend support to the specificity theory by demonstrating the existence of high-threshold populations of afferent fibers that only respond to noxious intensities of stimulation and that represent the recruitment of specific nociceptors. These studies identified a relatively large number of visceral afferent fibers that appear to respond only at levels of abdominal distention associated with pain. These fibers were found to make up approx 30% of all distention-sensitive fibers *(17,35)*. These observations have led proponents of both theories to acknowledge the existence of high-threshold fibers and silent nociceptors, and investigators have now begun attempts to incorporate them into more comprehensive integrative theories of pain transmission.

Cervero and Jaenig *(36)* have proposed a new model to account for afferent sensory innervation of visceral organs that also rely on three similar types of nociceptive neurons. Under normal circumstances, the low-threshold intensity coding afferent neurons (LTi) relay information about regulatory function and nonpainful stimulation through specific second order spinal neurons. These afferents are of the wide-dynamic range type described by Sengupta and respond to stimuli from very low through the high intensities. It has been suggested that these sensory fibers emanating from visceral organs such as the stomach and colon may provide information in a graded manner, such that sensations of mild distention can be distinguished from fullness or intense pain *(37)*.

If the stimulus intensity in the LTi exceeds a predefined level, these neurons participate in the transmission of nociceptive information to the CNS by activating different second order neurons in the spinal cord that results in the perception of pain. At this set point, dedicated nociceptors or high-threshold intensity coding neurons (HTi) are also activated and transmit nociceptive information to the CNS (Fig. 2A). A third type of neuron, called silent nociceptors, has recently been identified. These nociceptors are generally quiet and do not participate in the transmission of either vegetative or nociceptive information to the CNS, even during intense stimulation. However, these neurons can become activated through injury, inflammation, and central sensitization. Once sensitized, these fibers transmit pain signals to the CNS during even mild stimulation that occurs with normal regulatory activity in the viscera (Fig. 2B). These nociceptors may provide the physiologic mechanism for complaints of persistent or chronic abdominal pain in patients without underlying organic pathophysiology *(38–40)*.

In summary, the data currently available on visceral afferents and the transmission of innocuous and noxious signals to the CNS require a reevaluation of the functional categories of visceral afferents and nociceptors. The current encoding theories of intensity and specificity need to be integrated into a more realistic model of visceral afferent processing that

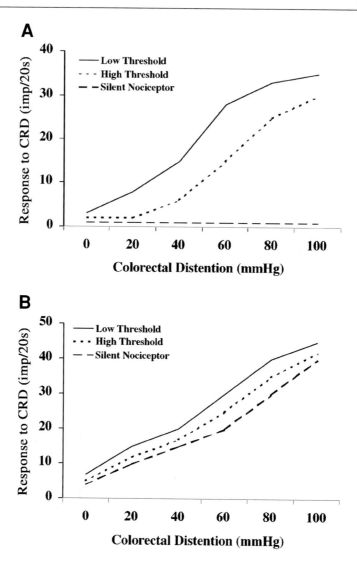

Fig. 2. When the stimulus intensity in the LTi mechanoreceptors exceed a predefined level, these neurons participate in the transmission of nociceptive information to the CNS by activating different second order neurons in the spinal cord that results in the perception of pain. At this set point, dedicated nociceptors or HTi are also activated and transmit nociceptive information to the CNS. Silent nociceptors are generally quiet and do not participate in the transmission of either vegetative or nociceptive information to the CNS, even during intense stimulation. However, these neurons can become sensitized and facilitate transmission of pain signals to the CNS during even mild stimulation.

accounts for chronic persistent pain. New models must incorporate recently recognized functional differences in sensory receptors and the coexistence of different neurophysiologic mechanisms in many visceral organs.

4. GATING MECHANISMS

Melzack and Wall *(41)* proposed the gate control theory of pain transmission, which states that the perception of pain is dependent on both the interaction of gating mechanisms within the spinal cord (dorsal horn) and in the brain stem. This model largely focuses on the interaction

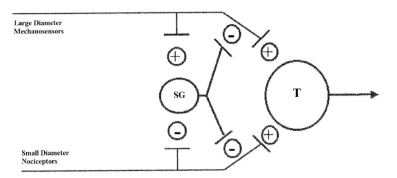

Fig. 3. The gate control theory proposes that large and small fiber sensory afferents converge on and activate transmission cell neurons in the dorsal horn, opening the gate for the transmission of nociceptive signals from the viscera to the brain stem. Large diameter mechanosensory afferents from visceral organs deliver excitatory signals to the interneurons and inhibit transmission cell neurons, whereas small diameter nociceptive sensory afferent fibers deliver inhibitory signals to the interneurons and facilitate the central transmission of nociceptive signals. Interneurons found in the substantia gelatinosa of the dorsal horn can inhibit transmission cell neurons resulting in analgesic effects.

of first order neurons from the viscera with second order neurons in the dorsal horn of the spinal cord. Figure 3 illustrates large and small fiber sensory afferents from the periphery converging on and activating transmission cell neurons in the dorsal horn. This activation opens the gate for the transmission of nociceptive signals from the viscera to the brain stem. Large diameter mechanosensory afferents from visceral organs deliver excitatory signals to the interneurons and inhibit transmission cell neurons, whereas small diameter nociceptive sensory afferent fibers deliver inhibitory signals to the interneurons and facilitate the central transmission of nociceptive signals *(42)*. Finally, interneurons found in the substantia gelatinosa of the dorsal horn can inhibit transmission cell neurons and produce analgesic effects.

The CNS may also directly modulate visceral pain. Descending inhibitory pathways, from the medulla and reticular formation converge in the substantia gelatinosa of the dorsal horn, interact with the interneurons, and inhibit transmission cell neurons. This can alter the perception of pain. Specific descending inhibitory inputs have been identified that are associated with abdominal visceral afferents. Additionally, stimulation of the cortex can activate these interneurons, which may be the neurologic basis for CNS modulation of pain. These observations may also partially explain the mechanisms responsible for the modulation of pain thresholds in patients with anxiety disorders and depression.

Empirical findings suggest that all spinal cord neurons that receive afferents from the viscera also receive afferents from muscle or cutaneous somatic receptors *(10)*. At the neuronal level, studies have shown that cutaneous stimulation has both facilitory and inhibitory effects on visceral afferents. Simultaneous stimulation of both receptive fields produces a greater response in the spinal neuron, and sequential stimulation produces inhibition in both directions *(43)*. Clinically, this may be important, because pain, which occurs simultaneously in both muscle and the colon, could produce a lower sensation of pain than would be expected.

The activation of modulatory circuits by somatic stimuli may significantly influence reflex and visceral sensory responses to distention. This hypothesis was recently evaluated in eight healthy human volunteers *(44)*. Graded isobaric distentions were performed in the stomach and duodenum while transcutaneous electrical stimulation was simultaneously applied to the hand at two different intensities. An intensity-dependent reduction in the perception of gut distention was observed. No significant effect was noted on reflex gastric relaxation to duodenal distention. The authors concluded that somatic stimulation reduces perception of gut distention without interfering with local reflex responses.

5. REFERRED PAIN

Clinical and experimental evidence have clearly shown that visceral pain is poorly localized and temporally dynamic. A stimulus producing pain, such as noxious balloon distention, within the hollow organs of the gastrointestinal tract may result in widely differing pain reports and referral sites in different patients. Pain may be reported at sites far removed from the organ distended (45). These observations are collectively defined as referred pain. The mechanisms of referred pain are complex and are thought to include both peripheral and central processes.

Sensation and perception of pain from the abdominal viscera is largely mediated by sympathetic mechanosensitive afferents. Compared to somatic structures, very few visceral sensory afferents enter the spinal cord at a given level. Additionally, the same splanchnic sensory neuron may originate from multiple visceral organs, and stimulation of a single splanchnic afferent entering the dorsal horn can activate up to 50% of second order neurons at that level (10). Consequently, a small number of sensory afferents can activate a significant number of spinothalamic tract neurons and result in poor localization of visceral pain.

As previously discussed, all spinal cord neurons that receive afferents from the viscera also receive afferents from muscle or cutaneous somatic receptors. Afferent fibers from various structures enter the dorsal horn of the spinal cord and then converge with second order neurons in common spinothalamic projection pathways. Therefore, activation of sensory afferents from different visceral or somatic structures may activate the same second order spinal neurons. This convergence–projection theory of pain transmission suggests that information from the periphery may be misinterpreted centrally and result in the inability to accurately differentiate the origination of certain nociceptive signals. Therefore, somatic structures, which are more densely innervated and more commonly stimulated than visceral structures, are more likely to be identified as the source of persistent pain. Cutaneous dermatomes offer a clinically useful method of isolating the origin of pain from the abdominal viscera.

Pain originating from the distal esophagus, stomach, proximal duodenum, liver, biliary tree, and pancreas (T5–T6 to T8–T9) is generally referred between the xiphoid process and the umbilicus. The midgut structures (small intestine, appendix, ascending colon, and proximal portions of the transverse colon) are innervated in spinal segments T8–T11 to L1, and have pain referred to the periumbilical region. The distal transverse colon, descending colon, and rectosigmoid (T11–L1) are generally referred to dermatomes located between the umbilicus and the pubis, and in the perineal regions (42). Although significant overlap is evident, knowledge of these characteristic landmarks of pain referral may be helpful in clinical practice.

6. TRANSMISSION AND CONTROL OF AFFERENT SIGNALS

6.1. Sympathetic and Parasympathetic Contribution to Pain

Although high concentrations of norepinephrine do not directly produce C-fiber activation, there is considerable data to suggest a role for the sympathetic nervous system in peripheral hyperalgesia (46). Sensitization of nociceptors may occur indirectly via adrenergically mediated release of prostaglandins from nearby cells (47). However, there are few, if any, studies that have examined the contribution of the sympathetic nervous system to the development of visceral sensitization.

Parasympathetic fibers from the mucosa can also modulate pain transmission, but do not appear to mediate pain directly. Of note, electrical stimulation of the abdominal vagus generally induces nausea and vomiting, but not pain (16). It has been shown that electrical stimulation of vagal afferents can activate descending pathways, which inhibit some, and facilitate other, spinothalamic tract neurons in the spinal cord (22). However, stimulation of vagal afferents more often inhibits, rather than facilitates, pain transmission (21).

6.2. Smooth Muscle Tone and Afferent Transmission

Although little correlation has been found between the presence of very high amplitude propagated contractions in the colon and reports of abdominal pain (48,49) some episodes of pain may be associated with discrete contractile events (50). Sensory neurons respond "in series" with smooth muscle fibers (51). Therefore, many of the neurons in the brain stem that fire in response to noxious colonic stimuli, also fire in response to spontaneous contractions (52). Atropine, which reduces smooth muscle tone in the gut and increases the distention volume required to produce pain, does not significantly alter the pressure required to produce pain (53). Consequently, smooth muscle tone and contractility may influence the threshold for excitation of receptors responsible for pain transmission either directly or indirectly.

Technological advances over the last few years have generated a renewed interest in the clinical evaluation of visceral sensation and perception. These advances have allowed researchers to investigate the influence of more dynamic properties of smooth muscle on visceral perception. Recent evidence has shown that adaptive relaxation of smooth muscle tone occurs in response to rectal balloon distention at a constant pressure (54). These data suggest that the healthy rectum actively adapts to chronic stretch of the rectal wall, which is a critical response for the normal short-term storage function of the rectum. Impaired adaptive relaxation may contribute to symptoms in patient populations with chronic recurrent abdominal pain and urgency. Crowell and Musial (55) compared changes in rectal volume in healthy controls and in patients with IBS during continuous rectal distention at pressures associated with first sensation and a moderate urge to defecate. They concluded that in IBS patients, symptoms of urgency and lower thresholds for abdominal pain might, in fact, be due to impaired adaptive relaxation of the rectum in response to chronic distention. This results in greater stimulation of visceral mechanoreceptors with luminal distention and increased levels of pain in patients with IBS as compared to normal volunteers.

6.3. Current Concepts

The complexity of visceral sensory afferent processing and the perception of abdominal pain are only partially revealed in the preceding discussion. Chronic visceral pain is directly influenced by temporal changes in both central and peripheral mechanisms. Primary hyperalgesia can be defined as a shift in the stimulus–response curve that results in a decrease in the stimulus intensity required to elicit or maintain nociceptor activation. The observed shift in the stimulus–response curve may lead to a primary hyperalgesia resulting from changes in the responsiveness of visceral afferent fibers with repetitive stimulation or inflammation. Electrophysiologic investigations of visceral sensory afferents following repetitive stimulation have yielded somewhat inconsistent results. Direct sensitization of nociceptors measured as changes in the discharge rates were not evident in studies of colonic or esophageal mechanosensitive afferents (56,57). However, Cervero and Sann (58) reported long-lasting post-discharges and increased background activity in high-threshold mechanosensitive afferents following repeated noxious stimulation of the ureter, which the authors interpreted as nociceptive sensitization. Evaluation of the stimulus–response curves of mechanosensitive afferents following the local administration of chemical irritants and the induction of local inflammation has more consistently demonstrated nociceptive sensitization *(58)*. Central mechanisms are also extremely important in the development of hyperalgesia. Sensitization of tissues adjacent to the area of immediate injury and central hyperexcitability result from secondary hyperalgesia *(59,61)*.

It has been suggested that both primary and secondary hyperalgesia play a role in chronic pain conditions, such as the IBS. Considerable clinical evidence exists to support this observation. For example, a significant number of patients with functional GI disorders experience pain at distension pressures or volumes that produce, at best, normal internal sensation in healthy volunteers *(38)*. Furthermore, IBS patients have a significantly lower threshold for the perception of non-noxious distension of the gut. Mechanisms for both primary (peripheral) and secondary (central) hyperalgesia have been proposed and may be explained through nociceptor sensitization and central plasticity *(62)*. These mechanisms may be different from, or in addition to, those described in the preceding sections, which were based on experiments lasting only up to several hours. More long-lasting or even permanent hyperalgesia, which typically accompanies functional bowel disorders, may occur due to a number of different reasons including: (i)tissue irritation which occurs in the neonatal state, which is a particularly vulnerable period; (ii)the loss of descending inhibitory modulation; (iii) the presence of inhibitory interneurons in the spinal cord; and (iv) the development of neuroplastic changes. An example of which is the enlargement of dorsal horn cells that occurs in response to chronic peripheral irritation.

How do these concepts tie in with what is known or assumed about conditions such as the IBS? Any acute or chronic mucosal inflammation can produce visceral hyperalgesia by both peripheral sensitization and central hyperexcitability *(38)*. These changes are usually transient in that they subside after the resolution of the original inflammation. Some patients, however, may be predisposed (possibly on a genetic basis) to a more permanent change in the central processing of pain. According to this theory, the lack of overt inflammation or disruption of tissue architecture in patients with IBS is explained by the fact that the initiating event was transient, but left persistent changes in its wake that resulted in central hyperalgesia. Although these hypotheses generally stress changes in the afferent system as the agent responsible for the generation of symptoms, they by no means exclude a role for other clinically relevant phenomenon. Thus, motor events in the gut, if prolonged and abnormally excessive, may also result in state of permanent sensitization akin to other forms of peripheral noxious stimulation. Repeated distension of the colon in humans (to 60 mm Hg) has been shown to increase the area of pain referral in the short term *(59)*, whereas less intense (< 40 mm Hg) stimuli do not alter sensation *(63)*. Similar findings were reported in a study that evaluated systematic changes in the volume and pressure profiles required to maintained a constant pain rating over 30 consecutive phasic distention trials *(55)*. In addition, of course, contractile events (normal or exaggerated) could be perceived as painful in patients with chronically sensitized nociception.

REFERENCES

1. Hertz AF. The sensibility of the alimentary canal in health and disease. *Lancet*, **1** (1911) 1051–1056.
2. Ray BS, Neill CL. Abdominal visceral sensation in man. *Ann. Surg.*, **126** (1947) 709–724.
3. Bentley FH, Smithwick RH. Visceral pain produced by balloon distension of the jejunum. *Lancet*, **i–ii** (1940) 389–391.
4. Sherrington CS. Cutaneous sensation. In *Textbook of Physiology*. Vol. 2., Shafer EA (ed.), Pentland, London, UK, 1900, pp. 920–1001.

5. Cervero F. Sensory innervation of the visceral: Peripheral basis of visceral pain. *Physiol. Rev.*, **74** (1994) 95–138.

6. Rang HP, Bevan S, Dray A. Chemical activation of nociceptive peripheral neurones. *Br. Med. Bull.*, **47** (1991) 534–548.

7. Ness TJ, Gebhart GF. Visceral pain: a review of experimental studies. *Pain*, **41** (1990) 167–234.

8. McMahon S, Koltzenburg M. The changing role of primary afferent neurons in pain. *Pain*, **43** (1990) 269–272.

9. Cervero F. Visceral nociception: peripheral and central aspects of visceral nociceptive systems. *Philos. Trans. R. Soc. Lond.*, **308** (1985) 325.

10. Cervero F, Tattersall JEH. Somatic and visceral sensory integration in the thoracic spinal cord. In *Visceral Sensation*. Cervero F, Morrison JFB (eds.), Elsevier, Amsterdam, 1986, p. 189

11. Willis WD, Coggeshall, RE. *Sensory Mechanisms of the Spinal Cord*. Plenum Press, New York, NY, 1991, pp. 153–215.

12. Fields HL. Pain from deep tissues and referred pain. In *Pain*. Fields HL (ed.), McGrawÄHill, New York, NY, 1987, pp. 133–169.

13. Cervero F. Neurophysiology of gastrointestinal pain. *Baillieres Clin. Gastroenterol.*, **2** (1988) 183.

14. Mayer EA, Raybould HE. Role of visceral afferent mechanisms in functional bowel disorders. *Gastroenterology*, **99** (1990) 1688–1704.

15. White JC, Sweet WH. Pain in abdominal visceral disease. In *Pain and the Neurosurgeon*. White JC, Sweet WH (eds.), Charles C Thomas, Springfield, IL, 1969, p. 560.

16. Grundy D. Mechanoreceptors in the gastrointestinal tract. *J. Smooth Muscle Res.*, **29** (1993) 37–46.

17. Sengupta JN, Saha JK, Goyal RK. Stimulus-response function studies of esophageal mechanosensitive nociceptors in sympathetic afferents of opossum. *J. Neurophysiol.*, **64** (1990) 796–812.

18. Cannon B. A method of stimulating autonomic nerves in the unanesthetized cat with observations on the motor and sensory effects. *Am. J. Physiol.*, **105** (1933) 366–372.

19. White JC. Sensory innervation of the viscera. Studies of visceral afferent neurones in man based on neurosurgical procedures for the relief of intractable pain. *Res. Pub. Assoc. Res. Nerv. Ment. Dis.*, **23** (1943) 373–390.

20. Stulrajter V, Pavelasek J, Strauss P, Duda P, Gorkin AP. Some neuronal, autonomic, and behavioral correlates of visceral Pain elicited by gall-bladder stimulation. *Act. Nerv. Sup. (Praha)*, **20** (1978) 203–209.

21. Ren K, Randich A, Gebhart GF. Effect of electrical stimulation of vagal afferents on spinothalamic tract cells in the rat. *Pain*, **44** (1991) 311–319.

22. Randich A, Thurston CL, Ludwig PS, Timmerman MR, Gebhart GF. Antinociception and cardiovascular responses produced by intravenous morphine: the role of vagal afferents. *Brain Res.*, **543** (1991) 256–270.

23. Fields HL. *Pain*. McGraw Hill, New York, NY, 1987, p. 41.

24. Melzack R, Wall PD. Brain mechanisms. In *The Challenge of Pain*. 2nd ed., Melzack R, Wall PD (eds.), Penguin Books, London, UK, 1988.

25. Giesler, Nahin RL, Madsen AM. Postsynaptic dorsal column pathway of the rat. *J. Neurophysiol.*, **51** (1984) 260–75.

26. Al-Chaer ED, Lawand NB, Westlund KN, Willis WD. Visceral nociceptive input into the ventral postero-lateral nucleus of the thalamus: a new function for the dorsal column pathway. *J. Neurophysiol.*, **76** (1996) 2661–2674.

27. Al-Chaer ED, Lawand NB, Westlund KN, Willis WD. Pelvic visceral input into the nucleus gracilis is largely mediated by the postsynaptic dorsal column pathway. *J. Neurophysiol.*, **76** (1996) 2675–2690

28. Gildenberg PL, Hirshberg RM. Limited myelotomy for the treatment of intractable cancer pain. *J. Neurol. Neurosurg. Psychiatry*, **47** (1984) 94–96.

29. Hirshberg RM, Al-Chaer ED, Lawand NB, Westlund KN, Willis WD. Is there a pathway in the posterior funiculus that signals visceral pain? *Pain*, **67** (1996) 291–305.

30. Hitchcock ER. Stereotactic cervical myelotomy. *J. Neurol. Neurosurg. Psychiatry*, **33** (1970) 224–230.

31. Sinclair DC. Cutaneous sensation and the doctrine of specific energy. *Brain*, **78** (1955) 584.

32. Jaenig W, Koltzenburg M. On the function of spinal primary afferent fibers supplying colon and urinary bladder. *J. Auton. Nerv. Syst.*, **30(Suppl)** (1990) 589–596.

33. Ness TJ, Gebhart GF. Characterization of superficial T13-L2 dorsal horn neurons encoding for colorectal distention in the rat: Comparison with neurons in deep laminae. *Brain Res.*, **8** (1989) 301–309.

34. Cervero F. Afferent activity evoked by natural stimulation of the biliary system in the ferret. *Pain*, **13** (1982) 137–151.

35. Cervero F, Sharkey KA. An electrophysiological and anatomical study of intestinal afferent fibers in the ra *J. Physiol.*, **401** (1988) 381–397.

36. Cervero F, Jaenig W. Visceral nociceptors: a new world order? *Trends Neurosci.*, **15** (1992) 374–378.

37. Mayer EM, Gebhart GF. Functional bowel disorders and the visceral hyperalgesia hypothesis. In *Basic an Clinical Aspects of Chronic Abdominal Pain.* Mayer EA, Raybould HE (eds.), Elsevier Science, New York NY, (1993) p. 3–28.

38. Mayer EA, Gebhart GF. Basic and clinical aspects of visceral hyperalgesia. *Gastroenterology*, **107** (1994 271–293.

39. Jaenig W, Koltzenburg M. The neural basis of consciously perceived sensations from the gut. In *Nerve and the Gastrointestinal Tract.* Singer MV, Goebell H (eds.), Kluwer, Dordrecht, The Netherlands, (1989 pp. 383–398.

40. Jaenig W, Koltzenburg M. Receptive properties of sacral primary afferent neurons supplying the colon. *J Neurophysiol.*, **65** (1991) 1067.

41. Melzack R, Wall PD. Pain mechanisms: a new theory. *Science*, **50** (1988) 971–979.

42. Klein KB. Approach to the patient with abdominal pain. In *Textbook of Gastroenterology.* 2nd ed., Yamad T (Ed.), JB Lippincott, Philadelphia, PA, 1995, p. 750–771.

43. Gebhart FR, Randich A. Brainstem modulation of nociception. In *Brainstem Mechanisms of Behavior* Klemm WR, Vertes RP (eds.), Wiley, New York, NY, 1990, 315–352.

44. Coffin B, Azpiroz F, Guarner, F, Malagelada JR. Selective gastric hypersensitivity and reflex hyporeactivity in functional dyspepsia. *Gastroenterology*, **107** (1994) 1345–1351.

45. Ruch TC. Pathophysiology of pain. In *Neurophysiology.* Ruch TC, Patton JD, Woodbury JW, Lowe AL (eds.) Saunders, Philadelphia, PA, 1961, p. 350–362.

46. Campbell JN, Mayer RA, Davis KD, Raja SN. Sympathetically maintained pain: a unifying hypothesis. I *Hyperalgesia and Allodynia.* Willis WD Jr (ed.), Raven, New York, NY, 1992, pp.141–150

47. Taiwo YO, Levine JD. Characterization of the arachidonic acid metabolites mediating bradykinin and nora drenaline hyperalgesia. *Brain Res.*, **458** (1988) 402–406

48. Crowell MD, Bassotti G, Cheskin LJ, Schuster MM, Whitehead WE. Method for prolonged ambulatory monitoring of high-amplitude propagated contractions from colon. *Am. J. Physiol.*, **26** (1991) G263-G268.

49. Bassotti, G., Crowell, M.D., & Whitehead, W.E. Contractile activity of the human colon: Lessions from 24-hour studies. *Gut*, **34** (1993) 129–133.

50. Holdstock DJ, Misiewicz JJ, Waller SL. Observations on the mechanism of abdominal pain. *Gut*, **10** (1969 19–31.

51. Iggo A. Gastrointestinal tension receptors with unmyelinated afferent fibers in the vagus of the cat. *Q. J. Exp Physiol. Cogn. Med. Sci.*, **42** (1957) 130–143.

52. Jaenig W. Spinal cord integration of visceral sensory systems and sympathetic nervous system reflexes. I *Visceral Sensation. Progress in Brain Research .* Cervero F, Morrison JFB (eds.), Elsevier, Amsterdam 1986, pp. 255–277.

53. Chapman WP, Jones CM. Variations in cutaneous and visceral Pain sensitivity in normal subjects. *J. Clin Invest.*, **23** (1944) 81–91.

54. Musial F, Crowell MD, Enck P. Effects of long-term rectal distention on rectal tone. *Gastroenterology*, **10€** (1994) A546.

55. Crowell MD, Musial F. Rectal adaptation to distention is impaired in the irritable bowel syndrome. *Am. J Gastroenterology*, **89** (1994) 1689.

56. Blumberg H, Haupt P, J„nig W, Kohler W. Encoding of visceral noxious stimuli in the discharge patterns o visceral afferent fibers from the colon. *Pfluegers Arch.*, **398** (1983) 33–40.

57. Sengupta JN, Saha KJ, Goyal RK. Differential sensitivity to bradykinin of esophageal distention-sensitive mechanoreceptors in vagal and sympathetic afferents of the opossum. *J. Neurophysiol.*, **68** (1992) 1053–1067

58 Cervero F, Sann H. Mechanically evoked responses of afferent fibers innervating the guinea-pig's ureter: ar in vitro study. *J. Physiol. Lond.*, **412** (1989) 345.

59. Ness TJ, Metcalf AM, Gebhart GF. A psychophysiological study in humans using phasic colonic distension as a noxious visceral stimulus. *Pain*, **43** (1990) 377–386.

60. Willis WD. Mechanical allodynia: a role for sensitized nociceptive tract cells with convergent input from mechanoreceptors and nociceptors? *Am. Pain Soc. J.*, **2** (1993) 23–33.

61. Willis WD Jr. Central sensitization and plasticity following intense noxious stimulation. In *Basic and Clinical Aspects of Chronic Abdominal Pain.* Mayer EA, Raybould HE (eds.), Elsevier, Amsterdam, 1993 pp. 202–217.

62. Cervero F. Mechanisms of peripheral and central sensitization. *Ann. Med.*, **27** (1995) 235–239.
63. Plourde V, Mertz H, Sytnik B, Tache Y, Mayer EA. Effects of somatostatin analogue on sensory perception to rectal balloon distension. *Dig. Dis. Sci.*, **37(Abstr)** (1992) 976.

II   INVESTIGATION OF DISEASE PROCESSES

12 Oxidative Stress

Emmanuel C. Opara

CONTENTS

1. INTRODUCTION

1.1. Free Radicals and Oxidative Stress

The electrons in an atom are arranged in pairs on shells or orbits that surround the nucleus where protons and neutrons coexist. In a stable atom, the number of protons in the nucleus is equal to the number of electrons on the shells, each of which can have no more than eight electrons. The chemical reactivity of a molecule is dependent upon the conformation of electrons on the outer shell. This conformation determines the ease with which the molecule can accept or donate one or more electrons. When a molecule has an unpaired or odd number of electrons in its atomic structure, it is referred to as a free radical, which is relatively unstable and, therefore, very reactive. For example, molecular oxygen (O_2) has two unpaired electrons in its outer shell, which makes it makes it possible for it to accept up to two electrons (one at a time) from another compound. When a single electron is added to O_2, it becomes the superoxide molecule (O_2^-), which is a free radical with an unpaired electron (Fig. 1). Other molecules, such as hydrogen peroxide (H_2O_2), are not necessarily free radicals, but are certainly very reactive. Such molecules along with free radicals are generally referred to as reactive oxygen species (ROS) [1]. H_2O_2 is formed when the superoxide radical accepts another electron and two hydrogen ions ($2H^+$). A combination of H_2O_2 with O_2^- results in the formation of the hydroxyl (OH^-) radical, the most toxic free radical in biological systems [1].

Reactive oxygen species have enormous ability to cause damage to cells and tissues because of their highly reactive nature [1–5]. There are both endogenous and exogenous sources of free radicals. The formation of ROS is a normal consequence of endogenous essential biochemical reactions [1,2]. The endogenous free radicals include those that are produced and act intracellularly, as well as those that are generated within the cell and released to the surrounding area [1,5]. They are derived from normal cellular metabolism and oxidative burst produced when phagocytic cells destroy invading microorganisms such as bacteria and viruses [2,5]. Some of the reactions include the autoxidation and consequent inactivation of small molecules, such as

From: *Colonic Diseases*
Edited by: T. R. Koch © Humana Press Inc., Totowa, NJ

$$
\begin{array}{rcl}
O_2 + 1e & \rightarrow & O_2^- \text{ (superoxide)} \\
O_2 + 2e + 2H+ & \rightarrow & H_2O_2 \text{ (hydrogen peroxide)} \\
H_2O_2 + O_2^- & \rightarrow & 2OH^- \text{ (hydroxyl radical)} \\
\text{where } e & = & \text{electron}
\end{array}
$$

Fig. 1. Formation of free radicals.

reduced flavins and thiols. Others involve the activity of certain oxidases, cyclooxygenases, lipoxygenases, dehydrogenases, and peroxidases *(1–5)*. Oxidases and the electron transport chain that is coupled to oxidative phosphorylation are primary and continuous sources of ROS. As shown in Table 1, the sites of generation of these toxic molecules encompass all cellular constituents, including the plasma membrane, mitochondria, lysosomes, peroxisomes, nucleus, endoplasmic reticulum, and other sites within the cytosol *(1,5)*. The exogenous sources of free radicals include tobacco smoke, air pollutants, organic solvents, anesthetics, pesticides, radiation, and high oxygen environment *(1,3,5)*. Under normal circumstances, there is a balance between the generation of ROS and the antioxidant defense systems that destroy them. When increased ROS levels are present in the face of a deficiency of antioxidant substances in the body, the situation is referred to as oxidative stress *(1–5)*, which has been associated with increase in age *(5–8)* and various chronic diseases *(1–5)*.

There are two interconnected systems of antioxidants, consisting of a micronutrient component and an enzymatic system of defense against free radical damage *(1–6)*. As shown in Table 2, the nonenzymatic micronutrient system involves small molecular weight molecules like glutathione (GSH) and vitamins, such as vitamin E (tocopherol), vitamin C (ascorbic acid), and previtamin A (β-carotene), as well as certain trace elements. While the vitamins act as donors and acceptors of ROS, the trace elements act as cofactors, which regulate the activities of antioxidant enzymes. These enzymes include metalloenzymes, such as the selenium-containing GSH peroxidase, the iron-containing catalase, and superoxide dismutase (SOD) with different isoenzymes that contain either copper, zinc, or manganese *(1)*. Paradoxically, a high intake of these trace elements, also referred to as transition metals, can promote the generation of reactive species from peroxides and cause significant morbidity *(5)*. In an analogous situation, animal tissues use the cytochrome P450 enzymes as primary defense systems against toxic chemicals ingested as dietary toxins. The induction of these enzymes not only protects against acute effects of the toxic chemicals, but also results in the production of ROS, which can cause oxidative damage to DNA leading to tissue neoplasia *(5)*. Of particular interest in the context of this discussion is the GSH transferase system of antioxidant defense. Cellular GSH levels can be depleted through the GSH transferase reaction, in which GSH is conjugated to foreign compounds and excreted. The loss of cellular GSH through this process has been implicated in the high susceptibility to malignancy of regions of the bowel, such as the colon and rectum, which inherently have low levels of GSH *(9)*.

2. ASSESSMENT OF OXIDATIVE STRESS

Oxidative stress causes oxidative damage because of the ROS with biological macromolecules such as lipids, proteins, and nucleic acids. Based on earlier studies, it was always held that the prime targets of free radical reactions are unsaturated bonds in membrane phospholipids. The consequence of these reactions, termed lipid peroxidation, is the loss of membrane fluidity, receptor alignment, and potential cellular lysis *(1–5)*. The results from later studies

Table 1
Sources of Reactive Oxygen Species

Endogenous	Biochemical reaction
Membrane lipid bilayers	Lipid peroxidation, lipoxygenase system, NADPH oxidase
Mitochondria	Lipid peroxidation, oxidative phosphorylation
Lysosomes	Oxidative burst, myeloperoxidase enzyme system
Endoplasmic reticulum	Xanthine oxidase, cytochromes P450 and b5
Peroxisomes	Catalase

Exogenous
Tobacco smoke
Industrial pollutants
Pesticides
Drugs
Radiation
High oxygen environment
Anesthetics
Organic solvents

Table 2
Components of the Antioxidant Network

Micronutrients		
Trace Elements	Vitamins	Other small molecules
Selenium	Vitamin A (retinol)	Glutathione (GSH)
Iron	β-Carotene (previtamin A)	Ubiquinone (CoQ$_{10}$)
Zinc	Vitamin C (ascorbic acid)	Carnosine
Copper	Vitamin E (tocopherol)	Uric acid
Manganese	Vitamin K (lipid quinones)	Bilirubin

Enzymes		
	Role as enzyme co-factor	
	Glutathione peroxidase	
	Catalase	
	Cytosolic superoxide dismutase	
	Cytosolic superoxide dismutase and ceruloplasmin	
	Mitochondrial superoxide dismutaset	

have led to the suggestion of a model composed of two possible sequences of reactions leading to oxidative damage *(4)*. According to this model, one sequence of reactions is the original theory, which states that oxidative stress causes lipid peroxidation, and this, in turn, results in cell damage. The alternative sequence is that oxidative stress causes cell damage, which leads to a secondary increase in lipid peroxidation of damaged cells *(4)*. In addition, free radical damage to sulfur-containing enzymes and other proteins results in their inactivation, cross-linking, and denaturation. In addition, nucleic acids can be attacked, and subsequent damage to the DNA can cause mutations that may be carcinogenic *(1–5)*. It has been proposed that increased levels of free Ca^{2++}, and damage to proteins and DNA are often more important events in cellular injury than lipid peroxidation. In other words, lipid peroxidation is frequently a consequence rather than a cause of final cell death (4). This hypothesis is supported by studies that show that ROS can interfere with various pathophysiological processes by activation of the ubiquitous protein kinase C (PKC) signal transduction system (10,11).

In spite of this ambiguity, it is well established that lipid peroxidation is associated with cellular injury and that lipid peroxides and their by-products are present in oxidative damage. Consequently, measurement of lipid peroxide levels and the levels of their degradative products are routinely used as indices of oxidative stress (4,12–17). One of the most common of these assays is the thiobarbituric acid (TBA) test (4,12). In this simple assay, sometimes referred to as the thiobarbituric reactive substances (TBARS) assay, the test sample is heated with TBA at low pH, usually around pH 3.5, generating a pink color, whose absorbance is measured at 532 nm (4,12). The TBA test appears to work well when applied to defined membrane systems, but has proven to be unreliable when used for assessment of oxidative stress in body fluids and tissue extracts owing to the presence of interfering substances in the latter (4). Halliwell and Chirico have evaluated the various assays used to measure the levels of lipid peroxides in samples, and have provided an excellent assessment of the inherent difficulties present in each of the assays (4). In summary, it seems highly unreliable to use a single assay to assess oxidative stress. It is advisable to perform two or more different assays on any given sample being evaluated for the presence of oxidative stress. Since free radicals have very short half-lives, in the order of seconds, it is very difficult to reliably determine the amounts present in a sample. However, attempts have been made to use spin trapping procedures to measure intermediate radicals in free radical chain reactions, and light emission methods for measuring excited carbonyls and singlet oxygen (4). It has become a routine procedure to simultaneously measure lipid peroxides, such as malodialdehyde (MDA), and their degradation products called 4-hydroxyalkenals. For this purpose, Calbiochem (San Diego, CA, USA) has produced a lipid peroxidation assay kit, which can be used to measure oxidative stress in plasma samples and tissue extracts. This assay specifically measures MDA and a 4-hydroxyalkenal called 4hydroxy-2(E)-nonenal (4HNE). We have routinely used this assay in our laboratory (18) and find it to be fairly reliable, but again, it is prone to interference by certain substances listed in the brochure provided with the kit. One class of products of lipid peroxidation that is increasingly gaining popularity for reliability of use to assess oxidative stress is the isoprostanes (14–16,19). Isoprostanes are prostaglandin-like compounds produced when free radicals cause peroxidation of arachidonic acid independent of the cyclooxygenase enzyme (14). Since isoprostanes possess contain F-type prostane rings, they are also referred to as F_2-isoprostanes (14,19).

As mentioned earlier, H_2O_2 is classified as reactive oxygen species because it is very highly reactive. The high propensity of this molecule to react with other compounds has often been employed in studies of oxidative stress. The reaction performed in this assay is based on the susceptibility of red blood cells to peroxidation by H_2O_2 (20,21). The level of formation of methemoglobin, a peroxidative product of hemoglobin, may then be assessed in a calibrated spectrophotometric assay (20). In spite of the protective effects of antioxidant, micronutrients, and enzymes, damage to cellular proteins, lipids, nucleic acids, and carbohydrates does occur, and consequently, there is a normal process of repair of some of the damaged macromolecules. However, in most cases, enzymatic degradation of unrepaired molecules is needed for the excretion of damaged elements, as the removal of the damaged materials appears to prevent or minimize the potential toxicity of oxidized macromolecules (2). Based on this phenomenon, an assay that estimates the urinary excretion of 8-oxo-7,8-dihydro-2'-deoxyguanosine (8-oxo-dG), a repair product of oxidative DNA damage, has been used to assess oxidative stress (22).

Another assay that was developed on the basis of the reactive nature of ROS with macromolecules is the polycyclic aromatic hydrocarbon-DNA adduct *(23)*. Polycyclic aromatic hydrocarbons (PAH) are formed by the pyrolytic process during cigarette smoking and are activated by the mixed function oxidases of various cells to electrophilic highly reactive compounds that can bind covalently to DNA. This assay is, therefore, particularly useful when cigarette smokers are evaluated for oxidative stress *(23)*.

One measurement that we routinely perform to determine oxidative stress in our laboratory is the trolox equivalent antioxidant capacity (TEAC) assay *(18,24)*. There are different variations of this type of assay available for the determination of total antioxidant capacity in samples. These include the total (peroxy) radical-trapping antioxidant parameter (TRAP) assay *(25)*, the ferric reducing/antioxidant power (FRAP) assay *(26)*, and the oxygen radical absorbance capacity (ORAC) assay *(27)*. In the TEAC assay performed in our laboratory, the total antioxidant capacity is estimated by the ABTS* (2,2'-azinobis(3-ethylbenzothiazoline-6-sulfonic acid) radical action decolorization assay involving preformed ABTS* radical cation and using trolox as standard *(28)*. In this assay, ABTS is made to react with potassium persulfate in the absence (blank) or presence of standards and samples, and the absorbance reading is taken at 734 nm. The total antioxidant capacity value in a sample is then assessed as TEAC. A value of 1 TEAC in a sample is defined as a concentration that is equivalent to 1 mmol/L of trolox, a water-soluble analogue of α-tocopherol (vitamin E). It is of interest that a recent study has shown that under standardized conditions, the estimated TEAC value reflects the additive value of the individual antioxidants present in a given sample *(29)*.

Since GSH plays a very important role as an antioxidant in the prevention of human disease *(9)*, another assay that we and other workers have frequently used as an index of oxidative stress is the measurement of tissue GSH levels *(9,30–33)*. There are various methods for measuring GSH, and most of them involve colorimetric assays. The procedure used in our laboratory for blood GSH measurement requires whole blood, which either has to be fresh or stored at 4°C for up to 1 mo if acid-citrate-dextrose (ACD) is added as preservative *(7)*. The blood sample is first hemolyzed with distilled water, and after treating the hemolysate with a precipitating solution of glacial metaphosphoric acid, disodium ethylene diamine tetra acetic acid(EDTA), and sodium chloride, it is filtered through Whatman #1 filter paper (Whatman, Clifton, NJ, USA); the clear filtrate is then used for the colorimetric GSH assay using 5,5' dithiobis-(2-nitrobenzoic acid) (DTNB) *(34)*. This colorimetric assay for GSH can also be performed on tissue extracts *(32)*, which can either be fresh or stored frozen at -70°C.

3. CONDITIONS ASSOCIATED WITH OXIDATIVE STRESS

The association of oxidative stress with a variety of pathophysiological situations has frequently presented the chicken or the egg type of dilemma to investigators, and the challenge has been to determine whether oxidative stress is the cause, consequence, or epiphenomenon in a growing number of conditions *(35–37)*. As shown in Table 3, some of these conditions include injury during radiation, burns, and ischemia–reperfusion. Others are cancer, inflammatory conditions, aging, neurodegenerative diseases, cigarette smoking-related illness, microbial infections, diabetic complications, and cardiovascular disease *(1–10,18, 31–33,35–38)*. Investigators have adopted different experimental approaches in the quest to determine if free radicals play any important role in the pathogenesis of human disease. In a significant number of studies, a common strategy has been to determine if antioxidant therapy, either through micronutrient supplementation or increased dietary intake of fruits and vegetables, has any impact on the disease process *(5,6,36,37)*. After considerable disappointment related to early studies that were poorly designed, the data from the newer well-controlled and carefully

Table 3
Conditions associated with Oxidative Stress

Diseases	Other conditions
Gastrointestinal disease	Cigarette smoking
Neurodegenerative disease	Chronic inflammation
(e.g., Parkinson's, Alzheimer's)	Chronic infection
Cardiovascular disease	Ischemia/reperfusion
Diabetes and its complications	Radiation
Cancer	Burns
Pulmonary disease	Aging
Cataract	

designed studies have been quite promising (5,36,37,39). Indeed, it does appear from these later studies that oxidative stress has been strongly implicated in as playing a significant role in the pathogenesis of neurodegenerative disease, chronic inflammatory disease, cardiovascular disease, certain neoplasms, and some forms of gastrointestinal disease (1,5,36–39).

Ischemia–reperfusion is inevitable in most surgical procedures and has been associated with significant morbidity in surgical patients (35,36). It has been proposed that the superoxide free radical generated from xanthine oxidase at reperfusion plays a significant role in postischemic injury in numerous tissues, including the intestine, stomach, pancreas, liver, lung, and the central nervous system among others (5,35,36,38,39,40). The vulnerability of almost all tissues to this type of injury is based on the widespread localization of the xanthine-oxidase system in the microvascular endothelium (36,40). It has been suggested that the sequence of events during ischemia–reperfusion starts with the generation of superoxide, followed by the adhesion and activation of specific endothelial and neutrophil adhesion molecules, resulting in microvascular injury mediated by ROS produced by neutrophils, elastase, and other proteases within the immediate environment (36,40). In most experiments designed to elucidate this pathway, the xanthine inhibitors, such as allopurinol and oxypurinol, were widely used to determine the role of xanthine oxidase in ischemia–reperfusion injury. These inhibitors caused dramatic reduction in both epithelial cell necrosis and increased microvascular permeability observed in ischemic bowel (40).

In chronic infections, bacteria, parasites, and cells infected by viruses are killed by a variety of ROS, which are produced by leukocytes and other phagocytes (5). Unfortunately, through this mechanism of defense, oxidative stress may become inevitable and result in oxidative damage to cellular macromolecules, such as DNA. Oxidative damage to DNA may cause mutations, which could lead to carcinogenesis (1–5). This scenario has been implicated in the processes by which chronic infections with hepatitis B and C viruses, and *Helicobacter pylori* lead to hepatocellular carcinoma and stomach cancer, respectively (5).

Exposure to radiation results in the production of free radicals within the exposed tissues, and it has been suggested that most of the biological alterations induced by radiation are attributable to the secondary generation of ROS, and hence the term, ionizing radiation (1,36,37). Another important cause of oxidative stress is cigarette smoking. Cigarette smokers are exposed to enormous quantities of free radicals with each puff that they inhale, and as a result, they become depleted of tissue antioxidant substances (1,3,5,41,42). Oxidative stress induced by cigarette smoking has been implicated in the pathogenesis of diseases most frequently associated with smoking, such as lung cancer, emphysema, and heart disease (3,5,41).

It is also important to point out that many drugs are also sources of ROS, and examples include quinones, as well as certain antibiotics and anticancer drugs, whose metabolism generates free radicals and oxidative stress *(39)*.

4. OXIDATIVE STRESS AND DISEASES OF THE COLON

Colon cancer and inflammatory bowel disease (IBD) are two colonic diseases commonly associated with oxidative stress *(5,9,31,33,39,40,43–48)*. It has also been proposed that oxidative stress may play a role in the pathogenesis of acquired megacolon, because it causes a loss of the neuroprotective effect of tissue antioxidants, resulting in altered colonic levels of inhibitory neurotransmitters seen in this disease *(49)*. It is noteworthy that acquired megacolon is seen most often in elderly subjects who are also prone to increased oxidative stress *(5–7,49)*. Necrotizing enterocolitis, a life-threatening condition associated with shock and infection, is another disorder in which oxidative stress appears to be implicated *(39)*. Numerous studies have been focused on the role of GSH in colonic disease induced by oxidative stress. The impetus for these studies was provided by the report that GSH deficiency, produced in the mouse by buthionine sulfoximine (BSO) administration, resulted in severe degeneration of epithelial cells of the jejunum and colon *(50)*. Simultaneous administration of GSH monoethyl ester to replenish tissue GSH levels in mice receiving BSO completely prevented any morphologic changes in their intestines *(50)*. This landmark study provided good evidence for the protective role of GSH in the integrity and function of the gastrointestinal tract. Furthermore, it has been shown that GSH levels are, by far, higher in the duodenum and ileum than the colon and rectum *(32,51)*, and the presence of low levels of GSH in the cells lining the mucosa of the colon and rectum have been linked to their higher susceptibility to malignancy than the other areas of the gastrointestinal tract with higher contents of GSH in the mucosa *(9,51)*. Still, it remains to be determined whether supplementation of GSH-enhancing substances have any therapeutic effect in patients suffering from colorectal cancers. It has recently been suggested that an elevated level of tissue GSH content at the time of diagnosis may indicate poor prognosis in colorectal cancer *(52)*. It is possible that an up-regulation of GSH synthesis may occur to meet the need for antioxidant defense against enhanced free radical production in this disease.

In general, the role of free radicals in the pathogenesis of cancer remains to be established. Some studies have shown that certain indices of oxidative stress are increased in tissues obtained from cancers of the large bowel. In one study, it was shown that MDA, phospholipase A_2, and myelopperoxidase activities were significantly increased in human colorectal cancerous tissues compared with macroscopically normal tissues *(39)*. In another study, increased levels of the highly reactive hydroxyl radical (OH^-) were detected in the feces of patients with colon cancer *(53)*. It has been suggested that the observation of free radical generation in feces may provide a missing link in our understanding of the etiology of colon cancer, because the oxidation of procarcinogens either by fecal OH^- or secondary peroxyl radicals may result in active carcinogens or mitogenic tumor promotors *(39)*.

Other studies have examined the role of GSH depletion in the pathogenesis of IBD using either the measurement of tissue GSH levels or supplementation of patients with substances that enhance tissue GSH levels, such as GSH esters and N-acetyl cysteine (NAC), as well as micronutrient, antioxidant vitamins *(31,33,44,46–48)*. While it has been consistently shown that tissue GSH levels are depleted in Crohn's disease *(31,33,44)*, the data have been inconsistent in ulcerative colitis *(31,33,47)*, leading to the suggestion that, although a change in GSH metabolism is associated with inflammation and active ulcerative colitis, it appears to be a consequence of inflammation rather than a pathogenic factor of the disease *(47)*. However, it has been reported that supplementation with NAC attenuates acute colitis through increased mucosal GSH levels *(48)*. Alternative approaches have also been used to determine the relationship between oxidative stress and IBD. In one study, mucosal biopsies were analyzed for protein carbonyl content (POPS), 8-oxo-dG, ROS, the trace elements, copper, zinc, and iron, as well as the antioxidant enzyme, SOD. The investigators found that biopsies from patients with Crohn's disease had increased levels of POPS, ROS, 8-oxo-dG, and iron, but decreased contents of zinc and copper compared to control subjects. They also found that there was an increase in the levels of POPS, ROS, and iron, but a decrease in the levels of zinc and copper in inflamed tissue obtained from patients with ulcerative colitis compared to normal control biopsies *(45)*. These data are consistent with observations from studies involving the use of sulfasalazine in patients with ulcerative colitis. Sulfasalazine is the most commonly prescribed drug for the treatment of ulcerative colitis, and although the drug was originally developed as an antibiotic, it apparently has no effect on the intestinal microflora, but appears to work by alternative mechanisms that may include antioxidant activity *(43)*. It is known that 5-aminosalicylate (5-ASA) is the active moiety of sulfasalazine *(54)*, and salicylates are very effective as hydroxyl radical scavengers *(43)*. There is also a possibility that 5-ASA may function as an Fe^{2++} chelator, thereby inhibiting the ability of this transition metal from taking part in free radical generation *(43)*. These observations have led to the suggestion that sulfasalazine, which is an effective drug in the empirical management of ulcerative colitis, may be a many faced antioxidant that is selectively concentrated in the colon and exerts its effect by chelating iron and by direct scavenging of free radicals *(43)*.

As previously mentioned, the data from studies based on determination of GSH status provide a stronger support for a role of oxidative stress in Crohn's disease than in ulcerative colitis. There is also good evidence from studies based on other approaches to determine the role of oxidative damage in the pathogenesis of Crohn's disease. It has been reported that there was a decrease in two antioxidant enzymes, SOD and metallothionein, in specimens of tissues obtained from patients with both ulcerative colitis and Crohn's disease compared with specimens from histologically normal control tissues *(55)*. It is, therefore, not surprising to find that an open label study, in which SOD encapsulated in liposomes was administered to patients suffering from Crohn's disease, resulted in significant improvement in the clinical course of the disease *(56)*. It has been proposed that ulcerative colitis and Crohn's disease converge as a syndrome that is secondary to different etiological factors with a common final pathway *(57)*. It is tempting to speculate that oxidative damage may be that common pathway leading to disease. According to this hypothesis, abnormalities in the immune system, such as activated lymphocytes and systemic local or humoral factors *(58)*, presence of activated neutrophils, and high levels of ROS in the inflamed colon *(43,45,46)* are secondary phenomenon but pivotal elements in maintaining the inflammatory cascade and tissue damage *(57)*. In a recent study of tissue extracts, we found no differences in total antioxidant capacity or lipid peroxide levels when normal colonic tissue was compared to tissues from inactive and active ulcerative colitis *(24)*. The observation may suggest that there may be specific decrements in the tissue levels of individual antioxidants, but not necessarily a global depletion of tissue antioxidants. It is also possible that in ulcerative colitis, there may be compensatory mechanisms by which the depletion of one or two antioxidants may lead to up-regulation in the production of other antioxidants to offset the deficit.

In conclusion, there are both endogenous and exogenous sources of reactive oxygen species. When high levels of these reactive molecules are present in the face of decreased levels of antioxidant substances, the situation is referred to as oxidative stress, which can result in oxidative damage to biological macromolecules and disease. There is a growing body of evidence that show an association between oxidative damage and the pathogenesis of a variety of human disease, including diseases of the colon. Based on the evidence from literature, it certainly appears that oxidative stress plays a role in the pathogenesis of inflammatory disease. Our inability to come to a consensus on this issue has been largely due to difficulties associated with reliable measurements of certain indices of oxidative stress and the scarcity of well-designed and controlled studies. There is immense opportunity for research in this area, and one hopes that future studies using appropriate techniques would finally clarify the role of oxidative stress in the pathogenesis of colon cancer and IBD.

REFERENCES

1. Machlin LJ, Bendich A. Free radical tissue damage: protective role of antioxidant nutrients. *FASEB J.*, **1** (1987) 441–445.
2. Pacifici RE, Davies KJ. Protein, lipid and DNA repair systems in oxidative stress: the free radical theory of aging revisited. *Gerontology*, **37** (1991) 166–180.
3. Cross CE, Halliwell B, Borish ET,et al. Oxygen radicals and human disease. *Ann. Intern. Med.*, **107** (1987) 526–545.
4. Halliwell B, Chirico S. Lipid peroxidation: its mechanism, measurement, and significance. *Am. J. Clin. Nutr.*, **57(Suppl)** (1993) 15S–25S.
5. Ames BN, Shigenaga MK. Oxidants, antioxidants, and the degenerative diseases of aging. *Proc. Natl. Acad. Sci. USA*, **90** (1993) 7915–7922.
6. Traber MG. Vitamin E, oxidative stress and healthy aging. *Eur. J. Clin. Invest.*, **27** (1997) 822–824.
7. Julius M, Lang CA, Gleiberman L, Harburg E, DiFranceisco W, Schork A. Glutathione and morbidity in a community-based sample of elderly. *J. Clin. Epidemiol.*, **47** (1994) 1021–1026.
8. Bales CW, Opara EC, Currie KL, Peterson BL, Lin PH. Interactions of age with oxidative stress and nutrient status. *FASEB J.*, **13** (1999) A701.
9. White AC, Thannickal VJ, Fanburg BL. Glutathione deficiency in human disease. *J. Nutr. Biochem.*, **5** (1994) 218–226.
10. Masters CJ. Cellular signaling: the role of the peroxisome. *Cell Signal*, **8** (1996) 197–208.
11. Gopalakrishna R, Jaken S. Protein kinase C signalling and oxidative stress. *Free Radic. Biol. Med.*, **28** (2000) 1349–1361.
12. Ohkawa H, Ohishi N, Yagi K. Assay for lipid peroxides in animal tissues by thiobarbituric acid reaction. *Anal. Biochem.*, **95** (1979) 351–358.
13. Janero DR. Malondialdehyde and thiobarbituric acid-reactivity as diagnostic indices of lipid peroxidation and peroxidative tissue injury. *Free Radic. Biol. Med.*, **9** (1990) 515–540.
14. Morrow JD, Roberts LJ. The isoprostanes: unique bioactive products of lipid peroxidation. *Prog. Lipid Res.*, **36** (1997) 1–21.
15. Alary J, Debrauwer L, Fernadez Y, et al. Identification of novel urinary metabolites of the lipid peroxidation product 4-hydroxy-2-nonenal in rats. *Chem. Res. Toxicol.*, **11** (1998) 1368–1376:
16. Montuschi P, Corradi M, Ciabattoni G, Nightingale J, Kharitonov SA, Barnes PJ. Increased 8-isoprostane, a marker of oxidative stress in exhaled condensate of asthma patients. *Am. J. Respir. Crit. Care. Med.*, **160** (1999) 216–220.
17. Chen JJ, Yu BP. Alterations in mitochodrial membrane fluidity by lipid peroxidation products. *Free Radic. Biol. Med.*, **17** (1994) 411–418.
18. Opara EC, Abdel-Rahman E, Soliman S, et al. Depletion of total antioxidant capacity in type 2 diabetes. *Metabolism*, **48** (1999) 1414–1417.
19. Murdeach R, Delanty N, Lawson JA, FitzGerald GA. Modulation of oxidant stress in vivo in chronic cigarette smokers. *Circulation*, **94** (1996) 19–25.
20. Giulivi C, Hochstein P, Davies KJA. Hydrogen peroxide production by red blood cells. *Free Radic. Biol. Med.*, **16** (1994) 123–129.
21. Brown KM, Morrice PC, Duthie GG. Erythrocyte vitamin E and plasma ascorbate concentrations in relation to erythrocyte peroxidation in smokers and nonsmokers: dose response to vitamin E supplementation. *Am. J. Clin. Nutr.*, **65** (1997) 496–502.
22. Prieme H, Loft S, Nyyssonen K, Salonen JT, Poulsen HE. No effect of supplementation with vitamin E, ascorbic acid, or coenzyme Q10 on oxidative DNA damage estimated by 8-oxo-7,8-dihydro-2'-deoxyguanosine excretion in smokers. *Am. J. Clin. Nutr.*, **65** (1997) 503–507.

23. Grinberg-Funes RA, Singh VN, Perera FP, et al. Polycyclic aromatic hydrocarbon-DNA adducts in smokers and their relationship to micronutrient levels and the glutathione-S-transferase M1 genotype. *Carcinogenesis*, **15** (1994) 2449–2454.
24. Koch TR, Yuan L-X, Stryker SJ, Ratliff P, Telford GL, Opara EC. Total antioxidant capacity of colon in patients with chronic ulcerative colitis. *Dig. Dis. Sci.*, **45** (2000) 1814–1819.
25. Wayner DDM, Burton GW, Ingold KU, Barclay LRC, Locke SJ. The relative contributions of vitamin E, urate,ascorbate and proteins to the total peroxyl radical-trapping antioxidant activity of human blood plasma. *Biochem. Biophys. Acta*, **924** (1987) 408–419.
26. Benzie IFF, Chung WY, Strain JJ. Antioxidant (reducing) efficiency of ascorbate in plasma is not affected by concentration. *J. Nutr. Biochem.,* **10** 1999, 146–150.
27. McKay DL, Perrone G, Rasmussen H, et al. The effects of a multivitamin/mineral supplement on micronutrient status, antioxidant capacity and cytokine production in healthy older adults consuming a fortified diet. *J. Am. Coll. Nutr.*, **19** (2000) 613–621.
28. Re R, Pellegrini N, Proteggente A, Pannala A, Yang M, Rice-Evans C. Antioxidant activity applying an improved ABTS radical cation decolorization assay. *Free Radic. Biol. Med.*, **26** (1999) 1231–1237.
29. Van den Berg R, Haenen GRMM, van den Berg H, Bast A. Applicability of an improved trolox equivalent antioxidant capacity measurements of mixtures. *Food Chem.*, **66** (1999) 511–517.
30. Ballard TC, Farag A, Branum GD, Akwari OE, Opara EC. Effect of L-glutamine on impaired glucose regulation during intravenous lipid administration. *Nutrition*, **12** (1996) 349–354.
31. Ruan EA, Rao S, Burdick JS, et al. Glutathione levels in chronic inflammatory disorders of the human colon. *Nutr. Res.*, **17** (1997) 463–473.
32. Koch TR, Fink JG, Ruan E, Petro A, Opara EC. Chronic glutathione depletion alters expression of enteric inhibitory neurochemicals in the mouse. *Neurosci. Lett.*, **235** (1997) 77–80.
33. Miralles-Barrachina O, Savoye G, Belmonte-Zalar L, et al. Low levels of glutathione in endoscopic biopsies of patients with Crohns colitis: role of malnutrition. *Clin. Nutr.*, **18** (1999) 313–317.
34. Beutler E. *Red Cell Metabolism. A Manual of Biochemical Methods*. Grune & Stratton, New York, NY, 1984.
35. Stein HJ, Oosthuizien MMJ, Hinder RA, Lamprechts H. Oxygen free radicals and glutathione in hepatic ischemia/reperfusion injury. *J. Surg. Res.*, **50** (1991) 398–402.
36. Bulkley GB. Free radicals and other reactive oxygen metabolites: clinical relevance and the therapeutic efficacy of antioxidant therapy. *Surgery*, **113** (1993) 479–483.
37. Halliwell B. Free radicals, antioxidants, and human disease: curiosity, cause or consequence? *Lancet*, **344** (1994) 721–724.
38. Rice-Evans CA, Diplock AT. Current status of antioxidant therapy. *Free Radic. Biol. Med.*, **15** (1993) 77–96.
39. Otamiri T, Sjodahl. Oxygen radicals: their role in selected gastrointestinal disorders. *Dig. Dis.*, **9** (1991) 133–141.
40. Zimmerman BJ, Granger DN. Oxygen free radicals and the gastrointestinal tract: role in ischemia-reperfusion injury. *Hepatogastroenterology*, **41** (1994) 337–342.
41. Church DF, Pryor WA. Free radical chemistry of cigarette smoke and its toxicological implications. *Environ. Health Perspect.*, **64** (1985) 111–126.
42. Lane JD, Opara EC, Rose JE, Behm F. Quitting smoking raises whole blood glutathione. *Physiol. Behav.*, **60** (1996) 1379–1381.
43. Babbs CF. Oxygen radicals in ulcerative colitis. *Free Radic. Biol. Med.*, **13** (1992) 169–181.
44. Iantomasi T, Marraccini P, Favilli F, Vincenzini MT, Ferretti P, Tonelli F. Glutathione metabolism in Crohns disease. *Biochem. Med. Metabol. Biol.*, **53** (1994) 87–91.
45. Lih-Brody L, Powell SR, Collier KP, et al. Increased oxidative stress and decreased antioxidant defenses in mucosa of inflammatory bowel disease. *Dig. Dis. Sci.*, **41** (1996) 2078–2086.
46. Thomson A, Hemphill D, Jeejeebhoy KN. Oxidative stress and antioxidants in intestinal disease. *Dig. Dis.*, **16** (1998) 152–168.
47. Holmes EW, Yong SL, Eiznhamer D, Keshavarzian A. Glutathione content of colonic mucosa. Evidence for oxidative damage in active ulcerative colitis. *Dig. Dis. Sci.*, **43** (1998) 1088–1095.
48. Ardite E, Sans M, Panes J, Romero FJ, Pique JM, Fernandez-Checa JC. Replenishment of glutathione levels improves mucosal function in experimental acute colitis. *Lab. Invest.*, **80** (2000) 735–744.
49. Koch TR, Schulte-Bockholt A, Otterson MF, et al. Decreased vasoactive intestinal peptide levels and glutathione depletion in acquired megacolon. *Dig. Dis. Sci.*, **41** (1996) 1409–1416.
50. Martensson J, Jain A, Meister A. Glutathione is required for intestinal function. *Proc. Natl. Acad. Sci. USA*, **87** (1990) 1715–1719.
51. Loguercio C, Di Pierro M. The role of glutathione in the gastrointestinal tract: a review. *Ital. J. Gastroenterol. Hepatol.*, **31** (1999) 401–407.

52. Barranco SC, Perry RR, Durm ME, et al. Relationship between colorectal cancer glutathione levels and patient survival. Early results. *Dis. Colon. Rectum.*, **43** (2000) 1133–1140.

53 Babbs CF. Free radicals and the etiology of colon cancer. *Free Radic. Biol. Med.*, **8** (1990) 191–200.

54. Mandell GL, Sande MA. Antimicrobial agents—sulfonamides, trimethoprim-sulfamethoxazole and urinary tract antiseptics. In *Goodman and Gilman's: The Pharmacological Basis of Therapeutics*. 6th ed., Gilman AG (ed.), Macmillan, New York, NY, 1980, pp. 1112–1113.

55. Mulder T, Verspaget H, Janssens A, de Bruin P, Pena A, Lamers C. Decrease in two intestinal copper/zinc containing proteins with antioxidant function in inflammatory bowel disease. *Gut*, **32** (1991) 1146–1150.

56. Niwa Y, Somiya K, Michelson A, Puget K. Effect of liposomal-encapsulated superoxide dismutase on active oxygen-related human disease. A preliminary study. *Free Radic. Res. Commun.*, **1** (1985) 137–153.

57. Keshavarzian A, Mobarhan S. Inflammatory bowel disease in the elderly. In *Digestive Diseases and the Elderly*. Vellas BJ, Russel R, Dyard F, Garry PJ, Albarede JL (eds.), Springer, New York, NY, 1996, pp. 35–52.

58. Schreiber S, Halstensen TS, Brandtzaeg P, MacDermott RP. Role of B-cell-dependent effect or mechanisms in inflammatory bowel disease. In *Inflammatory Bowel Disease from Bench to Bedside*. Targan SR, Shanahan F (eds.), Williams & Wilkins, Baltimore, MD, 1994, pp. 89–105.

13 Genetic Testing for Colon Cancer

Russell F. Jacoby and Carolyn E. Cole

Contents

1. INTRODUCTION

Colorectal cancer remains one of the most common cancers, with more than 130,000 cases diagnosed annually in the United States *(1)*. As a cause of cancer death, it is now second only to lung cancer. Although most colon cancer is sporadic, at least 15% of cases have some inherited component *(2)*. Colon cancer is perhaps the most familial of all cancers. By age 70, the risk of colorectal cancer is only 2% in the low-risk general population, but increases to 8% for a person with one affected first-degree relative, and to 17% when two relatives first-degree relatives are affected *(3)*. The risk increases further to about 60–80% for patients inheriting the genes that cause hereditary nonpolyposis colon cancer *(4)*, and 95–100% for patients with untreated familial adenomatous polyposis *(5)*. Awareness of genetic and other risk factors is important, because there are very effective means now available that could prevent most colon cancer morbidity and mortality.

Cancer genetics was among the earliest clinical applications of the techniques of molecular biology *(6–8)*. Advances in understanding the genetic basis of human diseases creates opportunities to make diagnostic and prognostic assessments based upon various types of analyses of variations in an individual's DNA. Molecular diagnosis involves the testing of DNA or RNA within a clinical context. The functions of nucleic acids and their encoded protein molecules are determined by the linear sequence of their monomers. Although the proteins they encode develop complex three-dimensional functional conformations as linear peptide chains become enfolded into helical or pleated sheets or higher-order structures, the simple primary amino acid sequences determine the ultimate structure and function. In modern molecular biology research, it is now much easier to obtain long nucleic acid sequence information to deduce the

From: *Colonic Diseases*
Edited by: T. R. Koch © Humana Press Inc., Totowa, NJ

Table 1
Screening for Cancer Risks in the Inherited Colon Tumor Syndromes *(17)*

Syndrome/Tumors	Lifetime risk	Recommended screening
FAP (*APC* gene mutation)		
Colon cancer	near 100%	Sigmoidoscopy q 1 yr after age 10–12 yr.
Duodenal/periampullary cancer	5–12%	Endoscopy/duodenoscopy q 1–3 yr after age 20–25yr.
Pancreatic cancer	Approx 2%	Possibly periodic abdominal US after age 20 yr.
Thyroid cancer	Approx 2%	Annual thyroid exam after age 10–12 yr.
Gastric cancer	Approx 0.5%	Same as for duodenal.
CNS cancer, usually cerebellar medulloblastoma (Turcot's syndrome)	RR 92	Annual physical exam, and possibly periodic head CT in affected families.
Hepatoblastoma	1.6% of children < 5 yr old	Possibly liver palpation, liver US, α fetoprotein; annually during age 1–10 yr.
HNPCC (MMR gene mutation)		
Colon cancer	about 80%	Colonoscopy q 1–2 yr after age 20–25 yr or earlier of 10 yr younger than earliest colon cancer in family.
Endometrial cancer	43–60%	Pelvic exam, transvaginal US and/or
Ovarian cancer	9–12%	Endometrial aspirate, q 1–2 yr after age 25–35 yr.
Gastric cancer	13–19%	Upper endoscopy q 1–2 yr after age 30–35 yr.
Urinary tract cancer	4–10%	Urinalysis and US q 1–2yr after age 30–35 yr.
Renal cell adenocarcinoma	3.3%	No screening recommendations given.
Biliary tract and gallbladder cancer	2–18%	No screening recommendations given.
CNS (usually glioblastoma)	3.7%	No screening recommendations given.
Small bowel cancer		No screening recommendations given.
Peutz-Jeghers syndrome (PJS) (*STK11* gene mutation)		
Colon cancer	2–13%	Colonoscopy q 3 yr after sx or late teens if no sx but interval may be more often if numerous polyps.
Stomach, duodenum	2–13%	Upper endoscopy q 2 yr after age 10 yr.
Small intestine	RR 13	Annual Hgb, SBFT X-ray q 2yr, after age 10 yr. Given capsule may be considered.
Breast cancer	RR 8.8	Breast exam q 1yr, mammograms q 2–3 yr, both start after age 30 yr.
Pancreatic cancer	RR 100	EUS or abdominal US q 1–2 yr after age 30 yr.
Uterine	RR 8	
Ovarian cancer	RR 13	
Adenoma malignum (cervix)	rare	
SCTAT tumors (females) (in almost all women with PJS, 20% become malignant)		
Sertoli cell tumor (males) unusual, 10–20% become malignant		Testicular exam q 1 yr after age 10 yr. Testicular US if feminizing features occur.
Juvenile Polyposis (*SMAD4* or *PTEN* mutation)		
Colon cancer	30–50%	Colonoscopy q 3 yr after sx or late teens if no sx interval may be more often if numerous polyps.
Gastric and duodenal cancer	rare	Upper endoscopy q 3 yr after early teenage years (mainly to avoid complications of benign polyps).
Cowden syndrome (*PTEN* mutation)		
Thyroid cancer	3–10%	Thyroid exam q 1 yr after early teenage years
Breast cancer	25–50%	Breast exam q 1 yr after age 25 yr and mammograms q 1 yr after age 30 yr.
Uterine and ovarian	? increase	No screening recommendations given.

Table above adapted from ref. *17*, used with permission.

CNS, central nervous system; US, ultrasonography; CT, computed tomography; q, every; SCTAT, sex cord tumor with annular tubules; RR, relative risk; Hgb, hemoglobin; Eus, endoscopic ultrasound; sx, symptoms.

sequence of proteins rather than determine them directly (9,10). The functional effects on the encoded protein of any mutations or sequence variations can then be discovered.

Molecular genetic discoveries in recent years have provided unequivocal evidence that cancer is a disease caused by mutations in a few critical genes, and in a significant number of colon cancer patients, at least one of these mutations is inherited. Inherited mutations cause cancer at a younger age and at a higher frequency. The genetic risk can be predicted by molecular diagnostic testing (11). The challenge to clinicians now is to apply this knowledge for the benefit of their patients. Unfortunately, despite the discovery in 1991 that the etiology of adenomatous polyposis is a mutation of the APC gene (12–14) and the obvious clinical phenotype of hundreds or thousands of colonic adenomas, the majority of these patients are not diagnosed until after they have developed metastatic cancer (5). Most of the resulting mortality could be prevented by earlier diagnosis, screening, and treatment. Hereditary nonpolyposis has a phenotype that is more difficult to recognize in the absence of a family history, but these patients similarly benefit from screening when the mutation causing the disease in their family is detected (15).

The current indications for genetic testing for inherited colon cancer are: (i) diagnostic confirmation in an individual or family by initially testing a patient already clinically manifesting the tumor(s) typical of that syndrome; and (ii) predictive molecular diagnostic testing for any individuals at risk for inheriting mutations known to cause colon tumors in a family.

The latter approach provides an opportunity to diagnose and intervene with effective management to benefit not just one patient but an entire family (16). Intensive measures can be efficiently targeted among children and other relatives as appropriate, depending on whether or not a particular individual has inherited a gene mutation of known clinical significance. However, when the mutation causing the disease in a family is not identified, the suspected syndrome is not ruled out, because current technology does not provide a complete search for all possibly relevant mutations even when the clinical diagnosis is certain. When the mutation affecting a family is known, a definitively negative molecular test allows an individual to revert to standard low risk screening (e.g., colonoscopy after age 50 yr), instead of the more frequent exams beginning at a much younger age recommended for mutation carriers (see Table 1)(17).

The standard family history obtained by primary care providers should remain an essential entry point for referral to a colon cancer genetics program for further evaluation (18,19). Molecular techniques may eventually become inexpensive enough to justify mass screening of the entire population, as is already being done in some states for another prevalent type of disease mutations, specifically those causing cystic fibrosis. All physicians can be helpful in initially recognizing any possible patients with hereditary colon cancer syndromes by obtaining a routine family history. The family history may reveal characteristics that suggest an inherited syndrome, such as multiple cancers or other typical clinical manifestations in a family or individual, particularly tumors diagnosed at an unusually early age.

2. BACKGROUND: CANCER GENETICS

2.1. Tumor Suppressor Gene Hypothesis

The interesting observation that tumors occur at an earlier age and more often in the inherited syndromes was first explained by Alfred Knudson's tumor suppressor gene hypothesis. Sporadic colon tumors are caused by somatic mutations in a few critical genes that accumulate in a single cell lineage. Hereditary colon tumor syndromes are caused by mutations in the same genes that cause sporadic tumors, but at least one of these is an inherited or germline mutation. Because the first mutational step has already occurred in every cell at the time of birth in the hereditary case, only one additional somatic mutation affecting a single cell is sufficient to inactivate that gene function. In contrast, sporadic cases require two distinct somatic mutational events to inactivate both the maternal and paternal copies of these genes in the same cell before a tumor develops.

The function of several more genes must be inactivated before an advanced cancer develops (20). Although these mutations are relatively rare events that may occur at random, many mutations can accumulate more rapidly if a genetic pathway important for maintaining normal DNA sequence or chromosomal structure is inactivated at an early stage during tumorigenesis.

2.2. APC Gene Mutations Cause Familial Adenomatous Polyposis

Familial adenomatous polyposis (FAP) is clinically characterized by a large number of adenomatous polyps in the colon and rectum. Patients with the classic severe form of the disease typically have more than 100 polyps (5). Adenomas develop in half of these patients by age 15 yr and 95% have adenomas by age 35 (21). If untreated, at least one of these adenomas will progress to cancer with an average age of colon cancer diagnosis of 39–42 yr (22). FAP is caused by germline mutation in the APC gene in the vast majority of cases (23,24). Extraintestinal lesions may include osteomas, odontomas, congenital hypertrophy of the retinal pigmented epithelium (CHRPE), epidermoid cysts, fibromas, and desmoid tumors. These manifestations in those patients with adenomatous colon polyps have been termed Gardner syndrome (25). Germline mutations in the APC gene also cause Gardner syndrome, but many of the phenotypic findings correlate with the specific type or location of mutation in the APC gene (26). Another phenotype–genotype correlation is the attenuated form of adenomatosis polyposis (AAPC), which manifests with a smaller number of polyps occurring at a later age in those patients with mutations located at the extreme 5' end of the APC gene (27).

2.3. DNA Mismatch Repair Gene Mutations
Are Responsible for Hereditary Nonpolyposis Colon Cancer

Hereditary nonpolyposis colon cancer (HNPCC) was first recognized more than a century ago by Dr. Warthin. During subsequent decades, this same family, and many others with HNPCC, were studied further by Dr. Henry Lynch (19). The molecular basis of this syndrome was elucidated in detail during the 1990s (28). Hereditary cancer registries have now been established at several medical centers throughout the world to provide appropriate diagnosis and care for families with HNPCC and a variety of other syndromes. These centers provide multidisciplinary consulting teams with expertise in gastroenterology, genetics, oncology, pathology and surgery.

As the name indicates, HNPCC is not associated with an increased number of adenomatous polyps. However, the colorectal polyps that do form in these patients are more likely to progress to malignancy, and both cancers and polyps occur at a younger age and in a more proximal distribution in the colon than the general population. The lack of an obvious early phenotype in contrast to APC (which has a profusion of polyps), makes presymptomatic genetic testing particularly helpful in HNPCC. HNPCC is characterized by an autosomal dominant inheritance pattern of colon cancer diagnosed at an average age of 45 yr, and colon cancer eventually occurs in 80% of mutation carriers (29). HNPCC survivors are at greatly increased risk for a second cancer. HNPCC patients have a 30% risk of a second cancer developing within 10 yr and risk increases to 50% after 15 yr (30,31), compared to the general population risks of 3 and 5%, respectively, after the same intervals. Mutations in MSH2 or MLH1 are also associated with a 42–60% risk of endometrial cancer in women before age 70 (29). Mutation carriers are

Table 2
Basic Elements of Informed Consent for Germline DNA Testing *(16)*

- Information on the specific test being performed.
- Implications of a positive and negative result.
- Possibility that the test will not be informative.
- Options for risk estimation without genetic testing.
- Risk of passing a mutation to children.
- Technical accuracy of the test.
- Fees involved in testing and counseling.
- Risks of psychological distress.
- Risks of insurance or employer discrimination.
- Confidentiality issues.
- Options and limitations of medical surveillance and screening following testing.

Table 3
Amsterdam Criteria for HNPCC *(83)*

(Family must have ALL of the following)

- At least three affected relatives with verified colorectal cancer.
- At least two successive generations affected.
- At least one is a first degree relative of the other two.
- At least one colon cancer < 50 yr of age.
- FAP is excluded.

at increased risk for other cancers, particularly malignancies of the upper gastrointestinal tract, urinary tract, and ovary (see Table 2).

HNPCC is caused by germline mutations in any one of the DNA mismatch repair (MMR) genes (*MLH1, MSH2, PMS1, PMS2, MSH6*) *(11)*. Mutations inactivating the protein products of these genes cause an accumulation of mutations in many other genes, causing a "mutator phenotype" leading to a higher risk for cancer *(32)*. Mutations in the DNA MMR genes may be suspected when the mutator phenotype is identified in the DNA of tumor tissue by detecting a phenomenon known as "microsatellite instability" *(33)*. Testing for microsatellite instability in tumors is useful to indicate the possibility of an inherited mutation in a DNA mismatch repair gene, since as expected, the vast majority of HNPCC tumors demonstrate this phenotype, but only about 15% of sporadic colon cancers have somatic mutations affecting these genes. Genetic testing is also indicated for affected individuals in families that meet the Amsterdam criteria (Table 3) or other criteria (Tables 4 and 5). Mutations in either *MLH1* or *MSH2* account for the majority of families with detectable gene mutation *(28)*. Mutations in *MSH6* have been reported in families with a later age of onset and lower frequency of colon cancer than typical for HNPCC *(34)*. Mutations in *PMS1* or *PMS2* have been implicated in a small number of families with HNPCC *(35)*.

2.4. Mutations in Other Genes Are Associated with Juvenile Polyposis, Peutz-Jeghers, and Other Hamartomatous Polyposis Syndromes

Alterations in several genes causing hamartoma syndromes have been identified (Table 6). Each syndrome is inherited in an autosomal dominant manner. The approach to management in these syndromes has not been defined as thoroughly as for APC or HNPCC, because fewer

Table 4
Bethesda Criteria for Testing of Colorectal Tumors for MSI (65)

(Patient should have ANY ONE of the following)

1. Individuals with cancer in families that meet the Amsterdam criteria.
2. Individuals with two HNPCC-related cancers, including synchronous and metachronous colorectal cancers or associated extracolonic cancers.
3. Individuals with colorectal cancer and a first-degree relative with colorectal cancer and/or HNPCC-related extra-colonic cancer and/or a colorectal adenoma; one of the cancers diagnosed at age <45 yr and the adenoma diagnosed at age < 40 yr.
4. Individuals with colorectal cancer or endometrial cancer diagnosed at age < 45 yr.
5. Individuals with right-sided colorectal cancer with an undifferentiated pattern (solid/cribiform) on histopathology diagnosed at age < 45 yr.
6. Individuals with signet-ring type colorectal cancer diagnosed at age < 45 yr.
7. Individuals with adenomas diagnosed at age < 40 yr.

Table 5
International Criteria for Determining MSI in Colorectal Cancer (65)

1. The form of genomic instability associated with defective DNA MMR in tumors is to be called MSI.
2. A reference panel of five microsatellites (BAT 25, BAT 26, D5S346, D2S123, and D17S250) has been standardized and is recommended for future research in the field. Tumors may be characterized as MSI-H if two or more of the five markers show instability (i.e., have insertion/deletion mutations), MSI-L if only one of the five markers show instability, or MSS if none of the five markers is unstable.
3. A unique clinical and pathological phenotype has been identified for the MSI-H tumors, which comprise about 15% of colorectal cancers, whereas MSI-L and MSS tumors appear to be phenotypically similar. MSI-H tumors are found predominantly in the proximal colon, have unique histopathological features, and are associated with a less aggressive clinical course than stage-matched MSI-L or MSS tumors. Preclinical models suggest the possibility that these tumors may be resistant to the cytotoxicity induced by certain chemotherapeutic agents. The implications of MSI-L are not yet clear.
4. MSI can be measured in fresh or fixed tumor specimens equally well. Microdissection of pathological specimens is recommended to enrich for neoplastic tissue, and normal tissue is required to document the presence of MSI.
5. The Bethesda Guidelines", which were developed in 1996 to assist in the selection of tumors for microsatellite analysis, were endorsed.
6. The spectrum of microsatellite alterations in noncolonic tumors was reviewed, and it was concluded that the above recommendations apply only to colorectal neoplasms.

patients have been followed for a significant time after predictive molecular diagnostic mutation testing. However, early diagnosis of this type of genetic predisposition to colon cancer may be expected to also have benefits, and the general principles of colon tumor risk management are similar in all these syndromes (Table 1). Although these polyps are hamartomas (normal tissue in an abnormal configuration), the risk of colon cancer is significantly elevated compared to the general population and may occur at a much younger age (5).

Table 6
Genes with Germline Mutations Associated
with Increased Colon Cancer Risk[a]

Hereditary syndrome	chromosome	gene(s)	
FAP	5q21	*APC*	
HNPCC	2p16	MSH2	
	3p21	*MLH1*	
	2q31–q33		*PMS1*
	7q11.2	*PMS2*	
		MSH6	
Juvenile polyposis	10q	*PTEN*	
		SMAD4/DPC4	
Cowden syndrome	10q	*PTEN*	
Peutz-Jeghers syndrome	19p	*STK11*	
HMPs	6q	unknown	

[a]Mutation detection may be commercially available, but availability does not imply that the sensitivity, specificity, or indications of such tests are known or validated.

Juvenile polyposis is defined as 10 or more juvenile polyps. These polyps have a normal epithelium (without dysplasia) and dilated mucus filled glands within an enlarged stroma that may appear to have a large number of inflammatory cells. Juvenile polyps are most common in the colon but may occur throughout the gastrointestinal tract. Juvenile polyposis is genetically heterogeneous. In different families, germline mutations occur in the *SMAD4 (DPC4) (36)* or the *PTEN* gene *(37,38)*. *PTEN* mutations have also been found in other syndromes with juvenile polyps and other manifestations, such as the Ruvalcaba-Myhre-Smith Syndrome or Bannayan-Zonana Syndrome *(39)*. Hereditary Mixed Polyposis Syndrome (HMPS) is a rare syndrome characterized by juvenile polyps, adenomas, and hyperplastic polyps *(40)*. HMPS has been linked to a genetic locus distinct from any other hamartoma syndromes, on chromosome 6q. Cowden syndrome includes juvenile polyps of the colon and entire gastrointestinal tract, pathognomonic skin lesions, and a substantial cancer risk in several other organs. Germline mutations in Cowden syndrome have been found in the *PTEN* gene *(39)*.

Peutz-Jeghers syndrome is characterized by perioral melanin spots and polyps with a distinctive arborizing pattern of the smooth muscle that may be adjacent to the epithelium without any intervening lamina propria. These polyps may be located throughout the gastrointestinal tract, but are most common in the small intestine. Cancers of the breast, pancreas, ovary, and/ or GI tract occur eventually in about half of these patients. Peutz-Jeghers syndrome is caused by germline mutations in the *STK11* gene *(41)*.

3. ESTIMATION OF GENETIC RISKS

3.1. Individual Personal Risk vs Mendelian Probability of Inheritance

The Mendelian probability is usually quite straight forward to calculate and usually represents the initial risk estimate available clinically. It reflects the average risk based on a pool of gametes from a parent with heterozygous mutation that have an equal probability of carrying the disease or normal allele *(42)*. Thus, for a single gene autosomal dominant disorder, any child of an affected person has a 50% chance of inheriting the disease allele. When two parents are both carriers of a recessive disorder the risk of inheritance of the disease alleles in a child is 25%. Since tumor suppressor gene mutations generally inactivate a normal function, they would be expected to act in a recessive manner on a cellular level. However, almost all cancer predisposition genes are inherited in an autosomal dominant manner. This may seem surprising at first glance, but the apparent paradox is resolved by considering these facts: (i) organisms consist of an extremely large number of cells;(ii) each cell in an affected individual carries a mutation inactivating one of the two parental alleles; (iii) somatic mutations inactivating the other normal allele are highly likely at least once during a lifetime; and (iv) tumors almost invariably develop when both alleles are inactivated within any one cell. Thus, although "recessive" on the cellular level, tumor suppressor genes act in a dominant manner on the level of the entire organism.

The Mendelian risk estimate of 50% inheritance for any child of an affected parent with an autosomal dominant disorder like cancer predisposition in some cases can be resolved into a more precise estimate of the actual personal risk of disease gene inheritance in a particular individual. Obviously, any one person actually either has the disease gene mutation or does not. When the chromosomal location of the disease gene is known, a generally useful method is linkage analysis. Genetic markers within 5 cM recombination distance from the disease gene could be used to obtain haplotypes for affected and unaffected members in the family resolving the risk estimates of inheritance to approx 5 vs 95%. Closely linked genetic markers (within 1 cM) would further refine the risk estimates in an individual relative to 1 vs 99%. Direct detection of the disease mutation by DNA sequencing or other techniques can diagnose inheritance at the absolute level of certainty (0 vs 100%).

These risks of course refer only to gene inheritance, which is not the same as the risk of developing the disease, unless penetrance and expressivity are both complete. For example, in patients with the *APC* gene mutations causing FAP, lifetime risk of colon cancer is indeed almost 100%, but in patients with DNA MMR gene mutations causing HNPCC, the lifetime risk of colon cancer is about 60–80%. The strongly predisposing alleles, because they are adverse to survival and selected against during evolution, are likely to be less frequent in the population than more common weaker alleles. An example of such a low penetrance allele in the *APC* gene, I1307K, converts an AAATAAAA sequence to AAAAAAAA. Although this germline variant is not in itself a cause of disease, it is more vulnerable to somatic mutations that can inactivate the *APC* gene. It has been reported to be present in 6% of all Ashkenazi vs 10% of Ashkenazi with colon cancer. The utility of genetic screening for this I1307K allele, which carries only a modest increase in risk for colon cancer is not as clear as for the clinically more severe syndromes *APC* and HNPCC, in which the difference in clinical management greatly depends upon gene inheritance *(43)*.

Physicians who refer their patients to a center or program specializing in colon cancer genetics will not need to be personally concerned about knowing many of the following complex issues in detail. Experienced referral centers are aware that some exceptions to the implicit assumption of simple Mendelian inheritance may complicate the analysis of genetic risks *(42)*:

1. Nonpaternity is often not disclosed during the family history, but technically is not a problem since direct mutation analysis will not be confounded, and it can also be detected easily during linkage analysis.
2. Uniparental disomy can mimic nonparentage, since two copies of a particular chromosome are inherited from only one parent (and no copies of that chromosome are contributed from the other parent).

3. Gene conversion occurs due to faulty correction of mismatched DNA strands, and might cause an error in linkage analysis since it could mimic an "impossible" double crossover in a short confined stretch of DNA.

4. Genomic imprinting is a phenomenon that causes a disorder to be inherited differently depending upon whether the paternal or maternal allele is mutant.

5. Mitochondrial inheritance is exclusively maternal, since these organelles are derived only form the ovum. Because there are many mitochondria, even in a single cell, and the proportion of mutant or normal mitochondria inherited can vary, it is difficult to predict the degree of affectation for disorders due to mutations of mitochondrial DNA.

Other assumptions are violated when one fertilized ovum does not develop into only one complete human:

1. Monozygotic twinning is usually not difficult to ascertain, and risk estimates are obviously 100% for an identical twin if the other has a diagnosed mutation.

2. Chimerism fuses two embryos into one and could be an alternative explanation for what appears to be somatic mosaicism.

3.2. Risk Assessment Modified by Knowledge of Clinical Phenotypes

Mutations in genes often reveal themselves in some manner that can be recognized as a characteristic or phenotype, but these may not be easily observable clinically prior to the development of cancer in some syndromes like HNPCC. Recognition of the tumor pattern among close relatives followed by an extended family history and then confirmation of the pathological diagnoses are the essential initial steps in the identification of new kindreds with cancer predisposition syndromes.

Various phenotypic criteria (Tables 3, 4, and 5) have been developed during the past few yr to guide genetic testing in HNPCC, because DNA sequencing analysis is expensive and has a lower yield in unselected cases with suspected hereditary cancer. The Amsterdam criteria (Table 3) were developed in 1991 to provide a clinical definition of HNPCC; they are also useful to select families for genetic testing of the DNA MMR genes associated with this syndrome. However, according to a population-based study, even the modified Amsterdam criteria would exclude at least one-third of families with demonstrable mutations in *MSH2* or *MLH1 (44)*. That study also demonstrated that germline mutations in *MSH2* or *MLH1* were responsible for at least 3.4% of all colon cancers in Finland. A more sensitive and less restrictive set of clinicopathological criteria to identify patients at risk for HNPCC were developed at a meeting in Bethesda in 1997 (Table 4). While the family history remains the primary method for identifying HNPCC, direct molecular diagnosis of individuals is now possible. The American Gastroenterological Association has recommended that direct molecular diagnosis be considered if patients meet any of the first three of the Bethesda criteria, but with the upper age limit raised from 45–50 yr. Mutations in *MSH2* or *MLH1* can be found in approx 40% of individuals who meet these criteria *(45)*.

Another method for risk assessment based on phenotype when HNPCC is suspected but the first three Bethesda criteria are not met, is the detection of the underlying abnormality that causes HNPCC, a form of genetic instability caused by mutations in DNA MMR genes. This phenomenon was serendipitously discovered in 1993, when microsatellite markers used for loss of heterozygosity (LOH) analyses were noted to have ubiquitous somatic variations in the number of repeat sequences that caused unexpected shifts in the size of alleles in tumors as detected by gel electrophoresis. The microsatellite instability phenotype is now generally known as MSI, but earlier papers used the alternative terminology "MIN" or "RER". Germline mutations in MMR genes have been linked to HNPCC and implicated in the pathogenesis of colon cancer. MSI testing requires DNA samples from normal and malignant tissue to compare their microsatellite alleles: extra alleles in the tumor, when compared to normal, is indicative of defective DNA repair. Pathology specimens such as formalin-fixed paraffin-embedded tissue blocks are sufficient if a margin of normal tissue is adjacent to the tumor. The results are reported as MSI-H (high) when at least two of the tested markers show instability, indicating an increased probability that the cancer arose due to an HNPCC-associated mutation. The results are reported as microsatellite stable (MSS) when no marker tested shows instability. In the absence of a compelling family history, this result is usually interpreted as ruling out HNPCC. MSI-L (low) is reported when instability is seen in only one of the markers, and does not indicate HNPCC. MSI-H is present in more than 90% of HNPCC cancers, compared to only 15–20% of sporadic cancers. Because MSI testing is a relatively inexpensive method compared to DNA sequencing, patients considered to have a lower prior probability of harboring a germline MMR mutation should initially have their colon cancers, if available, screened for MSI *(46)*. Under this suggested algorithm, patients at higher than 20% risk for having a MMR mutation would have MSH2 and MLH1 testing directly.

Although HNPCC generally has a better prognosis than sporadic colorectal cancer, the histology of HNPCC colon tumors tends to be poorly differentiated or undifferentiated. The 5-yr survival of HNPCC patients in a population-based study from Finland was reported as 65%, compared to 44% for those with sporadic colorectal cancers *(47)*. Tumors with undifferentiated cells growing in a solid pattern are most suggestive of underlying HNPCC, since this histology occurs in only 0.5% of sporadic cases, but 10% of HNPCC-associated colorectal cancers *(48)*. Abundant mucin production characterized by the presence of signet ring cells is another feature of HNPCC. There may also be a heightened immunologic reaction with a predominance of CD3+ T cells infiltrating the tumor and peritumoral nodules of B lymphocytes surrounded by T lymphocytes similar to the pattern seen in Crohn's disease *(49)*. However, these histological features are not sufficiently distinctive to be diagnostic of HNPCC. Immunohistochemical staining of colon tumors may indicate which gene (MSH2 or MLH1) should be targeted initially for germline mutation analysis by DNA sequencing in those patients suspected to have HNPCC.

3.3. Risk Assessment Based on Direct Molecular Testing for Genotype

The impact that genetic test results can have on medical decisions and outcomes has made molecular diagnostics an important new component of standard medical practice for certain familial syndromes. Molecular diagnosis is a potentially powerful method of cancer risk assessment for individuals inheriting mutant alleles of genes that have been identified as causing cancer predisposition (Table 6). Mutation detection is commercially available for the major genes causing colon cancer susceptibility, including *APC, MSH2, MLH1, PTEN, SMAD4*, etc. Some of these laboratories are listed on the GeneTests Web site (see Website: www.genetests.org). Genetic testing for syndrome diagnosis usually requires a blood draw, to obtain peripheral blood leukocytes to send to a laboratory for analysis of DNA or RNA, and is only available when ordered by a physician. These tests may cost several hundred dollars or more, and results may not be available for many weeks. Many other tests will be developed in the near future, but availability does not necessarily imply that their clinical indications, sensitivity, or specificity are adequately studied and thoroughly validated. Some laboratories are not approved under the United States Clinical Laboratories Improvement Act (CLIA). Any clinician ordering genetic tests should have a good understanding of all the complex issues involved. There are several possible sources of error in genetic testing, including clinical misdiagnosis of the suspected syndrome, inaccurate representation of relationships on the pedigree, and sample misidentification or contamination.

The process of evaluating a patient with suspected hereditary cancer should begin with a thorough family history and verification of pathological diagnoses to establish the most likely syndrome(s). Genetic counseling and informed consent (Table 2) are necessary before proceeding to molecular diagnostic testing, which should begin with a clearly affected member of the family. The diagnosis of a specific hereditary syndrome cannot be confirmed without identifying a mutation that functionally inactivates a gene known to cause the syndrome. Some laboratories will advise whether a sequence variation is of unknown significance, or on the other hand is indeed a mutation likely to have a deleterious effect because it causes a major change such as a truncated protein. Some missense mutations can interfere seriously with protein function, but interpretation of these mutations is more difficult if they cause minimal changes. Such indeterminate results should be communicated carefully to families with detailed genetic counseling. The significance of equivocal variants such as missense mutations may be clarified by testing other members of the same family to determine if the mutation correlates with cancer in several other individuals. Future research may further clarify the risk estimate by examining the effect of the same mutation in other families.

When a deleterious mutation is identified in an index case, any other relatives at risk can then be tested even if they are asymptomatic. Inheritance of the mutant allele would indicate a need for that relative to have intensive screening and preventive treatment, whereas inheritance of only normal alleles would indicate that only standard interventions the same as for the low-risk general population are sufficient. If the relative does not carry the mutation known to affect the family, they can be reassured that although their risk of cancer is not zero, it is no greater than the general population, and the mutation cannot be passed on to that patient's children.

4. MOLECULAR DIAGNOSTIC METHODS

4.1. DNA Sequencing Can Detect Previously Known or Unknown Mutations

Several techniques have been used to determine the precise order of nucleotide bases within a particular segment of DNA. Historically, the first technique invented by Allan Maxam and Walter Gilbert relied upon chemical cleavage of end-labeled DNA (50–52). The second technique, developed by Fred Sanger and colleagues, uses enzymatic synthesis to extend a short sequence of end-labeled primer DNA and modified dideoxy nucleotides to cause chain terminations that indicate the sequence (53,54). Modifications of the latter technique is now most widely used. Detection can be easily accomplished by incorporation of radioactive or fluorescent groups (55,56). Automated real-time detection of fluorescently labeled DNA fragments by laser-based instrumentation now makes possible very high-throughput generation of DNA sequence data (10,56). After such sequence data is obtained, it can be entered into computer databases and processed by sequence analysis programs to allow homology comparisons and identify possible functional domains of interest.

Several commercial and university laboratories perform DNA sequencing analysis for cancer susceptibility genes (Table 6). A blood sample is usually all that is needed to perform these genetic tests, since DNA can be simply extracted from leukocytes, or the leukocytes can be immortalized as a permanent source of DNA or RNA. The functional significance of a particular sequence variant is an important consideration for the proper interpretation of these test results, and is more in doubt if the mutation is not clearly deleterious and has not been observed previously in other families. Websites have been established to compile databases of mutations reported for some disease genes. However, in general, since the most up-to-date and complete information is not available from any one database, consultation with one or more of the few clinicians and researchers who have a special interest or focus on a particular syndrome should be obtained.

4.2. Linkage Analysis is Useful in Some Familial Colon Tumor Syndromes

Genome databases have been organized to store and analyze the large amount of complex gene mapping data (see Websites: www.gdb.org or www.ncbi.nlm.nih.gov). Genetic map data may be used to identify a mutant gene (allelic variant) associated with a human disease if a sufficient number of affected patients and families are available for study, and an easily analyzed genetic marker is closely linked (low probability of being separated by recombination). The utility of genetic markers relies upon their polymorphism, i.e., different variants that discriminate between homologous maternal and paternal chromosomal alleles. The restriction fragment-length polymorphisms (RFLPs) generally have only two variants (presence or absence of a restriction site), so are of limited usefulness compared to the highly polymorphic short tandem repeat or microsatellite markers, which can have a very large number of alleles because of variation in the number of repeat elements (57,58).

Linkage analysis can indicate which of several genes for a genetically heterogeneous syndrome may be mutated in a newly investigated family, particularly if these genes are located on different chromosomes and direct mutational analysis is expensive or difficult (e.g., MSH2 and MLH1 genes in HNPCC). Linkage analysis may also be useful in some families with disorders thought to be monogenic, if direct detection of a mutation is not possible by DNA sequencing or the protein truncation assay (e.g., APC) (59). Linkage analysis may be used to make predictions about disease status if there are at least two or more family members with a confirmed clinical diagnosis available to participate in DNA testing, along with the individual in question and unaffected relatives. The pedigree in question should be reviewed by the testing laboratory and informed consent obtained before submitting blood samples for analysis. APC gene testing by linkage analysis is performed at the University of Utah DNA diagnostic laboratory using polymerase chain reaction (PCR) markers or RFLP analysis. The pattern of highly polymorphic intragenic and flanking markers is compared in affected and unaffected family members. If evident, a pattern of inheritance indicating segregation of the affected haplotype is reported. In rare cases, a family is found to be "uniformative", since the affected allele cannot be distinguished from the unaffected allele, and no result can be reported.

4.3. Molecular Diagnosis of FAP by APC Protein Truncation Assay: In Vitro Protein Synthesis from RNA

The mechanism of inactivation of tumor suppressor genes may include frameshift, insertion, deletion, or nonsense mutations encoding a truncated protein that lacks an essential function. If research investigating a cancer predisposition gene frequently demonstrates germline mutations of this type, a clinical diagnostic test may be developed to detect the truncated polypeptides.

The molecular diagnosis of FAP involves an early example of the successful application of this method in clinical practice. The majority of FAP families have one of a variety of mutations scattered throughout the APC gene. However, most of these mutations result in truncation of the APC protein, since they encode novel stop codons due to single base pair substitutions or short deletions or insertions (5). Thus, an in vitro protein synthesis assay for truncated APC polypeptides can identify an APC gene mutation in about 80% of families with adenomatous polyposis (23,60). It was first introduced commercially in 1994 and is now available at several laboratories. Other methods for identifying the APC gene mutation, which may be useful in families negative by the protein truncation assay, are linkage analysis or DNA sequencing.

Molecular diagnostic testing is now approved for coverage by many insurers and managed care organizations. This acceptance may be enhanced because definitive negative results rule out disease inheritance and decrease the need for the otherwise necessary surveillance sigmoidoscopies, which, because they are performed annually, eventually cost much more than the fee charged for the protein truncation assay. The specialists most frequently ordering this test are gastroenterologists who account for 47% of patients, with only 18% of patients tested by medical geneticists and/or genetic counselors, and the remainder by a variety of other practitioners *(24)*. Consultation by a knowledgeable gastroenterologist is important, particularly one with a special interest in this problem who can appropriately counsel the patient and perform any necessary endoscopic procedures. Many physicians (32%) involved in the care of families with FAP are unfortunately unaware that a negative test in any patient is informative and useful only if a mutation has been detected in an affected relative *(24)*. Erroneously failing to institute endoscopic surveillance due to such a false negative test result could have devastating future consequences if polyps and cancer are not diagnosed early. The quality of care for patients with hereditary polyp and cancer syndromes should be improved by referral to specialized centers or physicians familiar with the complexity and manifold ramifications of genetic testing.

4.4. Mutation Detection by Other Methods

Mutations are changes in the DNA that may be inherited and thus affect the entire organism and perhaps its progeny (germline) or affect only a single clone of cells within the individual (somatic). Mutations range in magnitude from the entire genome (e.g., triploidy) to alterations of chromosomal structure (deletions, insertions, inversions, duplications, translocations of a portion of one chromosome to another), or single base changes (missense, nonsense, splice site, frameshift). Their functional impact may range from no effect at all (silent) to a complete lack of gene function (null), decrease of function (hypomorphic), or gain of a new function (neomorphic). Because of adverse selective pressures, mutations causing a severe phenotype (a greatly increased risk for cancer at a young age) are probably much less frequent in the population than those with a milder effect. These milder more common alleles are more difficult to detect by linkage analysis than classic syndromes like FAP, but could impact a much larger fraction of the population. Practically every human being has some mutations with potential clinical significance, but most of these are not detectable by current methods. Mutation analysis is also complicated by the fact that most disorders are not monogenic, but are determined by other major modifying genes and the environment (the latter etiologies are probably more likely for diseases with a later age of onset).

Mutation detection in the scanning mode searches a stretch of DNA for unknown mutations, in contrast to the diagnostic mode where specific tests are designed to detect known mutations *(61)*. Specific diagnostic tests can be developed using DNA sequencing, allele-specific oligonucleotide hybridization arrays, ligation detection, allele-specific amplification, and artificial introduction of restriction sites. Scanning methods include denaturing gradient gel electrophoresis, heteroduplex analysis, and single-stranded conformational analysis, and other techniques that cleave mismatched sequences chemically or by enzymes.

Denaturing gradient gel electrophoresis was able to identify mutations in the *MSH2* or *MLH1* genes in approx half of the families in one study who met the clinical diagnostic criteria for HNPCC *(46)*. This is similar to the proportion identified in other studies by in vitro transcription translation and direct sequencing. The failure to detect mutations in all HNPCC families may be due to mechanisms of inactivation of these genes that cannot be detected by the methods used, genetic heterogeneity, or other causes of the same phenotype.

PCR is a method of amplification that produces many copies of an entire sequence between any two known ends, even for very rare sequences in a complex DNA mixture (62–64). The DNA to be amplified is defined by two short single-stranded oligonucleotide primers (approx 20 bases) that anneal to complementary sequences on opposite strands of the template DNA target. The synthesized copies of the target DNA thus consists of the two oligonucleotide sequences and the sequence between them. Because the sequence between the primers can vary, it is possible to use this technique to diagnose germline or somatic mutations. Because it is rapid, specific, inexpensive, and amenable to automation, it is now routinely utilized in many research and clinical laboratories.

Multiple sequences can be tested simultaneously in one hybridization reaction by creating an array of different sequences located on one matrix. Affymetrix and other companies have extended this concept to include very large numbers of sequences on very high density arrays prepared by methods similar to those in semiconductor chip technology to produce "gene chips". Almost all of the mRNA coding sequences important in a particular cell or organism can be analyzed simultaneously on one array, making it possible to detect changes in the overall patterns of gene expression in response to experimental or therapeutic interventions or to compare normal to neoplastic development. Other types of arrays might, in the future, be used in the diagnostic rather than the scanning mode to economically identify the presence of particular gene mutations.

4.5. Colon Tumor Testing for Genetic Instability Associated with HNPCC

MSI testing is relatively inexpensive and may be a reasonable screening option prior to MMR gene mutation analysis. DNA from both normal and tumor tissue is needed for MSI analysis, since the phenotype is not observed in normal tissue and is recognized as a variation present only in the tumors. DNA for analysis can be obtained from either fresh or frozen tissue or from paraffin-embedded pathology specimens (even after many yr, archival blocks retain sufficiently intact DNA). The incidence of germline mutations detected in MMR genes in HNPCC kindreds selected by MSI or linkage analysis was 70% (28), but was only 25% in kindreds negative for MSI and linkage. The Bethesda criteria (Table 4) were developed in 1996 specifically to provide guidelines to select tumors for MSI testing (65). The large number of studies reporting MSI in colorectal cancer and other extra-colonic malignancies prior to 1998 lacked uniform criteria regarding which markers should be used and how many should be altered before a tumor is diagnosed with the instability phenotype. A National Cancer Institute workshop in December 1997 (Table 5) defined specific criteria and consensus guidelines for MSI testing (65). Other indications for MSI testing could be considered. These might include predicting differences in response to therapy related to the biology of this phenotype in the tumor itself, rather than implications at the level of organization of the patient or family regarding inherited cancer risk.

4.6. Stool Tests to Screen for Colon Cancers in Families with HNPCC

Testing for occult blood in the stool is a proven cost-effective method for reducing colon cancer mortality (66). However, this method has limited sensitivity because many early stage tumors do not bleed, and many cases of false positive results because trace amounts of blood may be present without the source being polyps or cancer. More direct methods of testing for tumor cells through mutant DNA shed in stool are now being developed. These methods test for mutations in the APC gene (67) and other genes that cause colon tumors and "nonapoptotic" human DNA that is a general feature of cancer. Clinical trials indicate that the performance characteristics of the EXACT stool test may be superior to Hemoccult, with possibly higher specificity and sensitivity *(68)*. Because some patients with hereditary syndromes are at risk for tumors of the small intestine that are difficult to detect by small bowel follow-through (SBFT) X-ray, use of the EXACT stool test or Given capsule endoscopy may allow earlier diagnosis.

5. IMPLICATIONS OF GENETIC TESTING FOR CLINICAL CARE

5.1. Clinical Applications of Molecular Diagnostic Methods

As the human genome project discovers inherited mutations causing disease, there will be new opportunities to develop preventive measures and treatments targeted against these specific molecular defects. Despite the exciting developments in the field of mutation detection in recent yr, there is no one best method with general utility and many have specific applications to a particular gene. Presymptomatic knowledge of an inherited cancer predisposing mutation has the benefit of indicating a need for increased surveillance to allow earlier diagnosis at a curable stage. The public will probably demand genetic testing for cancer susceptibility: 83% of respondents to a random survey expressed a moderate to strong interest in such testing. The expense of genetic testing may limit its acceptance by some patients if the laboratory costs are not covered by insurance. Third party payers have been encouraged by studies that have shown that the overall costs of colon tumor screening in a family are reduced to about half by molecular diagnosis, because endoscopic exams are not needed for the 50% of children and other relatives who test negative for a known mutation *(69,70)*.

5.2. Genetic Counseling and Informed Consent for Genetic Testing

Counseling regarding the possible risks and benefits of cancer early detection and prevention modalities and a discussion of the basic elements of informed consent (Table 2) should be obtained before offering germline DNA testing. Counseling should assist the patient and family understand the information provided, help them feel comfortable in the process of making an informed decision, and support them in choosing a course of action regarding management of their cancer risk and aid their psychosocial adjustment to the knowledge gained. The American Society of Clinical Oncology has recommended cancer predisposition testing if all these criteria are met *(16)*: (i) the prior probability of a positive result is high, because the patient has a strong family history of cancer or very early onset of disease; (ii) the test can be adequately interpreted; and (iii) the results will influence the medical management of the patient or family.

Genetic counselors in the past were focused on congenital defects and the pediatric population and did not have much training in the cancer-related aspects of genetics, because these clinical applications have only recently developed. Some other specialist physicians (oncologists, gastroenterologists, etc.) have met the needs of their patients by maintaining sufficient continuing education in molecular genetics, pedigree construction, and Bayesian analysis, so that they can directly deliver the necessary counseling services. Alternatively, practitioners could consult with other colleagues having expertise in cancer genetic testing *(16)*. Sensitivity to psychosocial issues is important. One study reported that patients with higher education levels were more than three times as likely to accept genetic testing when offered, and those with symptoms of depression were less likely to participate *(71)*. At least one center reports that they have relied solely on telephone rather than in-person counseling for some patients because they would otherwise need to travel a long distance *(72)*. However, this remote telephone-only method is controversial, and many other centers require at least one personal visit. The majority of patients tested for HNPCC mutations in one large series considered pretest counseling and support, during a test disclosure session, quite useful, but after 1 yr, only 2% of patients felt the greatest need for further counseling (73). These authors conclude that in HNPCC, perhaps limited resources can be directed more to the beneficial cancer surveillance aspect of care rather than to extensive psychological support. Another study (74) found that the primary motivations for participating in genetic testing were similar to previous reports and included: wanting to know if more cancer screening tests were needed, obtaining information about the risk for offspring and increasing certainty around their own risk. Psychosocial scores demonstrated that only a subgroup of patients exhibited distress, with greater distress for those individuals awaiting results or testing positive. Overall, there was a high level of satisfaction associated with the experience of testing.

5.3. Ethical, Legal, and Social Implications

The National Center for Human Genome Research at the National Institutes of Health, jointly with the Department of Energy, established the ELSI working group in 1990 to study the ethical, legal, and social implications of human genome research. This program has studied issues relating to the introduction of genetic testing into clinical practice, access to personal genetic information, and education of the public and professionals about human genetics. This effort may help to define the clinical validity and impact of several protocols for genetic testing.

5.2. Screening and Management

Colon cancer screening is recommended at more frequent intervals and beginning at a younger age for those at higher risk due to hereditary syndromes (Table 1). Because germline mutations are present in every cell, it is important to be aware of the increased risk for extra-colonic tumors in these syndromes, but each has a different spectrum of risk in other organs (Table 1). Screening is effective for preventing colon cancer in HNPCC, presumably by polypectomy. The rate of colon cancer diagnosis was reduced to 4.5% among HNPCC families screened at 3-yr intervals, compared to 11.9% among unscreened HNPCC families, and death rates were reduced by half for those screened (75). The more frequent intervals of screening now recommended would be expected to be even more effective at reducing cancer morbidity and mortality in HNPCC. Prophylactic colectomy has been considered an option for patients who are cancer phobic or may have poor compliance with annual colonoscopic screening (76).

5.5. Chemoprevention Research

Animal models with mutations in the same genes that cause colon tumor syndromes in humans have tremendous potential for the study of nutritional, pharmacological, or other interventions for cancer prevention and disease treatment (77–79). Researchers using a mouse model of adenomatous polyposis found that any drugs inhibiting cyclo-oxygenase profoundly prevented and regressed adenomas, but selective inhibitors of COX-2 had less gastrointestinal toxicity than nonspecific COX-1 and COX-2 inhibitors, like nonsteroidal anti-imflammatory drugs (NSAIDs) (80). These studies led to a clinical trial with celecoxib, resulting in its rapid approval by the U.S. Food and Drug Administration as the first drug for colon tumor prevention (81). The COX-2 inhibitor celecoxib is indicated for suppressing adenomas in FAP, but patients, when treated, must still continue annual surveillance and will eventually require colectomy. The approved dose of celecoxib in FAP is 400 mg twice daily (note this is more than the usual arthritis dose). Clinical trials are now in progress to investigate the potential benefits of celecoxib for chemoprevention of adenomas in the general population with a history of at least one colonic adenoma. However, there are as yet no clinical trials to support use of NSAIDs or any coxibs such as celecoxib or rofecoxib, for tumor prevention in those patients with HNPCC, a syndrome with important biological differences in tumor development. The preclinical trials in an animal model of HNPCC found no benefit from NSAID treatment, despite a very strong benefit of the same treatment in parallel experiments in an animal model of FAP. This chemopreventive drug treatment approach may be expected to be less effective in HNPCC, because of the biological differences in HNPCC tumors, which are less likely to overexpress COX-2, compared to adenomas and cancers in FAP or sporadic tumors in the general population.

6. SUMMARY

The American Gastroenterological Association has published a position statement and guidelines on genetic testing for hereditary colorectal cancer *(82)*. This document provides an excellent summary of the current status of the genetic testing approach: "The integration of genetic testing into clinical practice provides multiple benefits to individuals in families with histories of colorectal cancer. These benefits include earlier detection of colorectal neoplasms and prevention of cancer, removal of patient uncertainty, greater choice of surgical and other intervention options, elimination of unnecessary screening, and provision of information for planning family and career decisions. In hereditary colorectal cancer, genetic testing has been shown to be cost-effective."

7. RESOURCES FOR FURTHER INFORMATION

Resource	Website
Hereditary Colon Cancer Association	www.hcca.org.
A directory of some laboratories performing genetic testing	www.genetests.org.
Online version of the reference Mendelian Inheritance in Man	www3.ncbi.nlm.gov/Omim.
American Gastroenterological Association	www.gastro.org.
American Society for Gastrointestinal Endoscopy	www.asge.org.
American College of Gastroenterology	www.acg.gi.org.
National Cancer Institute information gateway	www.cancernet.nci.nih.gov
Centers for Disease Control and Prevention Office of Genetics	www.cdc.gov/genetics
Department of Health and Human Services,	
Secretary's Advisory Committee on Genetic Testing	www4.od.nih.gov/oba/sacgt
National Human Genome Research Institute	www.nhgri.nih.gov.

REFERENCES

1. American Cancer Society. In *Cancer Facts and Figures*. 2001.
2. Burt R, Petersen G. Familial colorectal cancer: diagnosis and management. In *Prevention and Early Detection of Colorectal Cancer*. Young GP, Rozen P, Levin B (eds.), Saunders, London, UK, 1996, pp. 171–194.
3. Feuer EJ, Wun LM. *DEVCAN: Probability of Developing or Dying of Cancer Software*, 4.0 ed., National Cancer Institute, 1999.
4. Aarnio M, Sankila R, Pukkala E, et al. Cancer risk in mutation carriers of DNA-mismatch-repair genes. *Int. J. Cancer*, **81** (1999) 214–218.
5. Jacoby RF, Burt RW. Polyposis syndromes. In *Textbook of Gastroenterology*. 3rd ed., Yamada T, Alpers DH, Laine L, et al. (eds.), Lippincott-Raven, Philadelphia, PA, 1999.
6. Antonarakis SE. Diagnosis of genetic disorders at the DNA level [erratum appears in *N. Engl. J. Med.*, **321** (1989) 56.]. *N. Engl. J. Med.*, **320** (1989) 153–163.
7. Green ED, Cox DR, Myers RM. The Human genome project and its impact on the study of human disease. In *The Genetic Basis of Human Cancer*. Vogelstein B, Kinzler KW (eds.), McGraw-Hill, New York, NY, 1998, p. 33.

8. Eisenstein BI. The polymerase chain reaction. A new method of using molecular genetics for medical diagnosis. *N. Engl. J. Med.*, **322** (1990) 178–183.

9. Hunkapiller MW. Protein sequence analysis: automated microsequencing. *Science*, **219** (1983) 650–659.

10. Hunkapiller T. Large-scale and automated DNA sequence determination. *Science*, **254** (1991) 59–67.

11. Giardiello FM. AGA technical review on hereditary colorectal cancer and genetic testing. *Gastroenterology*, **121** (2001) 198–213.

12. Kinzler KW, Nilbert MC, Su LK, et al. Identification of FAP locus genes from chromosome 5q21. *Science*, **253** (1991) 661–664.

13. Nishisho I, Nakamura Y, Miyoshi Y, et al. Mutations of chromosome 5q21 genes in FAP and colorectal cancer patients. *Science*, **253** (1991) 665–669.

14. Groden J, Thliveris A, Samowitz W, et al. Identifacation and characterization of the familial adenomatous polyposis coli gene. *Cell*, **66** (1991) 589–600.

15. Jarvinen HJ, Aarnio M, Mustonen H, et al. Controlled 15-year trial on screening for colorectal cancer in families with hereditary nonpolyposis colorectal cancer. *Gastroenterology*, **118** (2000) 829–834.

16. Anonymous. Statement of the American Society of Clinical Oncology: genetic testing for cancer susceptibility, Adopted on February 20, 1996. *J. Clin. Oncol.*, **14** (1996) 1730–1740.

17. Burt RW. Colon cancer screening. *Gastroenterology*, **119** (2000) 837–853.

18. Lynch HT, Shaw MW, Magnuson CW, Larsen AL, Krush AJ. Hereditary factors in cancer. Study of two large midwestern kindreds. *Arch. Intern. Med.*, **117** (1966) 206–212.

19. Lynch HT, Smyrk TC, Watson PT, et al. Genetics, natural history, tumor spectrum, and pathology of hereditary nonpolyposis colorectal cancer: an updated review. *Gastroenterology*, **104** (1993) 1535–1549.

20. Kinzler K, Vogelstein B. Colorectal tumors. In *The Genetic Basis of Human Cancer*. Vogelstein B, Kinzler KW (eds.), McGraw-Hill, New York, NY, 1998, pp. 565–590.

21. Bussey HJR. *Familial Polyposis Coli: Family Studies, Histopathology, Differential Diagnosis and Results of Treatment*. Johns Hopkins University Press, Baltimore, MD, 1975.

22. Jarvinen HJ. Time and type of prophylactic surgery for familial adenomatosis coli. *Ann. Surg.*, **202** (1985) 93–97.

23. Powell SM, Petersen GM, Krush AJ, et al. Molecular diagnosis of familial adenomatous polyposis. *N. Engl. J. Med.*, **329** (1993) 1982–1987.

24. Giardiello FM. The use and interpretation of commercial APC gene testing for familial adenomatous polyposis [see comments]. *N. Engl. J. Med.*, **336** (1997) 823–827.

25. Gardner E. Follow-up study of a group exhibiting dominant inheritance for a syndrome including intestinal polyps, osteomas, fibromas, and epidermal cysts. *Am. J. Hum. Genet.*, **14** (1962) 376–390.

26. Laurent-Puig P, Beroud C, Soussi T. APC gene: database of germline and somatic mutations in human tumors and cell lines. *Nucleic Acids Res.*, **26** (1998) 269–270.

27. Spirio L, Olschwang S, Groden J, et al. Alleles of the APC gene: an attenuated form of familial polyposis. *Cell*, **75** (1993) 951–957.

28. Liu B. Analysis of mismatch repair genes in hereditary non-polyposis colorectal cancer patients [see comments]. *Nat. Med.*, **2** (1996) 169–174.

29. Vasen HFA, Wijnen JT, Menko FH, et al. Cancer risk in families with hereditary nonpolyposis colorectal cancer diagnosed by mutation analysis. *Gastroenterology*, **110** (1996) 1020–1027.

30. Lynch HT, Harris RE, Lynch PM, Guirgis HA, Lynch JF, Bardawil WA. Role of heredity in multiple primary cancer. *Cancer*, **40** (1977) 1849–1854.

31. Mecklin JP, Jarvinen HJ. Clinical features of colorectal carcinoma in cancer family syndrome. *Dis. Colon Rectum*, **29** (1986) 160–164.

32. Aaltonen L, Peltomaki P, Leach F, et al. Clues to the pathogenesis of familial colon cancer. *Science*, **260** (1993) 812–816.

33. Boland CR. A National Cancer Institute Workshop on Microsatellite Instability for cancer detection and familial predisposition: development of international criteria for the determination of microsatellite instability in colorectal cancer. *Cancer Res.*, **58** (1998) 5248–5257.

34. Akiyama Y, Sato H, Yamada T, et al. Germ-line mutation of the hMSH6/GTBP gene in an atypical hereditary nonpolyposis colorectal cancer kindred. *Cancer Res.*, **57** (1997) 3920–3923.

35. Nicolaides NC, Papadopoulos N, Liu B, et al. Mutations of two pms homologues in hereditary nonpolyposis colon cancer. *Nature*, **371** (1994) 75–80.

36. Howe JR, Roth S, Ringold JC, et al. Mutations in the SMAD4/DPC4 gene in juvenile polyposis. *Science*, **280** (1998) 1086–1088.

37. Olschwang S, Serova-Sinilnikova OM, Lenoir GM, Thomas G. PTEN germ-line mutations in juvenile polyposis coli. *Nat. Genet.*, **18** (1998) 12–14.

38. Jacoby RF, Schlack S, Cole CE, et al. A juvenile polyposis tumor suppressor locus at 10q23 is deleted from non-epithelial cells in the lamina propria. *Gastroenterology*, **112** (1997) 1398–1403.

39. Wanner M, Celebi JT, Peacocke M. Identification of a PTEN mutation in a family with Cowden syndrome and Bannayan-Zonana syndrome. *J. Am. Acad. Dermatol.*, **44** (2001) 183–187.

40. Whitelaw SC, Murday VA, Tomlinson IP, et al. Clinical and molecular features of the hereditary mixed polyposis syndrome. *Gastroenterology*, **112** (1997) 327–334.

41. Jenne DE, Reimann H, Nezu J, et al. Peutz-Jeghers syndrome is caused by mutations in a novel serine threonine kinase. *Nat. Genet.*, **18** (1998) 38–43.

42. Bridge PJ. *The Calculation of Genetic Risks*. The Johns Hopkins University Press, Baltimore, MD, 1994.

43. White RL. Excess risk of colon cancer associated with a polymorphism of the APC gene? *Cancer Res.*, **58** (1998) 4038–4039.

44. Salovaara R. Population-based molecular detection of hereditary nonpolyposis colorectal cancer [erratum appears in *J. Clin. Oncol.*, **18** (2000) 3456.]. *J. Clin. Oncol.*, **18** (2000) 2193–2200.

45. Syngal S. Sensitivity and specificity of clinical criteria for hereditary non-polyposis colorectal cancer associated mutations in MSH2 and MLH1. *J. Med. Genet.*, **37** (2000) 641–645.

46. Wijnen JT. Clinical findings with implications for genetic testing in families with clustering of colorectal cancer. *N. Engl. J. Med.*, **339** (1998) 511–518.

47. Sankila R. Better survival rates in patients with MLH1-associated hereditary colorectal cancer [see comments]. *Gastroenterology*, **110** (1996) 682–687.

48. Jass JR. Pathology of hereditary nonpolyposis colorectal cancer. *Ann. NY Acad. Sci.*, **910** (2000) 62–73.

49. Alexander J, Watanabe T, Wu TT, Rashid A, Li S, Hamilton SR. Histopathological identification of colon cancer with microsatellite instability. *Am. J. Pathol.*, **158** (2001) 527–535.

50. Sambrook J, Fritsch EF, Maniatis T. *Molecular Cloning: A Laboratory Manual*. Cold Springs Harbor Laboratory Press, Cold Springs Harbor, NY, 1989.

51. Maxam AM. Sequencing end-labeled DNA with base-specific chemical cleavages. *Methods Enzymol.*, **65** (1980) 499–560.

52. Maxam AM. A new method for sequencing DNA. *Natl. Acad. Sci. USA*, **74** (1977) 560–564.

53. Sanger F. DNA sequencing with chain-terminating inhibitors. *Natl. Acad. Sci. USA*, **74** (1977) 5463–5467.

54. Sanger F. Determination of nucleotide sequences in DNA. *Science*, **214** (1981) 1205–1210.

55. Smith LM. Fluorescence detection in automated DNA sequence analysis. *Nature*, **321** (1986) 674–679.

56. Prober JM. A system for rapid DNA sequencing with fluorescent chain-terminating dideoxynucleotides. *Science*, **238** (1987) 336–341.

57. Weber JL. Human DNA polymorphisms based on length variations in simple-sequence tandem repeats. *Genome Anal.*, **1** (1991) 159–181.

58. Weber JL, May PE. Abundant class of human DNA polymorphisms which can be typed using the polymerase chain reaction. *Am. J. Hum. Genet.*, **44** (1989) 388–396.

59. MacDonald F, Morton DG, Rindl PM, et al. Predictive diagnosis of familial adenomatous polyposis with linked DNA markers: population based study. *BMJ*, **304** (1992) 869–872.

60. Powell SM, Petersen GM, Krush AJ, et al. Molecular diagnosis of familial adenomatous polyposis. *N. Engl. J. Med.*, **329** (1993) 1982–1987.

61. Forrest S. How to find all those mutations. *Nat.Genet.*, **10** (1995) 375–376.

62. Mullis K. Specific enzymatic amplification of DNA in vitro: the polymerase chain reaction. *Cold Spring Harbor Symp. Quant. Biol.*, **51** (1986) 263–273.

63. Mullis KB. Specific synthesis of DNA in vitro via a polymerase-catalyzed chain reaction. *Methods Enzymol.*, **155** (1987) 335–350.

64. Saiki RK, Schart S, Faloona F, et al. Enzymatic amplification of beta-globin genomic sequences and restriction site analysis for diagnosis of sickle cell anemia. 1985. *Biotechnology*, **24** (1992) 476–480.

65. Rodriguez-Bigas MA, Boland CR, Hamilton SR, et al. A National Cancer Institute Workshop on Hereditary Nonpolyposis Colorectal Cancer Syndrome: meeting highlights and Bethesda guidelines. *J. Natl. Cancer. Inst.*, **89** (1997) 1758–1762.

66. Mandel JS, Church TR, Ederer F, Bond JH. Colorectal cancer mortality: effectiveness of biennial screening for fecal occult blood. *J. Natl. Cancer Inst.*, **91** (1999) 434–437.

67. Traverso G, Shuber A, Levin B, et al. Detection of APC mutations in fecal DNA from patients with colorectal tumors. *N. Engl. J. Med.*, **346** (2002) 311–320.

68. Ahlquist DA, Skoletsky JE, Boynton KA, et al. Colorectal cancer screening by detection of altered human DNA in stool: feasibility of a multitarget assay panel. *Gastroenterology*, **119** (2000) 1219–1227.

69. Cromwell DM. Cost analysis of alternative approaches to colorectal screening in familial adenomatous polyposis. *Gastroenterology*, **114** (1998) 893–901.

70. Bapat B. Cost comparison of predictive genetic testing versus conventional clinical screening for familial adenomatous polyposis. *Gut*, **44** (1999) 698–703.
71. Lerman C. Genetic testing in families with hereditary nonpolyposis colon cancer. *JAMA*, **281** (1999) 1618–1622.
72. Lynch PM. Clinical challenges in management of familial adenomatous polyposis and hereditary nonpolyposis colorectal cancer. *Cancer*, **86** (1999) 2533–2539.
73. Aktan-Collan K. Evaluation of a counselling protocol for predictive genetic testing for hereditary nonpolyposis colorectal cancer. *J. Med. Genet.*, **37** (2000) 108–113.
74. Esplen MJ. Motivations and psychosocial impact of genetic testing for HNPCC. *Am. J. Med. Genet.*, **103** (2001) 9–15.
75. Jarvinen HJ, Mecklin J, Sistonen P. Screening reduces colorectal cancer rate in families with hereditary nonpolyposis colorectal cancer. *Gastroenterology*, **108** (1995) 1405–1411.
76. Lynch HT. Is there a role for prophylactic subtotal colectomy among hereditary nonpolyposis colorectal cancer germline mutation carriers? *Dis. Colon Rectum*, **39** (1996) 109–110.
77. Jacoby RF, Marshall DJ, Newton MA, et al. Chemoprevention of spontaneous intestinal adenomas in the Min/Apc mouse model by the nonsteroidal anti-inflammatory drug piroxicam. *Cancer Res.*, **56** (1996) 710–714.
78. Dove WF, Clipson L, Gould KA, et al. Intestinal neoplasia in the ApcMin mouse: independence from the microbial and natural killer (beige locus) status. *Cancer Res.* **57** (1997) 812–814.
79. Jacoby RF. Chemopreventive efficacy of combined piroxicam and difluoromethylornithine treatment of Apc mutant Min mouse adenomas, and selective toxicity against Apc mutant embryos. *Cancer Res.*, **60** (2000) 1864–1870.
80. Jacoby RF. The cyclooxygenase-2 inhibitor celecoxib is a potent preventive and therapeutic agent in the min mouse model of adenomatous polyposis. *Cancer Res.*, **60** (2000) 5040–5044.
81. Steinbach G, Lynch PM, Phillips RK, et al. The effect of celecoxib, a cyclooxygenase-2 inhibitor, in familial adenomatous polyposis. *N. Engl. J. Med*, **342** (2000) 1946–1952.
82. American Gastroenterological Association medical position statement: hereditary colorectal cancer and genetic testing. *Gastroenterology*, **121** (2001) 195–197.
83. Vasen HFA, Mecklin J-P, Meera Khan P, Lynch HT. The international collaborative group on hereditary nonpolyposis colorectal cancer. *Dis. Colon. Rectum*, **34** (1991) 424–425.

14 Inflammation

Cynthia A. Cunningham, Jonathan R. Fulton, and Christopher F. Cuff

1. INTRODUCTION

Despite the body's ability to maintain the integrity of the epithelium, the intestine is vulnerable to breaches that can result in inflammatory responses. Induction of a localized acute inflammatory response is necessary to contain disruption or invasion of the epithelial barrier. The onset and duration of an acute inflammatory response is limited, yet in some instances persistent immune activation promotes chronic inflammation, resulting in detrimental pathological consequences. The events and biological mediators involved in the inflammatory process of the gastrointestinal tract are discussed in this chapter.

2. ACUTE INFLAMMATION

Inflammation is defined as the sequence of immunologic events in response to a variety of damaging stimuli, including tissue injury and infection. The hallmark signs of acute local inflammation are swelling, heat, pain, redness, and loss of function. Intestinal inflammation is characterized by infiltration of the mucosa by leukocytes, damage to the epithelium and lamina propria matrix, and loss of normal nutrient absorptive function. Although acute inflammation is primarily focused on resolution of a local event, the process is also accompanied by a systemic acute phase response, which is mediated by the action of cytokines produced within the mucosa that diffuse through the vasculature. Overall, the sequence of events characteristic of inflammation involve local vasodilation of small vessels within the mucosa, chemotatic signaling and recruitment of circulating leukocytes, and subsequent leukocytic infiltration and activation that ultimately promotes resolution of the inciting event and promotes tissue healing.

From: *Colonic Diseases*
Edited by: T. R. Koch © Humana Press Inc., Totowa, NJ

The mucosa of the gastrointestinal tract contains diverse populations of leukocytes, including phagocytic cells such as macrophages and neutrophils, as well as lymphocytes, mast cells, and eosinophils; immune cells that primarily secrete soluble effector molecules. Upon stimulation, these cells initiate and promote an inflammatory response aimed at preventing further egress by foreign material. Soluble chemical mediators released by resident immune, epithelial, and stromal cells of the mucosa act to increase vascular permeability and up-regulate intercellular adhesion molecules both on endothelial cells and leukocytes circulating within local blood vessels. Some secreted inflammatory mediators act as chemotaxins necessary for the recruitment of leukocytes into the inflamed tissues, while others activate recruited leukocytes to release reactive oxygen species (ROS), proteases, cytokines, and other compounds that further promote inflammation.

An acute inflammatory response can be triggered by a variety of stimuli. In the gastrointestinal tract, stimuli include infectious pathogens, chemical irritation, and food allergy. In addition, important iatrogenic factors of mucosal inflammation include radiation damage, drug reactions, ischemia, and treatment-induced pathology, such as pseudomembranous colitis and ulceration induced by nonsteroidal anti-inflammatory (NSAID) agents. While the mechanisms of action of factors initiating intestinal inflammation are not entirely understood, several common features and mediators of acute intestinal inflammation have been identified.

2.1. Physiologic Stimulation of the Acute Inflammatory Response

Breaches of the gastrointestinal mucosa, whether by pathogens, toxins, or gastric acids, result in a sensory afferent nerve-mediated elevation of mucosal blood flow, known as the hyperemic response. The early onset of vasodilation characteristic of this response is generated by the release of calcitonin gene-related peptide (CGRP) and, perhaps to a lesser extent, other neurotransmitters including vasoactive intestinal peptide from sensory afferent nerves. This neural response augments the hyperemic response by releasing substance P, which induces mucosal mast cells to release histamine and promotes neutrophil recruitment into the lamina propria by up-regulating endothelial adhesion molecule expression, such as E- and P-selectin (1).

Initiation of the inflammatory response is enhanced by the contact activation system. This system is composed of four complex innate networks, known as the complement, coagulation, kinin, and fibrinolytic systems, and can be activated by exposure to foreign antigen, lipopolysaccharide, circulating immune complexes or vascular damage. Together, these interconnected networks regulate coagulation, vasodilation, and complement activation. The activated coagulation pathway factors kallikrein and factor XII attract neutrophils and stimulates their accumulation and degranulation. Production of bradykinin of the kinin system mediates vasodilation, pain, and increased capillary permeability. Cleavage of plasminogen into plasmin results in degradation of fibrin deposits, as well as cleavage and subsequent activation of complement components C1, C3, and C5. Collectively, these pathways contribute to initiation of an inflammatory response (Fig. 1).

2.1.1. INVOLVEMENT OF RESIDENT EPITHELIAL CELLS IN INITIATING EVENTS

Intestinal epithelial cells (IEC) have direct contact with the lumenal environment and, accordingly, are the first cells affected by damaging agents. Therefore, IEC are typically the initial activators of the inflammatory response and can play an active role in the subsequent immune responses. Stimulated IEC are capable of generating and transmitting signals via soluble factors and cell-bound molecules that result in increased leukocyte attraction and adherence at the site of tissue damage, as well as stimulating effector function.

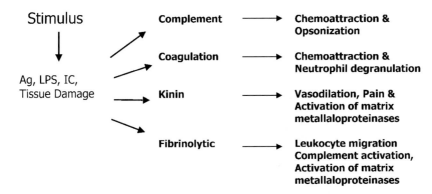

Fig. 1. Inflammatory signals initiate the contact activation system. Inflammatory stimuli such as antigens (Ag), bacterial LPS, immune complexes (IC), or tissue damage initiate the contact activation system. The active products of this system mediate a variety of responses that result in inflammation.

Activated mucosal epithelial cells secrete high levels of chemoattractant cytokines, known as chemokines, which promote the migration and subsequent adherence of leukocytes to the inflamed site. Chemokines are a family of small molecular weight cytokines that contain four conserved cysteine residues whose position is used to further classify them into four subfamilies designated C, CC, CXC, and CX_3C, where X represents another amino acid (2). The chemokines most relevant to mucosal inflammation belong to the CXC and the CC families (3,4). In humans, most CXC chemokines are more selective for neutrophils and T cells or B cells, but not monocytes (5). The CXC family include interleukin (IL)-8 and neutrophil attractant protein (NAP)-2, growth-related oncogene (GRO)-α, GRO-β, and GRO-γ, and extractable nuclear antigen (ENA)-78. In contrast, the CC subgroup contain four contiguous cysteine residues and include macrophage capping protein (MCP)-1, the macrophage inflammatory proteins (MIP) MIP-1β and MIP-1α, and regulated upon activation normal T cell expressed and secreted (RANTES). The CC chemokines secreted by IEC attract B lymphocytes and macrophages. During an acute response to mucosal insult, the chemokines initially secreted by distressed IEC are neutrophil attractants IL-8, the GRO family of chemokines, and ENA-78.

2.2. Adhesion and Infiltration of Effector Cells

2.2.1. Neutrophil Transmigration and Infiltration

Within the first 6 h of the inflammatory response, neutrophils begin to infiltrate from the post-capillary endothelial venules into the affected area. This influx of neutrophils is considered the fundamental histological feature of acute inflammation. Neutrophils normally travel through the vasculature in a process called neutrophil rolling, which allows the passing neutrophil to sample the endothelial cell surface for up-regulated intercellular adhesion molecules and chemokines indicative of local tissue damage. As the rolling neutrophils come in contact with chemoattractants, such as IL-8 and platelet activating factor (PAF), conformational changes occur in the surface integrin adhesion molecule leukocyte function-associated antigen (LFA)-1, allowing binding to intercellular adhesion molecule-1 (ICAM-1), which is up-regulated on the lumenal endothelial surface for subsequent transendothelial migration. At least during response to infection, transmigration of neutrophils across the intestinal epithelium appears to be stimulated by a recently described cytokine referred to as pathogen-elicited epithelial chemoattractant (PEEC) (6). PEEC is released into the gut

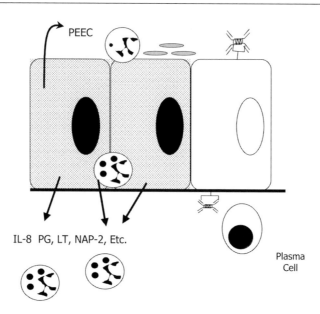

Fig. 2. Apical expression of chemoattractants drives neutrophil migration to the intestinal lumen. In response to inflammatory insult, IECs secrete a variety of chemoattractants including IL-8, PG, LT, NAP-2, and others, which produce a concentration gradient that leads to neutrophil influx into the site of tissue damage. In addition, during infection epithelial cells apically express PEEC, which promotes migration between the epithelial cells and into the intestinal lumen, where they can act against invading pathogens.

lumen following contact with pathogenic organisms to direct immigrant neutrophils directly to the pathogens (Fig. 2). Once extravascular within the inflamed mucosal stroma, neutrophils exhibit chemotaxis as a result of increased cell surface expression of receptors for chemoattractants, including IL-8, prostaglandins, leukotrienes, NAP-2, and complement products. Up-regulation of these cell surface molecules allow the neutrophils to migrate in the direction of increasing concentrations of chemokines deposited within the extracellular matrix until arriving at the distressed IEC layer.

2.2.2. LEUKOCYTE ADHESION

In addition to the chemokines, activated human epithelial cells up-regulate expression of surface molecules involved in adhesion and leukocyte activation. Perhaps most significant among these is ICAM-1. Increased expression of ICAM-1 on the apical cell surface can be correlated with an increase apical adhesion of neutrophils *(7)* and this interaction helps to retain neutrophils at the site of tissue damage. There are several other adhesion molecules that contribute to this process, albeit to a lesser degree. Such receptors include LFA-3, CD47, CD86, gp180, biliary glyoprotein (BGP) and E-cadherin *(7)*. E-cadherin is noteworthy in that while normally responsible for formation of adherence junctions, E-cadherin has been shown to exhibit co-stimulatory activity towards intraepithelial lymphocytes (IEL) via the integrin receptor $\alpha_E\beta_7$ *(8)*. Thus, increased E-cadherin expression also potentially stimulates IEL function. Gp180 also interacts with IEL via surface ligand CD8. Therefore, increased IEC gp180 expression potentially stimulates IEL functions (such as cytotoxicity and cytokine production) in conjunction with enhanced E-cadherin ligation, thus contributing to the inflammatory process.

2.3. Leukocyte Function in Inflammation

2.3.1. PHAGOCYTOSIS

2.3.1.1. Neutrophils. Upon entering the site of inflammation, the primary role for neutrophils is to destroy or neutralize the inflammatory agent. During the recruitment phase, neutrophils become functionally activated and, therefore, able to phagocytose and degranulate. These processes result in destruction of the inflammatory stimulus by both oxygen-dependent (respiratory burst) and oxygen-independent mechanisms. During phagocytosis, the inflammatory stimulus is engulfed into a cytoplasmic phagosome that fuses with granules containing lysosomes. These granules contain a diverse mixture of degradative components including enzymes (catalase, lysozyme, and serine proteases) and other effector proteins that exhibit antimicrobial activity such as α- and β-defensins. Granular contents mediate their function within the cytosol and are released into the extracellular space in a process known as extracellular degranulation or phagocytic regurgitation. Although serving a vital antimicrobial function, this extracellular release of granular components results in bystander damage of surrounding tissue. For example, activated neutrophils release elastase and cathepsin G. Human elastase degrades the extracellular matrix component elastin and, in conjunction with cathepsin G, proteolytically modifies collagen rendering it more susceptible to enzymatic digestion.

During phagocytosis, the respiratory burst results in the production of ROS. The effective end products responsible for pathogen destruction include superoxide radical (O_2^-), hydrogen peroxide (H_2O_2), hydroxyl radical (OH^-), and hypochlorous acid ($HOCl$). The highly reactive superoxide radicals, while effective biological oxidants, are short-lived and consumed in the immediate vicinity of their production. On the other hand, H_2O_2 and OH^- are capable of diffusing away from their initial site of release and enter other cells either by crossing plasma membranes (H_2O_2) or pass through anion channels (OH^-). Therefore, phagocytic cells can cause oxidant-dependent injury of susceptible target cells on both the plasma cell membrane and in intracellular sites. Unfortunately, bystander death of IEC or other cells can exacerbate tissue damage that accompany an inflammatory response. Additionally, ROS are capable of modulating the inflammatory response by inactivating various inflammatory mediators, including prostaglandins, complement C5a, and leukotriene (LT) C_4.

2.3.1.2. Monocytes and Macrophages. Macrophages are a prominent cell population located throughout the gastrointestinal tract, especially within the lamina propria and Peyer's patches. Macrophages and blood monocytes are attracted to the site of inflammation by the release of MIP-1 by activated IEC and neutrophils. While MIP-1 is considered the most potent chemoattractant, others include complement factor C5a and bacterial products such as endotoxin. Like the neutrophils, macrophages also are phagocytic and can kill using oxygen-dependent and -independent mechanisms. However, macrophages are not granulocytic and do not undergo degranulation and, therefore, do not exhibit the bystander toxicity associated with granulocytes. In addition to mediating pathogen destruction, monocytes and macrophages process and present antigen in the context of major histocompatibility complex (MHC) class I or class II molecules to CD8$^+$ and CD4$^+$ T lymphocytes, respectively. Activation of CD4$^+$ T helper lymphocytes is a key step in developing subsequent adaptive humoral and cell-mediated immune responses.

2.3.2. NON-PHAGOCYTIC INFLAMMATORY CELLS

Other granulocytic effector cells that migrate to the site of inflammation include mast cells and basophils. While morphologically distinct, these cell types each have a granular appearance and share similar functions. Mast cells and basophils are nonphagocytic cells usually associated with allergic responses due to their capacity to bind immunoglubulin (Ig)E. Mast cells residing in the mucosa are unique compared to those residing in connective tissue, in that they require T-cell derived IL-3 for proliferation, lack the major granule-associated enzyme chymase, and produce high levels of tumor necrosis factor-α (TNF-α). Upon stimulation, basophils degranulate in response to a number of signals including IgE, IL-1, IL-3, IL-8, and various inflammatory response products, such as complement components and neuropeptides (9). The granules contain proteolytic enzymes that directly affect their target and compounds that promote the inflammatory response such as histamine. Histamine induces contraction of intestinal smooth muscles, increases permeability of venules, and increases mucus secretion by goblet cells. Stimulated granulocytes further contribute to the inflammatory response by providing arachidonic acid metabolites, releasing PAF and chemotatic factors, and producing a number of cytokines, such as TNF-α, IL-3, IL-4, IL-8, granulocyte macrophage colony-stimulating factor (GM-CSF), and interferon-α (IFN-α).

2.3.2.1. Eosinophils. Eosinophils residing within the lamina propria provide important assistance for resolution of parasitic infections. Eosinophils express receptors for IgE, IgA, IgG, and complement factors C3b and C4, all of which are up-regulated upon exposure to basophil-derived histamine and eosinophil chemotatic factor of anaphylaxis. Although eosinophils have the potential to be phagocytic, they primarily produce and release granules that contain well-characterized enzymes, such as collagenase and histaminase. Probably one of the most important components produced by eosinophils is major basic protein, a secreted factor that exhibits multiple functions vital for parasite destruction and inflammation, including induction of histamine release from other granulocytes and heparin neutralization.

2.4. Soluble Mediators of the Acute Inflammatory Response

Soluble mediators of the inflammatory response are produced by IEC, leukocytes, and other resident cells including endothelial cells and fibroblasts. Many of the molecules are produced by more than one cell population, thereby promoting extension and amplification of their activity. While this approach may seem redundant, most of the mediators that act locally are rapidly inactivated either by direct inhibition or dilution.

2.4.1. Cytokines

While several cytokines are involved in the inflammatory process, the two most extensively characterized are IL-1β and TNF-α, both of which are released during the early stages of the inflammatory process. Several cell types produce IL-1, including macrophages and endothelial cells, while TNF-α is produced predominantly by macrophages and mast cells. Although these two cytokines are structurally unique and have separate receptors, they both elicit very similar effects. Both TNF-α and IL-1 can promote inflammation by causing neutrophil recruitment, inducing IEC to increase their prostaglandin production, and up-regulating the expression of adhesion molecules on endothelial cells. These two cytokines also modulate the inflammatory response by priming the cytolytic capabilities of macrophages and neutrophils. Despite the beneficial effects, TNF-α has been implicated as a major contributor to gastrointestinal damage, especially following infection with *Helicobacter pylori (10)* and exposure to NSAIDs *(11)* or bacterial endotoxin *(12)*.

In addition to the local and infiltrating leukocyte populations, it appears that the resident epithelial cells are an important source of cytokines. Human IEC lines T84 and Caco-2 constitutively express mRNA for a gamut of proinflammatory cytokines including IL-8, IL-15 (a cytokine that shares many of the biologic properties of IL-2, the classical T cell growth factor), and TNF-α. In addition, studies involving these cell lines and freshly isolated human

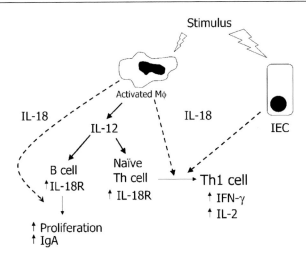

Fig. 3. Synergistic effect of IL-12 and IL-18 during inflammation. Following inflammatory stimulation, macrophages become activated and secrete various soluble effector molecules, including IL-12 and IL-18. Secretion of IL-12 induces naïve CD4+ Th cells to undergo differentiation into Th1 cells and up-regulate the expression of IL-18 receptor (IL-18R). Interaction with IL-18 potentiates IL-12-driven Th1 differentiation, and together IL-12 and IL-18 synergistically up-regulate IFN-γ and IL-2 production. Stimulation of B cells with IL-12 and IL-18 augment proliferation, class switching, and antibody production, however, just as with the T cells, B cells must interact with IL-12 prior to IL-18.

IEC indicate that upon stimulation with invasive bacteria or pretreatment with TNF-α and IL-1, these cell up-regulate expression of proinflammatory cytokines IL-8, monocyte chemotatic protein-1, GM-CSF, and TNF-α (4). Therefore, IEC contribute to initiating and potentiating an inflammatory response through cytokine production.

Macrophages serve as a key source for IL-10, IL-12, and IL-18. IL-10, along with IL-5 and IL-6, function to promote B cell activation and antibody isotype switching. Additionally, IL-10 elicits potent immunosuppressive effects, primarily by inhibiting IFN-γ production by T helper (Th)1 cells, by down-regulating the expression of class II MHC on antigen-presenting cells and suppressing production of various proinflammatory mediators, including nitric oxide, IL-1, IL-6, IL-8, GM-CSF, granulocyte colony-stimulating factor (G-CSF), and TNF-α. On the other hand, IL-12 and IL-18 exhibit positive effects on acute, and potentially chronic, inflammation. IL-12 acts synergistically with IL-2 to induce cytotoxic T lymphocyte (CTL) activation and, in turn, induces the expression of IL-18 receptor on T cells. Unlike IL-12, IL-18 alone is incapable of inducing Th1 differentiation, however IL-18 can augment IL-12-stimulated Th1 development. IL-12 and IL-18 directly affect Th1 responses individually and synergistically to activate T cells and induce proliferation and IFN-γ production (Fig. 3). This relationship is important for inflammation, in that concomitant administration of IL-12 and IL-18 induces intestinal inflammation in an IFN-γ-dependent but TNF-α-independent manner (13).

T cell-derived IL-16 and IL-17 have recently been shown to play important roles during intestinal inflammation. In fact, up-regulation of IL-16 has been documented in both Crohn's disease and ulcerative colitis (14). IL-16, which is also expressed by mast cells, is a strong chemoattractant for CD4+ T cells and, therefore, plays a role in accumulation and activation of CD4+ T cells recruited to sites of inflammation. In addition, IL-16 also functions to activate expression and production of proinflammatory cytokines such as IL-1β, IL-6, and

TNF-α in human monocytes. Although IL-17 expression is restricted to memory T cells, the IL-17 receptor is expressed on a variety of cell types including IEC. This cytokine induces a number of effects important to the inflammatory process including promoting maturation of neutrophils, inducing secretion of inflammatory mediators such as IL-6, IL-8, prostaglandin (PG) E_2, MCP-1, and G-CSF by adherent cells, up-regulating ICAM-1 expression, and promoting T cell proliferation. Exposure of a rat IEC cell line in vitro to IL-17 has been shown to augment IL-1β-induced cellular responses and elevate expression of the CC chemokine MCP-1 and CXC chemokine CINC, which is a cytokine that is closely related to human neutrophil attractant GRO (15).

2.4.2. ARACHIDONIC ACID METABOLITES

Upon activation, membrane phospholipids in various leukocytes including macrophages, neutrophils, and mast cells, are degraded into arachidonic acid and lyso-PAF. The latter compound is subsequently converted into PAF, a compound known to mediate inflammatory effects, including eosinophil chemotaxis, and the activation and degranulation of neutrophils and eosinophils. Arachonidic acid is further metabolized into PGs, LTs, and thromboxane; all of which are involved in the inflammatory process.

PGs are 20-carbon fatty acids produced from arachidonic acid that mediate an array of biological functions on the gut mucosa necessary for homeostasis and, more importantly, mucosal defense. PG synthesis is mediated by two, and potentially three (16), isoforms of the enzyme cyclooxygenase (COX). COX-1 is constitutively expressed, while COX-2 (and possibly COX-3) is induced during the initial and latent phases of inflammation, respectively. During inflammation, PG can mediate proinflammatory effects, such as fever, neutrophil chemotaxis, and increased vasodilation and vascular permeability.

Despite the proinflammatory effects, the major role of PG in the gut is to protect against acute mucosal injury (17) and down-regulate proinflammatory mediators. PGE$_2$, which is produced by several cell types, including neutrophils, monocytes, and macrophages, is a potent suppressor of TNF-α in macrophages and mast cells and also inhibits PAF and histamine (18). Furthermore, Barrera et al. (19) demonstrated that in vitro PGE$_2$ mediates reduction of IL-3 secretion from lamina propria mononuclear cells as well as IL-2 from activated T cells. In addition, PGE$_2$ is a major mediator of the epithelial crypt regeneration following chemical- or radiation-induced intestinal damage (20).

Although recently challenged (21), gastric ulceration as a result of NSAID therapy has been largely attributed to inhibition of PG production predominately by selective suppression of COX-1 (22). PGs produced by COX-1 mediate events necessary for normal gut function, such as stimulation of mucus and bicarbonate secretion, and maintenance of mucosal blood flow. COX-2 is expressed only at sites of inflammation and inhibition of this enzyme does not interfere with COX-1 and its products. Therefore, treatment with selective COX-2 inhibitors has become an important adjunct to NSAID therapy to avoid deleterious effects of PGE inhibition.

LTs are another group of metabolites of arachidonic acid and are categorized into two subclasses, LTB$_4$, and peptido-LTs (LTC$_4$, LTD$_4$, and LTE$_4$). LTs are produced predominantly by granulocytes; however epithelial and endothelial cells also produce measurable amounts of LTs. In the mucosa, neutrophils are the major source for LTB$_4$. LTB$_4$ is a potent leukocyte chemotaxin, especially for neutrophils, that up-regulates expression of LFA-1. Additionally, LTB$_4$ stimulates neutrophils to release oxygen species that contribute to local tissue damage. Mast cells are the major source for peptido-LTs, and unlike LTB$_4$, peptido-LTs exhibit no chemotatic activity. Instead, peptido-LTs potently stimulate smooth muscle contraction, increase vascular permeability, and increase endothelial expression of P-selectin promoting leukocyte rolling.

Thromboxane, produced predominantly by platelets and, to a lesser extent, neutrophils, stimulates LTB_4 release. In addition, because thromboxane is a potent vasoconstrictor, it has been suggested that it contributes to gastric ulceration by restricting blood flow (23).

PAF appears to regulate smooth muscle tone, activate neutrophils, and act as a chemotaxin for eosinophils. In addition, PAF up-regulates LFA-1 on leukocytes and can itself serve as an adhesion molecule on the surface of endothelial cells. PAF is a potent ulcerogenic factor at high doses (24) and has been shown to be responsible for most of the tissue injury observed in the gastrointestinal tract following administration of endotoxin (25) and other models of topical gastric irritation (26). Evidence suggests that this is most likely due to the ability of PAF to stimulate leukocyte adherence to the vascular endothelium and activate granulocytes to release ROS (27). Together, PAF and other arachidonic acid metabolites are potent regulators of discreet events in inflammation.

2.4.3. Nitric Oxide

In the gastrointestinal mucosa, physiological levels of nitric oxide (NO) influence mucus secretion, mucosal blood flow, and enteric nerve function. Several mucosal cell populations release NO upon stimulation. In addition to its role in physiologic maintenance, evidence for the role of NO in both promoting and limiting inflammation has been documented.

The role of NO in exacerbating intestinal inflammation is indirect. Rectal biopsies from ulcerative colitis patients indicate an increase in NO synthesis, which is believed to be predominantly produced by epithelial cells (28). However, the loss of NO either associated with acute shock-like states (e.g., soft tissue trauma and mesenteric ischemia-reperfusion) or artificial blockade of NO synthase leads to the activation of mast cells. This activation initiates an inflammatory response by up-regulating the adherence and subsequent infiltration by neutrophils. Likewise, decreased levels of NO production has been observed in other colonic disease states, including acquired megacolon (29). ROS of NO oxidation induces tissue toxicity. For example, NO can react with superoxide anion released by activated neutrophils forming peroxynitrite, a potent oxidant, and administration of peroxynitrite has been shown to cause injury and inflammation in the colon (30).

Despite the evidence suggesting a role for NO in mucosal dysfunction during inflammation, administration of large doses of NO does not induce mucosal injury (31), and in certain situations actually provides protection to the stomach from injury. NO inhibits PAF and histamine release from mast cells and likewise, enhancement of NO production by the blockade of the inhibitor of NO synthase (iNOS) appears to have a protective effect against chronic inflammation. Therefore, the role of NO in inflammation is unclear and is an important avenue of study.

2.5. Acute Phase Response

The local inflammatory response is accompanied by a systemic response known as the acute phase response characterized by induction of fever, transient increase in white blood cell counts, and release of acute phase proteins from the liver. Secretion of colony stimulating factors (macrophage colony stimulating factor [M-CSF], G-CSF, GM-CSF) stimulates hematopoiesis, accounting for the temporary increase in peripheral blood cell counts. Interaction of various proinflammatory cytokines, IL-1, IL-6, and TNF-α, with receptor bearing hepatocytes induces the production of an array of acute phase proteins, including C-reactive protein, serum amyloid A (SAA), fibrinogen, mannose-binding protein, lipopolysaccharide

(LPS) binding protein (LBP), and complement components to opsonize pathogens. Typically, these proteins function to enhance the immune response against pathogens. Activity of these proteins are concentration-dependent, and it is possible that effective levels of systemically produced LBP and SAA do not reach the gut. However, the liver is not the only source for these acute phase proteins. In vitro stimulation of human IEC lines with proinflammatory cytokines, such as TNF-α, IL-6, and IL-1, induces them to produce measurable amounts of LBP and SAA, suggesting a role for these proteins in local defense (32). Therefore, it is possible that IEC produced LBP and SAA that sensitize or enhance the local mucosal immune response to translocated endotoxin.

2.6. Adaptive Immunity

Typically, acute inflammatory responses are mediated by the innate branch of the immune system, but the acquired immune response directed by lymphocytes also plays a role in mediating and resolving inflammation. During an inflammatory response, activated T lymphocytes aid the containment of the antigenic stimuli by either releasing cytokines to promote the response or undertake direct cellular cytotoxicity. Depending on the stimulus, CD4[+] T cells promote macrophage activation and cytolytic T cell responses by secreting IL-2, TNF-α, and IFN-γ (referred to as a Th1 response), or support a humoral response through production of IL-5, IL-6, and IL-10 (a Th2 response). IL-2 promotes T cell proliferation, while IFN-γ is a strong activating factor for macrophages and augments many of the activities mediated by TNF-α. The Th2 cytokines IL-5, IL-6, and IL-10 function to permit B cell activation and antibody isotype switching. B cells serve an indirect, yet vital, role the inflammatory process by secreting antibody, especially IgA. Secreted into the gut lumen, IgA functions to bind antigen, thereby preventing interaction with, and potential invasion of, the epithelial barrier.

The Th2 cytokines, especially IL-10, function to inhibit Th1 responses. Likewise, IFN-γ down-regulates Th2 responses. This balance is of importance because most chronic inflammatory bowel diseases, such as Crohn's disease, exhibit characteristic skewing towards a Th1 response. Under normal conditions, most activated lymphocytes eventually undergo apoptosis, thereby limiting the response and any subsequent tissue damage. However, chronic inflammation results from untrammeled responses.

Intestinal inflammation is characterized by structural changes within the mucosa, including universal features such as shedding of IEC with blunting of the villi, which occurs simultaneously with either thickening of the lamina propria and hyperproliferative lengthening of the crypts or alternatively, with hypoproliferative atrophy of the crypts. The mechanisms governing the changes in the villous and crypt histoarchitecture of the mucosa are dependent on factors produced primarily by lamina propria mesenchymal fibroblasts (MSF), as well as factors produced by activated macrophages and T cells. In response to cytokines, such as TNF-α produced by activated macrophages and mast cells or IL-1 produced by macrophages, MSF produce large quantities of extracellular matrix degrading zinc-containing proteases known as matrix metalloproteinases (MMP). While MMPs are constitutively produced to facilitate normal tissue maintenance and remodeling, inflammation-induced overexpression can cause tremendous damage within the mucosa. Three key MMPs dominate this response: interstitial collagenase (MMP-1), gelatinase-A (MMP-2), and stromelysin-1 (MMP-3). These enzymes, and related MMPs secreted by activated T cells and macrophages, are activated extracellularly by proteolytic cleavage by activated plasmin or kallikrien, or by autolysis. Once activated, these enzymes degrade lamina propria collagen III and IV, and matrix proteoglycans, leading to dissolution of the matrix and shedding of the overlying epithelium (Fig. 4).

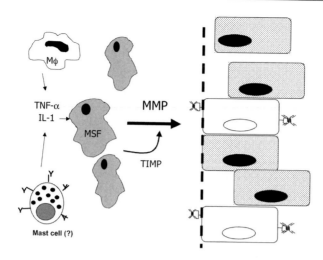

Fig. 4. MMP production by MSF results in digestion of the basement membrane and subsequent loss of the integrity of the intestinal epithelium. Under the influence of inflammatory cytokines, such as TNF-α produced predominantly by macrophages (and potentially mast cells), and IL-1 produced by macrophages (and other cells), MSF produce a number of MMPs. These MMPs degrade lamina propria collagen III and IV and matrix proteoglycans. MSF also produce TIMP to control their activity. In has been suggested that an imbalance of MMP and TIMP production is a major factor in massive tissue destruction during exacerbation of IBD.

The actions of MMPs are opposed by a family of inhibitory factors also derived from the MSF, known as tissue inhibitors of metalloproteinases (TIMP) as well as serum protease inhibitors such as α_2-antitrypsin. It has been speculated that disruption of a homeostatic balance in MMP and TIMP concentration is the major effector mechanism behind mucosal damage in chronic inflammation and may be either a primary cause in itself or a secondary effect of immune cell dysregulation (33). MMP-induced mucosal damage may also be indirectly opposed by the effects of immunosuppressive cytokines IL-10 and tumor growth factor-β (TGF-β) on the inflammatory cell axis. Indeed, MMP-2, -3, and -7 can proteolytically activate latent inactive TGF-β stores that are deposited within the extracellular matrix, which then serves as a negative feedback regulator on MMP producing cells and contribute to restitution.

3. RESOLUTION OF INFLAMMATION

The gastrointestinal mucosa is composed of a dynamic population of epithelial cells that constantly undergo turnover regeneration. Integrity of the mucosal barrier is maintained as cells derived from the crypts replace mature villus epithelial cells. This process requires coordination among the local cell populations by a regulatory network of cytokines and growth factors. Following inflammatory tissue damage, complete repair of the epithelial barrier occurs in two major stages that involve restitution followed by increased epithelial cell proliferation that results in functional restoration (34). Restitution occurs very early after initiation of damage and involves migration of immature epithelial cells from the mucosal crypts near the injured area to the exposed region. Once the denuded area has been sufficiently covered by the less mature crypt epithelial cells, epithelial cells proliferate and mature, thus promoting restoration of villous architecture characteristic of IEC.

The cytokines TGF-α, epithelial growth factor (EGF), IL-1β and IFN-α, promote restitution by increasing the local production of TGF-β *(35)*. TGF-β is secreted by macrophages, lymphocytes, IEC and platelets, and exhibits multiple effects on the epithelium and infiltrating leukocytes to down-regulate the inflammatory response and augment restoration of the epithelial barrier. In addition to inhibiting macrophage proliferation, TGF-β enhances tissue repair by promoting accumulation and proliferation of fibroblasts, whereas TGF-α enhances IEC proliferation. TGF-β also enhances IEC migration by promoting the deposition of extracellular matrix components fibronectin and collagen IV and promoting maturation of IEC. Several other cytokines and growth factors are involved in resolving inflammation, including basic fibroblast growth factor, keratinocyte growth factor and especially hepatocyte growth factor. IL-15 has also been shown to promote IEC growth *(36)*, and IL-10 appears to inhibit T cell proliferation and suppress cytokine production by macrophages.

Substantial in vitro data indicate that one of the most potent inducers of restitution is a group of constitutively expressed peptides characterized by a conserved motif of six cysteine residues collectively known as trefoil peptides *(37)*. Three known forms have been identified: pS2 in the proximal stomach, human spasmolytic polypeptide (HSP) in the distal stomach and biliary tree, and intestinal trefoil factor (ITF), which is produced throughout the small and large intestine. As one of the most abundant products secreted on the lumenal surface throughout the gastrointestinal tract, these highly conserved peptides have been recognized for their ability to induce IEC migration in a growth factor/TGF-β-independent manner *(38)*. Their activity can also be enhanced by interaction with gastrointestinal mucin glycoproteins *(39)*. These studies have led to the conclusions that during restitution, trefoil proteins in conjunction with mucin glycoproteins, act on the apical surface, while TGF-β repair of the epithelial barrier along the basolateral surface *(39)*.

Another group of important soluble factors needed for promoting tissue repair are the MMPs. Among other known biological activities, MMPs are thought to play a central role in tissue remodeling by initiating extracellular matrix degradation and turnover. For example, cleavage of type I collagen by MMP-1 (collagenase 1) initiates epithelial cell migration during epithelial recovery and is facilitated by stromelysin-1 (MMP-3), a type IV collagenase *(40)*. As discussed earlier, certain MMPs are capable of down-regulating the inflammatory response by cleaving IL-1 and allowing the release of TGF-β sequestered within the extracellular matrix.

4. CHRONIC INFLAMMATION

Chronic inflammation develops as a result of persistent immune response, either due to continual presence of an antigen or dysregulation of the immune response. While neutrophils play a central role in acute inflammation, accumulation and activation of T cells and macrophages is the hallmark of chronic inflammation. As the initial insult is contained, neutrophils are no longer recruited, and their presence is diminished. If the site becomes chronically inflamed, monocytes, macrophages, lymphocytes, and plasma cells predominate in the lesion. The monocytes and macrophages provide two important functions during the chronic state. First, they phagocytose remaining debris or pathogens unattended by the neutrophils, and second, they modulate T cell function through antigen presentation and cytokine secretion.

Cytokines, especially TGF-β, released by chronically activated macrophages stimulate fibroblast proliferation and collagen production. This can lead to a process of scar formation known as fibrosis. While fibrosis is normally associated with wound healing, it can interfere with normal intestinal function. Chronic inflammation also results in granuloma formation. Granulomas are tissue masses that consist of a central area of activated macrophages, which sometimes include multinucleated giant cells resulting from fusion of activated macrophages, surrounded by lymphocytes.

In the gut, pathological outcome of chronic inflammation include epithelial ulceration, villus atrophy, crypt hypertrophy, crypt abscesses, granuloma formation and fibrosis. Ample evidence exists implicating the involvement of events of both immune and nonimmune origin. With the notable exception of celiac disease, where the instigating antigen is wheat gluten, the initiating events or antigen for most chronic gastrointestinal diseases remains to be identified. Most chronic inflammatory gastrointestinal diseases display a characteristic polarization to a Th1 response. This paradigm is further demonstrated with the IL-10$^{-/-}$ mouse, which has a targeted deletion in the IL-10 gene. These mice spontaneously develop pathology reminiscent of human inflammatory bowel disease (IBD) unless kept in a germ-free environment and, thus, serves as a functional mouse model system for the human condition *(41)*. One notable exception to this concept is ulcerative colitis, which appears to be due to the overabundance of IL-5, which most likely contributes to the autoreactive antibody production characteristic of this disease *(42)*. In addition to this skewing, there is an aberrant increase in MMPs and EGF in local fibroblast cells. It has been hypothesized that the pathology associated with chronic gastrointestinal inflammation may be due to the overabundance of tissue remodeling factors *(43)*.

5. SUMMARY

Inflammation in the gut develops as a result of interactions between somatic intestinal cells, such as IEC and fibroblasts, and effector cells of the innate and adaptive arms of the immune system. These interactions are mediated by both soluble factors and cell-to-cell contact. Acute inflammation is either resolved or develops into chronic inflammatory reactions, which can result in fibrosis and loss of function. Understanding the molecular and cellular events in intestinal inflammation aids in efforts to develop new approaches to control the pathologic effects of inflammation.

ACKNOWLEDGMENTS

The work in our laboratory is supported by National Institutes of Health grant RO1 AI34544.

REFERENCES

1. Matis WL, Lavker RM, Murphy GF. Substance P induced the expression of an endothelial-leukocyte adhesion molecule by microvascular endothelium. *J. Invest. Dermatol.*, **94** (1990) 492–495.
2. Papadakis KA, Targan SR. The role of chemokines and chemokine receptors in mucosal inflammation. *Inflamm. Bowel Dis.*, **6** (2000) 303–313.
3. Yang SK, Eckmann L, Panja A, Kagnoff MF. Differential and regulated expression of C-X-C, C-C, and C-chemokines by human colon epithelial cells. *Gastroenterology*, **113** (1997) 1214–1223.
4. Jung HC, Eckmann L, Yang SK, et al. A distinct array of proinflammatory cytokines is expressed in human colon epithelial cells in response to bacterial invasion. *J. Clin. Invest.*, **95** (1995) 55–65.
5. Baggiolini M, Dewald B, Moser B. Human chemokines: an update. *Annu. Rev. Immunol.*, **15** (1997) 675–705.
6. McCormick B, Parkos CA, Colgan SP, Carnes DK, Madara JL. Apical secretion of a pathogen-elicited epithelial chemoattractant activity in response to surface colonization of intestinal epithelia by *Salmonella typhimurium*. *J. Immunol.*, **160** (1998) 455–466.
7. Huang GT-J, Eckmann L, Sacidge TC. Infection of human epithelial cells with invasive bacteria upregulates apical intercellular adhesion molecule-1 (ICAM-1) expression and neutrophil adhesion. *J. Clin. Invest.*, **98** (1996) 572–583.
8. Begue B, Sarnacki S, le Deist F, et al. HML-1, a novel integrin made of the beta 7 chain and of a distinctive alpha chain, exerts an accessory function in the activation of human IEL via the CD3-TCR pathway. *Adv. Exp. Med. Biol.*, **371** (1995) 67–75.

9. Wershil BK. Role of mast cells and basophils in gastrointestinal inflammation. *Chem. Immunol.*, **62** (1995) 187–203.

10. Beales IL, Post L, Calam J, Yamada T, Delvalle J. Tumour necrosis factor alpha stimulates gastrin release from canine and human antral G cells: possible mechanism of the *Helicobacter pylori*-gastrin link. *Eur. J. Clin. Invest.*, **26** (1996) 609–611.

11. Ding SZ, Lam SK, Yuen ST, et al. Prostaglandin, tumor necrosis factor alpha and neutrophils: causative relationship in indomethacin-induced stomach injuries. *Eur. J. Pharmacol.*, **348** (1998) 257–263.

12. Libert C, Van Molle W, Brouckaert P, Fiers W. Platelet-activating factor is a mediator in tumor necrosis factor/galactosamine-induced lethality. *J. Inflamm.*, **46** (1995) 139–143.

13. Chikano S, Sawada K, Shimoyama T, Kashiwamura S-I, Sugihara A, Sekikawa K, Terada N, Nakanishi K, Okamura H. IL-18 and IL-12 induce intestinal inflammation and fatty liver in mice in an IFN-γ dependent manner. *Gut*, **47** (2000) 779–786.

14. Seegert D, Rosenstiel P, Pfahler H, Pfefferkorn P, Nikolaus S, Schreiber S. Increased expression of IL-16 in inflammatory bowel disease. *Gut*, **48** (2001) 326–332.

15. Masaaki A, Andres PG, Li DJ, Reinecker H-C. NF-κB inducing kinase is a common mediator of IL-17, TNF-α and IL-1β induced chemokine promoter activation in intestinal epithelial cells. *J. Immunol.*, **162** (1999) 5337–5344.

16. Willoughby DA, Moore AR, Colville-Nash PR. COX-1, COX-2, and COX-3 and the future treatment of chronic inflammatory disease. *Lancet*, **355** (2000) 646–648.

17. Morteau O, Morham SG, Sellon R, et al. Impaired mucosal defense to acute colonic injury in mice lacking cyclooxygenase-1 or cyclooxygenase-2. *J. Clin. Invest.*, **105** (2000) 469–478.

18. Hogaboam CM, Bissonnette EY, Chin BC, Befus AD, Wallace JL. Prostaglandins inhibit inflammatory mediator release from rat mast cells. *Gastroenterology*, **104** (1993) 122–129.

19. Barrera S, Lai J, Fiocchi C, Roche JK. Regulation by prostaglandin E2 of interleukin release by T lymphocytes in mucosa. *J. Cell. Physiol.*, **166** (1996) 130–137.

20. Cohn SM, Schloemann S, Tessner T, Seibert K, Stenson WF. Crypt stem cell survival in the mouse intestinal epithelium is regulated by prostaglandins synthesized through cyclooxygenase-1. *J. Clin. Invest.*, **99** (1997) 1367–1379.

21. Lichtenberger LM. Where is the evidence that cyclooxygenase inhibition is the primary cause of nonsteroidal anti-inflammatory drug (NSAID)-induced gastrointestinal injury? Topical injury revisited. *Biochem. Pharmacol.*, **61** (2001) 631–637.

22. Vane JR, Botting RM. Mechanism of action of nonsteroidal anti-inflammatory drugs. *Am. J. Med.*, **104** (1998)2S–8S.

23. Whittle BJ, Oren-Wolman N, Guth PH. Gastric vasoconstrictor actions of leukotriene C4, PGF2 alpha, and thromboxane mimetic U-46619 on rat submucosal microcirculation in vivo. *Am. J. Physiol.*, **248** (1985) G580–G586.

24. Rosam AC, Wallace JL, Whittle BJ. Potent ulcerogenic actions of platelet-activating factor on the stomach. *Nature*, **319** (1986) 54–56.

25. Wallace JL, Steel G, Whittle BJ, Lagente V, Vargaftig B. Evidence for platelet-activating factor as a mediator of endotoxin-induced gastrointestinal damage in the rat. Effects of three platelet- activating factor antagonists. *Gastroenterology*, **93** (1987) 765–773.

26. Wallace JL, Hogaboam CM, McKnight GW. Platelet-activating factor mediates gastric damage induced by hemorrhagic shock. *Am. J. Physiol.*, **259** (1990) G140–G146.

27. Sun XM, Qu XW, Huang W, Granger DN, Bree M, Hsueh W. Role of leukocyte beta 2-integrin in PAF-induced shock and intestinal injury. *Am. J. Physiol.*, **270** (1996) G184–G190.

28. Kolios G, Wright KL, Linehan JD, Robertson DA, Westwick J. Interleukin-13 inhibits nitric oxide production in human colonic mucosa. *Hepatogastroenterology*, **47** (2000) 714–717.

29. Koch TR, Otterson MF, Telford GL. Nitric oxide production is diminished in colonic circular muscle from acquired megacolon. *Dis. Colon Rectum*, **43** (2000) 821–828.

30. Rachmielwitz D, Stamler JS, Karmeli F, et al. Peroxynitrite-induced rat colitis—a new model of colonic inflammation. *Gastroenterology*, **105** (1993) 1681–1688.

31. Kubes P, Reinhardt PH, Payne D, Woodman RC. Excess nitric oxide does not cause cellular, vascular, or mucosal dysfunction in the cat small intestine. *Am. J. Physiol.*, **269** (1995) G34–G41.

32. Vreugdenhil AC, Dentener MA, Snoek AM, Greve JW, Buurman WA. Lipopolysaccharide binding protein and serum amyloid A secretion by human intestinal epithelial cells during the acute phase response. *J. Immunol.*, **163** (1999) 2792–2800.

33. Saarialho-Kere UK. Patterns of matrix metalloproteinase and TIMP expression in chronic ulcers. *Arch. Dermatol. Res.*, **290(Suppl)** (1998) S47–S54.

34. Blikslager AT, Roberts MC. Mechanisms of intestinal mucosal repair. *J. Vet. Med. Assoc.*, **211** (1997) 1437–1441.

35. Podolsky DK. Review article: healing after inflammatory injury—coordination of a regulatory peptide network. *Aliment Pharmacol. Ther.*, **14** (2000) 87–93.

36. Reinecker HC, MacDermott RP, Mirau S, Dignass A, Podolsky DK. Intestinal epithelial cells both express and respond to interleukin 15. *Gastroenterology*, **111** (1996) 1706–1713.

37. Podolsky DK. Mechanisms of regulatory peptide action on the gastrointestinal tract: trefoil peptides. *J. Gastroenterol.*, **35** (2000) 69–74.

38. Dignass A, Lynch-Devaney K, Kindon H, Thim L, Podolsky DK. Trefoil peptides promote epithelial migration through a transforming growth factor beta-independent pathway. *J. Clin. Invest.*, **94** (1994) 376–383.

39. Kindon H, Pothoulakis C, Thim L, Lynch-Devaney K, Podolsky DK. Trefoil peptide protection of intestinal epithelial barrier function: cooperative interaction with mucin glycoprotein. *Gastroenterology*, **109** (1995) 516–523.

40. Nagase H, Woessner JF. Matrix metalloproteinases. *J. Biol. Chem.*, **274** (1999) 21,491–21,494.

41. Davidson NJ, Fort MM, Muller W, Leach MW, Rennick DM. Chronic colitis in IL-10$^{-/-}$ mice: insufficient counter regulation of a Th1 response. *Int. Rev. Immunol.*, **19** (2000) 91–121.

42. Fiocchi C. Inflammatory bowel disease: etiology and pathogenesis. *Gastroenterology*, **115** (1998) 182–205.

43. MacDonald TT, Bajaj-Elliott M, Pender SLF. T cells orchestrate intestinal mucosal shape and integrity. *Immunol. Today*, **20** (1999) 505–510.

15   Epidemiologic Studies and Outcomes Research in Colonic Diseases

John F. Johanson

CONTENTS

1. INTRODUCTION

The beginnings of epidemiology date to the time of Hippocrates in the 5th century BC *(1)*, although rigorous epidemiological studies have rarely been performed prior to the 20th century. In fact, only in the last 30 yr has a systematic body of principles been developed to guide the study of epidemiology *(2)*. Nevertheless, a burgeoning interest in epidemiology has established its foot hold as a scientific discipline. Where epidemiological data were previously greeted with skepticism, results are now openly accepted and represent the basis for many new hypotheses of disease etiology. One classic example is the Framingham Heart study which continues to provide valuable insights into the distribution, etiology, and natural history of coronary artery disease *(3)*.

Epidemiology can be defined as the study of the distribution and determinants of disease frequency in human populations *(1)*. This definition encompasses the three fundamental components of epidemiology; frequency, distribution, and determinants. The measurement of disease frequency involves the quantification of its occurrence. Terms such as incidence (the number of new cases of a disease over a specified period of time) or prevalence (the number of individuals with the disease at any one point in time) are utilized to describe the frequency of a disease *(2)*. The quantification of a disease's frequency assists the clinician in understanding its importance and aids in its diagnosis. For example, knowledge of disease prevalence may

From: *Colonic Diseases*
Edited by: T. R. Koch © Humana Press Inc., Totowa, NJ

help distinguish between common and rare diseases, which might present with similar symptoms. Disease distribution considers who, among a larger population, is more likely to contract a specific disease. This information is critical in identifying populations at risk and in formulating hypotheses as to potential factors contributing to disease development. Determinants represent potential causal factors. Epidemiology has been utilized most recently to identify potential environmental risk factors of chronic diseases. The description of the human genome will likely facilitate the examination of genetic risk factors for chronic diseases using the same epidemiologic methods.

The field of epidemiology is viewed as a scientific discipline based on the uniform methods used in its application. The systematic collection and analysis of data permits the application of statistical tools to determine the association between an exposure and the disease in question. That is, epidemiological methods allow the determination of the probability of developing a disease related to the presence of a specific factor or exposure compared to the probability of the same disease or outcome in the absence of this exposure. A number of factors, however, influence the association between disease and potential etiologic factor. These include chance, bias (a systematic error in data collection or interpretation), and confounding (the mixing of effects between an exposure, a disease, and an unrecognized factor[s], which might independently affect the risk of disease development) (1). Accordingly, judgments regarding cause and effect can be suggested by the results of epidemiological studies, but establishment of a cause and effect relationship requires inferences beyond the data from a single study. Additional information such as the strength of the association, its biologic credibility, the consistency of results with other studies, a compatible time sequence, and the presence of a dose—response relationship are essential in establishing a cause and effect relationship.

In practical terms, an understanding of epidemiology is useful for all medical practitioners, be they researchers or clinicians. The epidemiological distributions of specific disorders can often be helpful in suggesting potential etiologic agents or focusing upon relevant mechanisms of a disease's pathophysiology. By identifying environmental influences associated with its development, epidemiological studies can suggest new etiologic hypotheses, which may be tested in prospective studies or clinical trials. Similarly, clinicians benefit from a familiarity with the epidemiology of the diseases they regularly encounter, since knowledge of disease demographics can increase one's level of suspicion and aid in developing a differential diagnosis. Epidemiological studies may also identify new environmental risk factors, the avoidance of which may be helpful in preventing the development of specific disorders.

2. TYPES OF EPIDEMIOLOGY STUDIES

As the science of epidemiology has evolved, it has incorporated a variety of applications. When first employed, epidemiology was utilized to identify the source of infectious diseases. The term epidemiology is actually based on the root word epidemic. One of the first, and now classic, epidemiologic studies was performed in England in 1854, where John Snow, a London physician, was able to identify the cause of a cholera breakout based on death rates classified by geographic location within the city of London. Snow was able to chart the frequency and distribution of cholera based on location of the victim's residence and their resulting water supply. By doing so, he was able to identify the specific cause of this outbreak, contamination of drinking water by sewage (4). With the advances in public health, the significance of epidemics has diminished. Over the last century, the dominant causes of mortality and morbidity have shifted from predominantly infectious etiologies to chronic diseases. In the same way, the focus of epidemiology has shifted from determining the source of epidemics to identifying risk factors for the development of chronic diseases.

This is certainly true for colonic diseases, where the majority are not caused by recognized infectious agents.

Recent advances in the understanding of the genetic basis for disease has led to the development of a novel application of epidemiologic principles. This new discipline is called genetic epidemiology. Genetic epidemiology examines both environmental and genetic components of disease pathophysiology to better understand the cause of disease development. Examples of the application of genetic epidemiology in colonic diseases include inflammatory bowel disease, in which genetic origin (Askenazi Jews) seems to represent an increased risk for development. Likewise, the identification of the specific genes responsible for familial adenomatous polyposis and the description of the hereditary nonpolyposis colon cancer syndrome have opened up additional avenues for genetic eipidemiologic research.

3. EPIDEMIOLOGIC METHODS

A number of research design strategies have been utilized to examine the epidemiology of diseases. These can be classified as descriptive or analytic methods (1). Descriptive studies are the most common method employed to identify the frequency and distribution of colonic diseases. Descriptive techniques involve correlational studies, case reports or case series, and cross-sectional surveys. These studies examine the general characteristics of diseases based upon distributions related to person (demographics), place (geographic variation), and time (temporal trends). Most often, simple statistics such as rates (the number of individuals with the disease divided by the total population at risk) or proportions of the total population are used to describe the results. Examples of descriptive statistics include prevalence and incidence rates. In some cases, it is desirable to refine raw prevalence or incidence data to reduce distortion when comparing rates among different populations. This can be done using a statistical method called standardization (5). Put simply, standardization transforms an observed demographic distribution to a "standard" population. This serves to reduce distortion, which might otherwise result from the demographics of the specific population studied.

An example of standardization is the comparison of colorectal cancer rates among different countries. The unadjusted prevalence rates of colorectal cancer among populations living in underdeveloped countries are lower than rates identified among populations in the United States or other developed countries. On the surface, this observation would suggest the potential protective effects of some as yet unknown environmental factor. However, the observed differences between countries may also be the result of their differing age distributions; that is, patients living in underdeveloped countries have a reduced life expectancy. Since age seems also to be a risk factor for colorectal cancer, a developing country's lower prevalence rate may be the result of its younger population rather than a true difference in colon cancer prevalence. By standardizing prevalence rates of the different countries to the same population, the effects of confounding by age can be reduced, and a more precise comparison of potential environmental risk factors can be ascertained.

Analytic methods, which involve case-control and cohort studies, are traditionally employed to identify the determinants or risk factors for diseases. Case-control studies compare the association of a specific factor or exposure with the presence of the disease in question. Subjects are selected based on the presence (cases) or absence (controls) of the disease being studied. The two groups are then compared with respect to the proportion having the exposure or character of interest. Results are reported as an odds ratio, which can be thought of as the odds of developing a disease related to the particular exposure or factor compared to not having the exposure or risk factor (Fig. 1) (5). As might be suspected, the most difficult part of conducting this type of study is selecting appropriate controls. Case-control studies possess a

Disease

		Present	Absent
Risk Factor (exposure)	Present	A	B
	Absent	C	D

$$\text{Odds Ratio (OR)} = \frac{(A \times D)}{(B \times C)}$$

$$\text{Relative Risk (RR)} = \frac{[A / (A + B)]}{[C / (C + D)]}$$

Fig. 1. Two-by-two (2 x 2) table for calculating the association between risk factors and disease.

number of strengths. First, they are quick and relatively inexpensive. Second, they are well suited to analyze diseases with long latent periods because participants are selected based on already having contracted the disease. Third, case-control studies are optimal for diseases that are rare, because patients already having the disease are selected as cases. Finally, case-control studies can assess the influence of a number of different risk factors on the same disease. Case-control studies also have some limitations. Since individuals already having the disease in question are selected as cases, the influence of potential risk factors has already taken place. Consequently, these studies are almost always retrospective increasing the possibility of bias. A particularly common bias is recall bias, which means that those individuals with the disease are more likely to remember a specific exposure than would an individual without the disease. Another limitation of the retrospective nature of case-control studies is the difficulty in demonstrating a temporal relationship between disease and exposure. Finally, case-control studies are not suited to examining rare exposures.

The cohort design represents the other traditional analytic epidemiologic method used to study disease causality. In many ways, cohort studies are the opposite of case-control studies. Cohort studies select participants based on their exposure to a risk factor or other characteristic rather than a disease. By definition, all participants must be free of the disease of interest at the time the cohort is assembled. The study population is then followed to determine which participants develop the disease or diseases of interest. Cohort studies typically are prospective, although in rare cases they can be retrospective. The strengths of the cohort design lie in its ability to study a wide range of diseases associated with rare exposures and to elicit a temporal relationship between exposure and disease. The cohort design, however, is limited predominantly by its expense. The process of identifying a large number of subjects, particularly with a rare risk factor and then following them for long periods to determine disease development can be prohibitively costly. Moreover, cohort studies are not suited for the study of rare diseases, because the cohort would need to be extremely large to capture adequate numbers of patients with the disease. This leads to dramatically increasing costs. Finally, results of cohort studies rely heavily on all patients completing the study. This means that the reliability of studies with large dropout rates or large numbers of participants who are lost to

Table 1
Prevalence of Fecal Incontinence in the U.S.

Author	Reference	Study population	Prevalence rate
Nelson	11	Wisconsin, IL	2.2%
Drossman	9	USA	7.4%
Reilly	12	Olmsted County, MN	15.0%
Johanson	10	Rockford, IL	18.4%

follow-up may be questionable. Results of cohort studies are described in terms of relative risk (Fig. 1). The relative risk provides a measure of the actual risk associated with a disease and a particular exposure (5). As compared to an odds ratio, relative risk provides a more accurate indication of the likelihood of developing a disease in the exposed group. As the size of the study population increases, however, the odds ratio approximates the relative risk (1).

4. APPLICATION OF EPIDEMIOLOGIC PRINCIPLES

As discussed above, both descriptive and analytic methods are used to examine the frequency, distribution, and determinants of individual diseases. The application of these methods can be illustrated by a description of the epidemiology of fecal incontinence, a relatively common disorder of the distal colon.

4.1. Disease Definition

The first and most important step in examining the epidemiology of a disorder is to define the disease before starting. It is, likewise, important to use a generally accepted definition, when available, so that results of any study will be generalizable to other populations and will be applicable across a variety of clinical situations.

With regards to fecal incontinence, a number of related but distinct definitions of fecal incontinence have been utilized in epidemiologic investigations. Some have based their definition on the frequency of its occurrence. Thomas, for example, indicated in his definition, that leakage of stool is not incontinence unless it occurs two or more times per month (6,7). Others have defined incontinence based on the length of time it has been present. According to the Rome criteria for example, fecal incontinence is a "one month or longer history of continuous leaking or passage of stool at unwanted times" (8). Still others define incontinence by the amount of leakage; a small amount which stains the underwear is considered fecal soiling, whereas an amount "two teaspoons or more" is considered gross incontinence (9). Despite the disparity among definitions, the one unifying factor is that all incorporate the concept of leakage or unwanted passage of stool. Consequently, more recent epidemiologic studies have employed a definition in which any unwanted leakage of stool was considered to be incontinence regardless of its frequency or severity (10).

4.2. Clinical Epidemiology

Descriptive epidemiologic methods examine the prevalence and demographic distributions of disease. Prevalence data are often the easiest to assess and are presented as rates of patients with the disease divided by those without the disease. If the disease is relatively common, prevalence rates are presented as percentages, that is the number of patients with the disease per 100 population.

The prevalence of fecal incontinence has also been examined in the United States (Table 1). Nelson performed a random telephone survey of residents of southern Wisconsin identifying an overall prevalence rate of 2.2/100 respondents to his survey. Of these, half were incontinent of liquid stool, while a third were incontinent of solid stool corresponding to prevalence rates of 1.2 and 0.8%, respectively (11). Drossman and coworkers also examined the prevalence of fecal incontinence as part of a larger study of functional gastrointestinal disorders in the United States. They found an overall prevalence rate of 7.8%. When classified by severity of incontinence, fecal soiling was observed in 7.1% of respondents, while incontinence of solid stool occurred in only 0.7% (9). In a randomized community-based sample of 50–90-yr-old residents of Olmsted county, Reilly and coworkers found that 15% of responders admitted to incontinence of feces (12). In a study of ambulatory patients presenting to their physician for routine medical care, we found an even higher prevalence of fecal incontinence (10). Overall, 18% admitted to at least one episode of fecal incontinence. When categorized by type, incontinence of liquid stool was significantly more common then incontinence of either mucous or solid stool.

The wide variation in prevalence rates is probably due in part to differences in the definition of fecal incontinence. The prevalence rate of 18%, for example, was based on individuals who were visiting their physician. Since this was not truly population based, referral bias may have led to an overestimation of the true prevalence of fecal incontinence. Despite variation in study methods, however, prevalence rates among individual studies have been remarkably similar provided comparable definitions were utilized.

The demographic distribution of fecal incontinence consistently demonstrates a progressive increase in prevalence associated with age (9–12). Unfortunately, the distribution of fecal incontinence by gender is less clear. In our study of nearly 900 ambulatory persons presenting to their family doctor, fecal incontinence was 1.3 times more common in males than females (10). Drossman likewise identified a slightly higher prevalence of fecal soiling among males, although gross incontinence was more prevalent among females (9). By contrast, Nelson and Reilly both found fecal incontinence to be unequivocally more common in females than males (11,12). This discrepancy is probably due to differences in study populations and disease definition. Severe incontinence may be more common in females, while seepage of small amounts of liquid stool or mucous may be more common in males. Unfortunately, little data are available regarding the distribution of fecal incontinence by race or socioeconomic status. Nelson did not identify any association of incontinence with race, marital status, or work status (11). Similarly, no distinct geographic or temporal distributions have been identified.

4.3. Environmental Risk Factors

Analytic epidemiologic methods are necessary to study associations and suggest causality between potential environmental risk factors and diseases. Hypothetical etiologic risk factors must take into account known pathophysiologic mechanisms associated with the disease in question. For example, most patients who suffer from fecal incontinence experience one or more abnormalities of the internal anal sphincter, the external anal sphincter, or the pelvic floor muscles, leading to dysfunction of the mechanisms which typically maintain continence. Attempts to identify environmental risk factors, which are not plausible from a pathophysiologic standpoint, are not likely to be successful or clinically useful.

Obstetric trauma represents the most common cause of surgically treatable fecal incontinence. Risk factors include prolonged second stage of labor, large birth weight, use of forceps, and perineal tears (13). Early-onset of fecal incontinence is most often related to third or fourth degree lacerations with disruption of the internal and/or external anal sphincters. Approximately 3 to 4% of women with sphincter lacerations will develop incontinence of solid or liquid stool (14). Most major injuries to the anal sphincters are recognized immediately and repaired by the obstetrician.

Late-onset incontinence is thought to be related to passage of the baby through the birth canal stretching the pudendal nerves. A neuropraxic injury is believed to occur, which, in some women, causes a pudendal neuropathy and fecal incontinence many years later. This hypothesis is supported by studies of anal sphincter pressures and pudendal nerve terminal motor latency (PNTML) demonstrating an association between fecal incontinence, the number of vaginal deliveries, and abnormalities of PNTML (15–18).

Dementia appears to be one of the most important risk factor for fecal incontinence, particularly in nursing home residents (19,20). Dementia may lead to incontinence by a number of mechanisms. Demented individuals may not be able to understand or respond to an urge to have a bowel movement and, therefore, defecate in their clothing. Even if able to sense and respond, demented individuals may not be able to identify the toilet as the appropriate place to defecate. An inability to sense the urge to defecate may also lead to fecal impaction, with overflow diarrhea and incontinence (21). Alternatively, neurogenic sphincteric abnormalities may occur in association with fecal incontinence in demented patients. It is possible, for example, that disruption of cortical function may occur concomitantly with degeneration of the spinal pelvic nerves leading to coexistent dementia and neurogenic fecal incontinence. A similar phenomenon is thought to explain the association between neurologic disorders and constipation (22).

Diarrhea represents another important risk factor for the development of fecal incontinence with a five- to eightfold increased risk, depending upon how diarrhea is defined (12,19). This is not surprising since only minor decreases in internal anal sphincter function may result in leakage of liquid stool. Furthermore, incontinence of liquid stool may occur even with relatively normal sphincter function, particularly if rectal sensation is diminished (23–24).

Fecal impaction represents an important risk factor for fecal incontinence, particularly among institutionalized patients (21,25,26). Brocklehurst and coworkers examined 52 nursing home residents with fecal incontinence and found half of them to have fecal impactions. The remaining patients had "neurogenic" incontinence. Presumably, incontinence occurs as a result of overflow diarrhea in the presence of maximal rectal distention, thereby inhibiting internal anal sphincter contraction. The association between fecal impaction and incontinence has yet to be confirmed in the U.S. In a study of nursing home residents, we did not detect a significant association between constipation and fecal incontinence, regardless of how constipation was defined, whether by subjective complaint or by more objective findings of decreased stool frequency, straining, or hard stools. Moreover, laxative use was not associated with fecal incontinence (19).

Lack of mobility represents a final risk factor for fecal incontinence. This is not surprising, since individuals are more likely to be incontinent if they are not able to make it to the bathroom upon sensing an urge to defecate. Immobility is even more problematic, when combined with loose stools, providing even less time to get to the bathroom. This association was also observed by Nelson in a population-based survey of individuals with fecal incontinence (11). Physical limitations and poor general health were actually the most significant risk factors associated with fecal incontinence in his study demonstrating adjusted odds ratios of 1.82 and 1.64, respectively.

5. EPIDEMIOLOGY AND DISEASE PREVENTION

Disease prevention represents an application of epidemiologic principles. Once the frequency and distribution of a disease are established, attempts can be made to prevent the disease even if the specific etiologic risk factors may have not been completely elucidated. Disease prevention encompasses primary, secondary, and tertiary modalities. Primary prevention is true prevention, applied to a population considered to be physically and emotionally healthy before disease or dysfunction occurs, thus the need for information regarding disease distribution and frequency. The purpose of primary prevention is to reduce the vulnerability of an individual or population to illness through health promotion strategies, such as diet and exercise or by providing specific protection such as immunizations. Health promotion strategies may be directed toward the general health of individuals, families, or communities. These efforts may be public, such as adequate housing or smoking restriction in public places, or personal, examples of which might include exercise or weight control. Primary prevention strategies may also be described as active or passive. Active strategies would involve personal lifestyle choices, such as smoking cessation or dietary modification to reduce fat, a risk factor for colorectal cancer. Passive strategies would be represented by government enforcement of industrial waste rules to protect communities from toxic exposure.

Secondary prevention includes screening and early detection by defining and identifying high risk groups or people with precursor stages of disease. It may also involve treating early stages of disease to limit disability by averting or delaying the consequences of advanced disease. Examples of secondary prevention for colonic diseases include colorectal cancer screening among high risk populations or colonoscopic surveillance of ulcerative colitis to identify patients who would benefit from colectomy. Tertiary prevention takes place after the disease and disability are permanent and irreversible. The focus is on minimizing the effects of disease and disability by preventing additional complications or deterioration and emphasizes rehabilitation. Tertiary prevention attempts to optimize function in spite of the disabling condition.

Again, using fecal incontinence as an example, epidemiologic methods can be employed to help identify potential prevention strategies. The preponderance of risk factors associated with incontinence indicates that the pathogenesis of fecal incontinence is probably multifactorial. Although no studies have specifically tested the effectiveness of potential preventive measures, modification of known pathogenic risk factors would be expected to delay, if not prevent, the onset of fecal incontinence.

Nevertheless, prevention of fecal incontinence associated with obstetric injuries may be difficult. As described above, the known risk factors include prolonged labor, high birth weight, use of forceps, and perineal tears (13). Prompt delivery of babies with high birth weight or in cases of prolonged second stage of labor may decrease the risk of pelvic floor damage and subsequent weakening. This is probably best accomplished by cesarean section. Despite the potential reduction in long-term risk of developing fecal incontinence with cesarean section, the increased cost and hazards associated with cesarean section preclude its routine use simply for the prevention of fecal incontinence. Nonetheless, earlier cesarean section, rather than forceps delivery in patients with high birth weight or difficult labor, may reduce the risk of subsequent development of incontinence.

If dementia is a primary risk factor for fecal incontinence, prevention may, likewise, be difficult. Even though reversing dementia is probably unrealistic, incontinence may still be preventable in some demented patients (secondary–tertiary prevention). If incontinence results from loss of the cognitive ability to respond to an urge or to identify the toilet as the appropriate location to defecate, (a behavioral problem) fecal incontinence may be prevented by instituting a daily bowel program using rectal suppositories. Routinely placing a confused patient on the toilet after inserting a suppository would eliminate the problem of identifying the appropriate place to defecate. Sensing the urge would not be as important, since the suppository would stimulate the rectum to contract thus leading to defecation and concomitant evacuation of the rectum. Regularly emptying of the rectum should prevent the development of a fecal impaction, thereby eliminating another potential cause of incontinence. Unfortunately, if fecal incontinence is caused by degeneration of anal sphincter innervation, prevention of fecal incontinence is much more difficult. Nevertheless, implementation of these simple measures is likely to be successful in preventing at least some individuals from developing fecal incontinence.

By comparison, prevention of incontinence in patients with diarrhea or fecal impaction appears to be a more attainable goal. If the underlying cause of diarrhea can be identified, it should be specifically treated. Even if the underlying cause of diarrhea can not be identified or eliminated, symptomatic therapy with medications, such as loperamide, may improve stool consistency sufficiently to prevent incontinence, as solid stool is much easier to control. Similarly, fecal impaction can be treated symptomatically by routine use of laxatives or rectal suppositories to ensure that the rectum is emptied consistently. In light of the strong association between fecal incontinence and poor general health or physical disability, any additional measures directed to improving mobility may, likewise, forestall the onset of incontinence. Regular exercise, for example, may prevent incontinence by enabling one to maintain sufficient mobility providing ample time to make it to a bathroom. Regular exercise may also improve the strength of the pelvic floor muscles, thus augmenting external anal sphincter pressure.

The goal of secondary prevention is to identify groups at high risk for developing incontinence, in order to prevent more serious disease or complications. Early identification of sphincter injuries associated with birth trauma represents an important method of secondary prevention. Since the development of fecal incontinence frequently involves disruption of both internal and external anal sphincters, immediate recognition and prompt surgical repair of sphincter injuries related to birth trauma may prevent the onset of fecal incontinence. If there is any question whether sphincter damage has occurred, anal ultrasound should be performed. Routine use of Kegel exercises to maintain pelvic floor muscle tone represents another mode of secondary prevention, which has the additional benefits of being simple, safe, and inexpensive. It may be particularly beneficial among women who have had multiple childbirths.

6. OUTCOMES RESEARCH

6.1. Outcomes Research and Practice Guidelines

Outcomes research can be defined as the systematic study of clinical practice with special focus on patient-centered outcomes, including patient satisfaction, quality of life, functional status, and costs of medical care (27). Outcomes research is closely related to epidemiology, as it employs the same methods, namely descriptive studies, case-control studies, and cohort studies. The main difference between epidemiology and outcomes research, however, is focus. While epidemiology is used to elucidate the distribution and risk factors for disease development, outcomes research attempts to identify the optimal treatment or management strategy.

The most important distinguishing feature of outcomes research, when compared to traditional clinical research, is its emphasis on effectiveness rather than efficacy. Efficacy denotes the usefulness of a medical intervention tested under optimal conditions, typically in the framework of a randomized controlled clinical trial. Patient selection criteria are strict in clinical trials, and these studies are performed by highly trained physicians usually in academic centers of excellence. By comparison, effectiveness is the utility of an intervention in the real world, that is ordinary patients and physicians regardless of their training or practice situation (28). The third factor in determining the usefulness of a medical intervention is its efficiency or value to the patient. Stated another way, efficacy addresses the question of whether an intervention can work, effectiveness answers the question of whether it works in the routine practice setting, and efficiency determines whether it is worth doing. The distinction between these is important when the results of outcomes research are used to develop disease management guidelines. Interventions with proven efficacy may not necessarily perform as well in routine clinical practice, thus efficacy does not automatically equate with effectiveness. Furthermore, even if effective, an intervention may not be worth the cost.

Another unique feature of outcomes research is the widespread use of nonrandomized research designs. It is becoming increasingly apparent that the traditional randomized controlled trial may not be the optimal method to provide answers to common clinical questions. Accordingly, there has been a much greater reliance upon analysis of large databases to provide information on the effectiveness of routine medical care (29). These databases are populated with clinical data collected most often for billing purposes. Although database analyses provide a number of advantages, they are nonrandomized and, thus, limited by potential biases that might otherwise have been eliminated by randomization.

As the field of outcomes research evolves, controlled trials are becoming increasingly common and are now being called effectiveness trials. In contrast to the traditional clinical trial, effectiveness trials are much less restrictive. The most important difference between the two is the use of a heterogeneous mix of investigators chosen specifically to encompass practicing clinicians who may not necessarily be experts in the field. Other distinctions include, incorporation of community hospital or office settings and less rigorous exclusion criteria for study patients. Outcomes or effectiveness trials often involve patients who may be of advanced age, have multiple co-morbid diseases, or may not reliably take their medications. Finally, effectiveness trials collect data regarding patient satisfaction, quality of life, and economic data to assess both the effectiveness and efficiency of an intervention (30). By virtue of these differences, effectiveness trials provide more practical information about the patients that are seen in routine clinical practice.

7. ORIGINS OF OUTCOMES RESEARCH

Three factors have led to the emergence of the field of outcomes and effectiveness research. The first is the progressive increase in health care costs. In the 1960s the United States spent only 4% of gross national product (GNP) on healthcare, while current annual expenditures exceed 14%, a level far greater than any other developed nation. In this context, outcomes research provides a means to measure the relative effectiveness of different interventions, in order to identify those which may not provide sufficient benefit for worth considering their cost. Outcomes research also provides the framework to ensure that quality is not sacrificed in the enthusiasm to reduce expenditures. A second factor is the competition among providers. The number of managed care organizations has increased dramatically over the past 25 yr. Until recently, competition has been based predominantly on price. Outcomes research can provide an alternative method to compare providers by furnishing information on the quality of their practices. The third, and probably most influential reason for the evolution of outcomes research was the identification of significant geographic variation in the use of common medical procedures (including endoscopy) without any measurable difference in patient outcomes. A number of studies have been published identifying differences in resource utilization among different communities. Despite these differences, patient outcomes were comparable, raising the question of either overutilization of resources associated with increased costs or underutilization associated with suboptimal quality of care.

8. OUTCOMES AND DISEASE MANAGEMENT

Outcomes management is the application of outcomes research to clinical practice. It is based on two critical assumptions. First, an ideal disease management strategy exists, which can result in the lowest cost and highest quality of care. Second, this practice guideline can be identified by systematically measuring patient outcomes. Identification of an optimal management strategy, however, is a continuum. With the application of practice guidelines, patient outcomes are examined with the goal of a measurable improvement in quality. If outcomes are not improved, the guideline may need to be modified based on additional outcomes research in a process of continuous quality improvement (CQI) *(27)*.

The goal of disease management is also to reduce costs by decreasing practice variability by the use of practice guidelines. However, there are subtle differences between outcomes management and disease management. Outcomes management focuses on the individual physician–patient encounter and typically begins when the patient first seeks medical attention. This may occur well after the onset of symptoms or initiation of the disease process. Disease management, can be defined as a "systematic population-based approach, of identifying persons at risk, intervening with specific programs of care, and measuring clinical and other outcomes" *(27)*. Thus, disease management represents a population-based approach which is unlike the traditional patient–physician paradigm. Practice guidelines are applied to populations at risk even before they develop symptoms or present to their physician for evaluation and treatment. In this way, disease management employs elements of epidemiology, disease prevention, and outcomes research.

Disease management comprises a spectrum of care. The simplest and lowest cost interventions of a disease management program involve self-care, in which patients take responsibility for their own health. In doing so, disease management incorporates active primary prevention strategies as their first intervention. Examples in colonic diseases would include consumption of a high fiber diet in patients with diverticulosis to prevent diverticulitis or to reduce the risk of colon cancer development. The components of a disease management program increase in complexity from interventions by primary care physicians to those by specialists and from the outpatient to inpatient or chronic care setting. As the complexity of interventions increase, so does the cost of the program.

9. COMPONENTS OF OUTCOMES RESEARCH

The components of outcomes research are different when compared to traditional clinical research. Although both focus on the treatment of disease, outcomes research assumes the perspective of the patient and examines patient-centered outcomes, such as patient satisfaction, quality of life, and costs of medical care.

9.1. Patient Satisfaction

Although patient satisfaction is an important aspect of patient care, the relevance of this measure remains controversial. Critics suggest that patient satisfaction relies too heavily on subjective patient expectations and that in general, patients are not equipped to be able to judge the quality of healthcare provided. Nevertheless, patient satisfaction is becoming firmly established as a measure of health outcomes, as it can predict adherence to treatment recommendations, compliance with follow-up appointments, and level of resource utilization.

There are many ways to assess patient satisfaction. The easiest is to use a suggestion box or provide other informal opportunities for patients to comment on their health care. Unfortunately, the creditability and reproducibility of these methods are less than optimal. Consequently, a more reliable method should be employed to assess patient satisfaction in a consistent manner. The assessment process involves six steps *(31)*. The first step is to identify the survey population. Examples might include hospital inpatients or outpatients presenting to a multispecialty clinic. It is also important to ascertain who will be using the patient satisfaction data, be they hospital administrators, managed care plans, or the doctors providing care, since the survey may need to include different items depending upon who will use the results. In a similar manner, it is important to identify the goals of the process before beginning. A satisfaction survey, which is to be used to improve healthcare delivery to patients, might be quite different from one whose goal is for hospital marketing. The specific survey must then be selected or created, if none are available to meet the specific needs of the target audience. One of the most widely utilized patient satisfaction surveys can be found as part of the Medical Outcomes Study (32). This survey is easy to administer, since it consists of only seven questions and has been validated in varied outpatient settings. The frequency of administration must, likewise, be determined. Although these first five steps are important, the most significant aspect of surveying patient satisfaction is to use the results and implement changes to improve patient care. Without this last step, there is no reason to undertake the first five steps. Unfortunately, the importance of actually utilizing patient satisfaction data to modify physician behavior has been lost on many who track this outcome.

Patient satisfaction has become a critical outcomes measure, predominantly the result of forces outside the healthcare delivery process. As such, care must be exercised in collecting data and reporting results to accurately represent patients opinions. Caution must be exercised in interpreting patient satisfaction data, because it does indeed depend on patient expectations and knowledge of their own healthcare. Therefore, patient satisfaction data should not be interpreted in a vacuum, but must take into account other patient centered outcomes when assessing the quality of healthcare delivered.

9.2. Health Related Quality of Life

Health related quality of life (HRQoL) is a tool that is being used to supplement and, in some cases, improve upon traditional methods of assessing the effectiveness of various interventions. QoL can be defined as an individual's overall satisfaction with life and one's general sense of personal well-being (33). In other words, QoL represents the combination of physical, mental, and social well-being. When applied to healthcare, HRQoL attempts to elucidate areas of physical function, somatic sensation, psychological state, and social interaction, which are all affected by one's health status. These measures provide invaluable information regarding the overall impact of a disease and its treatment on the entire patient. Information on HRQoL is particularly useful in determining the optimal diagnostic or therapeutic management strategy in situations where: (i) the detection of psychosocial impairments will alter the care of individual patients; (ii) there is little difference in traditional treatment outcomes, such as mortality; and (iii) a number of effective strategies exist, and therapeutic tradeoffs are present between toxicity, survival, and cost (33).

One good example of a colonic disease, in which HRQoL measures are quite helpful, is irritable bowel syndrome (IBS), where few physiologic endpoints are available to assess changes in disease severity related to treatment. By employing a validated HRQoL instrument, a more objective assessment of treatment effect is possible, thereby rendering more appropriate therapy. The identification of significant psychosocial abnormalities might make it easier to apply a multidisciplinary team approach.

There are two basic types of HRQoL instruments; generic and disease-specific. The best known generic survey is the 36-Item Short Form Health Survey (SF 36) which was developed as part of the Medical Outcomes Study (34). This survey is comprised of 36 questions examining eight domains: (i) physical functioning; (ii) role limitations–physical; (iii) bodily pain; (iv) general health; (v) vitality; (vi) social functioning; (vii) role limitations—emotional; and (viii) mental health. It can be self-administered or administered by someone else and takes approx 3–5 min to complete. The SF 36 provides summary scores for physical and mental

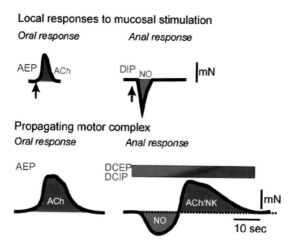

Local responses to mucosal stimulation

Oral response   Anal response

AEP   ACh   DIP   NO   mN

Propagating motor complex

Oral response   Anal response

AEP   DCEP
DCIP

ACh   ACh/NK   mN

NO

10 sec

Color Plate 1, Fig. 1. (*see* discussion and full caption in Chapter 3, p. 41.) Local responses to mucosal stimulation.

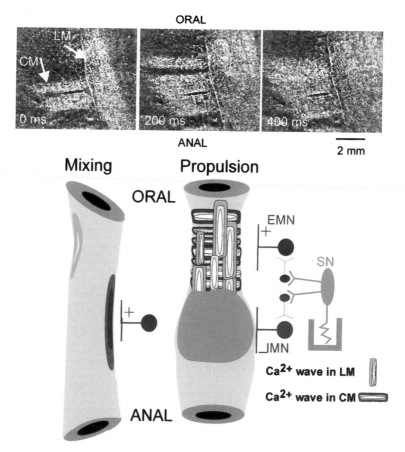

ORAL

LM
CM

0 ms   200 ms   400 ms

ANAL

2 mm

Mixing   Propulsion

ORAL

EMN

SN

JMN

Ca^{2+} wave in LM

Ca^{2+} wave in CM

ANAL

Color Plate 2, Fig. 2. (*see* discussion and full caption in Chapter 3, p. 46.) Calcium waves appear independently and spontaneously in both the LM and CM of the colon.

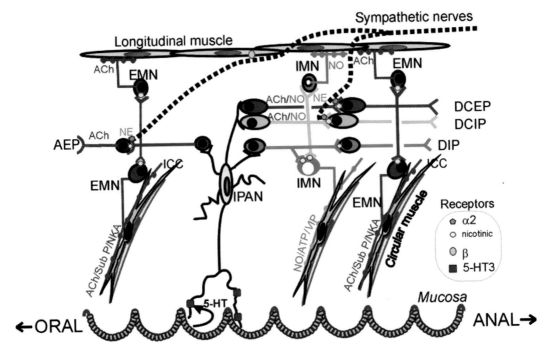

Color Plate 3, Fig. 3. (*see* discussion and full caption on in Chapter 3, p. 48.) Neural circuits underlying regulation of LM and CM layers during local reflexes and migrating motor complexes.

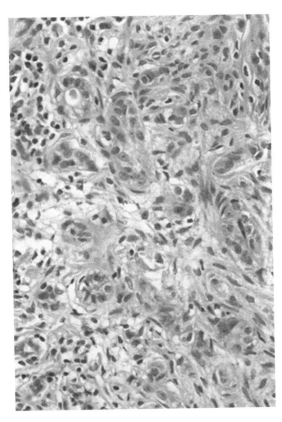

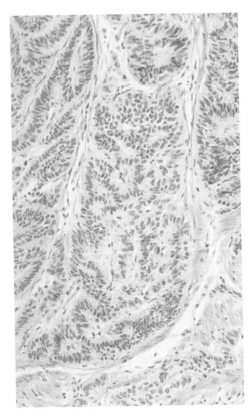

Color Plate 4, Fig. 3. (*see* discussion and full caption in Chapter 5, p. 78.) Appendicular carcinoid tumor. Adapted with permission from ref. *46*.

Color Plate 5, Fig. 4. (*see* discussion and full caption in Chapter 5, p. 79.) Carcinoid tumor of the rectum. Adapted with permission from ref. *46*.

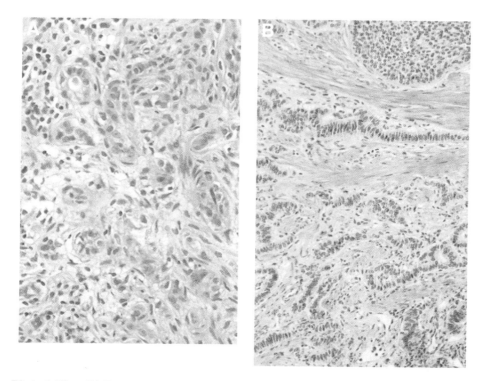

Color Plate 6, Figs. 5A,B. (*see* discussion and full caption in Chapter 5, p. 79.) Adapted with permission from ref. *46*.

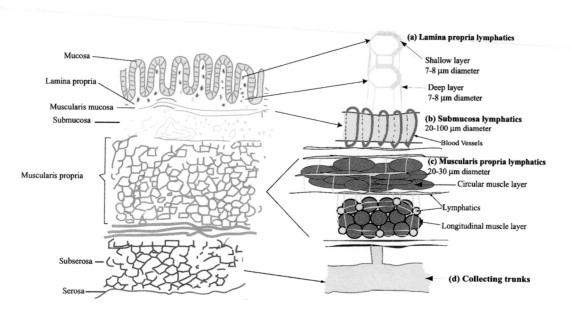

Color Plate 7, Fig. 1. (*see* discussion and full caption in Chapter 9, p. 124.)

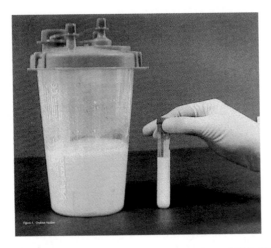

Color Plate 8, Fig. 4. (*see* discussion in Chapter 9, p. 133.) Chylous ascites.

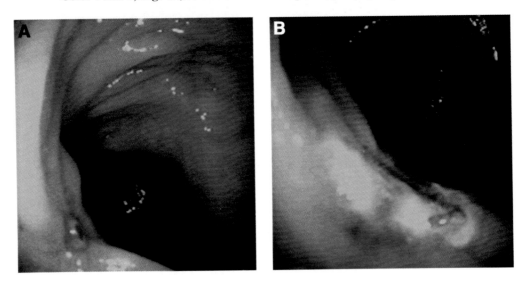

Color Plate 9, Fig. 1A,B. (*see* discussion and full caption in Chapter 16, p. 248.)

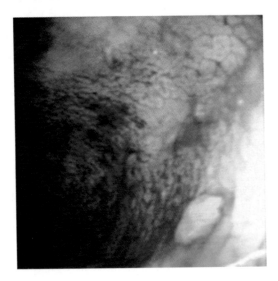

Color Plate 10, Fig. 2. (*see* discussion and full caption in Chapter 16, p. 251.)

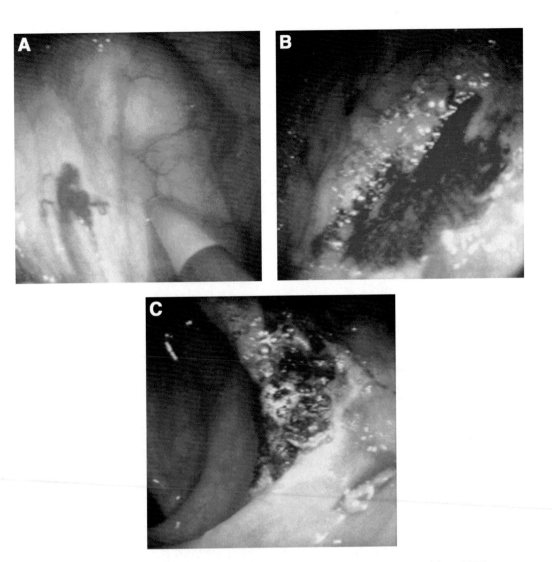

Color Plate 11, Fig. 3A–C. (*see* discussion and full caption in Chapter 16, p. 257.)

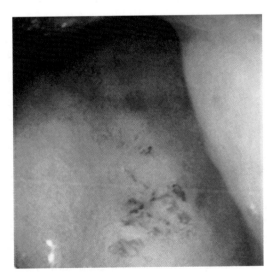

Color Plate 12, Fig. 4. (*see* discussion and full caption in Chapter 16, p. 259.)

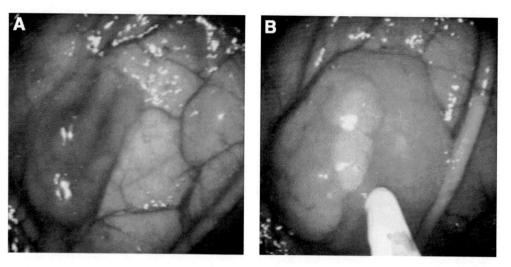

Color Plate 13, Fig. 6A,B. (*see* discussion and full caption in Chapter 16, p. 262.)

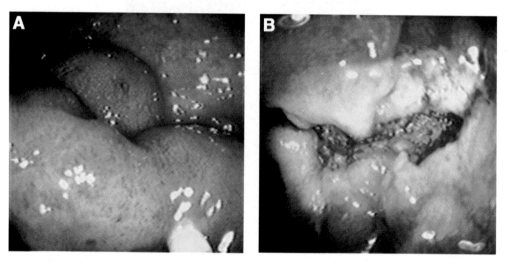

Color Plate 14, Fig. 7A,B. (*see* discussion and full caption in Chapter 16, p. 262.)

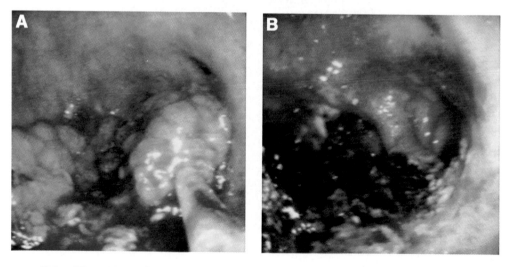

Color Plate 15, Fig. 8A,B. (*see* discussion and full caption in Chapter 16, p. 264.)

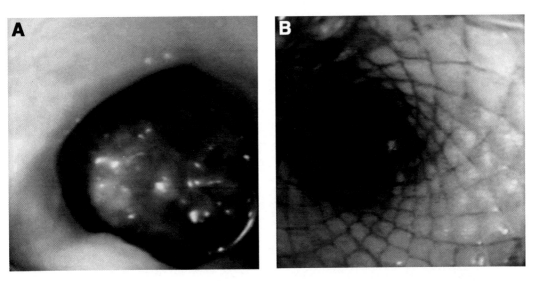

Color Plate 16, Fig. 9A,B. (*see* discussion and full caption in Chapter 16, p. 265.)

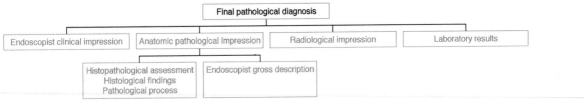

Color Plate 17, Fig. 1. (*see* discussion and full caption in Chapter 17, p. 276.)

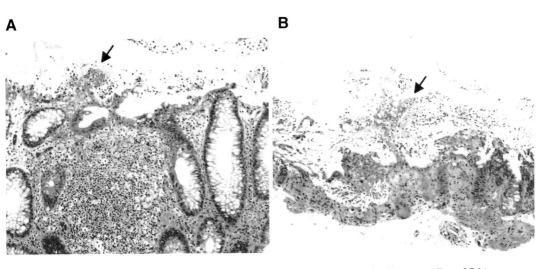

Color Plate 18, Fig. 2A,B. (*see* discussion and full caption in Chapter 17, p. 276.)

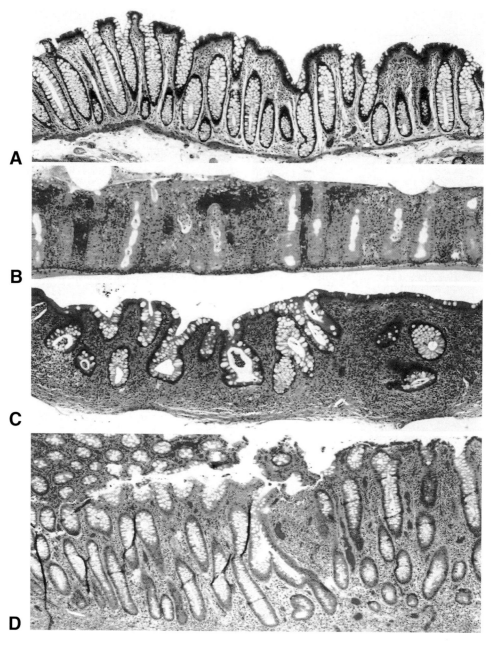

Color Plate 19, Fig. 3A–D. (*see* discussion and full caption in Chapter 17, p. 282.)

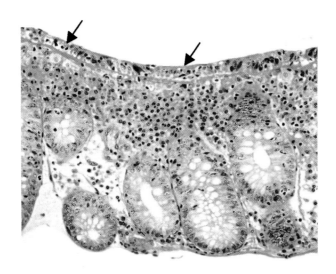

Color Plate 20, Fig. 4. (*see* discussion and full caption in Chapter 17, p. 289.)

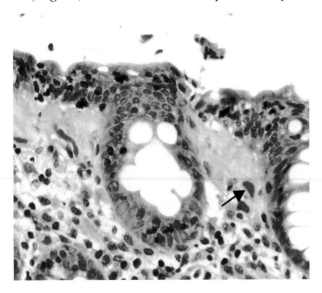

Color Plate 21, Fig. 5. (*see* discussion and full caption in Chapter 17, p. 291.)

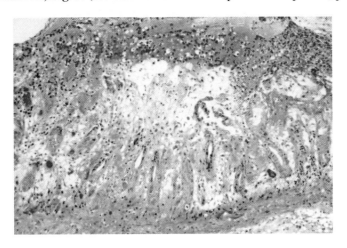

Color Plate 22, Fig. 6. (*see* discussion and full caption in Chapter 17, p. 292.)

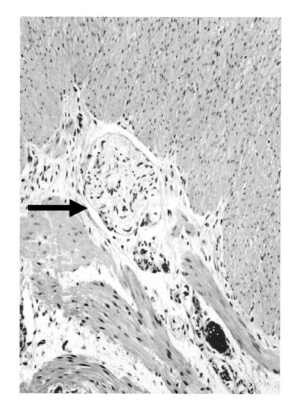

Color Plate 23, Fig. 4. (*see* discussion and full caption in Chapter 23, p. 390.)

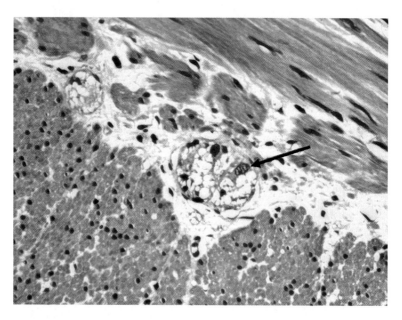

Color Plate 24, Fig. 5. (*see* discussion and full caption in Chapter 23, p. 391.)

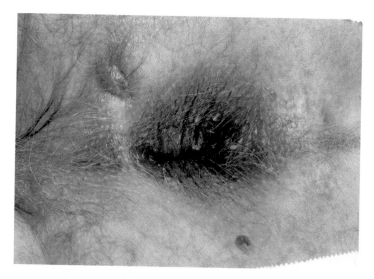

Color Plate 25, Fig. 5. (*see* discussion and full caption in Chapter 33, p. 541.)

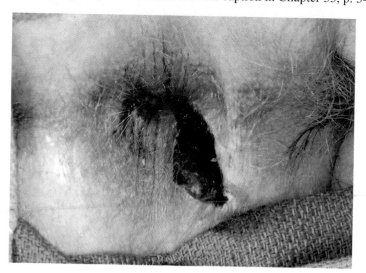

Color Plate 26, Fig. 6. (*see* discussion and full caption in Chapter 33, p. 541.)

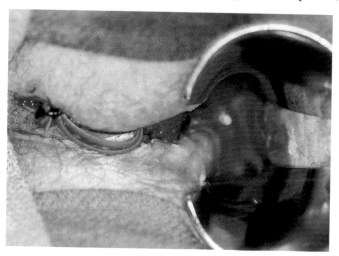

Color Plate 27, Fig. 7. (*see* discussion and full caption in Chapter 33, p. 541.)

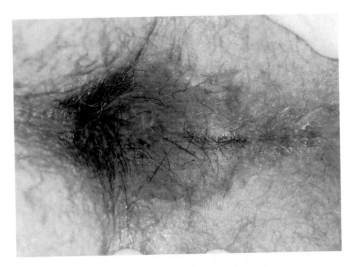

Color Plate 28, Fig. 8. (*see* discussion and full caption in Chapter 33, p. 542.)

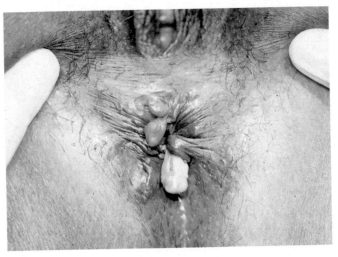

Color Plate 29, Fig. 9. (*see* discussion and full caption in Chapter 33, p. 543.)

health, and national norms are available for comparison. This instrument has been extensively tested for validity, reproducibility, and responsiveness (35).

Disease-specific or disease-targeted surveys were developed to better capture small, but clinically significant, changes in symptoms or disease states that might not be appreciated in the generic surveys. For example, the IBS-QoL queries the frequency and bothersomeness of IBS symptoms. Likewise, the inflammatory bowel disease (IBD)=QoL survey contains a number of questions regarding symptoms specific to IBD (36). There are few if any questions on the SF 36 regarding gastrointestinal (GI) symptoms, such as diarrhea, let alone the more specific questions relating to these particular diseases.

There are three main uses for HRQoL data (36). The first is descriptive. In descriptive studies, HRQoL surveys are utilized to identify domains that might be impaired in patients with specific diseases. Another use of descriptive measures might be the comparison of HRQoL in colonic diseases with that of noncolonic diseases. For example, comparing colon cancer with breast cancer. This type of application would require a generic instrument. The second potential use of HRQoL data is to discriminate between various disease subgroups. This is the most common application of HRQoL and is used to provide an indication of the severity of compromise of QoL among various disease populations. One example is the comparison of HRQoL among patients with IBS compared to patients with IBD or compared with the general population. The application of HRQoL surveys in a discriminative process most often requires generic instruments also, although recent development of disease-targeted surveys, such as the GI QoL Index, may improve the accuracy when comparing HRQoL among specific GI disorders. The final application of HRQoL is evaluative, which evaluates the response of an individual patient to an intervention. Instruments are employed in clinical trials to evaluate changes associated with specific treatments and are particularly useful in conditions where objective measures or responses are lacking. Again, IBS is a good example of this use.

9.3. Economic Analyses

In the current climate of progressively rising healthcare expenditures, the cost of a diagnostic test or treatment is becoming increasingly important. As the current rise continues, choices will have to made regarding the use of limited resources. Economic analyses provide the basis for identifying the most efficient interventions by providing the foundation upon which these decisions can be made. Two features characterize economic analyses. First, all economic analyses consider both the intervention and its subsequent outcome in terms of costs and consequences. Second, economic analyses make explicit the criteria most helpful in shaping the decision among different uses for the limited resources. In this regard, the fundamental tasks of any economic analysis are to identify, measure, value, and compare the costs and consequences of the interventions being considered (37).

There are a number of types of cost analyses, including cost-minimization, cost-effective, cost-utility, and cost-benefit analyses. Although each examines the costs of an intervention, their differences lie in how the results are analyzed and expressed. A cost-minimization analysis is performed when the outcomes of two or more interventions are equivalent and the economic evaluation is a search for the least costly alternative. In fact a cost minimization analysis is actually a form of cost-effective analysis. Few studies are designed to be cost-minimization studies initially, but when outcomes are found to be similar, they are simplified to this methodology.

A cost-effectiveness study measures the outcomes of an intervention in terms of a natural effect such as "life years saved". No attempt is made to value this measure economically, rather the reader is left to interpret the value of the natural measure based on their own circumstances. Even though the economic consequences of the outcomes are not examined explicitly, a cost-effectiveness analysis allows comparison of different disease states. For example, the cost per life year saved in screening for colon cancer can be compared with the cost per life year saved by mammography or cervical cancer screening to assess the effectiveness of various cancer prevention strategies.

A cost-utility analysis takes the cost-effectiveness methodology one step further by actually providing a quality measure of the consequence. In other words, a cost-effectiveness analysis might provide only a crude estimate of the life years saved, while the cost-utility analysis considers the value of each of those years by assigning a patient derived utility measure. Cost-utility studies are particularly useful in those instances when the intervention of choice is associated with significant side effects. Chemotherapy is one example where life years might be extended, but the quality of those life years might be significantly reduced if associated with constant nausea and vomiting.

The final form of economic study is the cost-benefit analysis. This method attempts to value the outcome or consequence of an intervention in economic terms, that is, the benefit is also expressed in dollars. This type of analysis provides a ratio of the net costs to the monetary benefits to facilitate a decision as to whether the beneficial consequences of an intervention justify its costs. The cost-benefit analysis tends to be the most helpful in making policy decisions, but problems in measuring costs often restrict the range of benefits that can be measured in monetary terms.

In practical terms, economic measures can be integrated into traditional randomized controlled trials or included into effectiveness studies. The benefit of employing economic measures as part of a clinical trial is the validity of its measurement resulting from the rigid nature of the clinical trial. Unfortunately, results are not often generalizable, since the randomized trial does not reflect real life situations. That is, frequent physician visits and additional tests are often included in randomized trials for safety reasons, potentially inflating the costs of the intervention in the real world. The costs identified using an effectiveness trial better reflect real life, but may be more difficult and more expensive to complete. A more detailed discussion of economic analyses can be found elsewhere *(37)*.

10. CONCLUSIONS

Epidemiology and outcomes research represent a continuum in the application of analogous research methods to study colonic diseases. Epidemiologic techniques provide the foundation for determining the frequency, distribution, and determinants of colonic diseases. Prevention strategies use the results of epidemiologic studies to identify patients at risk in an attempt to modify the development or severity of the disease. Outcomes research focuses on management once the disease is present, identifying the optimal treatment strategy of a disease; one that is effective and provides the most value for the patient. In contrast to traditional clinical research, outcomes research evaluates disease management from the perspective of the individual patient considering their satisfaction with healthcare, QoL, and the economic burden associated with the diagnosis and treatment of their illness.

Epidemiologic methods play a significant role in the diagnosis and treatment of colonic diseases. They can be employed to address the entire range of a colonic disease from diagnosis to treatment, providing data that can be used for developing hypotheses regarding its cause, prevention, and optimal therapy. Although originally thought to be of little use, the spectrum of epidemiology and outcomes research actually fulfills a key role in the study of colonic diseases, and their importance should not be underestimated.

REFERENCES

1. Hennekens CH, Buring JE. *Epidemiology in Medicine*. Little, Brown and Company, Boston, MA, 1987, pp. 3–30.
2. Rothman KJ. *Modern Epidemiology*. Little, Brown and Company, Boston, MA, 1986, pp. 1–34.
3. Dawber TR. *The Framingham Study: The Epidemiology of Atherosclerotic Disease*. Harvard University Press, Boston, MA, 1980.
4. Snow J. *On the Mode of Communication of Cholera* Churchill, London, 1855. Reproduced in *Snow on Cholera*. Haffner, New York, NY, 1965.
5. Kahn HA, Sempos CT. *Statistical Methods in Epidemiology*. Oxford University Press, New York, NY.
6. Thomas TM, Egan M, Walgrove A, Meade TW. The prevalence of feacal and double incontinence. *Community Med.*, **6** (1984) 216–20.
7. Thomas TM, Egan M, Meade TW. The prevalence and implications of feacal (and double) incontinence. *Br. J. Surg.* **72(Suppl)** (1985) S141.
8. Whitehead WE. Working Team for Functional Disorders of Anus and Rectum. Functional disorders of the anus and rectum. In *The Functional Gastrointestinal Disorders: Diagnosis, Pathophysiology, and Treatment* Drossman DA, Richter JE, Tallyu NJ, Thompson WG, Carazziari E, Whitehead WE (eds.), Little, Brown and Company, Boston, MA, 1994, pp. 217–263.
9. Drossman DA, Zhming L, Andruzzi E, et. al. U.S. householder survey of functional gastrointestinal disorders. *Dig. Dis. Sci.*, **38** (1993) 1569–1580.
10. Johanson JF, Lafferty J. Epidemiology of fecal incontinence: the silent affliction. *Am. J. Gastroenterol.*, **91** (1996) 33–36.
11. Nelson R, Norton N, Cautley E, Furner S. Community-based prevalence of anal incontinence. *JAMA*, **274** (1995) 559–561.
12. Reilly WT, Talley NJ, Pemberton JH, Schleck CD, Zinsmeister AR. Fecal incontinence: prevalence and risk factors in the community. *Gastroenterology*, **108** (1995) A32.
13. Snooks SJ, Swash M, Henry MM, Setchell M. Risk factors in childbirth causing damage to the pelvic floor innervation. *Int. J. Colorect. Dis.* **1** (1986) 20–24.
14. Harary AM. The anorectal complications of pregnancy and childbirth. *Practical Gastroenterology*, (1996) 24–38.
15. Snooks SJ, Swash M, Mathers SE, Henry MM. Effect of vaginal delivery on the pelvic floor: a five year follow-up. *Br. J. Surg.*, **77** (1990) 1358–1360.
16. Snooks SJ, Swash M, Setchell M, Henry MM. Injury to the innervation of the pelvic floor sphincter musculature in childbirth. *Lancet*, **2** (1984) 546–550.
17. Roberts PL, Coller JA, Schoetz DJ, Veidenheimer MC. Manometric assessment of patients with obstetric injuries and fecal incontinence. *Dis. Colon Rectum*, **33** (1990) 16–20.
18. Ryhammer AM, Bek KM, Laurberg S. Multiple vaginal deliveries increase the risk of permanent incontinence of flatus and urine in normal premenopausal women. *Dis. Colon Rectum*, **38** (1995) 1206–1209.
19. Johanson JF, Irizarry F, Doughty A. Risk factors for fecal incontinence in a nursing home population. *J. Clin. Gastroenterol.*, **24** (1997) 156–160.
20. Read NW, Celik AF, Katsinelos P. Constipation and incontinence in the elderly. *J. Clin. Gastroenterol.*, **20** (1995) 61–70.
21. Read NW, Abouzekry LA. Why do patients with fecal impaction have fecal incontinence. *Gut*, **27** (1986) 283–287.
22. Johanson JF, Sonnenberg A, Koch TR, McCarty DJ. Association of constipation with neurologic diseases: an epidemiologic study of the concordant occurrence of diseases in the Medicare population. *Dig. Dis. Sci.*, **37** (1992) 179–86.
23. Miller R, Bartolo DCC, Roe A, Cervero F, Mortensen NJ. Anal sensation and the continence mechanism. *Dis. Colon Rectum*, **31** (1988) 433–438.
24. Hoffman BA, Timmcke AE, Gathright JB, Hicks TC, Opelka FG, Beck DE. Fecal seepage and soiling: a problem of rectal sensation. *Dis. Colon Rectum*, **38** (1995) 746–748.
25. Barrett JA, Brocklehurst JC, Kiff ES, Ferguson G, Faragher EB. Anal function in geriatric patients with fecal incontinence. *Gut*, **30** (1989) 1244–1251.
26. Tobin GW, Brocklehurst JC. Fecal incontinence in residential homes for the elderly: prevalence, etiology and management. *Age Ageing*, **15** (1986) 41–46.
27. Epstein RS, Sherwood LM. From outcomes research to disease management: a guide for the perplexed. *Ann. Intern. Med.*, **124** (1996) 832–837.
28. Diamond GA, Denton TA. Alternative perspectives on the biased foundations of medical technology assessment. *Ann. Intern. Med.*, **118** (1993) 455–464.

29. Epstein AM. The outcomes movement—will it get us where we want to go? *N. Engl. J. Med.*, **323** (1990) 266–270.

30. Simon GE, Wagner E, Vonkorff M. Cost-effectiveness comparisons using real world" randomized trials: the case of new antidepressant drugs. *J. Clin. Epidemiol.*, **48** (1995) 363–373.

31. Schmitt CM. Patient satisfaction. *Clin. Perspect. Gastroenterol.*, **2** (1999) 324–328.

32. Rubin HR, Gandek B, Rogers WH, Kosinski M, McHorney CA, Ware JE. Patients' ratings of outpatient visits in different practice settings—results from the medical outcomes study. *JAMA*, **270** (1993) 835–840.

33. Eisen GM, Locke GR, Provenzale D. Health-related quality of life: a primer for gastroenterologists. *Am. J. Gastroenterol.*, **94** (1999) 2017–2021.

34. Ware JE Jr, Sherbourne CD. The MOS 36-item short-form health survey (SF 36): conceptual framework and item selection. *Med. Care*, **30** (1992) 473–483.

35. Stewart AL, Hays RD, Ware JE Jr. The MOS short-form general health survey: reliability and validity in a patient population. *Med. Care*, **26** (1988) 724–735.

36. Yacavone RF, Locke GR, Provenzale DT, Eisen GM. Quality of life measurement in gastroenterology: what is available. *Am. J. Gastroenterol.*, **96** (2001) 285–297.

37. Drummond MF, O'Brien B, Stoddart GL, Torrance GW. *Methods for the Economic Evaluation of Health Care Programs.* Oxford University Press, New York, NY, 1997.

16   Colonoscopy

Donald G. Seibert

CONTENTS

1. INTRODUCTION

There have been several steps in the evolution of the modern colonoscope from the Hirschowitz fiberoptic gastroscope. The tortuosity, variable anatomy, and acute angulation of the colon precluded successfully tolerated flexible fiberoptic colonic endoscopy until the design of an improved tip control and an insertion sheath that produced increased stiffness when torqued. Using silicon rubber casts of the rectum and sigmoid colon, Dr. Bergein Overholt optimized a prototype flexible sigmoidoscope. His initial clinical series of 40 patients was published in 1968 *(1)*. In parallel, Japanese investigators also designed longer gastrointestinal endoscopes with improved controls. By the early 1970s, patient colonoscopy series were being reported from several centers *(2–4)*. Image optical clarity, light source technology, and endoscope handling improved in an incremental manner until 1983 when Welch-Allyn announced that they had installed a charged-coupled device (CCD) video camera within an endoscope.

From: *Colonic Diseases*
Edited by: T. R. Koch © Humana Press Inc., Totowa, NJ

The video optics of a modern colonoscope now has a 120–130° wide angle view and an approx 30-fold magnification. Present tip controls allow for 180° up-down deflection and right-left controls of 160–180°. The insertion tube diameters vary between 11.3–12.8 mm, and instrumentation–suction tube channels vary between 2.7–4.2 mm. Double-channel colonoscopes are now available. Some models have variable stiffness in the shaft of the colonoscope. The tip irrigation systems have permitted better lens clearing. The modern colonoscope provides an excellent platform to travel the length of the colon and has permitted multiple advances in lesion recognition and treatment of specific colonic diseases. It has permitted access for electrocautery polypectomy, for Argon plasma cautery and laser photoablation of lesions. With an injection of India ink, specific sites in the colon can be located at the time of a repeat endoscopy or surgery. Inoperable strictures may be treated with laser ablation or by the placement of permanent stents. Colonoscopy in the setting of acute lower gastrointestinal hemorrhage is now the standard of care. Colonoscopy has been used to treat colonic pseudo-obstruction. Newer techniques of imagining, particularly with magnified video colonoscopy, vital dye staining of colonic mucosa, autofluorescence, and endoscopic optical coherence tomography may all evolve to provide ways of evaluating areas of bowel for dysplastic change.

2. BOWEL PREPARATION

An evaluation of the entire colonic mucosal surface can only be expected if the colon has been adequately prepared. The two most widely utilized preps are either 4 L of a polyethylene glycol (PEG)-based balanced electrolyte lavage or 3 oz of an oral sodium phosphate laxative.

The PEG-based lavage is arguably the safest type of prep, since there are minimal fluid or electrolyte shifts. Ingestion of the prep over 3–4 h the night before the procedure and an overnight dietary restriction results in adequate cleansing in 90% of patients (5). If there is an overnight dietary restriction, and the prep is taken the morning of the procedure, the proximal colon appears to be cleaner than if the prep is taken the night before (6). Because the ingestion of 4 L of a salty liquid is a significant hurdle in a subset of patients, attempts have been made to decrease the volume of the lavage with the addition of a laxative. A 4 L overnight PEG lavage has been compared to two liters PEG plus 20 mg bisacodyl or 2 L PEG 2 h after 296 mL magnesium citrate (7). The patients who took the laxative-bolstered preps had higher patient satisfaction scores and endoscopist's prep quality scores.

The buffered oral sodium phosphate prep (45 mL) is ingested along with 24 oz of a clear liquid the night before and morning of the procedure or as two doses the day before the procedure. A direct prospective comparison with PEG lavage suggested improved patient tolerance and similar efficacy (8,9). A cost comparison of the two preps, which calculated the costs of the prep and the relative risk for a reexamination due to an incomplete inadequate prep, demonstrated a clear cost-benefit with the use of sodium phosphate (10). This study, however, did not calculate patient care costs due to complications from preparation; there have been case reports of acute renal failure (11) and ischemic (12) colitis secondary to oral sodium phosphate. In up to 24% of patients, the oral sodium phosphate solution creates aphthoid-like erosions similar to that seen in Crohn's disease (13). This may cause diagnostic confusion if colonoscopy was performed because of gastrointestinal (GI) symptoms, and it could result in additional costs if biopsies are done to evaluate these lesions.

An alternative approach is to clear the bowel in a retrograde manner using a pulsed irrigation evacuation device. With this technique, a rectal speculum is inserted and microprocessor-timed pulses of warm tap water are periodically flushed in and out of the colon. A series of 20 consecutive patients that remained on clear liquids and consumed a bottle of magnesium citrate the day prior to their scheduled exam were cleansed with the pulse irrigator within 25 min immediately before colonoscopy. Cleansing was graded as acceptable or better in 100% of patients (14). While the result is good, it would appear that the need for instrumentation, privacy issues, and the nursing requirements for what is, in effect, a continuous enema would still make an oral lavage or sodium phosphate a more cost-effective approach to patient preparation.

3. SEDATION AND COLONOSCOPY

With the exception of a discreet subgroup of motivated patients that desire to undergo colonoscopy without medication, patients undergo colonoscopy with sedation if it is offered. This most commonly consists of a benzodiazepine (diazepam or midazolam) plus an opiate (meperidine or pentazocine). Patients need to be observed clinically and be monitored with continuous electrocardiography and pulse oximetry and intermittent blood pressure checks. The amount of medications given must be reduced in patients with pulmonary disease and in the elderly. The patient's response to medication is titrated throughout the procedure and if necessary, additional small doses are added to the initial dose for adequate anesthetic response. Since the only painful part of colonoscopy is the endoscope introduction, and since this is completed within a short period of time, there is no benefit to the use of neuroleptanalgesia (droperidol) which has a long half-life. In some hospital and outpatient endoscopy centers, all patients undergo sedation by an anesthetist and characteristically receive a low dose of pentazocine plus a propofol drip. The cost of the anesthesiologist was circumvented in two studies in which patients were attached to a patient-controlled analgesia (PCA) pump premixed with propofol and alfentanil and self-titrated their analgesia needs (15–16). Patients quickly recovered after the procedure and had no serious hemodynamic or respiratory complications. Nitrous oxide inhalation has been investigated for colonoscopy sedation, because of its excellent safety profile and quick post-procedure recovery time. Saunders et al. compared nitrous oxide to pethidine 50 mg plus diazepam 2.5 mg in a double-blinded placebo-controlled study of 89 patients. Both the nitrous oxide and conventional conscious sedation were considered to be an improvement over sedationless colonoscopy. Six of 29 patients in the diazepam–opiate group had oxygen desaturation, while none in the nitrous oxide group did. When Notini-Gudmarsson compared pain relief, patient satisfaction, and colonoscopy time in patients receiving nitrous oxide vs pethidine 1 mg/kg intramuscularly, the efficacy of both were considered to be equal, except that patients given nitrous were able to leave the hospital an average of 34 min earlier (17). More recently, Forbes and Collins randomized patients between inhaled nitrous oxide or intravenous midazolam, mean dose 4.7 mg, plus meperidine, mean dose 55 mg (18). The endoscopists did not note any difference in procedure performance with either medication, but both the endoscopists and the patients agreed that patient tolerance of the procedure was poorer with nitrous oxide. It would seem that nitrous oxide clearly provides some benefit compared to placebo and is similar to low dose sedation.

Some patients tolerate colonoscopy well with minimal or no analgesia. Wang Kim et al. reported on a series of 909 study patients who underwent colonoscopy by a single endoscopist (19). The completion rate was 98% with a mean insertion time to cecum of 6.9 min. The only analgesic given was meperidine 25 mg intramuscularly 10 min prior to the procedure. The factor that correlated with significant patient discomfort was insertion time, which, in turn, was related to prep quality. When the degree of discomfort was a level 4 or above (5 being the most severe), univariant analysis indicated that female gender and abdominal pain, as an indication for the colonoscopy, were related to significant procedure-related discomfort. S.D. Ladas also described 173 patients in whom colonoscopy was started without sedation (20). One hundred fifty-nine required no sedation during the exam, and a complete colonoscopy was achieved in 152 of the 173 patients. Multivariate logistic regression analysis showed that male sex and a prior segmental colonic resection were inversely associated with a need for sedation. Hoffman, Butler, and Shaver offered unsedated colonoscopy to 109 consecutive patients (21). Eighty patients consented to attempt colonoscopy without initial sedation, and sedation was required in five to complete the exam. Fifty-four percent had moderate or severe pain, but the majority of patients were willing to undergo a similar procedure in the future. Thiis-Evensen et al. reported a series of 451 patients between the ages of 50–59 undergoing unsedated screening colonoscopy (22). The cecum was intubated successfully in 82% of patients. Only 5% of patients found the exam to be uncomfortable, and over 90% of individuals stated that they would undergo a similar repeat colonoscopy in 5 yr. Sedation may not be needed in asymptomatic patients, particularly male patients, and patients with a prior colonic resection that are undergoing colonoscopy for colon cancer screening or surveillance. Sedation should, however, be available when needed during the procedure, so that the success rate of the procedure and the patient return rate in a surveillance program is not compromised.

4. TRAINING IN COLONOSCOPY

The trained colonoscopist must have a sufficient fund of medical knowledge for decision making before and during the procedure. The colonoscopist must be able to recognize abnormalities seen on endoscopy, be able to perform colonoscopy in a safe skillful manner, and be able to recognize and treat complications related to the procedure. Minimum training requirements suggested by the American Society for Gastrointestinal Endoscopy (ASGE) for trainees in GI endoscopy, as well as for non-gastroenterology colonoscopist, are 140 colonoscopies with training in polypectomy (23). Endoscopists should also be able to recognize mucosal findings and have a low miss-rate of lesions. Grading of trainees, both at the Hennepein County Medical Center (24) and at Case Western Reserve University (25), found that, after 100 procedures, the cecal intubation rate was only 84%. A training report on 135 fellows reported that the cecal intubation rate did not reach 95% until 200 colonoscopies were performed (26). These studies do not begin to address the adequacy of the exam or the success or complication rate of polypectomy. These issues are well discussed in a 1999 editorial by Bond and Frakes (27).

Because of the costs related to training, as well as patient concerns and concern for patients, there has been interest in colonoscopic simulators for teaching. These have evolved from simple tortuous tubes to computer simulators that recognize pressure and will graphically demonstrate loops that are being created with the colonoscope (28). It is not known whether this will only improve hand eye coordination of the endoscope controls, but also accelerate the more difficult aspects of colonoscopic training, namely sensation of proper torque, properly timed endoscope withdrawal and air suctioning, and loop management. These simulators do not appear to incorporate the effects that patient position change and application of external pressure have on endoscope advancement.

The magnetic imagining colonoscope could, theoretically, improve cecal intubation rates, patient tolerance, and accelerate learning in more advanced students. The magnetic colonoscope has 12 magnetic generator coils positioned along the shaft of the endoscope. An external sensor below the procedure cart determines the orientation of the endoscope based upon the position of these coils within the abdomen. As opposed to the occasionally helpful single projection radiographic fluoroscopic image (29), the anteroposterior (AP) and lateral view of the magnetic endoscope's configuration is continuously displayed without radiation exposure. An audit of looping using the magnetic imagining colonoscope in 100 complete colonoscopies was performed (30). Looping was seen in 91% of exams, with atypical loops being more common in women than men. Abdominal compression was most helpful in passing the hepatic flexure, and position change from a decubitus position to a supine position tended to assist the sigmoid to descending colon advancement as well as transverse colon advancement. A system such as this may assist training of the endoscopist, as well as the procedure assistant, in the management of loops.

5. IMPROVEMENT OF COLONOSCOPY SUCCESS RATE

5.1. Factors that Predict Incomplete Colonoscopy

Although some expert practitioners have had total colonoscopy success rates of greater than 98%, there are certain factors that appear to interfere with procedure success in some patients. Cirocco and Rusin reported a series of 1047 colonoscopies with a successful cecal intubation rate of 91% (31). The majority of incomplete exams were in women in which there was a history of abdominal hysterectomy. A history of diverticulitis did not affect completion rate. Anderson et al. Reported, in a series of 200 patients undergoing colonoscopy, that the success rate in men was 98.2%, while in women it decreased to 94.8% (32). The thinner women with a body mass index (BMI) index of less than 22 had an incomplete examination 49% of the time. They found that diverticular disease, history of constipation, or prior abdominal surgery did not relate to procedure success. Their conclusion was that thinner is not always better.

5.2. Choosing an Alternate Instrument to Improve Success Rate

Colonoscopes that have a fixed graduated stiffness and those with stiffness that can be varied have been evaluated. Odori et al. compared unsedated patients who underwent colonoscopy with a standard colonoscope to those who underwent colonoscopy with a variable stiffness instrument (33). Stiffening at the appropriate time assisted the procedure and lead to quicker insertion times. Dr. Doug Rex found little benefit to the endoscope, but had a a mean insertion time of 4 min and procedure complete exam rate of 99.2% with either type of instrument (34). For the moderately advanced practitioner and for the patient that is more likely to be a difficult colonoscopy, the variable stiffness instrument may be of some assistance.

The pediatric endoscope may also improve the success rate in those adult patients who are more likely to be difficult to complete colonoscope. A group of 150 outpatients were randomly assigned to colonoscopy with a standard vs a pediatric colonoscope (35). If the procedure was incomplete, there was then crossover to the other endoscope. In four of the seven patients where colonoscopy could not be completed with the adult colonoscope, the procedure could be completed with the pediatric instrument. In only one exam could the adult endoscope complete an exam unsuccessful with the pediatric one. If there was a prior hysterectomy 11 of 12 patients had complete colonoscopy with the pediatric colonoscope, but only 15 of 21 with the adult endoscope. The variable stiffness pediatric and adult colonoscopes have been compared to the standard pediatric and adult colonoscopes (36). A pediatric instrument reached the cecum 99% of the time compared to a 93% success rate with an adult endoscope.

In patients with fixed colonic loops, a gastroscope can occasionally be used for colonoscopy, although this frequently requires counter pressure and many position changes. The push enteroscope has also been employed successfully in 22 of 32 patients that had a prior incomplete exam with the standard colonoscope (37).

6. COMPLICATIONS RELATED TO COLONOSCOPY

Complications secondary to colonoscopy may be related to the prep, sedation, manipulation or overdistension of bowel, and instrument disinfection. Bowel perforations totaled 165 out of 99,539 (0.17%) diagnostic colonoscopies reported in 12 studies that were summarized

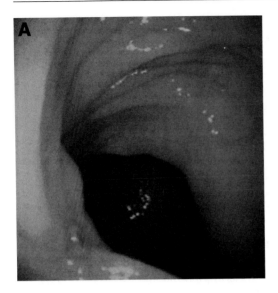
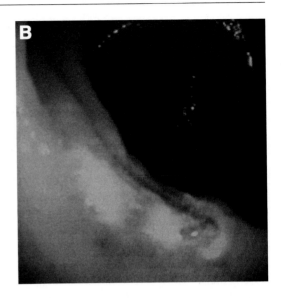

Fig. 1. (A) Delayed hemorrhage postpolypectomy with a central visible vessel. (B) The site has been treated with argon plasma coagulation without rebleeding.

by Waye et al. *(38)*. The mortality rate was 0.006%. The risks for perforation postpolypectomy rose nearly threefold to 76 of 18,659 patients, which is a rate of 0.41%. Postcolonoscopy bleeding, which is nearly unheard of, increases to 1.2% after a polypectomy has been performed. The manipulation of the endoscope may also cause laceration of the mesentery and splenic rupture *(39)*. Incarceration of the colonoscope within an inguinal hernia has also been reported *(40)*. Changes in blood pressure and pulse may occur, and oxygen desaturation may occur secondary to excessive sedation or to patient breathholding due to pain. Myocardial ischemia may occur *(41)*.

Postpolypectomy bleeding may occur immediately with transection of the polyp, with delayed bleeding occurring for up to 29 d post-procedure. The peak incidence appears to be during days 4–6 postpolypectomy. There is a higher risk when large polyps are removed *(42–43)* and if polyps are removed with the hot biopsy forceps *(44,45)*. The use of nonsteroidal antiinflammatory drugs and resumption of anticoagulation also appears to result in increased rates of post-polypectomy bleeding. Bleeding noted immediately post-polypectomy can be treated with a tightened cold snare around a bleeding pedicle, injection of 1:10,000 epinephrine into the base of the bleeding site, application of a band ligator, or application of an endoscopic clip. Alternatively, the heater probe, bipolar cautery, or Argon plasma coagulation may be used to stop early bleeding. Delayed postpolypectomy bleeding frequently is self-limited. If bleeding continues, treatment is needed. The site of bleeding will appear to be a visible vessel within an ulcer base and is readily treated. Treatment of four episodes of postpolypectomy hemorrhage with the use of bipolar electrocoagulation probe (BICAP) cautery was first reported by Grondin and Seibert in 1989 *(46)*. Rex, Lewis, and Waye reported a series of nine patients treated similarly in 1992 *(47)*. Delayed bleeding can also be treated with Argon plasma coagulation (see Fig. 1) or application of an endoclip. Postpolypectomy transmural burns are treated with antibiotics and observation. If frank perforation occurs, surgical management is recommended. The modern bowel preparations have been discussed in this manuscript. While osmotic preps with mannitol or sorbitol are well-tolerated, there is production of hydrogen and methane and there are case reports of explosion when electrocautery is used. If these preps are utilized, multiple air exchanges in the colon must be performed and, preferably, CO_2 insufflation should be used for colonic distension before electrocautery of a lesion is attempted. Colonic mucosal injury has been reported with both glutaraldehyde *(48)* and hydrogen peroxide *(49)*, resulting in symptomatic distal colitis. A breakdown in the protocol of endoscope disinfection has also caused patient-to-patient transmission of hepatitis C *(50)*.

7. IDENTIFICATION OF COLONIC NEOPLASIA

7.1. Colon Carcinoma Surveillance

The National Polyp Study Workgroup's study cohort of 1418 patients who had complete colonoscopy and the removal of one or more adenomas was noted during followp-up years to have a lower rate of colon cancer with respect to three referenced groups, the Mayo Clinic Cohort, the St. Mark's Cohort, and the Seer Program *(51)*. During follow-up, only five malignant polyps (early stage colorectal carcinomas) were detected by colonoscopy. Since the number of cancers one would have expected to find based upon the cancer rates in the three reference groups were 48.3, 43.4, and 20.7, the study group appears to have sustained a 76–90% risk reduction in colon cancer. Sigmoidoscopy appears to lead to a threefold reduction in colorectal carcinoma mortality *(52)*, but is not successful in preventing colorectal carcinoma. A left-sided sigmoidoscopy exam is, by definition, an incomplete examination of the colon, but its value as a stand alone screening exam is called into question when 44% of patients with proximal colonic adenomas have no index polyps within the range of a sigmoidoscope *(53)* and 46% of advanced proximal lesions have no distal lesions *(54)*. These two studies may overstate their case, since higher risk patients may have oversubscribed. The National Polyp Study and these colonoscopy studies do appear to validate the Lieberman cost-effectiveness model for colon cancer screening *(55)*, which suggested that one-time colonoscopy would make the greatest impact on colorectal cancer mortality. This model compared five screening programs: fecal occult blood test alone, flexible sigmoidoscopy alone, flexible sigmoidoscopy plus fecal occult blood testing, one-time colonoscopy, and air-contrast barium enema. The barium enema was not cost-effective, and fecal occult blood testing plus sigmoidoscopy were dependent upon yearly compliance of fecal occult testing to be cost-effective.

Colonoscopy, while treated as a gold standard in colonic cancer and polyp identification studies, still has a miss rate. Rex et al. reviewed medical records of 2193 colorectal cancer cases and found that colonoscopy identified the lesion in 95% of patients as opposed to 82.9% using barium enema *(56)*. In 941 patients, the initial study was a colonoscopy. A colon cancer was missed in 20 cases because the colonoscope failed to reach the level of the cancer, and in 27 cases, the cancer was likely to be within an area examined by the colonoscopist. The odds ratio of a missed cancer by a nongastroenterologist as opposed to a procedure performed by a gastroenterologist was 5.36, dropping the sensitivity of colonoscopy performed by nongastroenterologists to 87%. This, unfortunately, approached the sensitivity of a barium enema (83%) in this study. The National Polyp Study compared the yield of double contrast barium enema to a subsequent blinded colonoscopy exam in 580 patients undergoing surveillance after polypectomy *(57)*. Barium enema detected polyps in 26% of exams, while polyps were found on 39% of colonoscopies. Polyps with a diameter between 0.6–1 cm were not identified 47% of the time on barium enema but barium enema, did not miss any adenomas >1 cm. When the colonoscopist was unblinded as to the site of a barium enema-identified polyp, 20% of the time the lesion could be confirmed. Colonoscopy is not infallible. Back-to-back, same day colonoscopies by the same or different physicians, with the patient in the same or different body position found that the miss rate for the initial endoscopy was 24% overall. It was 13% for adenomas 6–9 mm and 6% for adenomas 1 cm or larger (58). Glick et al. reported 18 lesions >2 cm in diameter that were undetected by colonoscopy, even though these confirmed colonic neoplasms were identified on barium enema before the colonoscopy (59). These lesions tended to be relatively flat and had coloration similar to that of the surrounding mucosa. Thirty percent of the lesions contained a focus of cancer.

It is likely that the National Polyp Study and the back-to-back colonoscopy study by Rex had a similar miss rate of diminutive polyps. It is not known whether the rate of colon cancer would have been as drastically reduced in the National Polyp Study if only polyps >1 cm were resected. Polyp growth has been followed longitudinally in a group of 116 patients that had yearly colonoscopy and careful measurement of polyp size (60). Polypectomy was only performed if the polyp grew to more than 10 mm in size. Polyps >5 mm showed a tendency for growth, and polyps 5–9 mm tended to regress in size. After 3 yr, all polyps were removed. An intramucosal carcinoma was found in two polyps. One of these polyps had decreased from 9 to 7 mm in diameter, and the other had increased from 8 to 11 mm over 1 yr. Another three polyps had high grade dysplasia in adenomatous polyps that changed minimally over 3 yr. An additional patient with a polyp that increased from 8–12 mm over 2 yr had evidence for high grade dysplasia. Therefore six of 116 patients had polyps <1 cm in diameter containing high grade dysplasia or carcinoma. This would suggest that the cutoff for at risk polyps should perhaps be 6 mm and not 10 mm. Any imaging study, such as virtual colonoscopy, which may evolve for the screening of colon cancer, will need to identify lesions down to 6–8 mm in size for maximum impact in the prevention of colorectal carcinoma.

Not all neoplastic lesions need to be polypoid, and not all flat dysplastic lesions need to originate in the orient. Of 1000 consecutive United Kingdom patients who underwent a colonoscopy where the colonoscopist deliberately searched for flat or depressed lesions, 321 adenomas were found of which 117 were flat and 2 were depressed (61). Cancer was seen in 4% of the small flat lesions, in 29% of larger flat lesions, and in three of four depressed lesions. Mahsushita et al. have suggested that rather than hinder colonoscopy, a transparent cap on the tip of the endoscope actually increased the yield of the exam (62). Tandem colonoscopies were performed with or without the cap in random order. There were no additional polyps when the initial colonoscopy was performed with the cap. When the capped colonoscope followed a standard exam, an additional 15% of polyps were discovered.

8. ADVANCED IMAGING TECHNIQUES OF THE COLON

While standard colonoscopy is, at present, the best method for identification of colonic polyps, recognition of flat lesions, and discrimination between diminutive hyperplastic and adenomatous tissue without tissue biopsy has not been very successful. Adenomas tend to be somewhat redder, larger, and more proximal in the colon than hyperplastic polyps, but the endoscopist's initial assessment as to tissue type with a standard endoscope is incorrect in 30% of cases (63). Color alone is not a good marker to tissue type, since 24% of reddened polyps are hyperplastic, and 17% of whitish cap ones are adenomatous (64). To discriminate tissue type without a tissue biopsy new instrumentation is available.

Flat adenomas and depressed adenomas have been infrequently found in western series using standard endoscopic techniques, whether this is because they are not present, or unseen, is not known. Chromoendoscopy, which is endoscopy after the application of a stain to the mucosa, has improved lesion recognition, although this has not been widely practiced in the west (see Fig. 2). When coupled with high contrast or magnifying colonoscopy, there is improved recognition of diminutive lesions, recognition of dysplastic changes, and staging of

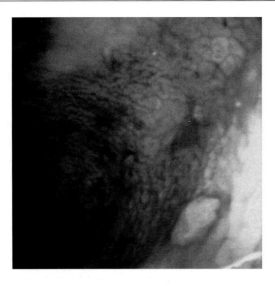

Fig. 2. Chromoendoscopy with 0.2% Indigo carmine stain displaying a normal colonic mucosal architecture with a diminutive polyp. It is difficult to characterize hyperplastic vs adenomatous polyps using a standard endoscope.

the depth of a mucosal tumor. Magnification endoscopes are available from Fujinion (Wayne, NJ) and Olympus (Melville, NY) with magnification of the viewed field between 100 and 170 times. The high resolution endoscope, which is also available from Fujinon and Olympus increases the pixels displayed on the monitor from 180,000–410,000, in effect making this a high definition television image. A magnifying lens can be used optionally.

Chromoendoscopy involves the ingestion or the direct spraying onto the colonic mucosa of a pigment or a stain, which in the colon enhances the surrounding crypt pattern as well as the surface pattern of any polyp or flat adenoma. Indigo carmine is purely a contrast stain, since it enhances the crypt pattern without any take up into cells. Patients ingest it as a capsule with their colonoscopy prep, or a 0.1–0.5% solution is sprayed directly over the mucosa to be examined during colonoscopy. Methylene blue is a vital stain, in that there is active absorption of the blue stain into intestinal cells. In the esophagus, it stains specialized epithelium, but in the colon, it appears to act like more of a contrast stain, as it pools in colonic microscopic crevasses. Congo red is a reactive stain that stains acidic cells. Excellent reviews in staining in GI endoscopy have been written by M.I. Canto *(65)* and C.S. Shim *(66)* in *Endoscopy* in 1999.

A mixture of Congo red and methylene blue was sprayed onto 51 raised colonic polyps of the colon *(67)*. When the polyps were examined using a standard colonoscope, neoplastic polyps were lighter than the surrounding bluish/red mucosa in areas that were tumor-free. In adenomas with severe atypia and adenocarcinoma, the degree of bleaching was greatest. Polyps that were not neoplastic (i.e., hyperplastic polyps) had the same coloration as the background mucosa. This method of chromoendoscopy could potentially assist differentiation of adenoma vs hyperplastic polyp and permit targeting of higher yield sites for biopsy in large polyps that are unremovable. The lighter coloration of the polyp compared to surrounding tissue should also facilitate the identification of small polyps, similar to the ease with which small polyps can be seen in patients that have marked melanosis coli in the background mucosa.

After Indigo carmine spraying of polyps, high contrast colonoscopy could discriminate the orderly arranged dotted pit pattern of a hyperplastic polyp from the surface groove or sulci pattern seen in adenomatous polyps (68). Sensitivity and specificity of discrimination was 93% and 95%, respectively. The endoscopist could identify the pit pattern with or without the additional magnification lens. Jaramillo et al. performed colonoscopy on 232 Swedish patients using a high resolution video endoscope and Indigo carmine staining (69). These patients did not have inflammatory bowel disease, a family history of hereditary nonpolyposis colorectal cancer, or a family history of familial adenomatous polyposis. In this western population, a total of 109 flat neoplastic lesions were found in 55 patients. Ninety-four lesions had low to high grade dysplasia, and 77 lesions measured 0.5 cm or less. When central depression was found, high grade dysplasia was present 43% of the time, as opposed to neoplastic lesions without central depression where high grade dysplasia was found in only 7%. Adenocarcinoma was seen in three flat lesions, each measured >1 cm. A Japanese population surveillance study with Indigo carmine chromoendoscopy and a magnifying colonoscope yielded 37 lesions <5 mm in diameter (70). Eighteen had mild atypia, 14 had moderate atypia and 5 had severe atypia. All of the lesions with extreme atypia and 11 of the moderate atypia had central depression. Minute lesions can, therefore, have severe atypia, and central umbilication should be sought. When flat early colorectal cancers are found, Saitoh et al. suggest that a surgical excision of the lesion is needed if chromoendoscopy of the lesion highlights deep central depression, an irregular bottom to the area of central depression, or convergence of colonic folds toward the tumor (71). A markedly abnormal colonic gland (pit) pattern within the lesion or a sharp margin to the polyp may suggest deeper local invasion when the area is examined with the magnifying colonoscope (72).

In western populations, the flat adenoma, which appears as a slightly raised plaque on the colon, is identified and appeared to have a higher rate of high grade dysplasia in retrospective series when compared to other small polyps. Wolber and Owen noted that of 340 adenomas, high grade dysplasia was seen in 12 of 29 flat adenomas (73). Muto et al. also found that 14 of 33 flat adenomas contained high grade dysplasia (74). In a prospective series of 148 patients and 66 adenomas, Lanspa et al. found 18 flat adenomas (75). In this series, no flat adenoma had high grade dysplasia. Flat adenomas are not likely to be a marker for hereditary nonpolyposis carcinoma, but they should be searched for, since they may be dysplastic. If multiple adenomas are found in the proximal colon, there may be a familial component that is also associated with gastric fundic gland polyps and duodenal adenomas.

Crypt foci aberrancies can be found in surgical specimens and are considered to be very early events in colon carcinogenesis. Crypt aberrancies are seen in familial adenomatous polyposis (76), in other areas of the colon in patients who have undergone colonic resection for colon cancer (77), and in animal models of carcinogen-induced colorectal carcinoma (78). Yokota et al. were able to detect in vivo aberrant crypt foci within the rectum with 0.1% methylene blue chromoendoscopy and a magnifying colonoscope (79). Fifty-one patients, 35 with a history of colorectal adenoma and/or cancer and 16 with no colonic lesion history had evaluation of the rectal mucosa. Crypt foci were defined as being more deeply stained with methylene blue with slight bulging of the crypt on the mucosal surface. In the 16 patients that had no history of a colonic lesion, 10 had no crypt foci and 6 had 1–10 foci per rectum. In the group that were higher risk, 19 had 1–10 aberrant crypts, 3 had a 11–30, and 11 had >31 aberrant crypts. Subsequent studies may use this assay to identify patients who are at greater risk for the development of colonic neoplasms. By contrast, such an assay could potentially detect a very early response to colon carcinoma chemoprophylaxis with anti-oxidants or cyclooxygenase (COX)-2 inhibitors. The pattern of colonic glands evaluated by magnifying endoscopy can also correlate with histological findings. Hayashi et al. showed excellent correlation between preoperative evaluation of 27 colonic cancers, 40 adenomas, and 10 specimens of normal mucosa *(80)*. The measured range in the irregularity of the colonic pits correlated with the degree of cellular atypia.

9. TECHNIQUES OF OPTICAL BIOPSY

Induced optical fluorescence appears to be a method that may improve detection and the determination of the degree of dysplasia of small colonic lesions. Tissue autofluorescence is based upon excitation of endogenous fluorophores by light. An exposure to a single wavelength of light emitted by a laser or a to broader band of color-filtered light is absorbed by these fluorophores and remitted at longer wavelengths as detectable fluorescence. The excitation wavelength is between 300–450 nm, and the emission wavelength is between 350–600 nm. Fluorophores include collagen, nicotinamide adenine dinucleotide (NAD/NADH), porphyrins, and several other compounds *(81)*. Colonic adenomas and cancer are less fluorescent than normal mucosa. This is due to a loss of autofluorescence remitted from underlying submucosal collagen due to thickening of the overlying mucosa from the polyp or due to replacement of submucosal collagen by invasive cancer *(82)*. The focal application of light with a probe has permitted analysis of a fluorescence signature from the identified lesion. Analysis of the fluorescence could correctly discriminate adenomas from hyperplastic polyps and normal mucosa nearly 90% of the time *(83–85)*. In addition to noting adenoma vs hyperplasia, a further change in fluorescence intensity from normal was seen in dysplastic epithelium *(86–87)*.

Exogenous fluorophores can also be given systemically or applied topically to enhance fluorescence changes. Both 5-aminolevulinic (5-ALA) and to a lesser degree porfimer sodium (Photofrin) enhance fluorescence of colonic neoplasias. In the abnormal tissue, the 5-ALA accumulates as protoporphyrin IX, which is very fluorescent because of a lack of ferrochelatase in tumors *(88)*. Photofrin also has preferentially higher levels within colonic tumors, but patients exhibit photosensitivity for more than a month after an infusion as opposed to 48 h with 5-ALA. Screening systems are now available in which large areas of mucosal surface can undergo endoscopic fluorescence imagining. Two systems that are commercially available are the D-Light (Storz, Germany) and the Life-GI (Xillix Technologies, Canada). Their potential use in screening of high risk populations, such as patients with a family history of familial polyposis or hereditary nonpolyposis colon cancer is apparent.

As with the esophagus and stomach, optical coherence tomography (OCT) within the colon can be used to evaluate found lesions or stage depth of invasion. In OCT, an endoscopic probe is inserted through a standard colonoscope, and at low power, a wavelength of 1270 nm is emitted. Back-scattered light is then mapped with an image that is similar to that seen with endoscopic ultrasound. OCT images demonstrate layers of histology as with endoscopic ultrasound, and small adenomatous foci within the mucosa can be identified. Small cancers exhibit surface irregularity, and malignant cells within the mucosa are more reflective than other areas *(89)*.

10. MUCOSAL BIOPSY ANALYSIS

In addition to histopathology, mucosal biopsies obtained via the colonoscope can be analyzed for abnormal DNA content, abnormal DNA methylation, and the presence of oncogenes or tumor suppressor genes. Mucosal biopsies incubated with tritiated thymidine identify proliferation of colonic crypts, which is increased in patients with sporadic adenomas, hereditary nonpolyposis colon cancer, and familial polyposis *(90)*. In 76 average risk patients, protein expression of p53 and bcl-2 within a rectosigmoid adenoma was indicative of an advanced proximal adenoma that had villous histology, severe dysplasia, or a diameter >1 cm *(91)*. This was true in 28 of 44 p53 positive and in 12 of 44 bcl-2 positive distal adenomas. If p53 was negative, only 2 of 59 patients had a proximal adenoma.

11. COLONOSCOPY AND INFLAMMATORY BOWEL DISEASE

The diagnosis of ulcerative colitis and Crohn's disease involving the colon is most frequently made by the endoscopic appearance of the mucosa and pathology seen on biopsy specimens. In ulcerative colitis, there is an increase in mucosal granularity, friability, loss of the undergoing vascular pattern, and a lack of any skip areas. In Crohn's disease, skip areas and asymmetric involvement of the colon is looked for, as are perivascular distribution of aphthoid lesions, fissuring within the colonic mucosa, and areas of deep ulceration. Small bowel follow through of a barium meal, ileoscopy *(92)*, and transvalvular enteroscopy using a mother-baby endoscope *(93)* may all increase diagnostic yield. Expected findings in the biopsies of ulcerative colitis include a uniform appearance, crypt branching and elongation, and goblet cell depletion. Crohn's disease may have goblet cell depletion and has similar crypt changes in involved areas, but has a variable degree and greater depth to the inflammatory response. Granulomata, which are only seen in Crohn's disease and not in ulcerative colitis, are found in a minority of Crohn's patients. These findings are separately discussed in the inflammatory bowel disease chapters in this text. When there is only colonic involvement by inflammatory bowel disease, there is considerable overlap, and in up to 20% of patients, discrimination between Crohn's colitis and ulcerative colitis cannot initially be made based on mucosal biopsies or endoscopic appearance. There is, therefore, certainly room for improvement in the endoscopic diagnosis of inflammatory bowel disease. In addition to diagnosis, colonoscopy is used to assess disease activity, and/or response to therapy, and for colon cancer surveillance.

A technique to evaluate for Crohn's disease recurrence or potentially help make the diagnosis in a symptomatic patient is fluorescence angiography. In this technique, 10% sodium fluorescein is injected intravenously, and during colonoscopy, an intermittently flashing blue light stimulates sodium fluorescein fluorescence. The submucosal vascularization is shown, and discrete fluorescent spots <2 mm in diameter are seen *(94)*. Occasionally, the mucosa in these areas will appear normal, and at other times, a subtle aphthous lesion can be found. Directed biopsies can then be performed since it is known that the highest yield for Crohn's-associated granulomata is within the central erosion of an aphthous lesion. Visualizing earlier aphthous lesions and directing biopsy sites may improve the sensitivity and specificity of the exam when assessing for early disease.

Disease activity of ulcerative colitis is usually determined by taking into account clinical symptoms, clinical signs, the endoscopic mucosal appearance, and the degree of inflammation seen in the colonic biopsies. Unfortunately, the severity based upon clinical signs and symptoms does not always match with the endoscopic interpretation. Other methods to assess mucosal disease severity are being developed. Magnifying chromoscopy appears to have a typical crypt pattern in patients with a lower clinical activity index and lower histology grade of inflammation *(95)*. Organ reflectance spectrophotometry performed during colonoscopy demonstrates that more severe ulcerative colitis has a higher index of mucosal hemoglobin concentration and a lower hemoglobin oxygen saturation *(96)*. This is indicative of mucosal congestion and mucosal hypoxia. Rather than biopsies to determine nitric oxide (NO) level, superoxide dismutase level, or total colonic antioxident potential *(97)*, NO can be directly measured by a NO-selective electrode *(98)* or by analysis of NO in suctioned colonic gas using a chemiluminescence technique *(99)*. NO concentrations measured with the microelectrode in patients with mild to severely inflamed mucosa were 12–72 times higher than normal controls. NO measured in colonic gas was 100 times higher in active disease patients compared to controls. Flow cytometry of biopsies confirmed that a greater number of colonic cells were in a synthetic phase of the cell cycle when there was increased disease activity *(100)*. It is readily apparent that any of these techniques could be applied to assess for a response to treatment or identification of early relapse in ulcerative colitis patients.

Colonoscopy is used to survey for the development of dysplasia or dysplasia associated lesion or mass (DALM) lesions in ulcerative colitis patients because the cumulative risk for colon cancer becomes significantly greater than the average risk background population after 8–10 yr of disease. The cumulative risk is 1.8% after 20 yr and 43% after 35 yr. The majority of patients do not undergo prophylactic proctocolectomy if they have inactive disease. This is the patient population who undergo colon cancer surveillance with colonoscopy at a 1- to 2-yr interval. This requires four quadrant biopsies from at least seven levels or at least 56 biopsies to have a 95% confidence of detection of dysplasia *(101)*. From ulcerative colitis colorectal cancer screening programs totaling 1463 patients that had an average number of screening exams per patient that ranged between 1.5 and 5.2, 66 cancers were eventually diagnosed *(102)*. Twenty-three were Duke's A, 16 Duke's B, and 17 Duke's C. Ten patients had metastatic disease. The majority of these cancers were diagnosed on the second or later surveillance endoscopy, and when cancer was diagnosed, 41% of patients had a Duke's C or higher cancer. This calls into question whether ulcerative colitis can be successfully and safely surveyed using standard surveillance as it is presently performed. High resolution colonic endoscopy with Indigo carmine chromoendoscopy was performed on a cohort of 85 Swedish ulcerative colitis patients *(103)*. Thirty-eight patients had polyps detected. Of the 104 polyps detected, 77 were flat, 21 were sessile, and 3 were pedunculated. In the remaining three, a descriptive morphology was not recorded. Low grade dysplasia was found in 21 of 23 neoplastic polyps and high grade dysplasia was seen in one flat tubular adenoma and in one sessile villous adenoma. If there is a correlation between flat adenomas and an increased risk for development of colorectal carcinoma this type of exam could potentially permit earlier recognition of patients at risk for colorectal carcinoma. One caveat to this statement is the fact that small sporadic adenomas are known to occur in ulcerative colitis and can be treated by polypectomy and shorter surveillance intervals without an underlying increase in colonic mucosal dysplasia *(104,105)*.

Rather than obtaining 56 distributed biopsies throughout the colon in order to assess randomly for dysplasia, it would be useful to have a better way of targeting sites that have a higher yield for dysplasia. Ott et al. used laser-induced fluorescence endoscopy (LIFE) to search for dysplastic mucosa in 15 ulcerative colitis patients either with or without 5-ALA ingestion *(106)*. This was compared to biopsies obtained during the conventional colonoscopy portion of the exam. Four suspicious lesions were noted and biopsied during conventional colonoscopy. None of the patients were found to have dysplasia on biopsy, and there was no false positives following autofluorescence and one false positive after 5-ALA administration. Because this study population had no dysplasia, the value of targeting biopsy cannot yet be assessed. Sialosyl-Tn antigen expression was screened for in specimens from 11 ulcerative colitis patients who developed colon cancer or dysplasia and compared to specimens in 11 ulcerative colitis patients who had no evidence of dysplasia on biopsy *(107)*. Earlier surveillance exams were also stained for sialosyl-Tn. Sialosyl-Tn antigen was found in 44% of the patient biopsies and in 11% of the control biopsies. Sialosyl-Tn positivity was also noted up to 7 yr prior to a colonic neoplasm. The frequency of surveillance exam or the number of biopsy specimens needed could potentially be increased if this antigen is expressed in colonic mucosa.

12. LOWER GI BLEEDING

Lower GI bleeding ranges from a minimal amount of blood seen after defecation to exsanguination from repeated passage of maroon stools. Minor episodes of overt lower GI blood loss consist of intermittent small quantities of bright red blood. Major episodes are frequently self-limited, in that they spontaneously stop bleeding or the rate of bleeding slows down enough to permit resuscitation with saline and packed red blood cells prior to colonoscopy. The few patients that have uncorrectable hypovolemia due to torrential hemorrhage should undergo an emergent preoperative upper endoscopy to exclude an upper GI source and a limited flexible sigmoidoscopy to exclude a rectal source immediately prior to laparotomy or angiography.

Patients with major bleeding that is self-limited should undergo urgent colonoscopy. An upper GI source should, at a minimum, be excluded with a nasogastric lavage, though this may miss intermittently bleeding duodenal lesions. Not all clinicians cleanse the colon prior to lower endoscopy if there is active hemorrhage. Chaudry et al. reported their experience of 126 colonoscopies on 85 patients for lower GI bleeding *(108)*. Though each of these colonoscopies was performed unprepped, fecal residue interfered with an adequate examination in only two patients. Bleeding spontaneously stopped in 68% of these patients. In 82 of 85 patients, it was felt that the source of bleeding was correctly identified or localized to the small bowel (in the cases of small bowel hemorrhage). In 17 of 27 actively bleeding lesions, treatment either with application neodyminum: yttrium-aluminum-garnet (Nd:YAG) laser photocoagulation or BICAP coagulation achieved hemostasis. The authors considered colonoscopy to be the initial diagnostic test. Though these patients had colonoscopy while unprepped and fecal residue did not pose a problem for these investigators, we would recommend a quick purge with PEG lavage to evacuate clotted blood as well as fecal residue. This facilitates an easier examination that can still be performed within 4–6 h of notification. The Center for Ulcer Research and Education (CURE) hemostasis study enrolled 100 patients prospectively for severe hematochezia *(109)*. Each patient had a negative nasogastric lavage, and rigid sigmoidoscopy and anoscopy did not identify a source of hemorrhage. After colonic cleansing, colonoscopy was performed. If bleeding was noted through the ileocecal valve, upper endoscopy was also performed. A colonic site of bleeding was found in 74% of patients. Angiodysplasia was most common and seen in 30% of patients, followed by bleeding diverticulosis in 17%, ulcerated polyps or cancer in 11%, focal ulcers or colitis in 9%, and rectal lesions not seen with rigid sigmoidoscopy in 4%. An upper GI site was found in 11%, and a small bowel source was inferred by negative colonoscopy and upper endoscopy in 9%. In only 6% of patients, no site could be found. Thirty-five percent of patients spontaneously stopped bleeding, 40% required endoscopic therapy during colonoscopy, and 24% required surgery. Treatment was primarily bipolar cautery. When a visible vessel could not be found in a bleeding diverticulum, the base and area around the diverticulum orifice were injected with 1:20,000 epinephrine with excellent success. When colonoscopy was instituted as a primary method of diagnosis and therapy, a drop in rate of angiography, days in the intensive care unit (ICU), emergency surgery, and days hospitalized realized a net savings of $10,065 per patient hemorrhage at University of California at Los Angeles (UCLA). This excellent study demonstrated the impact that colonoscopy has had on the treatment of this disease presentation. The only amendment regarding treatment approach is that I would advocate upper endoscopy before colonoscopy in this patient population, since 11% of patients had lesions that could be evaluated by upper endoscopy. Alternate methods of endoscopic treatment of the bleeding site would be 1:10,000 epinephrine injection, heater probe coagulation, argon plasma coagulation, application of an endoclip, or injection of a sclerosing agent, such as sodium morrhuate.

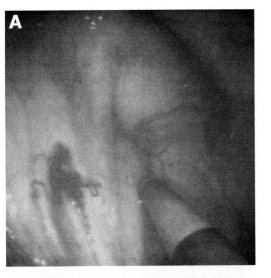

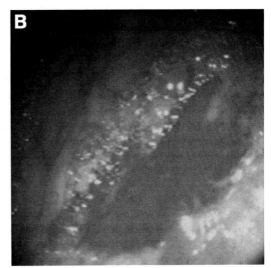

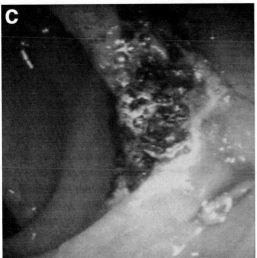

Fig. 3. (A) A proximal colonic angiodysplasia which presented with intermittent decreases in hemoglobin and limited lower gastrointestinal bleeding. The tip of the 7-Fr argon plasma coagulator probe is also seen. (B) A larger colonic angiodysplasia in the ascending colon. (C) The same angiodysplasia after argon plasma cautery. Four days later the patient sustained an overt hemorrhage, and the central vessel of this angiodysplasia required retreatment.

12.1. Angiodysplasia-Associated Colonic Bleeding

Angiodysplasias, which usually present with chronic gastrointestinal blood loss rather than with an acute major hemorrhage, appear as flat erythematous plaques up to 1.5 cm in diameter. A central feeder vessel can occasionally be seen. The majority of angiodysplasias, including nearly all that eventually bleed, are located within the right colon *(110)*. Identification requires a clean colon and occasionally a naloxone bolus if an opioid has been given for conscious sedation, since vascular contraction by a narcotic may lead to temporary disappearance of this vascular lesion *(111)*. Similarly, a cold water jet irrigation directly onto an angiodysplasia may cause temporary blanching *(112)*. Treatment by fulguration is started around the lesion periphery before the central vessel is ablated *(113)*. It is typical to have some active bleeding particularly of larger angiodysplasia during fulguration (see Fig. 3). This bleeding appears to be less frequent with the argon plasma coagulator than with contact bipolar cautery. Incomplete fulguration has a risk for delayed rebleeding. Upon reexamination after rebleeding, the lesion will appear ulcerated with a central visible vessel.

12.2. Diverticular Hemorrhage

Diverticular hemorrhage is either the first or the second most common source of acute lower GI hemorrhage in most series. Colonoscopic identification of a bleeding diverticulum or the actual bleeding vessel within the diverticulum is occasionally seen (114). Stigmata of recent diverticular bleeding include erosions in a diverticulum (115) and a sentinel clot (116). Though most diverticula are located in the sigmoid colon, the majority of diverticular hemorrhages appear to have a right colonic origin based upon scintigraphically tagged red blood cell exams. However, when colonoscopy identifies a diverticular hemorrhage, it is more often from a left colonic source (117). Out a series of 210 lower gastrointestinal hemorrhage patients, 83 diverticular bleed patients that did not have surgery or catheter emobolization had a cumulative hemorrhage recurrence rate of 11% at 1 yr, 15% at 2 yr, 19% at 3 yr, and 25% at 4 yr (118). It is not known whether endoscopic treatment of a diverticular hemorrhage impacts the hemorrhage recurrence rate.

12.3. Endoscopic Treatment of Radiation Proctitis

A medical response to the bleeding and tenesmus that accompanies radiation proctitis is variable. In those patients in which medical therapy fails, ablation of the friable neovascular sites (see Fig. 4) that are the source of bleeding has been attempted with BICAP cautery, heater probe (119), argon plasma coagulation (120,121), argon laser, Nd:YAG laser (123,124), and KPT laser (125) (see Table 1). In each of these studies, the blood product support needed post-treatment was less than what was before therapy. Rectal incontinence of blood and tenesmus were also frequently improved. Complications were minimal. The author has noted a surprising amount of symptomatic tenesmus when argon plasma coagulation is used for this entity as opposed as to what is seen with BICAP cautery and Nd:YAG. Perhaps the more focal treatment of the BICAP probe or the Nd:YAG laser and the greater number of neovascular sites treated at one time with the argon plasma are the cause of post-procedure tenesmus. After approx 2 wk this symptom resolves, and the patients are significantly improved with regard to rectal bleeding.

Other endoscopically treatable sources of hemorrhage are colonic neoplasms, isolated colonic ulcerations (126), Dieulafoy's lesions (127), stercoral ulcers (128), colonic varices (129), and postoperative hemorrhage from a stapled colorectal anastomosis (130). Colonic neoplasms can occasionally be removed with cautery snare, or the surface of an unresectable bleeding malignancy can be treated with cautery or laser to decrease the frequency of recurrent hemorrhages.

When patients pass small volumes of bright red blood per rectum, there is some question as to whether flexible sigmoidoscopy is an adequate study. Patient history regarding layering of blood within stool or blood restricted to the stool surface is notoriously unreliable, affecting the specificity of clinical history for lesion location. Segal et al. attempted to address this issue by performing colonoscopy after a detailed clinical history in 103 outpatients (131). Internal hemorrhoids were found in 78 patients and external hemorrhoids in 29 patients. Significant lesions were found in 36 patients including adenomas >8 mm, colitis, and carcinoma in four patients. Only seven lesions were thought to be proximal to the sigmoid colon. History did not discriminate between perianal bleeding and colonic pathology. In a similar study by Van Rosendaal et al., proximal lesions beyond the range of the sigmoidoscope were only found in the elderly (132). In both studies, even though most of the lesions were potentially within range of the sigmoidoscope, colonoscopy should be the initial procedure of choice, since patients who had a neoplastic lesion would need colonoscopy to exclude a proximal synchronous lesion; in addition, most older patients with a negative sigmoidoscopy would need a colonoscopy to exclude a proximal colonic lesion.

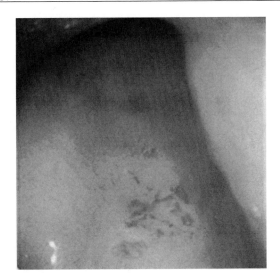

Fig. 4. Neovascular vessels in radiation proctitis.

Table 1
Endoscopic Treatment of Radiation Proctitis

Author (reference)	Rx Modality	No. Patients	Bleeding episodes	Hemoglobin	Tenesmus	Incontinence
Jensen et al. (119)	Heater Probe	12	Fewer	Rise	Less	Less
Jensen et al. (119)	BICAP	9	Fewer	Rise	Less	Less
Fantin et al. (120)	APC[a]	7	Absent	?	None	Less
Tam et al. (121)	APC[a]	15	Fewer	Rise	Less	Less
Taylor et al. (122)	Argon Laser	14	Fewer	?	?	?
Ahlquist et al. (123)	Nd:YAG Laser	4	Fewer	Rise	Less	Less
Barbatzas et al. (124)	Nd:YAG Laser	9	Fewer	Rise	?	Less
Taylor et al. (125)	KTP Laser	23	Fewer	Rise	?	Less

[a]Argon plasma coagulation.

13. EXCISION OF COLONIC NEOPLASMS

Most polyps found during colonoscopy are <1 cm in diameter and are removed with low power cautery snare (133). Because of the depth of the burn and risk for delayed hemorrhage, particularly in the right colon, hot biopsy forceps polypectomy should be restricted to polyps <5 mm in diameter (134). Hot biopsy of most diminutive polyps can usually be avoided, since nearly all polyps between 3 and 10 mm in diameter can be removed with the mini cautery snare. Cautery is optional with polyps between 3 and 5 mms, and polyps can be cut off with closure of a snare. Though there frequently is immediate visible bleeding with a cold polypectomy, rebleeding is extremely low when cautery is not used (135,136). Follow-up endoscopy has confirmed that the cold snare technique successfully removes all polypoid tissue when used on a diminutive polyp. This is in contradistinction to cold biopsy forceps of diminutive polyps, which have been shown to leave residual polyp tissue (137). When polyps are >5 mm, imme-diate post-cold polypectomy bleeding has been seen and may require injection therapy or topical cautery *(138)*. For this reason, the author personally uses cautery snare for all polyps >5 mm in diameter.

Pedunculated polyps are readily removed with slow stepwise transection of the stalk using a pure cautery current, or with a mixed cautery and cut current such as provided by the ERBE electrogenerator. A pure cut current for polypectomy has also been revisited and found to prevent delayed bleeding in one series, although it did predispose toward immediate postpolypectomy bleeding, which needed to be treated with endoclips *(139)*. The large pedunculated polyp poses an increased risk for delayed hemorrhage. As a method to prevent delayed hemorrhage, the application of a detachable endoloop before stalk transection was successful *(140)*; the initial success could not be duplicated by second investigator, who found that the loop would occasionally slip off the stalk, and in four cases, the loop itself caused transection of a thin stalk before polypectomy was performed *(141)*.

The newest technique, which permits relatively safe excision of large sessile polyps, is endomucosal resection (see Fig. 5). In this technique, there is needle injection of normal saline, hypertonic saline, 50% dextrose, or sodium hyaluronate into the colonic submucosa. The injectate expands the submucosa and lifts the overlying mucosa away from the muscularis propria (see Fig. 6). Normal saline diffuses relatively quickly after injection, therefore 1:10,000 epinephrine is frequently added to the injectate (see Fig. 7). The other materials, which are hyperosmotic or more viscous, do not diffuse nearly as quickly. If the lesion does not rise with injection this may indicate invasion of the submucosa and/or muscularis by the tumor *(142)*. Occasionally, there is difficulty getting a polyp to rise with injection when patients are referred for a total polypectomy after hot biopsy sampling of the center of the polyp during an initial colonoscopy. This is felt to be due to local fibrosis that is secondary to deep cautery during the hot biopsy.

After a cushion has been injected into the submucosa, the polyp can be removed in one piece or in several large fragments with snare polypectomy. If the snare continues to slide off the polyp, the edge of the polyp that the snare will not catch can be undermined a short distance with a needle knife so that the snare will now engage. If a double channel colonoscope is being used and the snare will not hold around a flat polyp as it is tightened, the snare can then be left loosely around the polyp, and after the tip of the polyp has been lifted with a biopsy forceps brought out the second channel, the snare will frequently catch the polyp's edge, permitting it to be transected. It is of course important not to be making contact between the snare and the biopsy forceps when current is applied. The problem of applying a snare to a relatively flat lesion can be entirely avoided using a transparent cap on the tip of the colonoscope. When the polyp is suctioned within the cap a snare that is held open at the tip of the cap can be closed with cautery removing the polyp that has been grasped with suction *(143,144)*. Injection technique also can bring a polyp, whose base is hidden behind a fold, into view by continuing to inject saline into the colonic submucosa until the polyp elevates into view.

Endomucosal resection is well described and referenced in the ASGE Technology Status Evaluation Bulletin *(145)*. It is clear that the technique provides a safe more superficial excision of large polyps. A retrospective review of colectomy specimens after endoscopic polypectomy compared postpolypectomy ulcers produced by endoscopic mucosal resection in 12 polyps vs the ulcer base of 16 polypectomy sites in which submucosal saline was not injected *(146)*. All ulcers after submucosal saline were confined to the submucosal layer, while 7 of 16, ulcers in which saline had not been injected prepolypectomy, reached the muscle layer or deeper. Although this is encouraging, there is a word of warning regarding the degree of protection that submucosal saline injection provides against a deep burn when argon plasma coagulation or a monopolar hot biopsy forceps are use to ablate residual polyp. In an animal

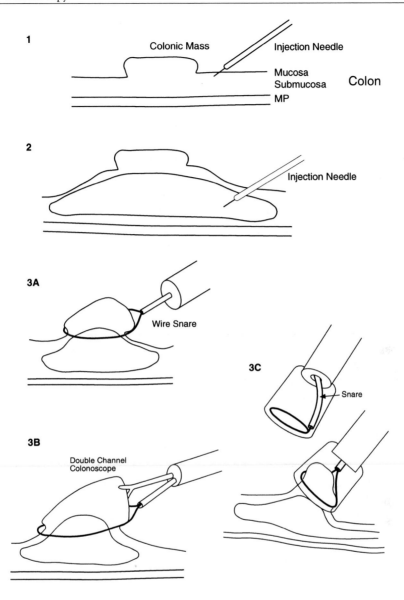

Fig. 5. Techniques of endomucosal resection. (1 and 2) After saline, saline mixed with epinephrine, or sodium hyaluronate is injected tangentially into the colonic submucosa, and the overlying polyp is lifted away from the muscularis propria. (3A) The majority of polyps can then be resected with a cautery snare. (3B) If the snare will not catch around the polyp, a pedicle can be created at the base of the polyp by lifting or tugging the polyp while the snare is being applied. This requires a two-channel colonoscope. After the polyp is caught within the snare, it is safest to open the biopsy forceps and retract them into the endoscope before cautery is applied. (3C) The polyp can also be held within a transparent suction cap on the tip of the colonoscope for application of the snare (see text).

model, the depth of burn was compared before and after saline injection *(147)*. Burns were made with a bipolar Gold probe for 2 s at 20 W, heater probe 30 J, a monopolar contact probe at 20 W for 2 s, and monopolar argon plasma coagulation at 45 W for 3 s. Without the saline, deep muscle injury occurred in 86% with argon plasma coagulation, 61% with monopolar contact, 50% with heater probe, and 18% with bipolar cautery. After saline, the argon plasma

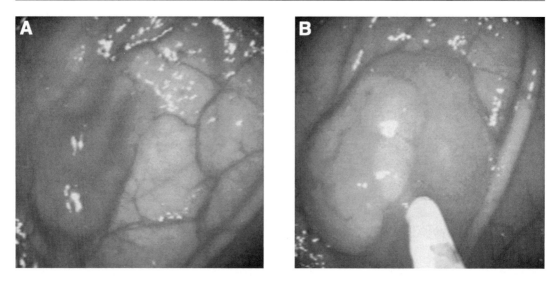

Fig. 6. (A) A 12-mm sessile polyp becomes in (B) easy to remove in one piece after saline is injected.

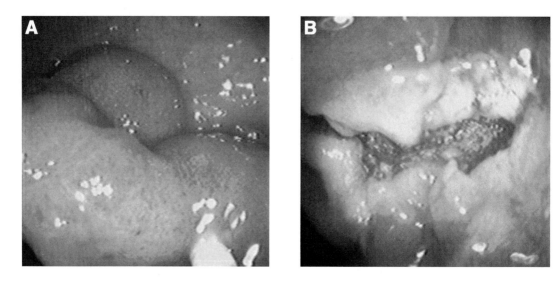

Fig. 7. A broad based 3-cm polyp found to have a large focus of high grade dysplasia is identified within the sigmoid colon. (A): Saline has been injected beneath the polyp demonstrating clear lifting of the entire polyp. (B) The polyp base is seen after removal with cautery effect identifiable around the rim of the polyp. As is commonly seen, there is no cautery change in the cut through the saline bleb under the center of the polyp.

coagulation deep burn rate decreased to 21%. After saline, the heater probe deep burn rate decreased from 50 to 0%, and the monopolar deep rate from 61 to 50%. Bipolar cautery, which has little depth to its burn, had a deep burn rate of 18% without saline injection. Therefore, after removing the majority of a polyp with a cautery snare, residual polyp should potentially not be removed with touch ablation using the tip of a monopolar snare or hot biopsy forceps. If argon plasma coagulation is used on very thin slivers of polypoid tissue, perhaps the pulses of energy should be less than 3 s.

After sessile polyps are partially removed, argon plasma coagulation has been safely used to treat visible and nonvisible residual adenomatous tissue. Zlatanic et al. reported a series of 77 patients with piecemeal polypectomy of polyps greater than 20 mm in size *(148)*. Polyp recurrence was compared in three groups. Group one had visible residual adenoma after the polypectomy and had the base of the site treated with argon plasma coagulator. The second group was thought to have a complete polypectomy and had no further treatment. The third had visible residual tissue left at the initial session and had no further treatment. This third group all had residual tissue on return visit 6 mo after the index procedure. If all of the visible tumor was removed without argon plasma coagulation, there was a 54% eradication rate (Group 2), and if visible tissue was identified and then the argon plasma coagulation used, there was 50% eradication rate (Group 1). Presumably, this residual tissue was then retreated. It would be interesting to know what the recurrence rate was after the second treatment. Brooker et al. used a similar approach, but included a group in which argon plasma coagulation was applied to the base of what was thought to be a complete polypectomy (invisible residual adenomatous tissue) *(149)*. In a series of 13 polypectomy patients, the endoscopist thought there was complete excision of the sessile polyp in eight polyps. Four patients then underwent argon plasma coagulation treatment to the base and margin of the polyp, and the remaining four patients received no argon plasma coagulation. In the five patients where there was known to be residual polyp, argon plasma coagulation was used to ablate visible residual tumor. In this group, recurrence was seen in two of the five. In patients with complete endoscopic removal that had no argon plasma coagulation, three of four had recurrence, and if argon plasma coagulation was applied on top of what appeared to be complete endoscopic removal, only one of four recurred. The location of these polyps is not described, but despite the warning in the animal model as to depth of an argon plasma coagulator burn, neither of these studies identified any problem with transmural burn or perforation.

Thermal photoablation of large polyps has also been reported with both the argon laser and the Nd:YAG laser (see Fig. 8). In a series of 196 patients with polyps treated with the Nd:YAG, complete long-term ablation with a mean 3-yr follow-up was achieved in 77% *(150)*. In Brunetaud et al.'s series of 264 patients with rectal and sigmoid villous adenomas, the only factor that led to an increased early complication rate, rate of recurrence, post-treatment stenosis, and growth of a subsequent carcinoma was the degree of circumferential involvement of the bowel by the base of the polyp *(151)*.

Though substantially larger polyps can now be safely excised assisted with submucosal saline injection, it should be remembered that larger polyps are more likely to contain high grade dysplasia or carcinoma compared to smaller polyps. A subset of these patients may need to have a colonic resection, although endoscopically the polyp has been entirely removed. In the case of an excised pedunculated polyp that contains invasive cancer, surgery is not needed if the cancer is well differentiated, if it has a peripheral location in the polyp, if there is no lymphatic or venous invasion, and if there is a clear margin between the polyp and the cautery site on the stalk. Sessile polyps are much more difficult to assess and if invasive cancer is seen in the polyp and if the patient is a good surgical candidate, they should undergo evaluation for surgery. Patients with carcinoma *in situ* do not have invasive cancer, and the decision as to whether they should undergo surgery or not is based upon whether the polyp has been totally removed or not *(152)*. When a polyp is ablated with the laser or with the argon plasma coagulator, the entire polyp cannot, by definition, be examined by the pathologist. Therefore, an island of carcinoma may be partially ablated rather than sampled and decision making regarding whether a patient should undergo surgery is not as accurate if the majority of a large polyp is ablated and not excised.

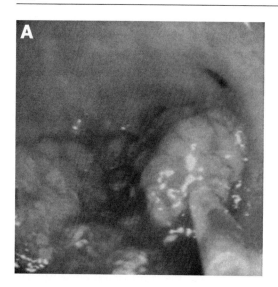 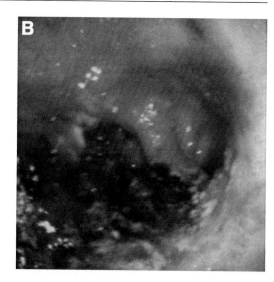

Fig. 8. (A) A large recurrent obstructing rectal carcinoma is being partially debulked with the cautery snare. (B) After Nd:Yag photoablation, the colorectal anastomosis can once again be identified and is widely patent.

14. PALLIATIVE ENDOSCOPIC TREATMENT OF COLON CARCINOMA

In patients that are not surgical candidates, laser photoablation can be utilized to maintain bowel lumen and occasionally, with small lesions, local laser extirpation can be a successful treatment modality. Brunetaud et al. also performed laser ablation therapy on 10 patients with colon cancers less than 3 cm in diameter that were polypoid and primarily exophytic *(153)*. After treatment, the biopsy base was negative for tumor. Two patients were lost to follow-up. Over a mean follow-up of 18.2 mo, there was one death due to known metastatic disease prior to treatment. The remaining patients remained free of disease. With larger lesions, the goal of laser therapy is to decrease bleeding and to normalize bowel habit. In a series of 104 patients, Escourrou et al. employed the Nd:YAG to establish and maintain rectal patency *(154)*. Rectal bleeding stopped in a third of patients, and eventually, 15 patients did require surgery because of bowel obstruction. Van Cutsem et al. had a similar finding, in that, initial palliation could be achieved in 82% of patients, however, by 1 yr, the treatment was no longer effective in 41% *(155)*. Treatment frequently requires more than one initial laser session to open the lumen and then retreatment is planned at a 2- to 3-mo interval for the rest of the patient's life. In those patients that are surgical candidates but present with a bowel obstruction, laser reestablishment of a lumen is an option for decompression of the bowel, thus obviating the need for a temporary decompressing colostomy. This was achieved by Eckhauser et al. in 11 patients with the Nd:YAG laser, permitting them to have primary resection and anastomosis *(156)*.

A decompression tube could be placed endoscopically proximal to the site of a colonic neoplastic obstruction in six of nine patients *(157)*. This permitted adequate bowel prep and a primary colonic resection with anastomosis. Neoplastic strictures have also been dilated with a balloon to temporarily open an obstructed lumen for a bowel preparation or to advance a small caliber endoscope to the proximal aspect of a neoplastic lesion and begin Nd:YAG treatment *(158)*. With the advent of self expanding metal stents this is infrequently utilized.

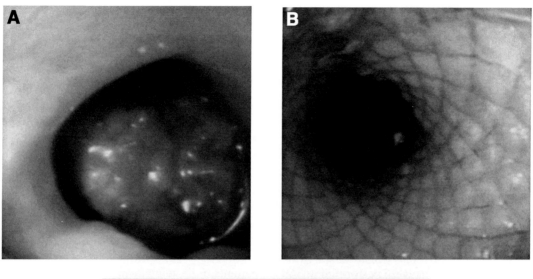

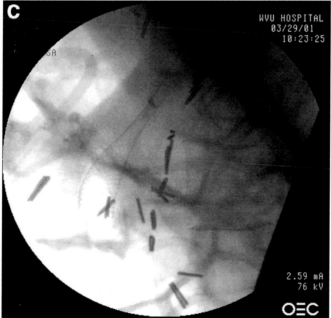

Fig. 9. (A) An obstructing recurrent carcinoma is identified immediately proximal to the colonic anastomosis (courtesy Lisa Gangarosa, MD). (B) Endoscopic view of this segment after a 22-mm diameter uncoated colonic wallstent has been placed. (C) Radiographic image of the deployed wallstent.

The expandable metal stents, are easy to deploy if a guide wire successfully bridges the site of obstruction (see Fig. 9). The stent may be placed with fluoroscopic guidance over a rigid wire without an endoscope. Since the newer stents will traverse a therapeutic channel endoscope, endoscopic retrograde cholangiopancreatography (ERCP)-type technique can be used for wire placement over which the metal stent is deployed, traversing the stricture. Baron et al. placed stents in 25 patients using endoscopic and radiologic techniques. Stent placement was successful in 94% of patients, and in 85%, obstruction could be relieved *(159)*. In the 10 patients in which stents were placed preoperatively, decompression occurred in 9, and in the 15 patients where the intent was palliation, this was successful in 82%. This type of approach yielded a 28.8% savings over traditional surgical management in a Swiss cost-effectiveness study (160).

15. DILATION OF BENIGN COLONIC STRICTURES

Through the endoscope, balloon dilation of colonic or ileal strictures has been successful (161). Benign distal colonic strictures have also been dilated with over-the-wire Savary-Gilliard polyethylene dilators (162). Dilations have been utilized to treat chronic ischemic strictures, non-neoplastic ulcerative colitis strictures, and nonsteroidal induced strictures (163). Postsurgical anastomotic strictures have been treated with over-the-wire dilators, endoscopic incision, hydrostatic balloon dilations, and achalasia dilators (164,165). Colonic and ileal strictures secondary to Crohn's disease have been treated with endoscopic dilation. A series of dilations in 85 consecutive Crohn's disease patients with anastomotic strictures in 63 patients and de novo ileal-cecal or colonic strictures in 22 patients has recently been reported by Brooker et al. (166). Forty percent of dilations in both groups had definite clinical improvement. Multiple dilatations were performed in 36% of patients. Following de novo stricture dilation, two patients sustained a left colonic perforation, and one patient experienced an episode of hemorrhage. In 13 patients treated by Ramboer et al. with de novo Crohn's disease, balloon dilation of enteral strictures was performed in the usual manner after which betamethazone was injected directly into the strictured site (167). This treatment resolved obstructive symptoms post-procedure without complications. Five patients did not require retreatment for 1 yr. No patient required surgery for obstructive disease.

16. MARKING SITES IN THE COLON

16.1. Colonic Tattooing

Prediction of the location of a lesion during colonoscopy is imprecise, unless it is within the rectum, rectosigmoid, ascending colon, or cecum (168). The transverse colon and a long tortuous sigmoid colon in particular provide difficulties to localization. This is important for planned hemicolectomy in the setting of a transverse colonic lesion or segmental resection with a sigmoid lesion. With the advent of laparoscopic surgery, palpation of lesions within the colon is difficult, and a marker that can be seen on the serosa is needed to direct a resection. The site of an endoscopically removed sessile neoplastic polyp will also occasionally need to be relocated, and identifying the site of cicatrization from a polypectomy burn is frequently impossible. A marker injected using colonoscopy must, therefore, be visible at a later date on repeat colonoscopy, as well as be visible on the external surface of the bowel. India ink appears to fill these criteria. Several case series have been compiled demonstrating efficacy of this technique (169,170). This has been performed in most cases using the technique published by Hyman and Waye (171). Though focal granulomas can later be found in resected colonic specimens, symptomatic complications of the procedure have been relegated to case report status (172,173). India ink is not sterile and must either be autoclaved or micropore-filtered. Filtering, however, may extract some of the larger carbon particles that, in turn, may make the tattoo less striking. A commercial-sterilized product of purified carbon particles is also available (SPOT; GI Supply, Camp Hill, PA). In an effort to standardize and validate the India ink technique, Price et al. injected concentrations of sterilized India ink, which varied from 1:10 to 1:10,000, in rabbits that were reexplored at days 1, 3, and 7 after injection (174). Severe ulceration was seen in the undiluted and 1:10 concentration, with little inflammatory response seen with the 1:100 and above dilutions. In a dog colonoscopy model, the 1:100,

1:1000, and 1:10,000 India ink concentrations were then injected, and dogs were reexamined with colonoscopy. Deep injection into the sclerosa was clearly visible on repeat endoscopy with injection volumes of 0.5 mL being adequate. Markings could also easily be seen with the 1:100 concentration at laparoscopy and laparotomy. It is, therefore, suggested that the 1:100 concentration and a deep injection of 0.5 mL be considered an optimal technique. They also cautioned that the needle placement and injection cannot be performed intramucosally, since the mucosa will slough over time, and there will be little tissue staining. This was noted in one of the dogs in this study.

Indocyanine green is another injectable stain. Hammond reported a series of 15 lesions in 12 patients that had 1% indocyanine green injected neighboring the lesions (*175*). There was still a clear marking of the lesions up to 36 h after the injection time. Indocyanine green 1% was also injected into the rabbit colon model in the previously referenced Price study, but could be seen in only one sacrificed animal the day after injection and in none of the animals days 3 or 7 after injection, questioning the utility of this stain (*176*). Unless surgery is planned for later the same day of the injection, methylene blue will diffuse from the colon submucosa without leaving adequate pigment and, therefore, does not function well as a long-term tattoo agent of the colon.

16.2. Clip Marking

If a metallic endoscopic clip remains hooked into the colonic wall, fluoroscopic localization of the clip and the lesion it is marking can be performed at the time of surgery. Unfortunately, clip migration is a problem. In 162 patients that had an endoscopic clip placed by Lehman et al. during a sigmoidoscopy study, to mark for a later radiologic review the proximal extend of a 60-cm examination, it was noted that 6% of the clips had dislodged within 4 h, 50% by 1 wk and 98% at 6 mo (*177*). This technique could, therefore, be misleading or ineffective depending on when a laparotomy is planned.

17. COLONIC DECOMPRESSION

Acute colonic pseudo-obstruction presents with progressive abdominal distension and usually mild abdominal discomfort over several days in the hospitalized patient. Though undoubtedly this entity may begin any day of the week, there appears to be a peak incidence of the endoscopist becoming aware of this problem on Friday afternoons. The diagnosis is confirmed with flat plate of the abdomen demonstrating a dilated colon with or without small bowel distension. A cecal diameter of 12 cm is considered to be a critical value for intervention, although patients may require intervention with lesser diameters or in the case of chronic megacolon may have a cecal diameter >12 cm with little risk of perforation. Many of the patients are postsurgical and have electrolyte abnormalities or use medications that effect gut motility. This topic is reviewed in Chapter 24.

Initial treatment should be conservative with the placement of a nasogastric tube and initiating patient rolling and possibly a rectal tube or small volume enemas. If there is no evidence for perforation, and the patient is symptomatic, or if the patient continues to have distension that has failed to respond to conservative measures, then colonoscopy and colonic decompression is warranted. After colonoscopy, another attempt is made to reverse any found precipitating factors with the knowledge that repeat colonoscopies may be required in up to 60% of patients (*178*). One may attempt to avoid repeat decompression colonoscopies by placement of a decompression colonic tube. Through-the-endoscope decompression tubes are very small and do not appear to aid in maintaining decompression. One has more success avoiding a second endoscopy if a modified 18-Fr Levine tube as per Dr. D. Rex (*179*) or a modified 24-Fr Edlich tube is introduced into the transverse colon over a stiff guidewire that is left in place while withdrawing the colonoscope. Using a similar wire exchange technique, Ell passed a 24-Fr decompression tube that was slid into place over a 12-Fr polyethylene guide catheter *(180)*. This technique successfully maintained colonic decompression in 14 of 16 patients and could be inserted between 4 and 16 min. Endoscopy does have a risk of bowel perforation, particularly if there is prolonged distension-induced ischemia, but the technique appears to be quite effective and avoids a cecostomy in most patients *(181)*.

REFERENCES

1. Overholt BF. Clinical experience with the fibersigmoidoscope. *Gastrointest. Endosc.*, **15** (1968) 27.
2. Wolff IW, Shinya H. Colonofiberoscopy. *JAMA*, **217** (1971) 1509–1512.
3. Williams CB, Tetsuichiro M. Examination of the whole colon with the fibreoptic colonoscope. *BMJ*, **3** (1971) 278–281.
4. Waye JD. Colonoscopy. *Surg. Clin. N. Am.*, **3** (1972) 278–281.
5. Thomas G, Brozinsky S, Isenberg J. Patient acceptance and effectiveness of a balanced lavage solution (Golytely) vs the standard preparation for colonoscopy. *Gastroenterology*, (1982) **82** 435–437.
6. Church JM. Effectiveness of polyethylene glycol antegrade gut lavage bowel preparation for colonoscopy—timing is the key! *Dis. Colon Rectum*, **41** (1998) 1223–1225.
7. Sharma VK, Chockalingham SK, Ugheoke EA, et al. Prospective, randomized, controlled comparison of the use of polyethylene glycol electrolyte lavage solution in four-liter versus two-liter volumes and pretreatment with either magnesium citrate or bisacodyl for colonoscopy preparation. *Gastrointest. Endosc.*, **47** (1998) 167–171.
8. Vanner SJ, MacDonald PH, Paterson WG, et al. A randomized prospective trial comparing oral sodium phosphate with standard polyethylene glycol-based lavage solution (golytely) in the preparation of patients for colonoscopy. *Am. J. Gastroenterol.*, **85** (1990) 422–427.
9. Clarkston WK. Oral sodium phosphate versus sulfate-free polyethylene glycol electrolyte lavage solution in outpatient preparation for colonoscopy: a prospective comparison. *Gastrointest. Endosc.*, (1996) **43** 42–48.
10. Hsu CW. Meta-analysis and cost comparison of polyehtylene glycol lavage versus sodium phosphate for colonoscopy preparation. *Gastrointest. Endosc.*, **48** (1998) 276–282.
11. Ahmed M, Raval P, Buganza G. Oral sodium phosphate catharsis and acute renal failure. *Am. J. Gastroenterol.*, **91** (1996) 1261–1262.
12. Oh JK, Meiselman M, Lataif LE Jr. Ischemic colitis caused by oral hyperosmotic saline laxatives. *Gastrointest. Endosc.*, **45** (1997) 319–322.
13. Zwas FR. Colonic mucosal abnormalities associated with oral sodium phosphate solution. *Gastrointest. Endosc.*, (1996) **43** 524–528.
14. Ayub K, Qureshi W, Brown R, Cole RA, Graham DY. *Gastrointest. Endosc.*, **51** (2000) AB88.
15. Heiman DR, Tolliver BA, Weis FR, O'Brien BL. Patient-controlled anesthesia for colonoscopy using propofol: results of a pilot study. *South Med. J.*, **91** (1998) 560–564.
16. Roseveare C, Seavell C, Patel P, Criswell J, Shepherd H. Patient-controlled sedation with propofol and alfentanil during colonoscopy: a pilot study. *Endoscopy*, **30** (1998) 482–483.
17. Notini-Gudmarsson. Nitrous oxide: a valuable alternative for pain relief and sedation during routine colonoscopy. *Endoscopy*, **28** (1996) 283–287.
18. Forbes GM, Collins BJ. Nitrous oxide for colonoscopy: a randomized controlled study. *Gastrointest. Endosc.*, **51** (2000) 271–277.
19. Kim HK, Cho YJ, Park JY, et al. Factors affecting insertion time and patient discomfort during colonoscopy. *Gastrointest. Endosc.*, **52** (2000) 600–605.
20. Ladas SD. Factors predicting the possibility of conducting colonoscopy without sedation. *Endoscopy*, **32** (2000) 688–692.
21. Hoffman MS, Butler TW, Shaver T. Colonoscopy without sedation. *J. Clin. Gastroenterol.*, **26** (1998) 279–282.
22. Thiis-Evensen E, Hoff GS, Sauar J, Vatn MH. Patient tolerance of colonoscopy without sedation during screening examination for colorectal polyps. *Gastrointest. Endosc.*, **52** (2000) 606–610.
23. American Society for Gastrointestinal Endoscopy. *Gastrointest. Endosc.*, **49** (1999) 845–850.
24. Cass OW. Objective evaluation of endoscopy skills during training. *Ann. Intern. Med.*, **118** (1992) 73–74.
25. Chak A. Prospective assessment of colonoscopic intubation skills in trainees. *Gastrointest. Endosc.*, **44** (1996) 54–57.

26. Cass OW, Freeman ML, Cohen J, et al. Acquisition of competency in endoscopic skills (ACES) during training: a multicenter study. *Gastrointest. Endosc.*, **43** (1996) AB308.

27. Bond JH, Frakes JT. Who should perform colonoscopy? How much training is needed? *Gastrointest. Endosc.*, **49** (1999) 657–659.

28. Williams CB, Saunders BP, Blade JS. Development of colonoscopy teaching simulation. *Endoscopy*, **32** (2000) 901–905.

29. Cirocco WC, Rusin LC. Fluoroscopy. A valuable ally during difficult colonoscopy. *Surg. Endosc.*, **10** (1996) 1080–1084.

30. Shah SG, Saunders BP, Brooker JC, Williams CB. Magnetic imaging of colonoscopy: an audit of looping, accuracy and ancillary maneuvers. *Gastrointest. Endosc.*, **52** (2000) 1–8.

31. Cirocco WC, Rusin LC. Factors that predict incomplete colonoscopy. *Dis. Colon Rectum*, **38** (1995) 964–968.

32. Anderson JC, Gonzalez JD, Messina CR, Pollack BJ. Factors that predict incomplete colonoscopy: thinner is not always better. *Am. J. Gastroenterol.*, **95** (2000) 2784–2787.

33. Odori T, Goto H, Arisawa T, et al. Clinical results and development of variable-stiffness video colonoscopes. *Endoscopy*, **33** (2001) 65–69.

34. Rex DK. Effect of variable-stiffness colonoscopes on cecal intubation times for routine colonoscopy by an experienced examiner in sedated patients. *Endoscopy*, **33** (2001) 60–64.

35. Saifuddin T, Trivedi M, King PD, Madsen R, Marshall JB. Usefulness of a pediatric colonoscope for colonoscopy in adults. *Gastrointest. Endosc.*, **51** (2000) 314–317.

36. Howell DA, Phyllidia MK, Desilets DJ, Campana JM. A comparative trial of variable stiffness colonoscopes. *Gastrointest. Endosc.*, **51** (2000) AB58.

37. Lichtenstein GR, Park PD, Long WB, Ginsberg GG, Kochman ML. Use of a push enteroscope improves ability to perform total colonoscopy in previously unsuccessful attempts at colonoscopy in adult patients. *Am. J. Gastroenterol.*, **94** (1999) 187–90.

38. Waye JD, Kahn O, Auerbach ME. Complications of colonoscopy and flexible sigmoidoscopy. *Gastrointest. Clin. N. Am.*, **6** (1996) 343–377.

39. Eller AA, Schiffman FJ. Splenic rupture: an unusual complication of colonoscopy. *Am. J. Gastroenterol.*, **92** (1997) 1201–1204.

40. Saunders MP. Colonoscope incarceration within an inguinal hernia: a cautionary tale. *Br. J. Clin. Pract.*, **49** (1995) 157–158.

41. Holm C, Christensen M, Rasmussen V, Schulze S. Hypoxaemia and myocardial ischaemia during colonoscopy. *Scand. J. Gastroenterol.*, **33** (1998) 769–772.

42. Walsh RM, Ackroyd FW, Shellito PC. Endoscopic resection of large sessile colorectal polyps. *Gastrointest. Endosc.*, **38** (1992) 303–309.

43. Van Gossum A, Cozzoli A, Adler M, et al. Colonoscopic snare polypectomy: analysis of 1485 resections comparing two types of current. *Gastrointest. Endosc.*, **38** (1992) 472–475.

44. Dyer WS, Quigley EMM, Noel SM, et al. Major colonic hemorrhage following electrocoagulating (hot) biopsy of diminutive colonic polyps: relationship to colonic location and low-dose aspirin therapy. *Gastrointest. Endosc.*, **37** (1991) 361–363.

45. Waye JD, Lewis BS, Yessayan S: Colonoscopy: a prospective report of complications. *J. Clin. Gastroenterol.*, **15** (1992) 347–351.

46. Grondin MV, Seibert DG. Treatment of delayed post-polypectomy bleeding using bipolar electrocoagulation. *Gastrointest. Endosc.*, **35** (1989) AB175.

47. Rex DK, Lewis BS, Waye JD. Colonoscopy and endoscopic therapy for delayed postpolypectomy hemorrhage. *Gastrointest. Endosc.*, **38** (1992) 127–129.

48. Rozon P, Somjen GJ, Baratz M, et al. Endoscope-induced colits: description, probable cause by glutaraldehyde, and prevention. *Gastrointest. Endosc.*, **40** (1994) 547–553.

49. Schwartz E, Dabezies MA, Krevsky B. Hydrogen peroxide injury to the colon. *Dig. Dis. Sci.*, **40** (1995) 1290–1291.

50. Bronowick JP, Venard V, Botte C, Monhoven N, et al. Patient-to-patient transmission of hepatitis C virus during colonoscopy. *N. Engl. J. Med.*, **337** (1997) 237–240.

51. Winawer SJ. Prevention of colorectal cancer by colonoscopic polypectomy. The National Polyp Study Workgroup. *N. Engl. J. Med.*, **329** (1993) 2028–2029.

52. Newcomb PA, Norfleet RG, Storer BE, et al. Screening sigmoidoscopy and colorectal cancer mortality. *J. Natl. Cancer Inst.*, **84** (1992) 1572–1575.

53. Lieberman DA, Weiss DG, Bond JH, et al. Use of colonoscopy to screen asymptomatic adults for colorectal cancer. *N. Engl. J. Med.*, (2000) **343** 162–168.

54. Imperiale TF, Wagner DR, Lin CY, et al. Risk of advanced proximal neoplasms in asymptomatic adults according to the distal colorectal findings. *N. Engl. J. Med.*, **343** (2000) 169–174.

55. Lieberman, DA. Cost-effectiveness model for colon cancer screening. *Gastroenterology*, **109** (1995) 1781–1790.

56. Rex DK, Rahmani EY, Haseman JH, et al. Relative sensitivity of colonoscopy and barium enema for detection of colorectal cancer in clinical practice. *Gastroenterology*, **112** (1997) 17–23.

57. Winawer SJ, Stewart ET, Zauber AG, et al. A comparison of colonoscopy and double-contrast barium enema for surveillance after polypectomy. *N. Engl. J. Med.*, **342** (2000) 1766–1772.

58. Rex DK, Cutler CS, Lemmel GT, et al. Colonoscopic miss rates of adenomas determined by back-to-back colonoscopies. *Gastroenterology*, **112** (1997) 24–28.

59. Glick SN, Teplick SK, Balfe DM, et al. Large colonic neoplasms missed by endoscopy. *Am. J. Radiol.*, **152** (1989) 513–517.

60. Hofstad B, Vatn MH, Anderson SN, et al. Growth of colorectal polyps: redetection and evaluation of unresected polyps for a period of three years. *Gut*, **39** (1996) 449–456.

61. Rembacken BJ, Fujii T, Cairns A, et al. Flat and depressed colonic neoplasms: a prospective study of 1000 colonoscopies in the UK. *Lancet*, **355** (2000) 1211–1214.

62. Matsushita M, Hajiro K, Okazaki K, et al. Efficacy of total colonoscopy with a transparent cap in comparison with colonoscopy without the cap. *Endoscopy*, **30** (1998) 444–447.

63. Norfleet RG, Ryan ME, Wyman JB. Adenomatous and hyperplastic polyps cannot be reliably distinguished by their appearance through the fiberoptic sigmoidoscopy. *Dig. Dis. Sci.*, **33** (1988) 1175–1177.

64. Norfleet RG, Ryan ME, Wyman JB. Adenomatous and hyperplastic polyps cannot be reliably distinguished by their appearance through the fiberoptic sigmoidoscopy. *Dig. Dis. Sci.*, **33** (1988) 1175–1177.

65. Canto MI. Staining in gastrointestinal endoscopy: the basics. *Endoscopy*, **31** (1999) 479–486.

66. Shim CS. Staining in gastrointestinal endoscopy: clinical application and limitations. *Endoscopy*, **31** (1999) 487–496.

67. Iishi H, Tatsuta M, Okuda S, Ishiguro S. Diagnosis of colorectal tumors by the endoscopic Congo red-methylene blue test. *Surg. Endosc.*, **8** (1994) 1308–1311.

68. Axelrad AM, Fleischer DE, Geller AJ, et al. High-resolution chromoendoscopy for the diagnosis of diminutive polyps: implications for colon cancer screening. *Gastroenterology*, **110** (1996) 1253–1258.

69. Jaramillo E, Watanabe M, Slezak P, Rubio C. Flat neoplastic lesions of the colon and rectum detected by high-resolution video endoscopy and chromoscopy. *Gastrointest. Endosc.*, **42** (1995) 114–122.

70. Mitooka H, Fujimori T, Maeda S, Nagasako K. Minute flat depressed neoplastic lesions of the colon detected by contrast chromoscopy using an indigo carmine capsule. *Gastrointest. Endosc.*, **41** (1995) 453–459.

71. Saitoh Y, Obara T, Ayabe T, et al. Invasion depth diagnosis of depressed type early colorectal cancers by combined use of videoendoscopy and chromoendoscopy. *Gastrointest. Endosc.*, **48** (1998) 362–370.

72. Kudo S, Tamura S, Nakajima T, et al. Diagnosis of colorectal tumorous lesions by magnifying endoscopy. *Gastrointest. Endosc.*, **44** (1996) 8–14.

73. Wolber RA, Owen DA. Flat adenomas of the colon. *Hum. Pathol.*, **22** (1991) 70–74.

74. Muto T, Kamaiya J, Zawada T, et al. Small "flat adenoma" of the large bowel with special reference to its clinicopathologic features. *Dis. Colon Rectum*, **28** (1985) 847–851.

75. Lanspa SJ, Rouse J, Smyrk T, et al. Epidemiologic characteristics of the flat adenoma of Muto. *Dis. Colon Rectum*, **35** (1992) 543–546.

76. Lane N, Lev R. Observation on the origin of adenomatous epithelium of the colon: serial section studies of minute polyps in familial polyposis. *Cancer*, **16** (1963) 751–764.

77. Pretlow TP, Barrow BJ, Ashton WS, et al. Aberrant crypts: putative preneoplastic foci in human colonic mucosa. *Cancer Res.*, **51** (1991) 1564–1567.

78. Sandforth F, Heimpel S, Balzer T, et al. Characterization of stereomicroscopically identified preneoplastic lesions during dimethylhydrazine-induced colonic carcinogenesis. *Eur. J. Clin. Invest.*, **18** (1988) 655–662.

79. Yokota T, Sugano K, Kondo H, et al. Detection of aberrant crypt foci by magnifying colonoscopy. *Gastrointest. Endosc.*, **46** (1997) 61–65.

80. Hayashi S, Ajioka Y, Suzuki Y, et al. A novel approach to detecting colorectal cancers: direct identification of histology by magnifying endoscopy. *Gastroint. Endosc.*, **51** (2000) AB148.

81. Sackmann M. Fluorescence diagnosis in GI endoscopy. *Endoscopy*, **32** (2000) 977–985.

82. Izuishi K, Tajiri H, Fujii T, et al. The histological basis of detection of adenoma and cancer in the colon by autofluorescence endoscopic imaging. *Endoscopy*, **31** (1999) 511–516.

83. Wang TD, Van Dam J, Crawford JM, et al. Fluorescence endoscopic imaging of human colonic adenomas. *Gastroenterology*, **111** (1996) 1182–1191.

84. Cothren RM, Sivak MV Jr, Van Dam J et al. Detection of dysplasia at colonoscopy using laser-induced fluorescence: a blinded study. *Gastrointest. Endosc.*, **44** (1996) 168–176.

85. Mycek MA, Schomacker KT, Nishioka NS. Colonic polyp differentiation using time-resolved autofluorescence spectroscopy. *Gastrointest. Endosc.*, **48** (1998) 390–394.

86. Wang TD, Van Dam J, Crawford JM, et al. Fluorescence endoscopic imaging of human colonic adenomas. *Gastroenterology*, **111** (1996) 1182–1191.

87. Cothren RM, Sivak MV Jr, Van Dam J, et al. Detection of dysplasia at colonoscopy using laser-induced fluorescence: a blinded study. *Gastrointest. Endosc.*, **44** (1996) 168–176.

88. Sackmann M. Fluorescence diagnosis in GI endoscopy. *Endoscopy*, **32** (2000) 977–985.

89. Jackle S, Gladkova N, Feldchtein F, et al. In vivo endoscopic optical coherence tomography of the human gastrointestinal tract—toward optical biopsy. *Endoscopy*, **32** (2000) 743–749.

90. Ho SB. The use of mucosal biopsy markers to predict colon cancer risk. *Clin. Gastrointest. Endosc. N. Am.*, **3** (1993) 623–638.

91. Papatheodoridis GV, Kapranos N, Tzouvala M, et al. p53 and bcl-2 protein expression in rectosigmoid adenomas. *Am. J. Gastroenterol.*, **93** (1998) 1136–1140.

92. Marshall JK, Hewak J, Farrow R, et al. Terminal ileal imaging with ileoscopy versus small-bowel meal with pneumocolon. *J. Clin. Gastroenterol.*, **27** (1998) 217–222.

93. Jakobs R, Benz C, Maier M, et al. Transvavular enteroscopy using a mother-baby endoscope system: a new approach to the distal ileum. *Gastrointest. Endosc.*, **45** (1997) 298–300.

94. Maunoury V, Mordon S, Geboes K, et al. Early vascular changes in Crohn's disease: an endoscopic fluorescence study. *Endoscopy*, **32** (2000) 700–705.

95. Matsumoto T, Kuroki F, Mizuno M, et al. Application of magnifying chromoscopy for the assessment of severity in patients with mild to moderate ulcerative colitis. *Gastrointest. Endosc.*, **46** (1997) 400–405.

96. Tsujii M, Kawano S, Tsuji S, et al. Colonic mucosal hemodynamics and tissue oxygenation in patients with ulcerative colitis: investigation of organ reflectance spectrophotometry. *J. Gastroenterol.*, **30** (1995) 183–188.

97. Koch TR, Yuan LX, Stryker SJ, et al. Total antioxidanct capacity of colon in patients with chronic ulcerative colitis. *Dig. Dis. Sci.*, **45** (2000) 1814–1819.

98. Iwashita E. Greatly increased mucosal nitric oxide in ulcerative colitis determined in situ by a novel nitric oxide-sensitive microelectrode. *J. Gastroenterol. Hepatol.*, **13** (1998) 391–395.

99. Lundberg JO, Hellstrom PM, Alving K. Greatly increased luminal nitric oxide in ulcerative colitis. *Lancet*, **344** (1994) 1673–1674.

100. Bortoluzzi F, Valentini M, Cernigoi C, et al. DNA flow cytometric evaluation of cell cycle distribution in ulcerative colitis: a proposed method for assessing severity of disease. *Gut*, **36** (1995) 50–54.

101. Rubin CE, Haggitt RC, Burmer GC, et al. DNA aneuploidy in colonic biopsies predicts future development of dysplasia in ulcerative colitis. *Gastroenterology*, **103** (1992) 1611–1620.

102. Lewis JD, Deren JJ, Lichtenstein GR. Cancer risk in patients with inflammatory bowel diseae. *Gastroenterol. Clin. N. Am.*, **28** (1999) 459–477.

103. Jaramillo E, Watanabe M, Befrits R, et al. Small flat colorectal neoplasias in long-standing ulcerative colitis detectected by high-resolution electronic video endoscopy. *Gastrointest. Endosc.*, **44** (1996) 15–22.

104. Schneider A. Differential diagnosis of adenomas and dysplastic lesions in patients with ulcerative colitis. *Z. Gastroenterol.*, **31** (1993) 653–656.

105. Medlicott SA, Jewell LD, Price L, et al. Conservative management of small adenomata in ulcerative colitis. *Am. J. Gastroenterol.*, **92** (1997) 2094–2098.

106. Ott SJ, Ochsenkuehn T, Stepp H, et al. Detection of colonic dysplasia by laser-induced fluorescence endoscopy with and without 5-aminolevulinic acid. *Gastrointest. Endosc.*, **51** (2000) AB95.

107. Itzkowitz SH, Young E, Dubois D, et al. Sialosyl-Tn antigen is prevalent and precedes dysplasia in ulcerative colitis: a retrospective case-control study. *Gastroenterology*, **110** (1996) 694–704.

108. Chaudhry V, Hyser MJ, Gracias VH, Gau FC. Colonoscopy: the initial test for acute lower gastrointestinal bleeding. *Am. Surg.*, **64** (1998) 723–728.

109. Jensen DM, Machicado GA. Colonoscopy for diagnosis and treatment of severe lower gastrointestinal bleeding. *Gastrointest. Endosc. Clin. N. Am.*, **7** (1997) 477–498.

110. Santos JCM, Aprilli F, Guimaraes AS, Rocha JJR. Angiodysplasia of the colon: endoscopic diagnosis and treatment. *Br. J. Surg.*, **75** (1988) 256–258.

111. Deal SE, Zfass AM, Duckworth PF, McHenry L. Arteriovenous malformations (AVMs): are they concealed by meperidine? *Am. J. Gastroenterol.*, **86** (1991) AB1352.

112. Brandt LJ, Mukhopadhyay D. Masking of colon vascular ectasias by cold water lavage [letter]. *Gastrointest. Endosc.*, **49** (1999) 141–142.

113. Krevsky B. Detection and treatment of angiodysplasia. *Gastrointest. Endosc. Clin. N. Am.*, **7** (1997) 509–524.

114. Jensen DM, Machicado GA. Colonoscopy for diagnosis and treatment of severe lower gastrointestinal bleeding. *Gastrointest. Endosc. Clin. N. Am.*, **7** (1997) 477–498.

115. Foutch PG. Diverticular bleeding: are nonsteroidal anti-inflammatory drugs risk factors for hemorrhage and can colonoscopy predict outcome for patients? *Am. J. Gastroenterol.*, **90** (1995) 1779–1784.

116. Foutch PG, Zimmerman K. Diverticular bleeding and the pigmented protuberance (sentinel clot): clinical implications, histopathological correlation, and results of endoscopic intervention. *Am. J. Gastroenterol.*, **91** (1996) 2589–2593.

117. Zuckerman GR, Prakash C. Acute lower intestinal bleeding PartII: etiology, therapy, and outcomes. *Gastrointest. Endosc.*, **49** (1999) 228–238.

118. Longstreth GF. Epidemiology and outcome of patients hospitalized with acute lower gastrointestinal hemorrhage: a population-based study. *Am. J. Gastroenterol.*, **92** (1997) 419–424.

119. Jensen DM, Machicado GA, Cheng S, et al. A randomized prospective study of endoscopic bipolar electrocoagulation and heater probe treatment of chronic rectal bleeding form radiation telangiectasia. *Gastrointest. Endosc.*, **45** (1997) 20–25.

120. Fantin AC, Binek J, Suter WR, Meyenberger C. Argon beam coagulation for treatment of symptomatic radiation-induced proctitis. *Gastrointest. Endosc.*, **49** (1999) 515–518.

121. Tam W, Moore J, Schoeman M. Treatment of radiation proctitis with argon plasma coagulation. *Endoscopy*, **32** (2000) 667–672.

122. Taylor JG, DiSario JA, Buchi KN. Argon laser therapy for hemorrhagic radiation proctitis: long-term results. *Gastrointest. Endosc.*, (1993) **39** 641–644.

123. Ahlquist DA, Gostout CJ, Viggiano TR, Pemberton JH. Laser therapy for severe radiation-induced rectal bleeding. *Mayo Clin. Proc.*, (1986) **61** 927–931.

124. Barbatzas C, Spencer GM, Thorpe SM, et al. Nd:YAG laser treatment for bleeding from radiation proctitis. *Endoscopy*, (1997) **28** 497–500.

125. Taylor JG, Disario JA, Bjorkman DJ. KTP laser therapy for bleeding from chronic radiation proctopathy. *Gastrointest. Endosc.*, **52** (2000) 353–357.

126. Rathgaber SW, Rex DK. Colonoscopy and endoscopic therapy of hemorrhage from viral colitis [letter]. *Gastrointest. Endosc.*, **39** (1993) 188–190.

127. Sone Y, Nakano S, Takeda S, et al. Massive hemorrhage from a dieulafoy lesion in the cecum: successful endoscopic management. *Gastrointest. Endosc.*, **51** (2000) 510–512.

128. Knigge KL, Katon RM. Massive hematochezia from a visible vessel within a stercoral ulcer: effective endoscopic therapy. *Gastrointest. Endosc.*, **46** (1997) 369–370.

129. Heaton ND, Davenport M, Howard ER. Symptomatic hemorrhoids and anorectal varices in children with portal hypertension. *J. Pediatr. Surg.*, **27** (1992) 833–835.

130. Cirocco WC, Golub RW. Endoscopic treatment of postoperative hemorrhage from a stapled colorectal anastomosis. *Am. Surg.*, **61** (1995) 460–463.

131. Segal WN, Greenberg PD, Rockey DC, et al. The outpatient evaluation of hematohezia. *Am. J. Gastroenterol.*, **93** (1998) 179–182.

132. Van Rosendaal GM, Sutherland LR, Verhoef MJ, et al. Defining the role of fiberoptic sigmoidoscopy in the investigation of patients presenting with bright red rectal bleeding. *Am. J. Gastroenterol.*, **95** (2000) 1184–1187.

133. Waye JD. New methods of polypectomy. *Gastrointest. Endosc. Clin. N. Am.*, **7** (1997) 413–422.

134. Williams CB. Small polyps: the virtues and dangers of hot biopsy [editorial]. *Gastrointest. Endosc.*, **37** (1991) 394–395.

135. Tappero G, Gaia E, Giuli P, et al. Cold snare excision of small colorectal polyps. *Gastrointest. Endosc.*, **38** (1992) 310–313.

136. McAfee JH, Katon R. Tiny snares prove safe and effective for removal of diminutive colon polyps. *Gastrointest. Endosc.*, **40** (1994) 301–303.

137. Woods A, Sanowski RA, Wadas DD, et al. Eradication of diminutive polyps: a prospective evaluation of bipolar coagulation versus conventional biopsy removal. *Gastrointest. Endosc.*, **35** (1989) 536–539.

138. Uno Y, Obara K, Zheng P, et al. Cold snare excision is a safe method for diminutive colorectal polyps. *Tohoku J. Exp. Med.*, **183** (1997) 243–249.

139. Parra-Blanco A, Kaminaga N, Kojima T, et al. Colonoscopic polypectomy with cutting current: Is it safe? *Gastrointest. Endosc.*, **51** (2000) 676–681.

140. Rey JF, Marek TA. Endo-loop in the prevention of the post-polypectomy bleeding: preliminary results. *Gastrointest. Endosc.*, (1997) **46** 387–389.

141. Matsushita M, Hajiro K, Takakuwa H, et al. Ineffective use of a detachable snare for colonoscopic polypectomy of large polyps. *Gastrointest. Endosc.*, **47** (1998) 496–499.

142. Uno Y, Munakata A, Tanaka M. The non-lifting sign of invasive colon cancer. *Gastrointest. Endosc.*, **40** (1994) 485–489.

143. Inoue H, Takeshita KI, Hori H, et al. Endoscopic mucosal resection with a cap-fitted panendoscope for esophagus, stomach and colon mucosal lesions. *Gastrointest. Endosc.*, **39** (1993) 58–62.
144. Tada M, Inoue H, Yabata E, et al. Colonic mucosal resection using a transparent cap-fitted endoscope. *Gastrointest. Endosc.*, **44** (1996) 63–65.
145. Anonymous. Technology status report evaluation. Endoscopic mucosal resection. *Gastrointest. Endosc.* **52** (2000) 860–863.
146. Iishi H, Tatsuta M, Kitamura S, et al. Endoscopic resection of large sessile colorectal polyps using a submucosal saline injection technique. *Hepatogastroenterology*, **44** (1997) 698–702.
147. Norton ID, Wang LN, Levine SA, et al. Efficacy of submucosal saline injection in the limitation of colonic thermal injury by electrosurgical devices. *Gastrointest. Endosc.*, **51** (2000) AB131.
148. Zlatanic J, Waye JD, Kim PS, et al. Large sessile colonic adenomas: use of argon plasma coagulator to supplement piecemeal snare polypectomy. *Gastrointest. Endosc.*, **49** (1999) 731–735.
149. Brooker JC, Shah SG, Williams CB, et al. Argon plasma coagulation assisted resection of large sessile colonic polyps: a randomized trial. *Gastrointest. Endosc.*, **51** (2000) AB109.
150. Malthus-Vliegen EM, Tytgat GN. The potential and limitations of laser photoablation of colorectal adenomas. *Gastrointest. Endosc.*, **37** (1991) 9–17.
151. Brunetaud JM, Maunoury V, Cochelard D, et al. Endoscopic laser treatment for rectosigmoid villous adenoma: factors affecting the results. *Gastroenterology*, **97** (1989) 272–277.
152. Cranley JP. Proper management of the patient with a malignant colorectal polyp. *Gastrointest. Endosc. Clin. N. Am.*, **3** (1993) 661–671.
153. Brunetaud JM, Maunoury V, Ducrotte P. Palliative treatment of rectosigmoid carcinoma by laser endoscopic photoablation. *Gastroenterology*, **92** (1987) 663–668.
154. Escourrou J, Delvaux M, deBellison F, et al. Laser for curative treatment of rectal cancer. Indications and follow-up. *Gastrointest. Endosc.*, **34** (1988) AB195.
155. Van Cutsem E, Boonen A, Geboes K, et al. Risk factors which determine the long term outcome of neodymium-YAG laser palliation of colorectal carcinoma. *Int. J. Colorect. Dis.*, **4** (1989) 9–11.
156. Eckhauser ML, Imbembo AL, Mansour EG. The role of pre-resectional laser recanalization for obstructing carcinomas of the colon and rectum. *Surgery*, **106** (1989) 710–76l.
157. Rattan J, Klausner JM, Rozenp, et al. Acute left colonic obstruction: a new nonsurgical treatment. *J. Clin. Gastroenterol.*, **11** (1989) 331–334.
158. Stone JM, Bloom RJ. Transendoscopic balloon dilatation of complete colonic obstruction. An adjunct in the treatment of colorectal cancer: report of three cases. *Dis. Colon Rectum*, **32** (1989) 429–431.
159. Baron TH, Dean PA, Yates MR 3rd, et al. Expandable metal stents for the treatment of colonic obstruction: techniques and outcomes. *Gastrointest. Endosc.*, **47** (1998) 277–286.
160. Binkert CA, Ledermann H, Jost R, et al. Acute colonic obstruction: clinical aspects and cost-effectiveness of pre-operative and palliative treatment with self-expanding metallic stents: a preliminary report. *Radiology*, **206** (1998) 199–204.
161. Johansson C. Endoscopic dilation of rectal strictures: a prospective study of 18 cases. *Dis. Colon Rectum*, **39** (1996) 423–428.
162. Triadafilopoulous G, Sarkisian M. Dilation of radiation-induced sigmoid stricture using sequential Savary-Gilliard dilators. *Dis. Colon Rectum*, **33** (1990) 1065–1067.
163. Gopal DV, Katon RM. Endoscopic balloon dilation of multiple NSAID-induced colonic strictures: case report and review of literature on NSAID-related colopathy. *Gastrointest. Endosc.*, **50** (1999) 120–123.
164. Hagiwava A, Togawa T, Yamasaki J, et al. Endoscopic incision and balloon dilatation for cicatrical anastomotic strictures. *Hepatogastroenterology*, **46** (1999) 997–999.
165. Virgilio C, Cosentino S, Favara C, et al. Endoscopic treatment of postoperative colonic strictures using an achalasia dilator. *Endoscopy*, **27** (1995) 219–222.
166. Brooker JC, Thomas-Gibson S, Shah SG, et al. Endoscopic dilatation of Crohn's strictures: longterm outcomes in 85 patients. *Gastrointest. Endosc.*, **51** (2000) AB98.
167. Ramboer C, Verhamme, Dhondt E, et al. Endoscopic treatment of stenosis in recurrent Crohn's disease with balloon dilation combined with local corticosteroid injection. *Gastrointest. Endosc.*, **42** (1995) 252–255.
168. Lam DT, Kwong KH, Lam CW, et al. How useful is colonscopy in locating colorectal lesions? *Surg. Endosc.*, **12** (1998) 839–841.
169. Fennerty MB, Sampliner RE, Hixson LJ, Garewal HS. Effectiveness of India ink as long-term colonic mucosal marker. *Am. J. Gastroenterol.*, **87** (1992) 79–81.
170. Botoman VA, Pietro M, Thirlby RC. Localization of colonic lesions with endoscopic tattoo. *Dis. Colon Rectum*, **37** (1994) 775–776.

171. Hyman N, Waye JD. Endoscopic four quadrant tattoo for the identification of colonic lesions at surgery. *Gastrointest. Endosc.*, **37** (1991) 56–58.

172. Park SI, Genta RS, Romeo DP, Weesner RE. Colonic abscess and focal peritonitis secondary to India ink tattooing of the colon. *Gastrointest. Endosc.*, **37** (1991) 68–71.

173. Dell'Abate P, Iosca A, Galimberti A, et al. Endoscopic preoperative colonic tattooing: a clinical and surgical complication. *Endoscopy*, **31** (1999) 271–273.

174. Price N, Gottfried MR, Clary E, et al. Safety and efficacy of India ink and indocyanine green as colonic tattooing agents. *Gastrointest. Endosc.*, **51** (2000) 438–442.

175. Hammond DC, Lane FR, Mackeigan JM, et al. Endoscopic tattooing of the colon: clinical experience. *Am. Surg.*, **59** (1993) 205–210.

176. Price N, Gottfried MR, Clary E, et al. Safety and efficacy of India ink and indocyanine green as colonic tattooing agents. *Gastrointest. Endosc.*, **51** (2000) 438–442.

177. Lehman GA, Maveety PR, O'Connor KW. Mucosal clipping—utility and safety testing in the colon. *Gastrointest. Endosc.*, **31** (1985) 273–276.

178. Rex DK. Colonoscopy and acute colonic pseudo-obstruction. *Gastrointest. Endosc. Clin. N. Am.*, **7** (1997) 499–508.

179. Rex DK. Colonoscopy and acute colonic pseudo-obstruction. *Gastrointest. Endosc. Clin. N. Am.*, **7** (1997) 499–508.

180. Ell C. Colon decompression using an anatomically adapted, large-caliber decompression probe. *Endoscopy*, **28** (1996) 456–458.

181. Geller A, Petersen BT, Gostout CJ. Endoscopic decompression for acute colonic pseudo-obstruction. *Gastrointest. Endosc.*, **44** (1996) 144–150.

17   Interpretation of Colonic Biopsies in Patients with Diarrhea

Sarah M. Dry, Galen R. Cortina, and Klaus J. Lewin

Contents

1. INTRODUCTION

1.1. Communication Between the Endoscopist and Pathologist

Accurate biopsy interpretation rests heavily on excellent communication between the endoscopist and the pathologist. We cannot overemphasize the importance of communication. Without proper clinical information, the pathologist may render an unhelpful or, worse yet, misleading diagnosis. Some pathologists prefer to arrive at an independent histopathologic diagnosis without first looking at the history or clinical question to avoid interpretation bias. However, the only approach for consistent, precise diagnoses in colonic biopsy pathology is the one that ultimately combines all pertinent information available from clinical, radiological, and laboratory sources, with the histopathogy to arrive at the final interpretation. A strikingly realistic study pitting histopathologic interpretation alone against a composite approach (clinical, radiologic, endoscopy, histopathology) in the diagnosis of colitis confirmed that the composite approach led to greater agreement and definitiveness (1). A schematic representation of the composite approach to diagnosis is given in Fig. 1.

Communication is especially critical in interpreting endoscopic biopsies, since clinically disparate diarrheal etiologies often show similar histopathologic features. For instance, pseudomembranes may be seen in ischemic colitis, acute self-limited (infectious) colitis, and

From: *Colonic Diseases*
Edited by: T. R. Koch © Humana Press Inc., Totowa, NJ

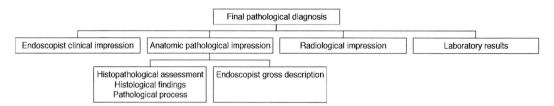

Fig. 1. Schematic for the interpretation of colonic biopsies. The composite approach to diagnosis is predicated on the pathological impression and the supplemental information. The anatomic pathological impression begins with the endoscopist's gross description and selection of biopsies, plus the histopathological findings and consideration of the pathological process (e.g., inflammation). The supplemental information includes the clinical impression, radiological impression, and the laboratory results. The order in which these are brought together is up to the individual pathologist, but to make a final pathological diagnosis, all of these should be integrated. The final clinical diagnosis lies with the gastroenterologist. In this scheme, the pathological information is in green and the clinical information is in blue (see color figure in insert following page 238).

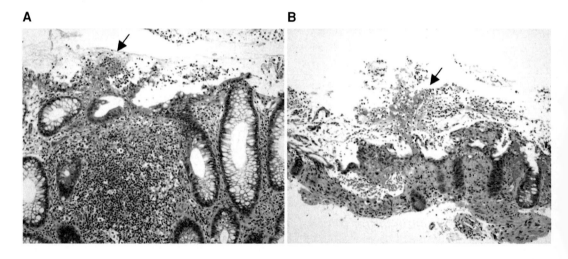

Fig. 2. Fibrinopurulent exudates (pseudomembranes), indicated by arrows, in *C. difficile* (A) and ischemic colitis (B). Other histologic features, including epithelial separation from the basement membrane (blebbing) without significant neutrophilic cryptitis, is very suggestive of ischemia, as is the etiology in the right panel, however, such features are not invariably present, especially in early lesions.

antibiotic-associated (*Clostridium difficile*) colitis (Fig. 2). Also, several factors, including prior or current drug therapy and duration of symptoms, can result in "atypical" findings and potentially lead to an incorrect diagnosis. This is described in more detail in Subheading 5.

While we pathologists (and many of our clinical colleagues as well) like to assume that "the tissue is the issue" and that clinical information is superfluous, this attitude is incorrect and dangerous, especially in the arena of gastrointestinal (GI) mucosal biopsies. Several excellent recent articles have addressed this topic *(2,3)*.

Critical information for the pathologist is listed in Table 1. Bloody diarrhea is characteristic of inflammatory bowel disease (IBD), infectious colitis, ischemic colitis, and some cases of drug-induced colitis, while nonbloody diarrhea is seen in microscopic–collagenous colitis (CC) and infectious colitis. Patients with IBD symptomatic for weeks to months will more

Table 1
Endoscopist–Pathologist Communication: Important Clinical Information

1. Nature of diarrhea (bloody vs nonbloody).
2. Duration of symptoms (d vs wk vs mo).
3. Current treatment (steroids, antibiotics, NSAIDs).
4. Other pertinent clinical history (i.e., upper GI disease, recent travel).
5. Location of biopsy (cecum, right colon vs left colon, sigmoid, etc.).
6. Endoscopic findings (i.e., diverticula, anastomotic line) and appearance (normal, erythematous, friable, etc.) at the biopsied site.
7. Pertinent radiographic data (e.g., strictures, thickening of bowel wall, mass lesions).
8. Pertinent laboratory data (e.g., stool cultures).
9. Clinical question: be specific (i.e., not "diarrhea" but "rule out microscopic colitis").

likely show changes of chronic injury (i.e., architectural distortion) than patients with only days to weeks of symptoms. Thus, the absence of features of chronic injury does not definitely rule out IBD *(3)*. Similarly, current or recent use of certain prescription drugs may create atypical findings in mucosal biopsies, including features identical to lymphocytic colitis *(4–6)*. Following treatment, patients with ulcerative colitis (UC) may show "skip" lesions (inflamed alternating with uninflamed mucosa) *(7)*, rectal sparing *(8)* or even normal mucosa *(7)*, and such findings could be misinterpreted as supportive of Crohn's disease (CD). Non-steroidal anti-inflammatory drugs (NSAIDs) can lead to a wide variety of lesions throughout the GI tract (see Table 15).

Both oral contraceptives *(9)* and cocaine use *(10)* have been associated with ischemic colitis in young healthy adults. Finally, other clinical history, such as upper GI manifestations of CD or a history of recent travel, can greatly help the pathologist in making a diagnosis of "most consistent with" CD (vs UC) or infectious colitis, respectively.

Endoscopic information, including anatomic site biopsied and findings and/or appearance at that site are equally important. The anatomic location of the biopsy is critical in evaluating the degree of lamina propria inflammation. The cecum and right colon normally have a denser lamina propria lymphoplasmacytic infiltrate, which should not be over interpreted by the pathologist as "mild chronic colitis". Second, mucosa adjacent to diverticula frequently shows atypical histology, including mild neutrophilic cryptitis or features of chronic mucosal injury *(11)*. Without the appropriate clinical history, such a finding could be interpreted as infectious colitis or IBD. Perianastomotic site biopsies may show features of acute colitis or of chronic ischemic injury. Third, the endoscopic appearance at each site, and at times of the colon generally, can help the pathologist make a diagnosis of lymphocytic–microscopic–collagenous colitis and may help distinguish among UC and CD (discussed in Subheadings 5 and 6).

Finally, a specific directed question from the endoscopist to the pathologist is critical. The more informed we are about your patient, the more likely we are to be able to render a definitive, accurate diagnosis, or at least a relevant differential diagnosis. Brief questions, such as "bloody diarrhea × weeks, stool cultures negative ?IBD" or "watery diarrhea × months, normal endoscopy, ?microscopic–collagenous colitis" are excellent. Do not ask broad, unfocused questions in an effort to cover all possible diagnoses. For instance, in a patient with long-standing UC undergoing routine surveillance biopsies for dysplasia, the question should be "long-standing UC, rule out dysplasia" not "long-standing IBD, rule out CD, rule out dysplasia". The second question, especially in a patient currently on drug therapy, may result in a diagnosis of "cannot rule out CD" due to the presence of drug-induced skip lesions or rectal sparing.

Table 2
One Approach to a Systematic Evaluation of Mucosal Biopsies

1. Low power impression:
   a. Does the surface epithelium appear intact, reactive (mucin depletion, inflammatory cell infiltrates), eroded, or ulcerated?
   b. Are the crypts generally perpendicular to the surface epithelium, and do they reach straight down to the muscularis mucosa, or do they show irregular outlines, branching, or failure to reach the muscularis mucosa?
   c. Does crypt epithelium appear intact, reactive (mucin depletion, inflammatory cell infiltrates, crypt abscesses) or focally and/or completely missing?
   d. Does the lamina propria appear to contain normal or increased numbers of inflammatory cells?
   e. Does the lamina propria appear to be edematous, congested, or fibrotic, or do the lymphatics appear unusually dilated?
   f. Is submucosa present? If so, do the vessels appear normal in caliber? Is there increased fibrosis or significant inflammation (other than lymphoid aggregates)?
   g. Is there evidence for a mass lesion (carcinoma, lymphoma, carcinoid, or submucosal neoplasm, including a stromal tumor)?
2. Intermediate power impression:
   a. Are there increased numbers of inflammatory cells within the surface epithelium?
   b. Is there evidence of reactive surface or crypt epithelial changes not appreciated on low power?
   c. Is the subepithelial collagen band (SCB) normal in appearance and thickness?
   d. If excess inflammatory cells are present in the epithelium or lamina propria, are they composed of neutrophils, eosinophils, lymphocytes, plasma cells, or granulomas?
   e. Are focal lesions (i.e., neutrophilic cryptitis, granulomas) present that were not appreciated on low power examination?
   f. Is there evidence of epithelial regeneration (i.e., increased crypt mitoses)?
   g. If submucosa is present, do its constituent parts (vessels, mesenchymal tissue) still appear normal, or is there evidence of amyloid deposition, increased fibrosis or increased inflammation?
3. High power impression:
   a. Is a specific etiology present (i.e., CMV inclusions, spirochetes)?

Table 3
Factors that May Lead to Inaccurate Mucosal Biopsy Interpretation

1. Lack of adequate clinical, endoscopic, and radiographic data (see Table 1).
2. Lack of adequate sampling within the colon.
3. Poor technical preparation of the slide.
4. Pathologist misinterpretation of normal mucosa as showing features of disease.
5. Failure of the pathologist to recognize that treatment effects may alter or reverse "typical" histopathologic features.
6. Failure of the pathologist to recognize that histopathologic features may be shared by clinically disparate diseases.
7. Failure to seek expert pathologic opinion, when appropriate.

What are the responsibilities of the pathologist when interpreting and reporting an endoscopic biopsy? Clearly, each biopsy must be evaluated in a systematic fashion so as not to miss any critical histologic features of disease; Table 2 lists one approach to biopsy interpretation. Table 3 lists the most common factors that lead to inaccurate interpretation of mucosal biopsies. First, normal mucosa should be reported as such. The normal colon contains a certain degree of lymphoplasmacytic inflammation in the lamina propria, greater in the cecum and right colon. To report normal lamina propria inflammation as "mild chronic inflammation" is misleading to both the clinician and patient. This may be especially true if the biopsies were obtained to rule out lymphocytic–microscopic colitis (L/MC)or IBD.

Second, the pathologist (and endoscopist) must accept that definitive clinical disease diagnosis is not always possible, especially in biopsies showing features of acute colitis (is it infectious, ischemic or drug injury?) or in some cases of IBD (CD or UC?). We believe pathologists should provide accurate diagnoses with associated comment sections listing the relevant differential diagnosis, rather than rushing to label patients with a specific disease. Ultimately, it falls on the gastroenterologist to accumulate relevant laboratory (i.e., stool cultures) and radiology data, as well as the follow-up (possibly including rebiopsy) that may eventually allow precise disease classification. As a corollary, pathologists must be aware of the clinical implications of their diagnoses. A diagnosis of CD has very different implications for surgical and medical management than does a diagnosis of UC. A diagnosis of chronic colitis, of any type, has far different implications than a diagnosis of acute self-limited colitis in terms of medical management, as well as for the patient. Pathologists also must be clear in their terminology; the phrase "reactive atypia" should not raise a concern about neoplasia, whereas using only the term "atypia" may be interpreted as suggesting the possibility of malignancy.

Pathologists must be willing to obtain specialist opinion in areas outside of their expertise. All pathologists occasionally face diagnostically difficult cases and benefit from the opinions of specialists. Finally, as we have stressed above, pathologists should answer, either in the body of the report or in the comment section, any questions asked by the endoscopist.

In turn, endoscopists must have reasonable expectations of their pathologists. This requires a basic understanding of the histologic features of different diseases, how histology can (or cannot) distinguish among diseases in the differential diagnosis, and where to biopsy to obtain the most informative histology. We hope that the remainder of this chapter will provide the readers with this information.

2. TECHNIQUES: ENDOSCOPY AND HISTOLOGY

Before we begin discussion of the histopathologic features of diarrheal diseases, we would like to review endoscopy and histology techniques that can aid (or hinder) the interpretation of colonic biopsies. First and foremost, we are ardent supporters of the jumbo biopsy forceps. The endoscopists at University of California at Los Angeles (UCLA) have used these forceps, as opposed to the pinch biopsy forceps, routinely for almost 20 yr and they seem to be as safe as other forceps. Jumbo biopsy forceps obtain tissue with two to three times greater surface area than the pinch forceps, but do not generally obtain a deeper biopsy (2). We prefer the jumbo forceps, because it is easier for histotechnologists to properly orient, embed, and section larger strips of tissue. As a result we receive high quality tissue sections that increase the probability that we can make a definitive and accurate interpretation.

Second, we encourage all endoscopists to limit the number of tissue samples in a single fixative bottle to three or four. While placing more tissue samples in a single fixative bottle may decrease pathology costs for the patient, the resulting tissue sections typically are markedly suboptimal for interpretation. Why is this? First, it is nearly impossible for a histotechnologist to properly orient and line up more than three or four strips of mucosa. Further complicating this is that many biopsies submitted in this manner are obtained with the pinch biopsy forceps, resulting in numerous small tissue fragments. As a result, many tissue strips are tangentially sectioned, while other tissue fragments are "cut through" and disappear from the paraffin block prematurely. Potentially helpful endoscopic information (i.e., thickened fold or sigmoid) gets lost when multiple biopsy sites are placed in one jar. Finally, it is very difficult for a pathologist to keep track of so many fragments of mucosa, especially over the course of 9–20 levels typically cut for a GI mucosal biopsy. A quick review of slides with greater than five tissue

Table 4
Colonic Diseases with Inflammation and/or Diarrhea

General process	Selected examples
Infectious	
Viral	CMV, adenovirus
Bacterial	E. coli, Shigella, Salmonella, Campylobacter, Clostridia, Mycobacteria
Protozoal	E. histolytica
Parasitic	Helminths
Iatrogenic	
Drug	Antibiotic-associated, NSAID, cathartic
Radiation	Acute, chronic
Inflammatory	
Acute self-limited colitis	? Infectious
IBD	CD, UC
Allergic	Food intolerance
Systemic	Behcet's syndrome
Local	Diverticulitis, microscopic colitis
Other	
Amyloidosis	Systemic amyloidoses
Ischemic	Vasculopathy, hypotension
Neoplasm	Carcinoid tumor (with syndrome), lymphoma

samples will confirm that increasing the number of tissue fragments in a bottle reduces the overall interpretability of the biopsy.

Third, for reading the slides we prefer the tissue to be sectioned in a "ribbon" rather than "checkerboard" fashion. In a ribbon of tissue, multiple levels of the biopsy are placed contiguously in a single line from one end of the slide to the other. This allows ready comparison of histologic findings between sequential levels of the biopsy, which can be critical in trying to identify poorly formed granulomas or rare neutrophilic cryptitis in a patient suspected of having CD. In the checkerboard arrangement, the levels from the tissue block are placed in rows and columns on the glass slide, typically with three rows and up to eight columns of tissue. In the checkerboard arrangement, it is not readily apparent whether sequential levels proceed by rows or by columns. As a result, it can be extremely difficult, if not impossible, to follow sequential levels within a slide.

3. FEATURES OF COLONIC MUCOSA IN PATIENTS WITH DIARRHEA

Multiple possible etiologies exist for diarrhea; a partial list can be found in Table 4. Complete discussion of the histopathology of all these entities is beyond the scope of this chapter, and the reader is referred to several excellent pathology textbooks (12–19). The remainder of this chapter will focus on the most common diseases resulting in diarrhea, including IBD, lymphocytic–microscopic–collagenous colitis, acute self-limited (infectious) colitis, and ischemic colitis. Since it is understood that diarrheal disease can originate outside the colon (e.g., celiac disease, carcinoid syndrome) extra-colonic sources of diarrhea are not further mentioned (other than stressing the importance of recognizing normal colonic mucosa, so as not to confuse the clinical picture with an erroneous diagnosis of mild nonspecific colitis). A brief discussion of histologic features associated with drug intake (such as NSAIDs) and various artifacts is also included.

To understand colonic mucosal disease, features of normal mucosa must be appreciated. Normal colonic mucosa has a thin straight muscularis mucosa with straight tubular crypts running perpendicular to it. Crypts may bend adjacent to lymphoid follicles. Normally present innominate grooves or glands show a complex structure with multiple crypts opening into a common apical lumen; these may be mistaken for the branched crypts seen in chronic mucosal injury. Importantly, branched crypts in young children (<9 yr old) may be seen and likely reflect normal colonic growth (3). The intervening stroma (lamina propria) has a very delicate supportive structure of small caliber vessels and stromal cells. A resident physiologic population of inflammatory cells, consisting primarily of lymphocytes, plasma cells, eosinophils, and macrophages, is present. Their density is low, and generally, they remain uncrowded and superficial, unless they are in physiologic lymphoid follicles (mucosa-associated lymphoid tissue). Lymphocytes minimally penetrate the epithelial zone (approx 1 per 20 epithelial cells) (20) and are not associated with injury. Neutrophils are not normally found in colonic mucosa. The epithelium has a small zone of crypt regeneration in the lower third of the crypt, and there is progressive maturation toward the surface. Maturation is typified by cytoplasmic development of goblet mucus cells or columnar absorptive cells, and small basally oriented nuclei Fig. 3 (21). Following endoscopy, lamina propria edema and fresh hemorrhage may be seen (12).

4. ACUTE COLITIS

Acute colitis may result from a variety of etiologies, such as infection (viruses, bacteria, protozoa), drugs, or radiation, and often no precise etiology is uncovered. Commonly implicated drugs include NSAIDs, hypertonic enemas, and bisacodyl (3). In cases without a history of offending drug use or of radiation, the phrase "acute self-limited (infectious) colitis" is often employed to signify findings that presumably are infectious in etiology and transient in most cases. Mucosal injury in infectious colitis may be due to toxin production or to microbial invasion. In this country, common bacterial agents include *Salmonella*, *Campylobacter* and *Escherichia coli*, with *Shigella* and *Yersinia* less frequently cultured (12); protozoal (amebiasis) and viral (cytomegalovirus [CMV]) infections are seen less often than bacterial diseases in immunocompetent patients. Acute infectious colitis may be diffuse, patchy, or even focal within the colon (13). Infectious colitis is often part of an enterocolitis, and the small intestine may be more involved than the colon. On endoscopic exam, the colon may appear normal, edematous, erythematous, friable, or ulcerated and may be indistinguishable from IBD (3,13). Clinically, patients may present with either watery or bloody diarrhea, or may initially have watery diarrhea that later turns bloody.

While the pathologist can easily diagnose acute colitis, uncovering a precise etiology based on histopathology typically is elusive. If an infectious agent is identified, it is usually through stool culture. Only infrequent pathogens such as spirochetes, Mycobacterium avium-intracellulare or CMV inclusions are seen microscopically. Also, certain pathological descriptions such as pseudomembranes are not specific for *C. difficile* toxin, as identical features have been reported in staphylococcal and shigella infections (13). Pseudomembranes also may be seen in ischemia (Fig. 2), though frequently other histologic findings favor ischemia over infection (see Subheading 8).

Drug-induced acute colitis may show identical histopathologic features to those seen in infectious colitis (3,13). Thus, at UCLA, we typically sign out cases as "acute colitis without features of chronic injury, see comment" and, in the comment section, note "the differential diagnosis for these findings includes acute self-limited (infectious) colitis and drug injury".

Histopathologic findings in acute colitis are listed in Table 5 and are illustrated in Fig. 3. A key finding is of active colonic inflammation imposed on normal colonic mucosa without

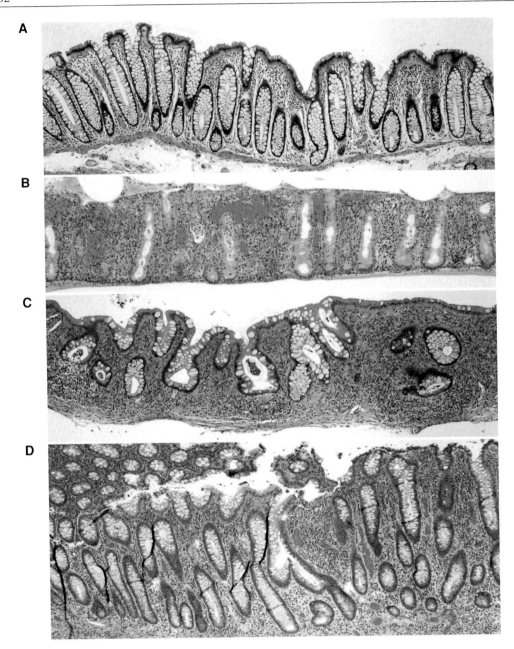

Fig. 3. Colonic mucosa in four different states of inflammation. The goal here is to show how important architecture is as a guide to normal acute colitis and chronic colitis like UC and CD. In addition, it is illustrated that there can easily be overlap in pathology among different diseases, such as UC and CD. (A) Normal colonic mucosa with straight crypts, sparse lamina propria mononuclear cells in the upper third, and no congestion or reactive crypt changes. (B) Acute colitis with preserved crypt architecture, but with neutrophilic infiltration of the lamina propria and crypts, congestion and reactive crypt changes are abundant. (C) Typical features of UC with short and branched crypts, basilar lymphoplasmacytosis, but also with neutrophilic activity. (D) Architecturally distorted and chronically and actively inflamed colonic mucosa (similar to panel C), however it is from a case of Crohn's colitis (elsewhere in the specimen there is fistulating, segmental, and granulomatous disease). These panels serve to demonstrate both the similarities and distinctions in normal, acutely inflamed, and chronically inflamed colonic mucosa.

Table 5
Key Microscopic Features of Acute Colitis

1. Preserved crypt architecture (generally).
2. Lamina propria congestion (with or without hemorrhage) and edema.
3. No significant amount of lymphocytes and plasma cells in the basal portion of the lamina propria, below crypt bases (basal lymphoplasmacytosis).
4. Neutrophilic invasion of crypts (neutrophilic cryptitis) with or without crypt abscesses, usually affecting the mid to upper crypt area, with epithelial mucin depletion.
5. Neutrophilic invasion of surface epithelium with reactive changes (including mucin depletion) and possibly erosions, ulcerations, or regeneration.
6. Fibrinopurulent surface exudates (pseudomembranes) variably present.
7. Lamina propria expansion, largely within the superficial to mid portion, by a mixed inflammatory cell infiltrate with numerous neutrophils.
8. Diffuse, patchy, or focal involvement of the colon.

Table 6
Histologic Differential Diagnosis for Acute (Presumed Infectious) Colitis

Disease	Why might there be similarity?	What can the endoscopist do?
1. IBD	1. Patchy acute colitis often seen. 2. Ulcers variably present. 3. Chronic mucosal injury rarely present. 4. Epithelioid granulomas rarely present. 5. Terminal ileal acute inflammation rarely present.	1. Provide results of stool cultures. 2. Provide recent travel history. 3. Provide history of immunosuppression.
2. Drug injury	1. Features in drug injury may be identical to acute infectious colitis.	1. Provide history of therapeutic drug use (e.g., NSAIDs).
3. Radiation injury	1. Features in radiation may be identical to acute infectious colitis.	1. Provide history of recent or current radiation therapy.

hallmarks of chronic injury (3). An actively inflamed mucosa shows congestion, edema, plump vascular endothelium, neutrophilic infiltration, mild lymphocytic and plasmacytic infiltration, reactive crypt epithelial changes, such as nuclear enlargement, and loss of cytoplasmic constituents, such as mucin. Crypts often show regenerative activity, including increased mitotic figures. There is marked variation in histology depending on the severity or etiology of the disease. The mucosa is the main target in acute colitis, although fulminant disease may show deeper extension, even rarely transmural with colonic perforation (13).

The differential diagnosis for acute colitis is listed in Table 6. Acute colitis is often infectious in origin, but infectious colitis can also lead to chronic injury. Chronic mucosal injury may occur in the setting of severe infection with destruction of the mucosa; implicated bacterial agents have included *Shigella, Salmonella, Chlamydia, Aeromonas*, syphilis, and *Campylobacter (3,13)*. Findings in these cases include crypt dropout, crypt branching, and failure of crypts to reach the muscularis mucosa, and these features may persist beyond the acute infection (13). Clearly, such findings can lead to an incorrect diagnosis of IBD. Importantly, patients with IBD may also get superimposed acute infectious colitis. This is another example where communication between the pathologist and their endoscopist is critical to establish the correct diagnosis or differential diagnosis. Epithelioid granulomas or epithelioid histiocytes may be seen in infectious colitis, particularly in *Mycobacteria*, *Chlamydia*, *Campylobacter*, *Salmonella*, and *Yersinia* infections, and severe patchy ulcers may be seen in the terminal ileum with *Yersinia*, *Salmonella typhi*, and *Mycobacteria tuberculosis* infections (13). The finding of epithelioid granulomas, terminal ileal ulcers or patchy acute neutrophilic cryptitis may lead to a misdiagnosis of CD. CMV primary or recrudescent infection may be associated with ulcers, although the diagnostic nuclear and cytoplasmic inclusions are easily missed (13).

5. CHRONIC IBD (UC/CD)

In the past, IBD was more commonly referred to as idiopathic IBD, since there was no clear etiology for the chronic or recurrent bouts of inflammatory activity. The etiology of IBD still remains a matter of debate, with varying scientific support for genetic factors, altered mucosal permeability, chronic infection, and vasculitis. Clearly, there is genetic susceptibility, with as many as 25% of both CD and UC patients having an affected family member. Both CD and UC affect males and females approx equally, Caucasians more frequently than nonCaucasians, and people of Jewish descent more frequently than nonJews. The highest incidence for both diseases is in the third decade, but may occur anytime between the ages of 5 and 75 (less commonly younger or older) (13).

Classic clinical symptoms at presentation are slightly different for CD and UC. Bloody diarrhea is characteristic of UC, while the diarrhea in CD is often nonbloody. CD more often presents with right lower quadrant pain, sometimes accompanied by a palpable mass; these symptoms may be mistaken for acute appendicitis. In classic UC, the endoscopic exam shows rectal involvement with diffuse mucosal erythema, friability, and variably present pinpoint ulcerations that extend continuously along the mucosa proximally, either to involve only the rectum, the left side, or at times the entire colon with sparing of the terminal ileum. In contrast, classic CD shows terminal ileal disease, with mucosal erythema, friability, and apthous ulcers, and variable involvement of the colonic mucosa with clearly demarcated areas of normal mucosa intervening with diseased mucosa (skip areas); the rectum is often spared. Radiographic or endoscopic studies in CD may also show evidence of extracolonic disease, such as strictures or fistulas.

Unfortunately, not all cases of CD and UC show classic features. It has become apparent that with treatment, UC may show many endoscopic and histopathologic features of CD, including skip lesions (7) and rectal sparing (8). Areas previously involved by active UC even have been reported to show normal mucosa without evidence of chronic mucosal injury (7). Also, UC at times shows a "backwash ileitis", which consists of active inflammation that should be restricted to the distal few centimeters of ileum adjacent to the ileocecal valve. Some cases of CD have been reported to be largely restricted to the mucosa and to diffusely involve the colonic mucosa, in a manner simulating UC (12). Extreme variability exists in CD with respect to organ involvement, magnitude, depth, distribution, and granulomatous inflammation. These examples again emphasize the need to incorporate clinical, radiographic, and histologic data into the final diagnosis and the importance of excellent communication between the endoscopist and pathologist.

Histologic features seen in IBD are listed in Table 7. A prevailing histologic finding is architectural distortion (1,3,13,16). This is essentially colonic mucosa that has been injured by prolonged inflammation, to such an extent that it does not remodel normally and becomes scarred, as evidenced by crypt loss, crypt branching, abnormal crypt shapes, and at times crypt displacement into the submucosa. Increased numbers of lymphocytes and plasma cells in the lamina propria, especially in the basal portion adjacent to or beneath crypt bases, is another

Table 7
Key Microscopic Features of Chronic IBD

1. Distorted crypt architecture, including branched crypts and irregular crypt outlines, crypt loss, and shortened crypts that do not reach the muscularis mucosa.
2. Lamina propria expansion by chronic inflammatory cells, especially plasma cells and lymphocytes, with variable numbers of neutrophils.
3. Lymphocytes and plasma cells in the basal portion of the lamina propria, below crypt bases (basal lymphoplasmacytosis).
4. Multifocal neutrophilic cryptitis and crypt abscesses (variable, based on degree of activity).
5. Reactive epithelial changes, including mucin depletion (with active disease).
6. Surface villiform change.
7. Epithelial cell metaplasia (Paneth cell, pyloric gland type).
8. Lamina propria, muscularis mucosa, and submucosal fibrosis (primarily CD).
9. Dense submucosal inflammatory cell infiltrate.
10. Granulomas infrequently present (primarily CD).
11. Muscularis mucosa hyperplasia and splaying of the muscular fibers.

important feature; besides IBD, this is seen only in chronic infectious colitis. Chronic mucosal damage like that seen in chronic crypt destructive colitis of UC is illustrated in Fig. 3.

UC is overwhelmingly a mucosal disease that is highly amenable to diagnosis on mucosal biopsy by an anatomic pathologist in the appropriate clinical setting. The advantage in UC over CD is that the pathologic changes are limited to the mucosa and superficial submucosa and, therefore, should appear in the biopsies. Cases of UC will show the features of chronic mucosal injury described above, as well as variable amounts of neutrophilic cryptitis and crypt abscesses, depending on activity and treatment. In untreated cases, chronic mucosal injury and inflammatory activity should be relatively uniform within all biopsies from the same anatomic site; in treated cases (as noted above), both of these features may be patchy within and between biopsies. If there is fibrosis, it should be subtle and often seen just at the muscularis mucosa (13). An important variant of classic UC is fulminant UC, which may show full thickness inflammation (predominately plasma cells) and necrosis with bowel perforation. When fulminant colitis complicates a case of established UC, the diagnosis is apparent. However, when the initial presentation is of fulminant colitis, it may be difficult to make a definitive diagnosis of UC. The challenge for the pathologist in these cases is to avoid jumping to the diagnosis of CD, due to the presence of full thickness disease, variably accompanied by perforation (13).

In contrast, CD is characteristically patchy in distribution. Histologic patchiness is most obviously manifested by marked variation in chronic mucosal injury or active disease within strips of biopsied mucosa obtained from the same biopsy site. For example, three strips of mucosa taken from "60 cm" will show acute and chronic changes completely involving one strip, partially involving a second and completely sparing the third. Such patchiness also may be seen in treated UC, or at the proximal most edge of the UC zone, but is extremely uncommon in untreated UC. Granulomas in the mucosal biopsy are considered by many clinicians and pathologists to be diagnostic of CD, or at least essential to that diagnosis. However, true epithelioid granulomas are seen in a minority of mucosal biopsies from CD patients; only 15–36% of cases will have an epithelioid granuloma, depending on the number of biopsies and levels examined (13). Our experience with resection specimens indicates that the epithelioid granulomas of CD are much more commonly located in the deep submucosa or muscularis propria, which are areas not typically sampled in a mucosal biopsy. Furthermore, epithelioid granulomas may be seen in infectious colitis (see Subheading 4), sarcoid (3), and are a non-

Table 8
Histologic Differences Between Classic UC and CD

Histologic feature	UC (classic features)	CD
Site most often affected	Rectum, with variable proximal disease.	Terminal ileum, right colon.
Extent of disease	Diffuse, from rectum proximally.	Patchy involvement (skip areas).
Depth of disease	Mucosa, superficial submucosa.	All layers may be affected, with bowel wall perforation and/or fistulas.
Broad ulcers	Frequent (varies based on activity).	Uncommon—apthous ulcers seen.
Inflammatory polyps pseudopolyps	Frequent.	Uncommon.
Submucosal inflammation	Rare (typically superficial submucosa only, contiguous with mucosal disease).	Common (often extensive).
Submucosal fibrosis	Rare, except in severe disease.	Common.
Granulomas	Absent.	Uncommon on biopsies (see text).
Fissures	Absent.	Common.
Patchy inflammation	Rare in untreated cases (see text).	Common.
Rectal involvement	Common (see text).	Uncommon.

specific finding in IBD when they are intimately associated with a ruptured crypt. Table 8 compares histologic features of CD and UC.

It is much more difficult to diagnose CD, unequivocally, on mucosal biopsies. Histologic descriptions of CD are based on resection specimens (16), and, thus, include features, such as submucosal fibrosis, fistulas, neuronal hyperplasia within submucosa–muscularis propria, and muscularis propria fibrosis. However, these areas are not seen in a mucosal biopsy, which samples only as deeply as the superficial submucosa (if one is lucky, more commonly, the biopsy includes only mucosa). For a diagnosis of CD, it is more likely that the bulk of the evidence is not found in the pathological specimens obtained by endoscopy, but that the biopsies will be supportive of the clinical impression. In addition, biopsy is essential to exclude a non-CD process. The greatest pathological support in mucosal biopsies would be in the form of a chronic granulomatous colitis with a distribution inconsistent with UC and a clear-cut skip area. In addition, some colitis is not definable and carries the term indeterminate colitis; for more information on this area, the reader is directed to several excellent pathology textbooks (12–19). The chronic mucosal damage, such as that seen in chronic crypt destructive colitis of CD, can be identical to that in UC and is illustrated in Fig. 3. To repeat, it is necessary to have the many other features of CD present to distinguish the two colitides.

We would be remiss if we did not remind our readers that features of chronic mucosal injury are not specific to IBD (Table 9). As mentioned in other sections within this chapter, features of chronic mucosal injury may be seen in chronic infection (especially *Campylobacter*, *Aeromonas*, *Shigella*, and *Yersinia*) (3,13), in "diverticula colitis" (11,22), in "diversion colitis" (23,24), and in drug injury, such as NSAIDs (3). Chronic infectious colitis, in addition to crypt architectural distortion, often shows basal lymphoplasmacytosis (3,13), which is common in IBD and uncommonly seen in diversion colitis, diverticular colitis and drug injury. Chronic mucosal injury is strongly associated with IBD, but ultimately, clinicians must

Table 9
Other Conditions that Histologically Mimic Chronic IBD

Disease	Why might there be similarity?	What can the endoscopist do?
1. Chronic infectious colitis	1. Crypt architectural distortion may be seen. 2. Basal lymphoplasmacytosis may be seen. 3. Granulomas variably present.	1. Stool cultures, if not already done. 2. Clinical history (travel, immunosuppression, etc.).
2. Diverticula colitis	1. Crypt architectural distortion may be seen. 2. Neutrophilic cryptitis may be seen. 3. Paneth cell metaplasia may be seen.	1. Note biopsy was adjacent to diverticula, or taken from sigmoid in patients with diverticular disease.
3. Diversion colitis	1. Crypt architectural distortion may be seen.	1. Note biopsy taken from diverted segment of colon.
4. Chronic ischemia[a]	1. Crypt architectural distortion may be seen.	1. Note risk factors for ischemia.
5. Drug injury	1. Crypt architectural distortion may be seen.	1. Note medications (e.g., NSAIDs).

[a]Other histologic features often suggest ongoing ischemia over IBD (see Table 13)

exclude other possible etiologies, not the pathologist. This is especially true in CD, where mucosal pathology is less sensitive and specific than in UC.

As evidenced by the above discussion, excellent endoscopist–pathologist communication, including radiologic, laboratory and clinical data, is critical for accurate interpretation of mucosal biopsies in suspected IBD. Evidence of extracolonic disease, including small bowel strictures, fistulas and upper GI disease should be given to the pathologist. A sufficient number of biopsies should be taken from normal and abnormal areas and target lesions and should be accompanied by endoscopic descriptions of each site biopsied. Ideally, minimum areas to biopsy include the terminal ileum, cecum, ascending, transverse, descending, sigmoid, and rectum; this may vary based on disease duration, symptoms at the time of diagnosis, and clinical certainty of the diagnosis of UC or CD. For a diagnosis of CD, biopsies that include endoscopically normal and abnormal mucosa at the same site (i.e., an apthous ulcer and the adjacent normal mucosa) can be invaluable in helping to confirm the diagnosis.

6. LYMPHOCYTIC-MICROSCOPIC COLITIS

There has been much debate within the literature regarding the most appropriate nomenclature for this entity. Proponents of both terms generally agree on the histologic features listed in Table 10. However, advocates of the term "lymphocytic" colitis emphasize that the intraepithelial inflammatory cells should be predominantly lymphocytes and believe the term "microscopic" colitis is an overused diagnostic term for any patient with diarrhea, normal endoscopy, and a histologically abnormal mucosa. They argue that the term "lymphocytic colitis" is more precise, since other diseases may have diarrhea, normal endoscopy, and abnormal histologic findings (20,25). For simplicity, we will refer to it by the two most common names, L/MC. It is not yet clear if and how L/MC is related to CC (25,26)). With the exception of the distinctive subepithelial collagen band (SCB), the histologic features of the two entities are identical (Tables 10 and 11). Likewise, the clinical presentation, endoscopic findings and possible etiologies are similar.

Table 10
Key Microscopic Features of L/MC

1. Diffuse infiltration of the surface epithelium by lymphocytes.
2. Reactive epithelial changes (generally), including mucin depletion.
3. Lamina propria chronic inflammatory infiltrate, primarily lymphoplasmacytic.
4. Preserved crypt architecture (generally).
5. No significant neutrophilic component; none or rare neutrophilic cryptitis.
6. Uniform diffuse involvement of both right and left colon (generally).

Table 11
Key Microscopic Features of CC

1. Nos. 1–5 as for L/MC, Table 10.
2. Patchy increased thickness of the SCB often associated with lifting off of the overlying surface epithelium. Note: this finding may be extremely focal, occurring only in one out of seven or eight biopsies and more often in the right colon.
3. Diagnostic features usually found proximal to the rectosigmoid, especially in the right colon.

L/MC clinically is suspected in a patient with chronic watery diarrhea and normal mucosa on endoscopic exam. Occasionally, subtle endoscopic changes are encountered, including erythema, decreased vascular markings, and congestion (3,12,20). This entity has been described to occur in children (27) as well as adults, with an equal sex distribution (25,26). Several studies have noted concurrent small bowel abnormalities such as celiac disease (25) or tropical sprue(28). L/MC has been reported to occur in Western countries, and there are even cases reported from India and Pakistan (28,29). This is unlike CC, which seems to occur primarily in Western countries. Various drugs, including carbamazapine (26), ranitidine (5), ticlopidine (6), and Cyclo 3 Fort (4) have been associated with classic colonic mucosal changes of L/MC. The etiology of L/MC is not clear and is most likely multifactorial. Some report elevated titers of autoimmune markers (26), and various associated autoimmune conditions, including Sjogren's syndrome and scleroderma (25).

Classic histologic features of L/MC colitis are listed in Table 10. The most striking features in this disorder are the surface epithelial injury associated with diffuse marked intraepithelial lymphocytes and the increased lamina propria chronic inflammation (Fig. 4). Greater than 10 lymphocytes per 100 surface epithelial cells typically are seen, with many cases showing more than 20:100. This contrasts markedly to the ratio of 4 to 5:100 seen in normal colon, infectious colitis and IBD (20). Occasional intraepithelial eosinophils or neutrophils may be seen (20). The surface epithelium shows moderate to marked mucin depletion, and the epithelium is often cuboidal or flattened, rather than columnar (20). The lamina propria shows a heavy chronic inflammatory infiltrate, with a predominance of lymphocytes; eosinophils and neutrophils may be present (20,26,30). Crypt epithelium often shows lymphocytic inflammation, but neutrophilic cryptitis is infrequently seen (20), in contrast to acute self-limited (infectious) colitis and IBD. Whereas the features of CC tend to be more prominent in the right colon, features of L/MC typically are distributed diffusely throughout right and left colon.

The differential diagnosis for L/MC colitis is listed in Table 12, along with histologic explanations. The features of collagenous colitis are discussed further below. Patients taking various drugs, including NSAIDs, carbamazepine, ranitidine, ticlopidine, and Cyclo 3 Fort, have been reported to develop diarrhea and histologic findings identical to those seen in

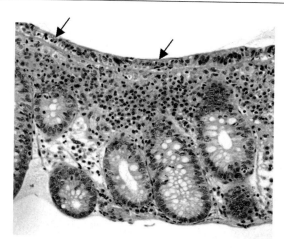

Fig. 4. L/MC. This photomicrograph demonstrates numerous surface intraepithelial lymphocytes (some indicated by arrows), accompanied by reactive epithelial changes, including mucin depletion. Also note the surface epithelium does not show the normal columnar shape, but is instead cuboidal. The superficial half of the lamina propria is expanded by lymphocytes and plasma cells, without significant inflammation below the crypt bases (compare with Fig. 3C). Crypt architecture is intact, with straight crypt outlines.

Table 12
Histologic Differential Diagnosis for L/MC

Disease	Why might there be similarity?	What can the endoscopist do?
CC	1. SCB typically patchy in distribution.	1. Biopsy right colon (more common site of SCB). 2. Biopsy four to six sites, rather than one to two.
Drug-induced injury	1. Histology may be identical to that seen in L/MC.	1. Provide a detailed medication history, including NSAIDs.
Brainerd (epidemic) diarrhea	1. Similar numbers of surface intraepithelial lymphocytes. 2. Surface epithelial degenerative changes generally absent.	1. Provide history of epidemic diarrhea.
Diverticula or polyps (adenomas or hyperplastic)	1. Surface inflammation may be present in areas immediately adjacent to or within polyps or diverticula.	1. Provide endoscopic findings of diverticula or polyps.
Normal colon	1. Surface epithelium overlying lymphoid follicles and/or aggregates often shows lymphocytic infiltration and reactive epithelial changes. 2. Right colon may have mildly increased numbers of intraepithelial lymphocytes compared to remainder of colon.	1. Pathologist should be able to distinguish.

L/MC (3–6). "Brainerd" or epidemic diarrhea (often without an identifiable microbiologic agent) produces similar marked intraepithelial lymphocytosis, with 18–22:100 epithelial cells reported in one study. However, the same study failed to find the surface epithelial damage and lamina propria chronic inflammatory infiltrate typical of L/MC (31).

Pathologists must be aware that the surface epithelium overlying normal lamina propria lymphoid aggregates or follicles may show infiltration by lymphocytes, with reactive changes, including loss of mucin and a cuboidal (as opposed to columnar) shape (20,21). In addition, cecal and ascending mucosa may show slightly more intraepithelial lymphocytes than the remainder of the colon (20). In order to recognize these changes as within normal limits, the pathologist must recognize that the surface inflammation is intimately associated with lymphoid follicles or aggregates and is patchy, as opposed to the diffuse inflammation seen in L/MC. Similarly, mucosa adjacent to diverticula or polyps (adenomatous or hyperplastic) may show increased lamina propria inflammation and surface inflammatory infiltration with reactive changes (11,32). An endoscopic description of a polyp, diverticula, or biopsy of the sigmoid colon should alert the pathologist to the correct differential diagnosis. It is our personal experience that in the sigmoid colon, endoscopic small polyps (2 to 3 mm) or thickened folds are frequently associated with diverticular disease. These probably represent the reactive mucosal lip of tissue adjacent to the diverticulum ostia.

Also listed in Table 12 are recommendations for how the endoscopist can help the pathologist eliminate entities in the differential diagnosis. For instance, multiple biopsies of both right and left colon that show histologic features of L/MC without a SCB or history of offending drug use would, at UCLA, result in a diagnosis of L/MC. However, the same features seen in a single biopsy of the left colon, without a medication history, would be more likely to result in a diagnosis of "suggestive of L/MC, see comment". The comment section would then list the above differential diagnosis.

7. COLLAGENOUS COLITIS

As noted above, the clinical findings, endoscopic findings and possible etiologies are highly similar to L/MC, and will not be discussed in significant additional detail here. Interestingly, CC predominantly affects women (20:1 female to male ratio) (26,30). As with L/MC, CC has been reported to occur in children (30). Again, associations have been noted with small bowel disease, including collagenous gastritis (33), celiac sprue (30) and refractory sprue (34), as well as with various autoimmune diseases (30).

Histologically, the key difference between L/MC is the presence of a thickened SCB. Otherwise, CC shows the same features of increased intraepithelial lymphocytes with associated surface epithelial damage and increased lamina propria chronic inflammatory infiltrate as seen in L/MC (35) (Table 11 and Fig. 5). On hematoxylin and eosin (H&E) stains, the SCB appears as a band of lightly eosinophilic material immediately below the epithelial surface, frequently with collagen tendrils extending down into the lamina propria in an irregular fashion. The collagen often entraps capillaries in the upper lamina propria. Overall, this makes the lower border of the epithelial basement membrane indistinct (30,35). Trichrome stains can help confirm the presence of collagen. How thick should this band be before it becomes significant? In the proper clinical and endoscopic context, most pathologists currently argue that the presence of an abnormal collagen band, as described above, is sufficient, regardless of the measured thickness, which can vary greatly from case to case (26,30,35).

Pathologists may misdiagnose CC by focusing exclusively on the thickness of the SCB. Hyperplastic polyps, tangential sections of normal mucosa, peripheral sections of a crypt sheath, and mild nonspecific variations in basement membrane thickness all may suggest a thickened SCB. Importantly, the lower border of the SCB in these conditions will be smooth and sharp, as opposed to the irregular lower border seen in CC (26,35). Inflammation within the mucosa and surface epithelium, in addition to the SCB, is necessary to consider the diagnosis of CC. However, the presence of a SCB in the appropriate clinical, endoscopic and

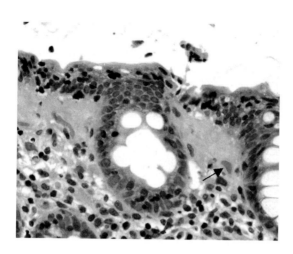

Fig. 5. CC. In addition to increased numbers of surface intraepithelial lymphocytes accompanied by reactive epithelial changes, this photomicrograph demonstrates a thickened abnormal SCB. Entrapped capillaries are present (arrow), and the lower border is indistinct.

histologic setting has essentially no diagnosis other than CC. Other diseases (i.e., ischemia or NSAID injury) may show hyalinization of or increased fibromuscular tissue in the lamina propria, but these changes usually involve the majority or all of the lamina propria, and are not restricted to a band-like pattern immediately below the surface epithelium. If a SCB is not seen, the differential diagnosis is the same as that for L/MC, see Table 12.

8. ACUTE REVERSIBLE ISCHEMIC COLITIS

Ischemic colitis has multiple and widely diverse etiologies. Low-flow states and hypovolemia, such as occur in cardiovascular disease or shock, are a common cause. Areas of poor vascular collateral circulation ("watershed areas"), such as the splenic flexure and rectosigmoid, are often affected. However, ischemic colitis also occurs in otherwise healthy young women on oral contraceptives *(9)*, in cocaine users *(10)*, in certain fungal *(36)* or viral (especially CMV) infections, and with certain enteroinvasive (i.e., *Shigella*) or toxin-producing (i.e., *E. coli* O157:H7 or *C. difficile*) bacteria *(3)*. Vascular disease, including atherosclerotic disease, thromboembolic disease, radiation injury, or vasculitis *(3,37)* can also produce colonic ischemia. We have personally seen changes in mucosal biopsies taken at or near surgical anastomotic sites that are identical to those seen in chronic ischemia. The portion(s) of colon involved in these varied etiologies may not correspond to the classic watershed areas described above.

Ischemic injury to the colon may be acute and reversible, acute and fulminant, or chronic. Classic histologic features of acute, reversible ischemic colitis are listed in Table 13 and illustrated in Fig. 6. We must emphasize that there may be significant histologic overlap between acute reversible ischemic colitis and acute infectious colitis, especially in cases with fibrinopurulent pseudomembranes (Fig. 2). The major differential diagnosis is infectious colitis. In fact, at UCLA, we often diagnose such cases as "(mild, moderate, or severe) acute colitis with pseudomembranes, see comment." In the comment section, we note, "the differential diagnosis for these findings includes ischemia and infection". Both entities may show

Table 13
Key Microscopic Features of Acute Reversible Ischemic Colitis on Mucosal Biopsies

1. Epithelial separation from the basement membrane (blebbing), with associated reactive epithelial changes, including mucin depletion.
2. Variable epithelial necrosis, either full-thickness or surface epithelial and superficial crypts only, with or without associated lamina propria necrosis and mucosal ulceration.
3. Patchy involvement (affected next to normal mucosa in the same biopsy) often seen.
4. Crypt outlines preserved without architectural distortion, although crypt epithelium may be lost.
5. Crypts may be filled with mucus and inflammatory cells.
6. Mixed lamina propria and crypt inflammatory infiltrate, often with many neutrophils; neutrophilic cryptitis variably present.
7. Fibrinopurulent surface exudates (pseudomembranes) often seen.
8. Lamina propria hemorrhage and/or edema may be present.
9. Lamina propria fibrosis variably present. In chronic ischemia, fibrosis is typically present, but it is not seen in patients presenting with an initial acute attack.
10. Intravascular thromboses may be present in the lamina propria or submucosa.

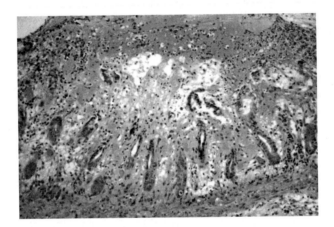

Fig. 6. Acute reversible ischemic colitis. Crypt outlines are visible and show intact architecture, with straight crypts extending to the level of the muscularis mucosa without crypt branching. Surface and crypt epithelial necrosis is seen, as well as reactive epithelial changes. Lamina propria hemorrhage and edema are seen, and a fibrinopurulent exudate (pseudomembrane) covers the epithelial surface.

neutrophilic cryptitis, fibrinopurulent pseudomembranes, markedly increased lamina propria neutrophilic inflammation, and surface and/or crypt epithelial necrosis. However, acute ischemic change often shows epithelial separation from the basement membrane ("blebbing"), allowing one to favor ischemia over infection.

Fulminant acute ischemic colitis shows transmural infarction, often with perforation *(12,13)*. In chronic ischemia, the lamina propria becomes fibrotic and chronic inflammation, often band-like, as well as fibrosis may be seen in the submucosa. Crypt architectural distortion (including crypt loss and crypt branching) is often present, along with epithelial cell metaplasia *(12)*. These changes may resemble CD, however, features of ongoing acute ischemic injury, such as epithelial blebbing, will often be seen and will alert the pathologist to the correct diagnosis. Again, communication between the endoscopist and pathologist will also help establish the correct diagnosis.

Table 14
Histologic Differential Diagnosis for Acute Reversible Ischemic Colitis

Disease	Why might there be similarity?	What can the endoscopist do?
Infectious colitis	Histology similar to acute reversible ischemic colitis.	1. Provide pertinent clinical data, i.e., immunosuppression (CMV, fungal), sepsis, cardiac failure, known vasculitis and/or autoimmune disease or atherosclerotic disease. 2. Provide results of stool cultures and toxin screens (*C. difficile*).
Radiation injury	Histology similar to acute reversible ischemic colitis.	1. Provide history of recent radiation therapy or of history of cancer within the pelvis.

The differential diagnosis for acute reversible ischemic colitis is given in Table 14. As noted earlier in this chapter, several infectious agents, including *Yersinia* and CMV, can produce extensive full thickness epithelial necrosis and ulceration along with lamina propria hemorrhage and edema. Radiation may produce both acute and chronic mucosal injury, histologically similar to acute and chronic ischemic injury. Neutrophilic cryptitis, mucosal ulceration, and lamina propria edema may all be seen in acute radiation damage; in chronic injury, crypt architectural distortion and lamina propria hyalinization are present. Key features that distinguish radiation injury include atypical fibroblasts and myointimal proliferation within vessels. Atypical fibroblasts consist of cells with enlarged and somewhat atypical appearing nuclei; however, a key accompanying feature is enlarged amounts of cytoplasm, such that the normal nuclear to cytoplasmic ratio is maintained. Myointimal proliferation within vessels is highly characteristic of ischemic injury, but typically is seen in the submucosa or below, and thus may not be sampled in a routine endoscopic mucosal biopsy *(12)*.

9. MISCELLANEOUS HISTOLOGICAL FINDINGS IN PATIENTS WITH DIARRHEA

The etiologies mentioned earlier in the chapter account for a large proportion of patients with diarrhea, however, some patients with diarrhea have normal or near normal histologic findings. In some patients, histologic findings may suggest disease that is not actually present. We wish to end this chapter with Table 15, which presents a list of such findings and their histologic features. Drug injury, diverticula colitis, and diversion colitis have been discussed in earlier sections on chronic IBD (see Subheading 5) and L/MC (see Subheading 6). For more information on bowel prep effect (artifacts), the reader is directed elsewhere *(12,13,38)*.

Our intent in this chapter was to educate our nonpathologist colleagues about the challenges pathologists may have in interpreting colonic mucosal biopsies in patients with diarrhea. We believe that we have stressed adequately the following three key points. First, communication between the endoscopist and pathologist is critical for accurate biopsy interpretation. Second, clinically disparate diseases may share the same histologic features. Third, because there is great overlap in histologic features among different diseases, an experienced GI pathologist may not rush to label a patient with one disease, but may instead list the differential diagnosis. We hope we have achieved our objectives, and that this chapter will help you to interact more effectively with pathologists.

Table 15.

Conditions with Abnormal Histology that May Be Encountered in Mucosal Biopsies

Disease	Why might there be similarity?	What can the endoscopist do?
1. Bowel prep effect	1. Patchy neutrophilic invasion of crypt epithelium; may be seen at one or at several different biopsy sites with or without reactive epithelial changes. 2. Features of ischemic colitis, UC pseudomembranes. 3. Lamina propria edema.	1. Often seen after hypertonic phosphate bowel preparations, including Fleet enemas and bisacodyl laxatives. 2. Seen following hydrogen peroxide enemas or contamination of endoscopes by cleaning solutions. 3. Seen following osmotic enema preparations.
2. Diverticula colitis	1. Crypt architectural distortion may be seen. 2. Neutrophilic cryptitis may be seen. 3. Paneth cell metaplasia may be seen.	1. Note biopsy was adjacent to diverticula or from sigmoid in patients with diverticular disease.
3. Drug injury	1. Variety of lesions, including ulcers, crypt architectural distortion, features of ischemic colitis, eosinophilic colitis, features identical to L/MC, and pseudomembranes. 2. Isolated terminal ileal involvement maybe seen, mimicking CD.	1. Provide history of all medications, including NSAIDs and over-the-counter preparations. 2. May be seen with NSAIDs.
4. Diversion colitis	1. Crypt architectural distortion may be seen.	1. Note biopsy taken from diverted segment of colon.

REFERENCES

1. Shivananda S, Hordijk ML, Ten Kate FJ, Probert CS, Mayberry JF. Differential diagnosis of inflammatory bowel disease: a comparison of various diagnostic classifications. *Scand. J. Gastroenterol.*, 26 (1991) 167–173.
2. Weinstein WM. Mucosal biopsy techniques and interaction with the pathologist. *Gastrointest. Endosc. Clin. N. Am.*, 10 (2000) 555–572.
3. Carpenter HA, Talley NJ. The importance of clinicopathological correlation in the diagnosis of inflammatory conditions of the colon: histological patterns with clinical implications. *Am. J. Gastroenterol.*, 95 (2000) 878–896.
4. Beaugerie L, Luboinski J, Brousse N, et al. Drug induced lymphocytic colitis. *Gut*, 35 (1994) 426–428.
5. Beaugerie L, Patey N, Brousse N. Ranitidine, diarrhoea, and lymphocytic colitis. *Gut*, 37 (1995) 708–711.
6. Berrebi D, Sautet A, Flejou JF, Dauge MC, Peuchmaur M, Potet F. Ticlopidine induced colitis: a histopathological study including apoptosis. *J.Clin. Pathol.*, 51 (1998) 280–283.
7. Kleer CG, Appelman HD. Ulcerative colitis: patterns of involvement in colorectal biopsies and changes with time. *Am. J. Surg. Pathol.*, 22 (1998) 983–989.
8. Odze R, Antonioli D, Peppercorn M, Goldman H. Effect of topical 5-aminosalicylic acid (5-ASA) therapy on rectal mucosal biopsy morphology in chronic ulcerative colitis. *Am. J. Surg. Pathol.*, 17 (1993) 869–875.
9. Deana DG, Dean PJ. Reversible ischemic colitis in young women. Association with oral contraceptive use. *Am. J. Surg. Pathol.*, 19 (1995) 454–462.
10. Boutros HH, Pautler S, Chakrabarti S. Cocaine-induced ischemic colitis with small-vessel thrombosis of colon and gallbladder. *J. Clin. Gastroenterol.*, 24 (1997) 49–53.
11. Makapugay LM, Dean PJ. Diverticular disease-associated chronic colitis. *Am. J. Surg. Pathol.*, 20 (1996) 94–102.
12. Fenoglio-Preiser CM, Noffsinger AE, Stemmermann GN, Lantz PE, Listrom MB, Rilke FO. *Gastrointestinal Pathology: An Atlas and Text.* 2nd ed., Lippincott-Raven, Philadelphia, PA, 1999.
13. Lewin KJ, Riddell RH, Weinstein WM. *Gastrointestinal Pathology and Its Clinical Implications.* Igaku-Shoin, New York, NY, 1992.

14. Ming SC, Goldman H. *Pathology of the Gastrointestinal Tract,* 2nd ed., W.B. Saunders, Baltimore, MD, 1998.

15. Lockhart-Mummery HE, Morson BC. Crohn's disease (regional enteritis) of the large intestine and its distinction from ulcerative colitis. *Gut,* **1** (1960) 87–105.

16. Kleer CG, Appelman HD. Surgical pathology of Crohn's disease. *Surg. Clin. N. Am.,* **81** (2001) 13–30.

17. Price AB, Morson BC. Inflammatory bowel disease: the surgical pathology of Crohn's disease and ulcerative colitis. *Hum. Pathol.,* **6** (1975) 7–29.

18. Mottet NK. *Histopathologic Spectrum of Regional Enteritis and Ulcerative Colitis.* Saunders, Philadelphia, PA, 1971.

19. Geller SA. Pathology of inflammatory bowel disease: a critical appraisal in diagnosis and management. In *Inflammatory Bowel Disease: From Bench to Bedside.* Targan SR, Shanahan F (eds.), Williams and Wilkins, Baltimore, MD, 1994.

20. Lazenby AJ, Yardley JH, Giardiello FM, Jessurun J, Bayless TM. Lymphocytic ("microscopic") colitis: a comparative histopathologic study with particular reference to collagenous colitis. *Hum. Pathol.,* **20** (1989) 18–28.

21. Levine DS, Haggitt RC. Colon. *Histology for Pathologists.* Sternberg SS (ed.), Lippincott-Raven, Philadelphia, PA, 1997.

22. Goldstein NS, Leon-Armin C, Mani A. Crohn's colitis-like changes in sigmoid diverticulitis specimens is usually an idiosyncratic inflammatory response to the diverticulosis rather than Crohn's colitis. *Am. J. Surg. Pathol.,* **24** (2000) 668–675.

23. Ma CK, Gottlieb C, Haas PA. Diversion colitis: a clinicopathologic study of 21 cases. *Hum. Pathol.,* **21** (1990) 429–436.

24. Haque S, Eisen RA, West AB. The morphologic features of diversion colitis: studies of a pediatric population with no other disease of the intestinal mucosa [see comments]. *Hum. Pathol.,* **24** (1993) 211–219.

25. Jawhari A, Talbot IC. Microscopic, lymphocytic and collagenous colitis [see comments]. *Histopathology,* **29** (1996) 101–110.

26. Giardiello FM, Lazenby AJ. The atypical colitides. *Gastroenterol. Clin. N. Am.,* **28** (1999) 479–490.

27. Mashako MN, Sonsino E, Navarro J, et al. Microscopic colitis: a new cause of chronic diarrhea in children? *J. Pediat. Gastroenterol. Nutr.,* **10** (1990) 21–26.

28. Puri AS, Khan EM, Kuman M, Pandey R, Choudhuri G. Association of lymphocytic (microscopic) colitis with tropical sprue. *J. Gastroenterol. Hepatol.,* **9** (1994) 105–107.

29. Hamid S, Jafri W, Abbas Z, et al. Microscopic colitis: a diagnosis to consider. *J. Pak. Med. Assoc.,* **43** (1993) 203–205.

30. Zins BJ, Sandborn WJ, Tremaine WJ. Collagenous and lymphocytic colitis: subject review and therapeutic alternatives. *Am. J. Gastroenterol.,* **90** (1995) 1394–1400.

31. Bryant DA, Mintz ED, Puhr ND, Griffin PM, Petras RE. Colonic epithelial lymphocytosis associated with an epidemic of chronic diarrhea. *Am. J. Surg. Pathol.,* **20** (1996) 1102–1109.

32. Mills LR, Schuman BM, Thompson WO. Lymphocytic colitis. A definable clinical and histological diagnosis. *Dig. Dis. Sci.,* **38** (1993) 1147–1151.

33. Pulimood AB, Ramakrishna BS, Mathan MM. Collagenous gastritis and collagenous colitis: a report with sequential histological and ultrastructural findings. *Gut,* **44** (1999) 881–885.

34. Robert ME, Ament ME, Weinstein WM. The histologic spectrum and clinical outcome of refractory and unclassified sprue. *Am. J. Surg. Pathol.,* **24** (2000) 676–687.

35. Lazenby AJ, Yardley JH, Giardiello FM, Bayless TM. Pitfalls in the diagnosis of collagenous colitis: experience with 75 cases from a registry of collagenous colitis at the Johns Hopkins Hospital. *Hum. Pathol.,* **21** (1990) 905–910.

36. Hosseini M, Lee J. Gastrointestinal mucormycosis mimicking ischemic colitis in a patient with systemic lupus erythematosus. *Am. J. Gastroenterol.,* **93** (1998) 1360–1362.

37. Okada M, Konishi F, Sakuma K, Kanazawa K, Koiwai H, Kaizaki Y. Perforation of the sigmoid colon with ischemic change due to polyarteritis nodosa. *J. Gastroenterol.,* **34** (1999) 400–404.

38. Ryan CK, Potter GD. Disinfectant colitis. Rinse as well as you wash [editorial]. *J. Clin. Gastroenterol.,* **21** (1995) 6–9.

18 Anorectal Manometry

Devang N. Prajapati and Walter J. Hogan

CONTENTS

1. INTRODUCTION

Anorectal disorders are common and among the most distressing experienced by patients in primary and referral practice, yet often go unreported. A quarter of the population suffers from anorectal symptoms, but less than one in five seek medical attention for this *(1)*. Constipation is experienced by 3–20% of the population, while incontinence is experienced by 3–8% of the adult population, both conditions with a higher prevalence in the elderly *(2)*. Anorectal pain syndromes, including proctalgia fugax and levator ani syndrome, though less common, are a source of significant disability. Anorectal manometry plays an important role in the evaluation of patients with anorectal disorders. In this chapter, we review the basics of anorectal manometric assessment and its clinical correlates.

2. BACKGROUND

2.1. Normal Anorectal Physiology

The anorectal area is richly supplied with sensory and motor nerves that act in concert to maintain continence and facilitate defecation. Although a complete review of the physiology is beyond the scope of this chapter, an understanding of the main continence mechanisms will aid in understanding the utility of anorectal manometry. The main continence mechanisms consist of the internal and external sphincters, the puborectalis muscle, and the rectum, which acts as a reservoir for feces and appropriately senses distention *(3)*. Failure of any of these components can cause significant problems with incontinence or constipation. The internal sphincter is composed of smooth muscle, is tonically contracted, and acts as a passive barrier to passage of liquid feces or gas from the rectum *(4)*. The main stimulus for relaxation is rectal

From: *Colonic Diseases*
Edited by: T. R. Koch © Humana Press Inc., Totowa, NJ

distention and is mediated by enteric nerves. On the other hand the external sphincter is composed of striated muscle, which is also tonically contracted but is inhibited or augmented by higher cortical input, mediated through the sacral nerves and pudendal nerve. The puborectalis acts as a sling to maintain an acute rectal anal axis to maintain continence, but can relax to allow defecation, and usually acts in concert with the external sphincter.

Normally, when feces are presented to the rectum, the rectal distention results in a reflex relaxation of the internal anal sphincter as a sampling mechanism followed by a reflex external sphincter contraction, which can be modulated by higher cortical centers to relax if appropriate to defecate. The rectum relaxes to accommodate the stool, which is important as the voluntary external sphincter contraction fatigues after a few seconds. Dysfunction of any of these well coordinated actions, may result in defecation difficulties, most commonly constipation or incontinence. Anorectal manometry allows the clinician to assess the function of each of the components of the continence and defecatory mechanism in patients with anorectal complaints.

2.2. Anorectal Manomtery

Anorectal manometry today is a refinement of many years of research into anorectal physiology. In the 19th century, Gowers (5) demonstrated the rectoanal inhibitory reflex, which started the development of techniques to evaluate the defecatory process. Schuster et al. (6) in 1963 demonstrated a method of assessing this reflex and subsequently described a technique of assessing the internal and external sphincter dynamics. Since then, there have been many changes in the techniques of measurement, however, the basic principles of anorectal manometry remain the same: measurement of anorectal pressures, reflexive activities of the anal sphincters, and sensation of the rectum.

Although there is no question as to the usefulness of anorectal manometry in understanding anorectal physiology, there has been some concern expressed in the past about the relevance of the multitude of associated anorectal tests used in clinical practice. While it has been suggested that manometry adds little to an experienced examiner's physical (digital) examination (7), it is generally accepted that anorectal manometry is more accurate and provides important additional information regarding the defecatory mechanism. Several studies have shown that manometry is both accurate and reproducible (8,9), and there is evidence that anorectal manometry can be helpful in the evaluation and treatment of anorectal disorders (10–12). The clinician must however, be cognizant of the fact that manometry is a diagnostic tool and the results of this study must always be taken in the context of the individual patient's clinical problem.

2.3. Basic Principles

Manometry is a technique of measuring pressures, whether in the esophagus, sphincter of Oddi, or the anorectal area. The pressures of the rectum and anal canal, both active and passive, are measured, using anorectal manometry. Although there are various different types of manometric pressure recording machines, the basic equipment essentially consists of a catheter device, inserted into the rectum, to record the pressures applied by the rectum and anal canal, and a transducer to convert this pressure into electrical units and represent it numerically or graphically on a computer or polygraph recorder (Fig. 1).

Placing a device in the rectum to measure pressures, is by nature artificial, and some compromise must be made in the physiologic accuracy of the measurements. To minimize this inherent bias however, various different types of pressure recording catheters have been developed over the years. One of the first types of catheters developed is the balloon-type

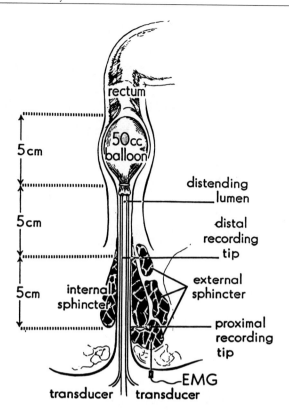

Fig. 1. Schematic drawing illustrating the position of an anorectal manometry catheter within the rectum. The manometric assembly shows the position of the water-perfused open tipped pressure recording port in relation to the anal sphincters. A 50-mL latex balloon is attached to the distal tube for rectal distention for sensory testing and evaluation of rectoanal inhibitory reflex. An EMG needle is shown in the location where external sphincter activity is evaluated. The catheter has multiple recording sites in a radial array providing a circumferential and longitudinal profile of the anal sphincters.

catheter, which consists of two inflatable balloons attached to a central tube and is connected distally to pressure transducers. A polygraph records pressure changes within these balloons when they are inserted into the rectum and inflated with air or water. While this device is effective in measuring sphincter pressures, there are certain drawbacks. Firstly, the balloon catheter is large, bulky to insert, and hence, there is concern that the recordings are affected by the measuring device itself (although in patients with anal fissures this has not been shown to be the case) *(13)*. Secondly, this technique does not provide a sphincteric pressure profile or a circumferential assessment of the sphincteric musculature.

Currently, there are two other major types of catheters used for anorectal manometry. The first is a water-perfused catheter, with a variable number of recording sites. In this catheter, water is perfused through multiple fine tubes at a constant rate via a external pump. Since water is relatively incompressible, resistance to the outflow of water is proportional to the pressure applied to the recording site, and this can be transmitted, via external transducers, to electrical energy and charted on polygraph form. Attached to this catheter is a balloon for inflation, which is used to assess rectal sensation and internal sphincter responses to distention. A photograph of this type of catheter and the water perfusion pump are shown in Figs. 2 and 3.

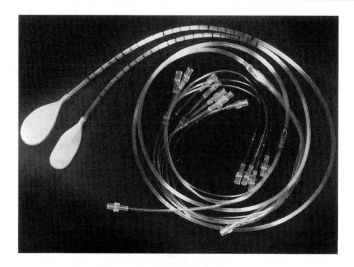

Fig. 2. Water-perfused anorectal manometry catheter (Arndorfer, Greendale, WI) with a radial array of recording sites. The catheter diameter is (2 to 3 mm), and the black marks are spaced at 1.0-cm intervals. A latex balloon is attached to the distal portion of the catheter over a pressure recording port, to assess sensory response and rectal inhibitory reflex during distention.

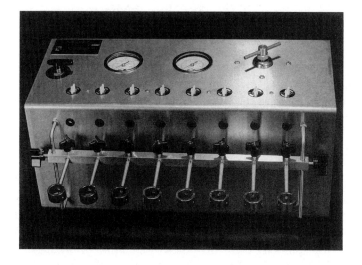

Fig. 3. Anorectal manometry water perfusion pump system. The microcapillary infusion pump (Arndorfer, Greendale, WI) is a low compliance system, which is used to continually infuse the catheter with water at a rate of 0.6 mL/min/tip.

There are many advantages to this type of water perfused device: (i) it can give a profile of sphincter pressures radially as well as longitudinally; (ii) it is relatively easy to set-up and use; and (iii) it is not as costly as some of the other techniques. One disadvantage concerns the possibility that the perfused water may cause stimulation of the anorectal musculature itself.

The other major type of catheter is the microtransducer, or solid state, catheter (14,15). With this catheter, a variable number of recording ports are covered with a thin, pressure-sensitive membrane, which is deformed proportional to the external pressure applied by the overlying anorectal musculature. This pressure change is quantified on the strain gauge transducer, located at the recording site in the catheter itself, and is charted on a polygraph-type device, or computer program. A balloon is attached to the catheter for rectal distention. The microtransducer catheter has a number of the advantages over the water-perfused system, particularly since it avoids the theoretical risk of perfused water stimulating the anal musculature. Unfortunately, these catheters develop more baseline drift, are more prone to breakage, and hence more costly. Studies have shown neither catheter to be clinically superior to the other in clinical practice, and their use is largely based on local institutional expertise and choice. Unfortunately, the lack of standardization of the various types of anorectal manometry catheters makes comparisons of results of different studies quite difficult. As a result of the different catheters and measuring techniques, each individual laboratory should develop its own set of normal parameters for the device it uses, prior to evaluating patients with anorectal abnormalities.

3. CLINICAL ASSESSMENT

3.1. Indications

Although anorectal manometry has been performed as part of the evaluation of a wide range of anorectal and defecatory disorders, in many circumstances, there is little prospective data to substantiate the clinical utility of this test. Generally accepted clinical indications include, evaluation of patients with fecal incontinence or patients with constipation suspected to be related to pelvic floor dysynergy who may benefit from biofeedback therapy. Other less common indications are the detection of Hirshprung's disease, particularly in the adult, and pre- and/or postsurgical evaluation of patients with sphincter trauma.

3.2. History and Physical Examination

Anorectal manometry provides a portion of the total evaluation of a patient with a defecatory disorder. A relevant history and physical examination of the patient will provide important information that will allow focused testing of the individual patient and a more accurate interpretation of the manometric data. The clinical history should determine if the patient's primary problem is constipation or incontinence. This may not be as easy as it sounds. In patients presenting with suspected incontinence, specific questions such as, "Do you lose stool with lifting or straining?", suggest external sphincter dysfunction and may help narrow the diagnostic direction. Childbirth is a strong risk factor for fecal incontinence in women and related information concerning the birth and any associated trauma should be noted. Patients who present with constipation, should be questioned about the frequency of bowel movements, nature and timing of stool, and the need for self-digitations to evacuate stool, which may suggest different categories of constipation (16). Determining what the patient considers abnormal bowel movements, is important. For example, clustered stooling may be interpreted by some patients as constipation and diarrhea by others. In this context, a stool diary is very helpful, since there is often a discrepancy between the patient's reported symptoms and their actual stooling pattern (17).

In addition to a detailed history, physical examination can give a significant amount of useful information in patients with anorectal disorders. Although the techniques of examination of the perineum vary among clinicians, the basic tenets remain the same. Usually the patient is examined in the left lateral decubitus position, with knees and hips flexed. While this position is not physiological, it is most comfortable for both the examiner and patient. On inspection, structural abnormalities such as external hemorrhoidal tissue, fistulae, and previous operative scars are important to observe. On retraction of the buttocks, gaping of the anus is highly suggestive of sphincteric weakness and is sometimes seen in patients with rectal prolapse (18). Asking the patient to bear down and observing the extent of pelvic descent may suggest a cause of incontinence or indicate pelvic floor dysynergia.

Perineal descent has traditionally been quantified radiologically, although a perineometer (19) can be used to approximate this value during physical examination. However, there may be a discrepancy between the values of descent obtained by these two techniques (20). Accepted normal values for perineal descent are between 1–4 cm. Values of perineal descent >4 cm, particularly with ballooning of the perineum with straining, are associated with the descending perineum syndrome, an uncommon cause of incontinence or constipation (21). Perineal descent <1 cm has been associated with pelvic floor dysynergia (22). Rectal prolapse can also be observed but may require sustained valsalva by the patient.

Digital rectal examination is performed to ensure the rectum is free of stool and will allow some assessment of sphincter tone. However the correlation with manometric findings is not very strong (7,23). By asking the patient to squeeze around the examining digit, augmentation of basal pressure by the external sphincter can be assessed. In a study of patients with incontinence, Read et al. (24) showed that there was no significant relationship between clinical assessment of sphincter tone and the maximal squeeze pressure. Another study (25) suggested some correlation between both basal and squeeze pressures measured by manometry and estimated by digital examination, but the authors concluded that digital palpation was a rough approximation of the anal sphincter pressures, and anorectal manometry was required in many clinical situations. An estimation of the propulsive forces of the rectum can be assessed by having the patient attempt to expel the examining digit. The digital examination, is an ideal time to instruct patients on "how" to squeeze the anal sphincter, while avoiding a valsalva maneuver, so they will know what is expected when asked to perform this action during the manometric examination.

3.3. Anorectum: Motility–Manometry

Anorectal manometry records anorectal pressures, both at rest and during activity, both reflexive and voluntary. Although the potential number of tests associated with anorectal manometry is large, many have not been standardized nor prospectively validated. With all these different tests available, it is very important for the clinician to have a specific diagnostic or therapeutic question to answer. Although there is a lack of standardization of manometric techniques, the basic manometric evaluation consists of assessment of basal sphincter pressure, augmented sphincter pressure, rectal sensation and compliance to balloon distention, and demonstration of the rectoanal inhibitory reflex.

3.3.1. RESTING ANAL PRESSURE

Resting anal pressure is measured by either a pull through of the sphincter zone with the manometric catheter, or by a stationary recording of the sphincter with the catheter placed at the "high pressure point". Both methods supply information about the internal (involuntary) anal sphincter. While these techniques largely record the internal anal sphincter pressure, a quarter to half of the pressure may, in fact, be contributed by the external anal sphincter (4,26). Both rapid and station pull through have been used to assess the resting sphincter, depending on the speed of withdrawal of the catheter from the rectum. Our laboratory uses a station pull through technique, starting approx 15 cm from the anal verge, and subsequently withdrawing the catheter in 0.5 cm segments at 30-s intervals. The other

INTERNAL ANAL SPHINCTER PRESSURE PROFILE
Station Pull Thru without Voluntary Squeeze

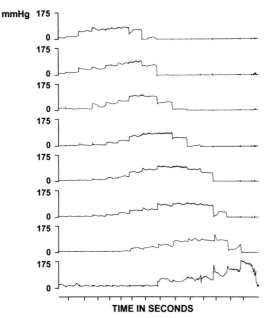

TIME IN SECONDS

Fig. 4. Internal anal sphincter pressure profile by a catheter station pull through without squeeze. This manometric tracing demonstrates the basal (internal) sphincter pressure profile by a station pull through technique. The basal pressure is determined as the arithmetic mean of the maximal pressures in each recording channel. The length of the "high pressure zone" can approximate anal sphincter length. Radial asymmetry of the anal sphincter tracing may suggest "keyhole" sphincteric defects.

anorectal manometry techniques, including the stationary method, also give reasonable resting pressure measurements *(27)*.

Using a catheter with a radial array of recording sites, allows for an assessment not only of the maximal pressure in the anal sphincter zone, but also provides an approximation of the radial profile of the sphincter (Fig. 4). Low pressures recorded from one site in the circumferential pressure profile may indicate weakness in this sphincter location, which can be fully assessed by endoscopic ultrasonography. An estimate of the relative sphincter length can also be obtained by performing a pull-through of the sphincter zone. In general, men appear to have a longer anal canal and higher sphincter pressures compared to women, which may reflect greater muscle mass *(28)*. Our laboratory values obtained by anorectal manometry are shown in Table 1.

3.3.2. VOLUNTARY CONTRACTION

Manometric testing provides some objective evidence of the ability of the patient to augment basal sphincter pressure (voluntary contraction of the external sphincter [Figs. 5 and 6]). During this portion of testing, the patient is asked to augment resting sphincter pressure by squeezing the external sphincter around the indwelling manometric catheter. This maneuver measures the strength of the external sphincter, which is tonically contracted at rest, (like the orbicularis oculi). The external sphincter undergoes reflexive phasic contraction with increases in intrabdominal pressure, and reflexive relaxation with balloon distention *(4)*.

Table 1
Normal Anorectal Manometry Values[a]

Parameter		
Basal sphincter pressure		95.9 ± 21.2 (mmHg + SD)
Augmented (squeeze) sphincter pressure	Male	108.2 ± 47.2 (mmHg + SD)
	Females	45.0 ± 20.0 (mmHg + SD)
Length of anal canal		4.02 ± 0.57 cm
Threshold for sensation to rectal distention		33 ± 21.0 (mL + SD)
Rectal compliance		15 – 30.0 (mL/mmHg)

[a]Manometric values measured with a low compliance water perfused catheter system (from the author's laboratory). SD, standard deviation.

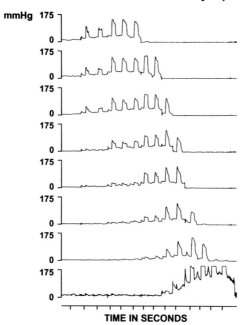

INTERNAL ANAL SPHINCTER PRESSURE PROFILE
Station Pull Thru with Voluntary Squeeze

TIME IN SECONDS

Fig. 5. Augmented (external) sphincter pressure during station pull through technique. Augmented (squeeze) station during pull through of the anal sphincter is performed by asking the patient to maximally squeeze the anal sphincter at each station. The difference between the augmented pressure and basal pressure is assumed to be the contribution of the external sphincter to the continence mechanism. However, the clinical utility of this test is limited, because it is solely dependent upon the patient's understanding and effort (see text).

While studies have shown that measurement of voluntary contraction gives a reasonable estimate of the patient's external sphincter function (and possibly the puborectalis muscle), the test is definitely effort-dependent. Often the patient may not comprehend the instructions to "squeeze" or may be socially inhibited from performing the maneuver. Sometimes the external sphincter contraction is augmented during balloon distention, or when the patient coughs, to a "higher" sphincteric pressure amplitude than that recorded during the testing period when the patient is "requested" to squeeze.

MAXIMAL VOLUNTARY SQUEEZE (EXTERNAL) SPHINCTER PRESSURE

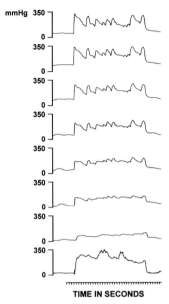

TIME IN SECONDS

Fig. 6. Maximal augmented (squeeze) sphincter pressure. This test is performed with the maximal number of recording channels in the anal canal and demonstrates the patient's ability to augment basal sphincter pressure by maximally squeezing the voluntary sphincter. The test is highly effort-dependent and, uniformly, will demonstrate fatigue with a decline in pressure over time.

There is evidence that the external sphincter pressure decreases with age, particularly in women *(29)*. The reason for this is not entirely clear, but it has been hypothesized that chronic injury or stress, possibly related to childbirth or chronic straining due to constipation *(30)*, adversely affects the pelvic nerves. The pudendal nerve in particular is susceptible to injury, in these patients, and impairment is demonstrated as an increase in pudendal nerve terminal motor latency. As a result of this nerve injury, there is increased perineal descent and external sphincter muscle weakness *(31)*.

3.3.3. RECTAL ANAL INHIBITORY REFLEX

Balloon distention is performed to assess the sensitivity of the rectum to pressure; this method illicits an anorectal inhibitory reflex. This reflex was first described by Gowers in 1877 *(5)* and is a reflexive relaxation of the internal sphincter with rectal distention. The rectal anal inhibitory reflex can be elicited with as little 5 mL of balloon distention, and the relaxation increases as the volume of distention increases *(32)*. In order to maintain continence, the external sphincter contracts while the internal sphincter relaxes, during which time the internal sphincter spontaneously recovers its basal tone. It is hypothesized that the reflex is a sensing mechanism to determine if gas or stool is the cause for the rectal distention. The rectal anal inhibitory reflex is a true reflex in the sense that it is present in patients with spinal cord transection and, in fact, is likely enteric, because patients who have undergone sacral rhizotomy, have this reflex, though it may be modified by descending spinal pathways *(33)*. Importantly it has been shown that this reflex is absent in patients with Hirshprung's, and may be useful in detecting adults with a short segment aganglionosis *(34)*.

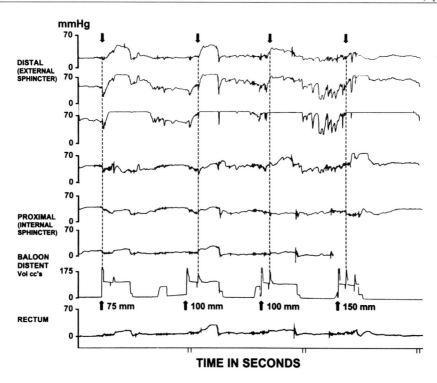

Fig. 7. Anorectal pressures during balloon distensions. The manometric catheter is positioned with the maximal number of recording sites in the anal canal and the rectal balloon is inflated with progressively larger vol. Key assessments during this phase of testing include: (i) the relaxation of the internal sphincter or rectoanal inhibitory reflex (RAIR); and (ii) sensory testing by eliciting patient's sensory response to distention (i.e., gas, urge to move bowels, pain). The arrows at the top of this figure demonstrate paradoxical sphincter contraction with balloon distention, which may be seen in patients with anismus.

3.3.4. RECTAL BALLOON DISTENTION: RECTAL COMPLIANCE

An important test performed during anorectal manometry is evaluation of anorectal responses to rectal balloon distention (Fig. 7). In addition to eliciting the rectal anal inhibitory reflex (described in Subheading 3.3.3.), assessment of the patient's sensory response to rectal distention, and calculations of rectal compliance can be obtained. In our laboratory, we perform balloon inflations, in duplicate, with vol ranging from 5–150 mL, in stepwise increments, and ask patients to describe their initial and subsequent sensations, and to indicate when they experience an urge which would prompt them to consider defecation. The majority of our normal volunteers will have an urge to eliminate when balloon vol between 30–50 mL are attained. Patients with constipation often do not have an urge to stool until much higher balloon vol are reached. On the other hand, some patients with incontinence or irritable bowel syndrome *(35)*, appear to have a hypersensitive rectum with sensory responses to low volumes of balloon distention. Patients with spinal cord injury, or diabetes may have impaired sensation as a result of sensory neuropathy, and this may contribute to their problems of incontinence or constipation.

Rectal compliance is routinely assessed in patients with anorectal disorders during our manometric assessment. In physical terms, compliance is the change in pressure per unit change in vol, and in the rectum, gives some indication of the distensibility of the rectum

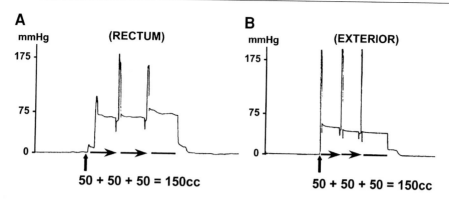

Fig. 8. Intraballoon pressures recording inside and outside rectum to determine rectal compliance measurements. Rectal compliance is assessed by calculating the difference between the intraballoon pressure (A) inside and (B) outside the patient's rectum at various inflation volumes. In this tracing, the rectal compliance is 25 mL/mmHg. The mathematical correction is made for the resistance of the balloon itself. Values of rectal compliance obtained by this method reflect the intrinsic distensibility of the rectal walls and surrounding tissues.

(Fig. 8). The greater the compliance, the more accommodating the rectal ampulla and vice versa. Rectal tone is a measure of the contractile state of the rectum. Conditions associated with decreased compliance include inflammatory bowel disease and radiation proctitis, whereas conditions with increased compliance include severe constipation associated with megacolon. Rao et al. *(36)* showed that patients with active ulcerative proctitis could not tolerate intrarectal balloon pressures that were tolerated by patients with quiescent colitis or normal individuals. In the patient group with active colitis, only half of the patients could tolerate vol of 150 mL while all of the normal subjects and 76% of the patients with quiescent colitis could tolerate this.

While this intuitively makes sense, reported values of normal rectal compliance vary considerably (6–20 mL/cm H_2O *[37]*) and there appears to be considerable overlap in rectal compliance measurements associated with different disorders. Somewhat counterintuitive findings, such as decreased rectal compliance in patients with constipation or increased rectal compliance in patients with incontinence can cause diagnostic confusion as to the underlying defecatory disorder and lack clear physiologic explanation.

Clearly intrarectal balloon pressure is a surrogate marker of presumed wall tension of the rectum, and it is based on certain assumptions that may or may not be valid. Anatomic variations in the rectum, the intrinsic compliance of the balloon, the contribution of the various structures that comprise the rectal wall, and the rectum's intrinsic ability to accommodate changes in vol with time, all may have an influence on the measured value of rectal pressure with balloon distention *(38)*. For example, a long cylindrical rectum vs a short more spherical rectum may have different compliance values, if the same type of balloon is used in each study. Factors, such as the rate of inflation and the order of balloon distention, may also alter the patient's sensory response, as well as the compliance measurements *(39)*. Currently, the value of rectal compliance assessed manometrically has not been evaluated prospectively in patients with various noninflammatory conditions. The overall role of rectal compliance obtained by manometric balloon studies in clinical management of patients with anorectal disorders remains unclear.

4. OTHER TESTS

In addition to the routine investigations outlined above, a number of other tests can be performed during manometric study. In many cases, these clinical tests have not been shown to be universally useful, though they are often utilized in research studies, or in special clinical circumstances.

4.1. Balloon Expulsion Tests

Rectal balloon expulsion tests assess the ability of the patient to coordinate muscle contraction and relax the anal sphincters in order to pass a partially inflated balloon, i.e., a substitute for stool. This test is most often performed in patients with a history of constipation. The balloon expulsion test may also be helpful in identifying patients with obstructive defecation who would benefit from biofeedback therapy. Barnes and Lennard-Jones (40) evaluated 39 patients with both slow and normal transit constipation and compared the results to those of normal control subjects, in their ability to pass balloons inflated with 50, 100, and 150 mL of water. While all of the controls could successfully pass these balloons, most of the patients with constipation were not able to expel the balloon. In another study of patients with functional obstructed defecation determined by defecography, more than half (57%) of the patients could not pass a 60 mL filled balloon. Interestingly, there was no difference in manometric values between these patients and those who could not pass the balloon (41). In another investigator's experience, a 60 mL balloon could be expelled by most healthy patients within 60 s, with minimal elevation of abdominal pressure (42).

Other studies suggest that the balloon expulsion tests do not discriminate as well between patients with constipation and normal controls. Rao et al. (43) reported that 89% of patients with obstructed defecation, 23% of patients with nonobstructive defecation, and 16% of normals could not expel a 50 mL inflated balloon from the rectum. In our experience however, many patients referred for anorectal evaluation are unable to expel a 50 mL balloon, regardless of their diagnosis, so that this maneuver is not a very discriminatory test in our hands.

4.2. Saline Continence Test

Assessment of the ability of the anal sphincter to remain competent during the stress of a stool filled rectum bearing down from above has been approximated in patients with suspected anorectal incontinence, initially with a solid sphere and attached weights (44) and subsequently with a rectal saline load, to simulate a watery load (diarrhea) (24). A catheter is placed in the rectum, and with the patient in the seated position, isotonic saline is infused into the rectum at a rate of 60 mL/min. The patient is asked to retain the saline until a total of 800–1500 mL is infused. Measurements of the time and vol to first leakage, and the total vol retained are obtained. The saline continence test is used largely to assess patients who have incontinence only when stressed with large amounts of liquid stools. An abnormal saline continence test with leakage before 500 ml of saline is infused occurs in the majority of patients with anorectal incontinence. The ability to retain a saline load within the rectum is also reduced with advancing age and in women. However, patients with normal anal sphincter function in the appropriate situation can develop incontinence with diarrhea, suggesting that anal sphincter muscle weakness is not the only factor in determining whether or not a patient will develop incontinence when a large amount of liquid stool is rapidly presented to the distal colon. The saline continence test does not differentiate which factors may be responsible for liquid incontinence, and its usefulness as a clinical test is questionable.

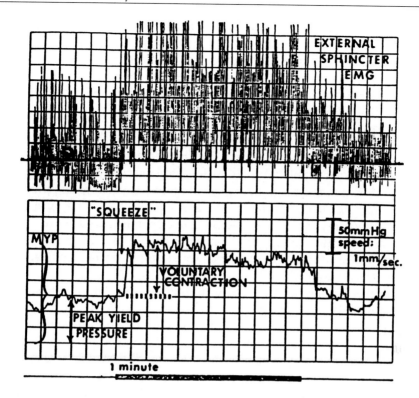

Fig. 9. External sphincter EMG tracing. Simultaneous cutaneous EMG and anorectal manometry of the anal canal during voluntary squeeze.

4.3. Nonmanometric Tests

4.3.1. ELECTROMYOGRAPHY–NERVE LATENCY STUDIES

Electrophysiologic techniques for evaluation of anal continence have been used for over half a century (45). These techniques have found use in assessing the function of the striated muscle of the external sphincter and pudendal nerve (46). Conventional needle electromyography (EMG) can be used to assess the external sphincter and puborectalis muscle by inserting the needle percutaneously to the side of the anal canal and recording basal muscle electrical activity and changes that occur with cough, strain, and voluntary contraction (Fig. 9). Using a similar technique, single fiber EMG is able to assess fiber density, a marker of muscle denervation, which is decreased in some patients with incontinence (47). Pudendal nerve terminal motor latency (PNTML) measurements assess the response of this nerve to electrical stimulation. This study is done with a specially designed finger device comprised of a stimulating electrode at the tip and a recording plate at the base, which is inserted into the anal canal, to record the time required for the impulse to travel this fixed distance. Slowed conduction has been demonstrated in patients with idiopathic fecal incontinence (48), particularly those patients with both urinary and fecal incontinence (49). Nerve stimulation tests can be uncomfortable for the patient (46), and the overall clinical usefulness of these tests has been questioned. In fact in a study by Wexner et al. (50), 13% of the incontinent patients studied with EMG/PNTML had normal testing, while 32% of constipated patients had normal testing. Similarly, 15% of patients with abnormal EMG and up to 43% of patients with abnormal PTNML measurements had normal basal or squeeze sphincter pressures. In another study, severity of striated anal sphincter muscle denervation did not correlate with significant abnormalities in anorectal manometry testing or fecal incontinence *(51)*. On the other hand, a study by Sorensen et al. *(52)* showed good correlation between EMG and manometric finding of the external sphincter. As a result of these inconclusive findings and with newer technologies, including endoanal ultrasound, to "map" out the anatomy of the anal sphincter, the exact role of EMG/PTNML measurements in anorectal physiologic evaluation remains elusive.

4.3.2. DEFECOGRAPHY: EVACUATION PROCTOGRAPHY

Defecography is a radiologic technique for evaluating defecatory morphodynamics *(53)*. The technique involves the use of 150 mL of barium paste inserted into the rectum. The patient is instructed to sit on a commode while cineradiography is performed during the patient's attempt to defecate *(54)*. Defecography may be useful in detecting a physical cause of outlet obstruction that occurs only during defecation. The main parameters assessed are the anorectal angulation, perineal descent, and the development of rectoceles, enteroceles, or intussusception formation *(55)*. Rectoceles are often discovered on physical examination and may be confirmed with defecography *(56,57)*.

Unfortunately, there is significant overlap in the findings with defecography in patients with abnormal defecation and those with normal defecation. Certain findings such as small rectoceles are often seen in normal patients, therefore, the significance of this finding is questionable. Similarly, perineal descent > 3 cm, which is considered the upper limit of normal *(58)* can been seen in about a quarter of normal women during straining *(57)*. Another study showed significant variation in the measurement of perineal descent and anorectal angle measurements that has been reported in the literature *(59)*. A separate study showed that, while increased pelvic floor descent correlated with childbirth, there was no difference in descent between patients with obstructed defecation, incontinence, or idiopathic pain *(60)*. Due to the variability in findings, defecography is often used in conjunction with anorectal manometry.

4.3.3. ENDOSCOPIC ULTRASOUND

Endoanal ultrasound is a relatively new device used in evaluation of anorectal disorders *(61)*. In many respects it has revolutionized our ability to assess the structure and integrity of the internal and external sphincters. The detail of this technology is beyond the scope of this chapter. Endoanal sonography detects unsuspected abnormalities in many patients *(62)*. The findings on endoanal sonography correlate well with concentric EMG, which has traditionally been the "gold standard" for assessment of functional sphincter muscle defects *(63)*. The technique is useful in detecting abnormalities in patients with sphincter hypertrophy, fistulae, incontinence, or myopathies. The endoanal ultrasound procedure has dramatically improved our ability to characterize structural anorectal abnormalities in patients with fecal incontinence. In many instances there is good correlation between the findings on endosonography and anorectal manometry. However, the morphology of the anal sphincters seen on ultrasound does not always correlate with manometric findings obtained in incontinent patients; hence both diagnostic modalities are often complementary *(64,65)*.

5. CLINICAL ISSUES TO BE EVALUATED BY ANORECTAL MANOMETRY

5.1. Constipation

Constipation is a difficult condition to define. In various patients, infrequency of bowel movements, hard stools, straining at stool, or a feeling of incomplete evacuation may all be referred to as "constipation". Traditionally, idiopathic constipation has been categorized into three separate categories depending on the predominant mechanism: slow transit or colonic inertia, pelvic floor dysfunction, and a combination of the two. Differentiation between these categories is important, particularly since the treatment regimens for each can be very different. Symptoms of excessive straining, difficulty passing liquid or soft stool, and self-digitations for evacuation are suggestive of pelvic floor dysfunction, which can be further evaluated with anorectal manometry. Anorectal manometry is also useful in excluding Hirschprung's as a cause of chronic constipation. Patients with Hirschprung's do not demonstrate a rectoanal inhibitory reflex, and this finding can be diagnostic of this condition in the appropriate clinical presentation *(66)*.

The majority of patients with constipation will not have any significant abnormality demonstrated by anorectal manometry. Most constipated patients do not have significantly different basal and augmented sphincter pressures compared to normals *(67,68)*. Even at a tertiary center, up to a quarter of patients referred for evaluation of constipation did not have any sphincteric abnormalities *(69)*. Studies suggest that constipated patients, particularly those with slow transit, have diminished sensitivity to rectal balloon distention in producing a defecatory urge *(67,70–72)*.

The other manometric finding in patients with constipation is that of pelvic floor dysynergia. In this situation, when the patient strains to have a bowel movement, relaxation of the pelvic floor and external sphincter and puborectalis in particular, fails to occur normally. This phenomenon is referred to as anismus or obstructed defecation pattern. In patients with anismus, a paradoxical contraction of the external sphincter is present, which results in a functional obstruction to normal defecation *(73)* (Fig. 6). While this phenomenon can be demonstrated by various methods, including EMG and defecography, it can be shown manometrically as a demonstrable pressure increase in the anal canal with attempted defecation and inability to pass a inflated balloon. Rao et al. *(43)* have attempted to quantify this problem by means of a defecatory index, which is the ratio of the rectal pressure with straining to the anal residual pressure. Index values of <1 or 1.5 are seen in patients with obstructed defecation. This index takes into account three potential mechanisms of anismus; weak propulsive force of the rectum, paradoxical anal sphincter contraction, and failure of normal anal canal relaxation, all of which can be seen in both constipated and normal patients to varying degrees. Identifying patients with anismus is important, since they may not respond to laxatives *(74)*, but may benefit from biofeedback.

Patients who may be undergoing colectomy for management of severe constipation should have anorectal manometric study prior to surgery to evaluate slow transit vs obstructed defecation. However, results of this test are not always predictive of a successful postoperative outcome *(75)*. Patients who fail to respond after colectomy often have severe obstructive defecation or significant psychologic overlay associated with their constipation symptoms *(75,76)*.

5.2. Anal Pain

There are two types of anorectal pain syndromes; a levator ani syndrome and proctalgia fugax. In the levator ani syndrome, a dull aching pain is described in the rectum, which can last for hours to days with no obvious pathology. Proctalgia fugax is a sudden pain in the anal area that lasts for brief periods of time and is also not associated with any obvious pathology. In general, most patients with these complaints are evaluated with anorectal manometry to rule out other diseases. However, anorectal manometry does not play a significant role in elucidating the cause of pain in these patients *(77)*. A unique group of patients with obstructed defecation and proctalgia fugax were described by Kamm et al. *(78)*. These patients had an elevated anal canal pressure and a thickened internal anal sphincter on anal endosonography, thought to be secondary to a hereditary myopathy. A subsequent study of patients with obstructed defecation showed a thickened internal anal sphincter in a small subset of the group *(79)*.

5.3. Incontinence

Fecal incontinence is probably the condition in which anorectal manometry has its greatest diagnostic usefulness. Fecal incontinence has been reported in 3–8% of the population *(1,80,81)*, although this must be elicited on individual questioning, as patients are often reluctant to divulge this information on their own. Since the maintenance of continence is a complex process, many different abnormalities can impact on the continence mechanism and lead to this symptom.

The etiology of fecal incontinence can be classified into structural and functional abnormalities of the pelvic floor. Diarrheal states, and fecal impaction can overwhelm normal anal continence mechanisms resulting in "overflow" fecal incontinence. Patients with structural sphincteric abnormalities, e.g., accidental trauma, obstetric injury, or anorectal surgery, have weakness of the anal sphincters, which can lead to incontinence. Various neurologic conditions, for example diabetes mellitus and spinal cord injuries, can impair not only the muscular function of the anal sphincters, but can also alter anorectal sensation, resulting in incontinence due to a combination of disorders.

Idiopathic fecal incontinence affects females primarily and is thought to result from pelvic floor denervation. The cause for pelvic floor denervation is hypothesized to be trauma to the pelvic nerves during vaginal delivery, chronic straining at stool, and rectal prolapse. The injury to the pelvic nerves may result in weakness of the external anal sphincter, and hence, episodes of incontinence. Recently, there is evidence that chronic straining may not result in eventual external sphincter weakness. In a study by Womack et al. *(82)* evaluating patients with increased perineal descent, the only difference between patients with and without incontinence was the basal anal sphincter pressure and rectal compliance, questioning whether chronic traction on the pelvic nerves is responsible for external sphincter weakness and incontinence.

Although patients with an obvious cause for their incontinence, i.e., sphincteric trauma, typically have weak sphincter tone confirmed on anorectal manometry study, those patients with idiopathic incontinence often have diverse manometric findings. The mechanism of fecal incontinence in the majority of patients with idiopathic fecal incontinence is frequently multifactorial, encompassing both sensory and motor deficits *(83,84)*. A study by Allen et al. *(85)* compared 14 normal age- and sex-matched controls with 14 incontinent patients and 14 younger normals. They found no significant difference in the squeeze pressures between continent and incontinent patients. However, they did note a significantly decreased vol at first leak to a saline load in incontinent patients compared with continent subjects. The incontinent patients also appeared to sense rectal distention at higher balloon inflation vol than did the continent patients, suggesting that impaired rectal sensation may be an important factor in their disorder. In a study of 350 patients by Felt-Bersma and Klinkenberg-Knol *(85)*, incontinent patients had lower mean basal and squeeze pressures compared to continent patients, but there was significant overlap in the pressures recorded from both groups. In the same study, it was demonstrated that the saline continence test did not accurately discriminate between the continent and incontinent patients. Interestingly, in this report, the best test to differentiate continent from incontinent patients was the maximal squeeze pressure. In a study by Mchugh and Diamant *(30)* 43% of patients complaining of incontinence had normal anal resting and squeeze pressures, although there was a wide range of normal values.

In patients with fecal incontinence and normal anal sphincter pressures, the rectum has lower vol in response to isobaric distention, suggesting there is some abnormality in the reservoir capacity of the rectum, possibly through aberrant sensory mechanisms *(87,88)*. Some patients with incontinence, who have normal anorectal pressures, may, in fact, have abnormally high pressure peaks in the rectum, which exceed the normal anal canal pressures resulting in incontinence. This increased rectal pressure is independent of rectal compliance or tone *(89)*.

6. SPECIAL CLINICAL SITUATIONS

6.1. Spinal Cord Injury

Patients with spinal cord injuries suffer from significant defecatory difficulties. Most commonly the major problem is chronic constipation. Not uncommonly, fecal impaction occurs with overflow incontinence. Isolated fecal incontinence is less common, but equally distressing. Although the exact pathophysiology is not entirely clear, most spinal cord patients are not able to defecate voluntarily, and rely on reflexive mechanisms and digital manipulation to have a bowel movement. Slow colonic transit, inability to increase abdominal pressure, loss of anal sphincter function all have been implicated as complicating causes of constipation in these patients *(90)*. Tjandra et al. *(91)* showed that spinal cord injury patients not only have lower basal and squeeze anal pressures compared to healthy controls, but have prolonged pudendal nerve terminal motor latency. The combination of these findings, along with fecal impaction with overflow incontinence may account for the major causes of incontinence.

The manometric findings in spinal cord patients depend, to a certain extent, on the location of the spinal cord lesion. In patients with a high spinal cord lesion, impaired rectal sensation and impaired voluntary contraction of the external sphincter are the major abnormalities, although reflexive contraction of the external sphincter remains intact. In patients with a low spinal lesion, low basal pressure and impairment of reflexive contraction of external sphincter account for many episodes of incontinence *(92)*.

6.2. Post Partum Anal Function

Childbirth is a well recognized risk factor for anorectal incontinence. The mechanisms may be both mechanical injury to the anal sphincter or neurologic *(93)* damage during vaginal delivery. With the development of anal endosonography, there is evidence that mechanical injury to the internal and external sphincter, is fairly common, upwards of 90% in one study. Mechanical injury is not always the cause of symptoms however *(94)*. Damon et al. *(95)* showed that even after the first vaginal delivery sphincteric defects are common, but may not be evident symptomatically. In a prospective study by Sultan et al. *(96)*, 35% of primiparous and 44% percent of multiparous women had evidence of a sphincteric deficiencies upwards to 6 mo postpartum. At the same time 13% of primiparous women and 23% of multiparous women had incontinence, most of whom continued to have symptoms. Forceps delivery, prolonged second stage of labor, and high birth weight infants appear to be major risk factors for pelvic floor injury and incontinence in postpartum females *(96–98)*.

Neurologic injury, as suggested by an increase in pudendal nerve terminal motor latency, is fairly common immediately postpartum. However, at 6 mo, this damage improves or returns to normal in many patients. In most cases, this neurologic injury, does not lead to sphincter weakness; structural sphincteric defects are the primary cause of incontinence postpartum. Because the peak incidence of incontinence in women occurs past the reproductive years, clearly, other structural factors are involved, including age-related weakness of the sphincter with aging, and possibly deficient hormonal production associated with menopause *(99)*.

6.3. Biofeedback

Biofeedback is a technique of retraining a learned behavior through reinforcement, or operant conditioning *(100–102)*. There are a wide range of biofeedback techniques and training regimens for both incontinence and constipation, although most involve retraining the patient's defecatory response to anorectal sensory stimuli. The efficacy of biofeedback is difficult to determine, due to the variety of techniques used in different published studies.

In patients with fecal incontinence, a 50–92% reduction in episodes of incontinence have been reported in various studies, although there are some studies that show no benefit from biofeedback *(103)*. A study by Rao et al. *(104)* showed that 1 yr after biofeedback therapy, there was an increase in anal squeeze pressure, duration of squeeze, improved capacity to retain liquids, and a reduction in incontinence episodes. Key parameters in determining success with biofeedback appears to be enhanced anorectal sensation with improvement in the anal sphincter pressures. Often there is no change in the anal sphincter pressures with biofeedback, but decreased is incontinence secondary to improved rectal sensation *(105)*.

Biofeedback has been used to treat patients with constipation considered to be secondary to functional outlet obstruction or pelvic floor dysynergy *(106–108)*. Unlike fecal incontinence, where objective evidence of reduced numbers of episodes of fecal incontinence can be used as a marker of assessing treatment response, constipation often involves more subjective patient responses to treatment. As a result, there is a wide range of published treatment response rates, varying from 18–100%. In patients with constipation, improving the response to certain sensory cues, is as important as changes in anorectal pressures. Rao et al. *(109)* showed that, following biofeedback treatment, there was evidence of improvement in symptoms and improvement of anorectal defecatory dynamics in three-quarters of the patients with obstructed defecation.

In our experience, biofeedback may be helpful in select patients with pelvic floor dysynergy and those with fecal incontinence with intact sensation. However, the durability of the treatment effect is a major drawback. Although many of our patients symptoms improve while undergoing biofeedback, a year or two later they relapse to the pattern of impaired defecation. The long-term results of maintaining constipated patients off laxatives, has been mixed in our experience.

6.4. Diabetes and Fecal Incontinence

Fecal incontinence frequently occurs in patients with diabetes mellitus, particularly those with diarrhea *(110)*. This incontinence is also multifactorial in most patients and complicated by diabetic neuropathy. Abnormal findings in diabetics with fecal incontinence include, impaired rectal sensation, failure of phasic contraction of the external anal sphincter to rectal distention, weak basal and augmented squeeze pressures, and decreased rectal compliance *(37,111,112)*. Treating the diarrhea of diabetics often helps, and in some patients with impaired anorectal sensation, biofeedback has been shown to be useful *(75)*.

7. SUMMARY

Anorectal disorders are socially embarrassing to the patient and are more common than previously suspected. Anorectal manometry is a useful diagnostic tool in the evaluation and management of patients with anorectal disorders. Patients with fecal incontinence and those with pelvic floor dysynergia can benefit from manometric investigation, either to confirm a specific diagnosis or determine those patients who may benefit from biofeedback therapy. Less common indications for anorectal manometry include, detection of adults with Hirshprung's disease and pre- and/or postsurgical evaluation of sphincteric injuries.

A number of different catheters and recording devices are available to perform anorectal manometry. All of these instruments are acceptable for most basic manometric evaluation. Although there are a multitude of potential manometric tests available, many of these tests are useful only in research studies and have not been rigorously validated for routine clinical application. A significant drawback to current manometric evaluation of anorectal function is the lack of standardization of techniques, resulting in different reference ranges of normal. As a result of this variability, comparing results of anorectal manometry studies is difficult. Agreement by investigators on the appropriate standardized equipment and recording techniques for studying anorectal function should be a future priority to eliminate this dilemma.

Besides the further computerization of manometric data recording, the subsequent advances in the clinical usefulness of anorectal manometry will likely occur with combining manometry with some morphologic evaluation of the anal sphincters during simulated defecation, either with endosonography or cineradiography. There remains much to be learned about the defecatory process and the disorders that involve this complex mechanism. Until this information becomes available, the anorectal manometry test is the only key available to unlock a portion of the box which holds the mysteries of constipation and anorectal incontinence.

REFERENCES

1. Drossman DA, Li Z, Andruzzi E, et al. U.S. householder survey of functional gastrointestinal disorders. Prevalence, sociodemography, and health impact. *Dig. Dis. Sci.*, **38** (1993) 1569–1580.
2. Diamant NE, Kamm MA, Wald A, Whitehead WE. American gastroenterologic association medical position on anorectal testing techniques. *Gastroenterology*, **116** (1999) 732–760.
3. Wald A. Fecal incontinence: effective nonsurgical treatments. *Postgrad. Med.*, **80** (1986) 123–130.
4. Whitehead WE, Schuster MM. Anorectal physiology and pathophysiology. *Am. J. Gastroenterol.*, **82** (1987) 487–497.
5. Gowers WR. The automatic action of the sphincter ani. *Proc. R. Soc. Lond.*, **26** (1877) 77–84.
6. Schuster MM, Hendrix TR, Mendeloff AI. The internal anal sphincter response: manometric studies on its normal physiology neural pathways, and alteration in bowel disorders. *J. Clin. Invest.*, **42** (1963) 196–207.
7. Hallan RI, Marzouk DE, Waldron DJ, Womack NR, Williams NS. Comparison of digital and manometric assessment of anal sphincter function. *Br. J. Surg.*, **76** (1989) 973–975.
8. Rogers J, Laurberg S, Misiewicz JJ, Henry MM, Swash M. Anorectal physiology validated: a repeatability study of the motor and sensory tests of anorectal function. *Br. J. Surg.*, **76** (1989) 607–609.
9. Varma JS, Smith AN. Reproducibility of the proctometrogram. *Gut*, **27** (1986) 288–292.
10. Rao SS, Patel RS. How useful are manomteric tests of anorectal function in the management of defecation disorders? *Am. J. Gastroenterol.*, **92** (1997) 469–475.
11. Wexner SD, Jorge JM. Colorectal physiologic tests: use or abuse of technology? *Eur. J. Surg.*, **160** (1994) 167–174.
12. Vaizey CJ, Kamm MA. Prospective assessment of the clinical value of anorectal investigations. *Digestion*, **61** (2000) 207–214.
13. Horvath KD, Whelan RL, Golub RW, Ahsan H, Ciricco WC. Effects of catheter diameter on resting pressures in anal fissure patients. *Dis. Colon Rectum*, **38** (1995) 728–731.
14. Vela AR, Rosenberg AJ. Anorectal manometry: a new simplified technique. *Am. J. Gastroenterol.*, **77** (1982) 486–90.
15. Schouten WR, van Vroonhoven TJ. A simple method of anorectal manometry. *Dis. Colon Rectum*, **26** (1983) 721–724.
16. Mertz H, Naliboff B, Mayer EA. Symptoms and physiology in severe chronic constipation. *Am. J. Gastroenterol.*, **94** (1999) 131–138.
17. Ashraf W, Park F, Lof J, Quigley EM. An examination of the reliability of reported stool frequency in the diagnosis of idiopathic constipation. *Am. J. Gastroenterol.*, **91** (1996) 26–31.
18. Madoff RD, Williams JG, Caushaj PF. Fecal incontinence. *N. Engl. J. Med.*, **326** (1992) 1002–1007.
19. Henry MM, Parks AG, Swash M. The pelvic floor musculature in the descending perineum syndrome. *Br. J. Surg.*, **69** (1982) 470–472.
20. Oettle GJ, Roe AM, Bartolo DC, Mortensen NJ. What is the best way of measuring perineal descent? A comparison of radiographic and clinical methods. *Br. J. Surg.*, **72** (1985) 999–1001.

21. Harewood GC, Coulie B, Camilleri M, Rath-Harvey D, Pemberton JH. Descending perineum syndrome: audit of clinical and laboratory features and outcome of pelvic floor retraining. *Am. J. Gastroenterol.*, **94** (1999) 126–130.

22. Pezim ME, Pemberton JH, Levin KE, Litchy WJ, Phillips SF. Parameters of anorectal and colonic motility in health and severe constipation. *Dis. Colon Rectum*, **36** (1993) 484–491.

23. Eckardt VF, Kanzler G. How reliable is digital examination for the evaluation of anal sphincter tone? *Int. J. Colorectal Dis.*, **8** (1993) 95–97.

24. Read NW, Harford WV, Schmulen AC, Read MG, Ana CS, Fordtran JS. A clinical study of patients with fecal incontinence and diarrhea. *Gastroenterology*, **76** (1979) 747–756.

25. Felt-Bersma RJ, Klinkenberg EC, Meuwissen SG. Investigation of anorectal function. *Br. J. Surg.*, **75** (1988) 53–55.

26. Wong RF, Bonapace ES, Chung CY, Liu JB, Parkman HP, Miller LS. Endoluminal sonography and manomtery to assess anal sphincter complex in normal subjects. *Dig. Dis. Sci.*, **43** (1998) 2362–2372.

27. McHugh SM, Diamant NE. Anal canal pressure profile by reappraisal as determined by rapid pull-through technique. *Gut*, **28** (1987) 1234–1241.

28. Taylor BM, Beart RW, Phillips SF. Longitudinal and radial variations of pressure in the human anal sphincter. *Gastroenterology*, **86** (1984) 693–697.

29. McHugh SM, Diamant NE. Effect of age, gender and parity on anal canal pressures. Contribution of impaired anal sphincter function to fecal incontinence. *Dig. Dis. Sci.*, **32** (1987) 726–736.

30. Laurberg S, Swash M. Effects of aging on the anorectal sphincters and their innervation. *Dis. Colon Rectum*, **32** (1989) 737–742.

31. Snooks SJ, Barnes PR, Swash M, Henry MM. Damage to the innervation of the pelvic floor musculature in chronic constipation. *Gastroenterology*, **89** (1985) 977–981.

32. Sagar PM, Pemberton JH. Anorectal and pelvic floor function. Relevance to continence, incontinence and constipation. *Gastroenterol. Clin. N. Am.*, **25** (1996) 163–184.

33. Sun W, Macdonagh R, Forster D, Thomas DG, Smallwood R, Read NW. Anorectal function in patients with complete spinal transection before and after sacral posterior rhizotomy. *Gastroenterology*, **108** (1995) 990–998.

34. Faverdin C, Dornic C, Arhan P, et al. Quantitative analysis of anorectal pressures in Hirschprung's disease. *Dis. Colon Rectum*, **24** (1981) 422–427.

35. Bradette M, Delvaux M, Staumont G, Fioramonti J, Bueno L, Frexions J. Evaluation of colonic sensory thresholds in IBS patients using a barostat. Definition of optimal conditions and comparison with healthy subjects. *Dig. Dis. Sci.*, **39** (1994) 449–457.

36. Rao SS, Read NW, Davison PA, Bannister JJ, Holdsworth CD. Anorectal sensitivity and responses to rectal distention in patients with ulcerative colitis. *Gastroenterology*, **93** (1987) 1270–1275.

37. Wald A, Tunuguntla K. Anorectal sensorimotor dysfunction in fecal incontinence and diabetes mellitus: modification with biofeedback therapy. *N. Engl. J. Med.*, **310** (1984) 1282–1287.

38. Madoff RD, Orrom WJ, Rothenberger DA, Goldberg SM. Rectal compliance: a critical reappraisal. *Int. J. Colorectal Dis.*, **5** (1990) 37–40.

39. Kendall GP, Thompson DG, Day SJ, Lennard-Jones JE. Inter- and intra-individual variation in pressure-volume relations of the rectum in normal subjects and patients with irritable bowel syndrome. *Gut*, **31** (1990) 1062–1068.

40. Barnes PR, Lennard-Jones JE. Balloon expulsion from the rectum in constipation of different types. *Gut*, **26** (1985) 1049–1052.

41. Fleshman JW, Dreznik Z, Cohen E, Fry RD, Kodner IJ. Balloon expulsion test facilitates diagnosis of pelvic floor outlet obstruction due to non-relaxing puborectalis muscle. *Dis. Colon Rectum*, **35** (1992) 1019–1025.

42. Meunier PD, Gallavardin D. Anorectal manometry: the state of the art. *Dig. Dis.*, **11** (1993) 252–264.

43. Rao SS, Welcher KD, Leistikow JS. Obstructed defecation: failure of rectoanal coordination. *Am. J. Gastroenterol.*, **93** (1998) 1042–1050.

44. Diamant NE, Harris LD. Comparison of objective measurement of anal sphincter strength with anal sphincter pressures and levator ani function. *Gastroenterology*, **56** (1969) 110–116.

45. Cheong DM, Vaccaro CA, Salanga VD, Wexner SD, Phillips RC, Hanson MR. Electrodiagnostic evaluation of fecal incontinence. *Muscle Nerve*, **18** (1995) 612–619.

46. Henry MM. Neuorophysiological assessment of the pelvic floor. *Gut*, **29** (1988) 1–4.

47. Neill ME, Swash MS. Increased motor unit fiber density in the external anal sphincter in ano-rectal incontinence: a single fiber EMG study. *J. Neurol. Neurosurg. Psychiatry*, **43** (1980) 343–347.

48. Kiff ES, Swash M. Slowed conduction in the pudendal nerves in idiopathic (neurogenic) fecal incontinence. *Br. J. Surg.*, **71** (1984) 614–616.

49. Snooks SJ, Barnes PR, Swash M. Damage to the innervation of the voluntary anal and periurethral sphincter musculature in incontinence: an electrophysiologic study. *J. Neurol. Neurosurg. Psychiatry*, **47** (1984) 1269–1273.

50. Wexner SD, Marchetti F, Salanga VD, Corredor C, Jagelman DG. Neurophysiologic assessment of the anal sphincters. *Dis. Colon Rectum*, **34** (1991) 606–612.

51. Infantino A, Melega E, Negrin P, Masin A, Carnio S, Lise M. Striated anal sphincter electromyography in idiopathic fecal incontinence. *Dis. Colon Rectum*, **38** (1995) 27–31.

52. Sorensen M, Tetzschner T, Rasmussen OO, Christiansen J. Relation between electromyography and anal manometry of the external anal sphincter. *Gut*, **32** (1991) 1031–1034.

53. Ekberg O, Mahieu PHG, Bartram CI, Piloni V. Defecography: Dynamic radiological imaging in proctology. *Gastroenterol. Int.*, **3** (1990) 63–69.

54. Mahieu P, Pringot J, Bodart P. Defecography: I. Description of a new procedure and results in normal patients. *Gastrointest. Radiol.*, **9** (1984) 247–251.

55. Mahieu P, Pringot J, Bodart P. Defecography: II. Contribution to the diagnosis of defecation disorders. *Gastrointest. Radiol.*, **9** (1984) 253–261.

56. Bartram CI, Turnbull GK, Lennard-Jones JE. Evacuation proctography: an investigation of rectal expulsion in 20 subjects without defecatory disturbance. *Gastrointest. Radiol.*, **13** (1988) 72–80.

57. Shorvon PJ, McHugh S, Diamant NE, Somers S, Stevenson GW. Defecography in normal volunteers: results and implications. *Gut*, **30** (1989) 1737–1749.

58. Parks AG, Porter NH, Hardcastle J. The syndrome of the descending perineum. *Proc. R. Soc. Med.*, **59** (1966) 477–482.

59. Felt-Bersma RJ, Luth WJ, Janssen JJ, Meuwissen SG. Defecography in patients with anorectal disorders. which findings are clinically relevant? *Dis. Colon Rectum*, **33** (1990) 277–284.

60. Hiltunen KM, Kolehmainen H, Matikainen M. Does defecography help in diagnosis and clinical decision-making in defecation disorders? *Abdom. Imaging*, **19** (1994) 355–358.

61. Law PJ, Bertram CI. Anal endosonography: technique and normal anatomy. *Gastrointest. Radiol.*, **14** (1989) 349–353.

62. Felt-Bersma RJ, Cuesta MA, Koorevaar M, et al. Anal endosonography: relationship with anal manometry and neurophysiologic tests. *Dis. Colon Rectum*, **35** (1992) 944–949.

63. Enck P, Von Giesen HJ, Schafer A, et al. Comparision of anal sonography with conventional needle elec-tromyography in the evaluation of anal sphincter defects. *Am. J. Gastroenterol.*, **91** (1996) 2539–2543.

64. Schafer R, Heyer T, Gantke B, et al. Anal endosonography and manometry: comparison in patients with defecation problems. *Dis. Colon Rectum*, **40** (1997) 293–297.

65. Gantke B, Schafer A, Enck P, Lubke HJ. Sonographic, manometric and myographic evaluation of the anal sphincters morphology and function. *Dis. Colon Rectum*, **36** (1993) 1037–1041.

66. Tobon F, Reid NC, Talbert JL, Schuster MM. Nonsurigcal test for the diagnosis of Hirschprung's disease. *N. Engl. J. Med.*, **278** (1968) 188–194.

67. Read NW, Timms JM, Barfield LJ, Donnelly TC, Bannister JJ. Impairment of defecation in young women with severe constipation. *Gastroenterology*, **90** (1986) 53–60.

68. Glia A, Lindberg G, Nilsson LH, Mihocsa L, Akerlund JE. Constipation assessed on the basis of colorectal physiology. *Scand. J. Gastroenterol.*, **33** (1998) 1273–1279.

69. Mertz H, Naliboff B, Mayer E. Physiology of refractory chronic constipation. *Am. J. Gastroenterol.*, **94** (1999) 609–615.

70. De Medici A, Badiali D, Corazziari E, Bausano G, Anzini F. Rectal sensitivity in chronic constipation. *Dig. Dis. Sci.*, **34** (1989) 747–753.

71. Waldron D, Bowes KL, Kingma YJ, Cote KR. Colonic and anorectal motility in young women with severe idiopathic constipation. *Gastroenterology*, **95** (1988) 1388–1394.

72. Preston DM, Lennard-Jones JE. Severe chronic constipation of young women: "idiopathic" slow transit constipation. *Gut*, **27** (1986) 41–48.

73. Preston DM, Lennard-Jones JE. Anismus in chronic constipation. *Dig. Dis. Sci.*, **30** (1985) 413–418.

74. Turnbull GK, Lennard-Jones JE, Bartram CI. Failure of rectal expulsion as a cause of constipation: why fiber and laxatives sometimes fail. *Lancet*, **1** (1986) 767–769.

75. Kamm MA, Hawley PR, Lennard-Jones JE. Outcome of colectomy for severe idiopathic constipation. *Gut*, **29** (1988) 969–973.

76. Leon SH, Krishnamurthy S, Schuffler MD. Subtotal colectomy for severe idiopathic constipation. *Dig. Dis. Sci.*, **32** (1987) 1249–1254.

77. Whitehead WE, Wald A, Diamant NE, Enck P, Pemberton JH, Rao SS. Functional disorders of the anus and rectum. *Gut*, **45** (1999) II55–II59.

78. Kamm MA, Hoyle CV, Burleigh DE, Law PJ, Swash M et al. Hereditary internal anal sphincter myopathy, causing proctalgia fugax and constipation. *Gastroenterology*, **100** (1991) 805–810.

79. Nielsen MB, Rasmussen OO, Pedersen JF, Christiansen J. Anal endosonography findings in patients with obstructed defecation. *Acta Radiol.*, **34** (1993) 35–38.

80. Talley NJ, O'Keefe EA, Zinsmeister AR, Melton LJ 3d. Prevalence of gastrointestinal symptoms in the elderly: a population based study. *Gastroenterology*, **102** (1992) 895–901.

81. Drossman DA, Sandler RS, Broom CM, McKee DC. Urgency and fecal soiling in people with bowel dysfunction. *Dig. Dis. Sci.*, **31** (1986) 1221–1225.

82. Womack NR, Morrison JFB, Williams NS. The role of pelvic floor denvervation in the etiology of idiopathic fecal incontinence. *Br. J. Surg.*, **73** (1986) 404–407.

83. Sun WM, Donnelly TC, Read NW. Utility of a combined test of anorectal manometry, electromyography and sensation in determining the mechanism of "idiopathic" fecal incontinence. *Gut*, **33** (1992) 807–813.

84. Rogers J, Henry MM, Misiewicz JJ. Combined sensory and motor deficit in primary neuropathic fecal incontinence. *Gut*, **29** (1988) 5–9.

85. Allen ML, Orr WC, Robinson MG. Anorectal functioning in fecal incontinence. *Dig. Dis. Sci.*, **33** (1998) 36–40.

86. Felt-Bersma RJ, Klinkenberg-Knol EC, Meuwissen SG. Anorectal function investigations in incontinent and continent patients. Differences and discriminatory value. *Dis. Colon Rectum*, **33** (1990) 479–486.

87. Siproudhis L, Bellissant E, Pagenault M et al. Fecal incontinence with normal anal canal pressures: where is the pitfall? *Am. J. Gastroenterol.*, **94** (1999) 1556–1563.

88. Siproudhis L, Bellissant E, Juguet F, Allain H, Bretagne J-F, Gosselin M. Perception of and adaptation to rectal isobaric distention in patients with fecal incontinence. *Gut*, **44** (1999) 687–692.

89. Read NW, Haynes WG, Bartolo DC, et al. Use of anorectal manometry during rectal infusion of saline to investigate sphincter function in incontinent patients. *Gastroenterology*, **85** (1983) 105–113.

90. De Looze DA, De Muynck MC, Van Laere M, De Vos MM, Elewaut AG. Pelvic floor function in patients with clinically complete spinal cord injury and its relation to constipation. *Dis. Colon Rectum*, **41** (1998) 778–786.

91. Tjandra JJ, Ooi B, Han WR. Anorectal physiologic testing for bowel dysfunction in patients with spinal cord lesions. *Dis. Colon Rectum*, **43** (2000) 927–931.

92. Sun WM, Read NW, Donnelly TC. Anorectal function in incontinent patients with cerebrospinal disease. *Gastroenterology*, **99** (1990) 1372–1379.

93. Snooks SJ, Setchell M, Swash M, Henry MM. Injury to innervation of pelvic floor musculature in childbirth. *Lancet*, **2** (1984) 546–550.

94. Burnett SJ, Spence-Jones C, Speakman CT, Kamm MA, Hudson CN, Bartram CI. Unsuspected sphincter damage following childbirth revealed by anal sonography. *Br. J. Radiol.*, **64** (1991) 225–227.

95. Damon H, Henry L, Bretones S, Mellier G, Minaire Y, Mion F. Postdelivery anal function in primiparous females. *Dis. Colon Rectum*, **43** (2000) 472–477.

96. Sultan A, Kamm MA, Hudson CN, Thomas JM, Bartram CI. Anal-sphincter disruption during vaginal delivery. *N. Engl. J. Med.*, **329** (1993) 1905–1911.

97. Donnelly V, Fynes M, Campbell D, Johnson H, O'Connell PR, O'Herlihy C. Obstetric events leading to anal sphincter damage. *Obstet. Gynecol.*, **92** (1998) 955–961.

98. Snooks SJ, Swash M, Henry MM, Setchell M. Risk factors in childbirth causing damage to pelvic floor innervation. *Br. J. Surg.*, **72** (1985) S15–S17.

99. Haadem K, Dahlstrom JA, Ling L. Anal sphincter competence in healthy women: clinical implications of age and other factors. *Obstet. Gynecol.*, **78** (1991) 823–827.

100. Engel BT, Nikoomanesh P, Schuster MM. Operant conditioning of rectosphincteric responses in the treatment of fecal incontinence. *N. Engl. J. Med.*, **290** (1974) 646–649.

101. Enck P. Biofeedback training in disordered defecation: a critical review. *Dig. Dis. Sci.*, **38** (1993) 1953–1960.

102. Wald A. Biofeedback therapy for fecal incontinence. *Ann. Intern. Med.*, **95** (1981) 146–149.

103. Loening-Baucke V. Efficacy of biofeedback training in improving fecal incontinence and anorectal physiologic function. *Gut*, **31** (1990) 1395–1402.

104. Rao SS, Welcher KD, Happel J. Can biofeedback therapy improve anorectal function in fecal incontinence? *Am. J. Gastroenterol.*, **91** (1996) 2360–2366.

105. Miner PB, Donnelly TC, Read NW. Investigation of mode of action of biofeedback in treatment of fecal incontinence. *Dig. Dis. Sci.*, **35** (1990) 1291–1298.

106. Kawimbe BM, Papachrysostomou M, Binnie NR, Clare N, Smith AN. Outlet obstruction constipation (anismus) managed by biofeedback. *Gut*, **32** (1991) 1175–1179.

107. Bleijenberg G, Kuijpers HC. Treatment of spastic pelvic floor syndrome with biofeedback. *Dis. Colon Rectum*, **30** (1987) 108–111.

108. Wexner SD, Cheape JD, Jorge JM, Heymen S, Jagelman DG. Prospective assessment of biofeedback for the treatment of paradoxical puborectalis contraction. *Dis. Colon Rectum*, **35** (1992) 145–150.

109. Rao SS, Welcher KD, Pelsang RE. Effects of biofeedback therapy on anorectal function in obstructed defecation. *Dig. Dis. Sci.*, **42** (1997) 2197–2205.

110. Feldman M, Schiller LR. Disorders of gastrointestinal motility associated with diabetes mellitus. *Ann. Intern. Med.*, **98** (1983) 378–384.

111. Sun WM, Katsinelos P, Horowitz M, Read NW. Disturbances in anorectal function in patients with diabetes mellitus and fecal incontinence. *Eur. J. Gastroenterol. Hepatol.*, **8** (1996) 1007–1012.

112. Caruana BJ, Wald A, Hinds JP, Eidelman BH. Anorectal sensory and motor function in neurogenic fecal incontinence: a comparison between multiple sclerosis and diabetes mellitus. *Gastroenterology*, **100** (1991) 465–470.

19 Endoanal and Endorectal Ultrasound

Lisa M. Gangarosa

Contents

1. INTRODUCTION

Ultrasound (US) has long been used as a noninvasive medical imaging technique. In 1957, Wild and Reid introduced the concept of endoluminal sonography by using a mechanical rotating transducer to evaluate the rectum *(1)*. DiMagno and colleagues introduced the first endoscope with an US transducer incorporated into the tip in 1980 *(2)*. Over the last 20 yr, there have been considerable advancements in technology and equipment, and there are now several instruments available for gastrointestinal (GI) tract US, with or without simultaneous endoscopic capability. The purpose of this chapter is to introduce the basics of US as well as some of the most commonly used instruments currently available for endoanal and endorectal US, to review indications for endoanal and endorectal US, and finally to review results of endoanorectal US in major areas of clinical use.

2. ULTRASOUND

US utilizes sound energy. Audible sound for humans is in the 20 Hz to 20 KHz frequency range *(3)*. Medical diagnostic US is typically in the 2–25 MHz range. The higher the frequency, the greater the image resolution. However, frequency varies inversely with depth of penetration. Scanning at 5 MHz allows penetration of about 12 cm; scanning at 10 MHz allows about 6 cm of penetration.

Transmission and reflection of US are required for image formation. A transducer emits the US, which travels in waves through tissue. Each tissue has an inherent property called acoustic impedance. When US travels through a junction of two tissues with differing acoustic impedance, some of the US is reflected. Reflected US, which reaches the transducer, is then converted by a processor into an image. US travels through most human tissues (except bone) at the same speed (1540 m/s). This allows depth to be assessed.

From: *Colonic Diseases*
Edited by: T. R. Koch © Humana Press Inc., Totowa, NJ

There are two types of transducers, which are actually composed of piezoelectric crystals. A mechanical sector scanning transducer has a rotating crystal which produces radial images (180–360°). Linear array transducers have a series of stationary crystals, which produce sector or linear images. Linear array transducers are capable of providing color-flow Doppler information. Real-time US-guided fine-needle aspiration (FNA) is possible with linear array imaging.

US interpretation is both subjective and operator-dependent.

3. EQUIPMENT

There are currently several choices for US equipment that are capable of imaging the anus and/or rectum, and some of those most commonly used will be discussed. Some instruments allow for simultaneous endoscopic viewing (endoscopic US or EUS), while others do not. To best image the anal canal, radial imaging (7–12 MHz) is required. In the rectum, radial and/or linear array imaging (5–12 MHz) can be utilized.

Olympus (Olympus America, Melville, NY) has many products available for EUS, including a forward viewing mechanical sector scanning echocolonoscope (CF-UM20-7.5 or -12) with frequency capability of 7.5 or 12 MHz. These provide a 360° radial US image. The CF-UM20 features a distal tip with a diameter of 17.4 mm and forward viewing capabilities allowing for a 120° field of view. Olympus also has a video echoendoscope (GF-UMQ130), which offers a small distal end diameter of only 12.7 mm. Two models, both radial scanners, with different frequency options are available (7.5/12 MHz or 7.5/20 MHz). Olympus also markets the processor for these instruments (EU-M30). Olympus markets radial scanning ultrasonic probes, UM-2R/3R (12 MHz/20 MHz), which can be passed through any endoscope with a channel diameter of 2.8 mm or more. With these probes, the US exam can be performed during routine endoscopy. Recently Olympus introduced two rigid nonendoscopic rectal US probes, which provide 360° mechanical radial scanning at either 7.5 or 12 MHz (RU-75M-R1 and RU-12M-R1). The latter is designed for evaluating the anus. These are compatible with the Olympus US processor. The company also markets a linear array echoendoscope that scans at 7.5 MHz (GF-UC30P), which must be used with a processor (AI-5200S) made by Acoustic Imaging (Phoenix, AZ). Olympus is in the process of updating all of their EUS scopes.

Pentax (Pentax Precision Instruments, Orangeburg, NY) first introduced a forward oblique viewing linear array echoendoscope in the early 1990s. Scanning can be done at 5 or 7.5 MHz (FG-36UX). Hitachi (Hitachi Medical, Tarrytown, NY) manufactures the compatible US processor (EUB 525).

Bruel and Kjaer (Naerum, Denmark) produces a rigid, nonendoscopic anorectal probe system (probe Type1850, scanner Type 1846 or 3535), which provides 360° mechanical radial scanning at 7 or 10 MHz.

Fuginon (Fuginon, Wayne, NJ) produces a series (SP-501) of ultrasonic probes (of varying frequencies) that can be passed through the working channel of colonoscopes, as well as a 7.5 MHz "front loaded" probe (SP-701 PL B-7.5). These can scan both radially and linearly.

4. NORMAL US IMAGING OF THE RECTUM AND ANUS

The rectal wall is composed of mucosa, submucosa, muscularis propria, and perirectal fat–serosa. When imaged at 5–12 MHz, five layers of alternating hyper- and hypo-echogenicity are seen (Fig. 1).

The anal canal and sphincters are more complex (Fig. 2). The anal canal is 2.5–4 cm long and is typically divided into three areas: the upper part, with 6–12 longitudinal folds called anal columns; the lower portion, with internal and external sphincters, and the opening itself. The

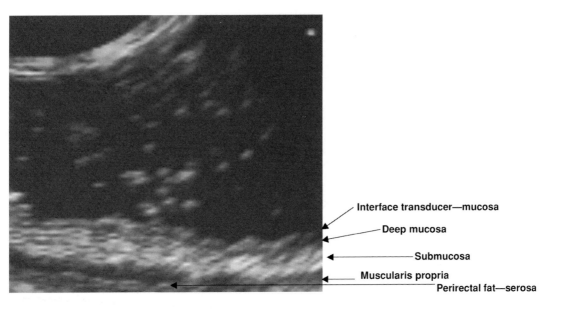

Interface transducer—mucosa

Deep mucosa

Submucosa

Muscularis propria

Perirectal fat—serosa

Fig. 1. Normal layers of rectal wall seen with linear array echoendoscope at 7.5 MHz.

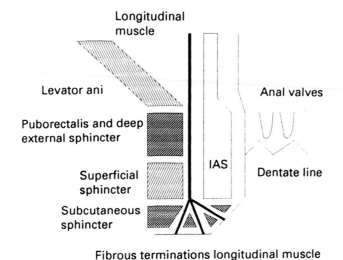

Longitudinal muscle

Levator ani

Puborectalis and deep external sphincter

Superficial sphincter

Subcutaneous sphincter

Anal valves

IAS

Dentate line

Fibrous terminations longitudinal muscle

Fig. 2. Diagram of coronal view of anal canal. Reproduced with permission from ref. *4.*

anal canal connects with the rectum at the point where it passes through the levator ani muscles. The upper region's columns contain the internal hemorrhoidal plexus. The lower portions of the anal columns are joined by small concentric circular folds of skin to form anal valves just above the dentate line. Below the dentate line, the anal canal is lined by squamous epithelium that lacks hair follicles or glands. The epithelium then becomes a keratinized layer of squamous mucosa containing hair follicles and glands and is continuous with the skin of the rest of the body. The lower anal canal and the anal opening are composed of two muscular sphincters. The

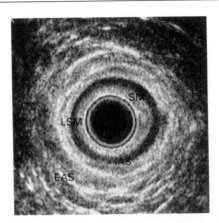

■ EAS (heterogenous) = External anal sphincter   ■ IAS = Internal and sphincter
□ SM =Subepithelial layer   □ LSM = Longitudinal muscle

Fig. 3. Normal layers of anal canal seen with radial probe. Reproduced with permission from ref. *4.*

internal anal sphincter (IAS) is composed of concentric layers of circular smooth muscle continuous with the muscularis propria of the rectum. The external anal sphincter (EAS) is composed of striated muscle encircling the outside wall of the anal canal and anal opening and is innervated by the pudendal nerve *(4)*.

US imaging of the anal canal also results in an alternating pattern of hyper- and hypo-echogenic layers (Fig. 3).

In a study comparing endoanal US in cadavers with anatomic cross sections *(5)*, the IAS was seen as an asymmetric hypoechoic ring, thickest ventrally. The EAS was heterogenous and thickest dorsally. In four out of seven cadavers, a thin hyperechoic layer felt to represent the "intersphincteric" space separated the two sphincters. Histologically, no intersphincteric space was identified. Longitudinal (smooth) muscle was found between the IAS and EAS. No significant difference in IAS volume was found between US measurements and anatomic measurements (105.76 ± 14.22 mm^3 vs 110.88 ± 13.45 mm^3). However, US overestimated the EAS volume, which the authors felt was secondary to the inability to clearly delineate the longitudinal muscle layer on US.

5. INDICATIONS FOR ANORECTAL US IN PRACTICE

Despite the fact that most published studies on endoanal US involve small numbers of patients, the following have become widely accepted indications for endoanal US: (i) evaluating the sphincters for defects in patients with fecal incontinence; (ii) evaluating peri-anal fistulas and abscesses; and (iii) staging anal neoplasia. Indications for rectal EUS are the following: (i) preoperative rectal cancer staging with or without perirectal lymph node FNA; (ii) evaluation of a submucosal rectal lesions; and (iii) evaluation of perirectal pelvic disease. Contraindications to endoanorectal US are the following: (i) lack of patient cooperation; (ii) known or suspected perforated viscus; (iii) acute diverticulitis; (iv) fulminant colitis; (v) lack of experienced endosonographer; and (vi) unstable cardiac or pulmonary conditions *(6)*. Endoanorectal US is safe. In an international retrospective survey of 4190 lower EUS exams, two bleeding (0.05%) complications were reported *(7)*.

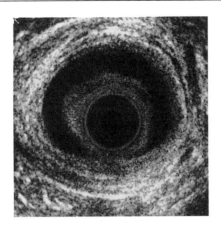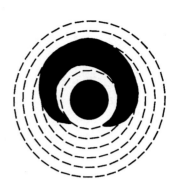

Fig. 4. A lateral sphincterotomy results in the defect seen on the left side of the internal sphincter. Reproduced with permission from ref. *4*.

5.1. Fecal Incontinence

Fecal incontinence can be due to anatomic sphincter abnormalities, including those resulting from obstetrical trauma, surgery, or perineal injury. Endoanal US can image both sphincters simultaneously, detect anatomic abnormalities if present, and, thus, identify potentially correctable injuries. Defects are recognized by replacement of the normal echogenic pattern by a segment of altered echogenicity (Fig. 4).

Endoanal US has largely replaced needle electromyography as test of choice to delineate sphincter defects because of efficacy and patient comfort *(8–10)*. Sensitivity and specificity for detection of defects with endoanal US (as compared to either surgical or histological findings) are 95–100% and 75–100%, respectively *(11–15)*. In a prospective study of 53 Australian patients with fecal incontinence, 42 were found to have abnormal sphincteric appearance on endoanal US *(16)*. Of these, two-thirds were found to have anterior EAS (± IAS) defects consistent with obstetrical trauma. Other causes of sphincter abnormalities that were identified included sphincterotomy (14%), fistula (10%), abscess, fissure excision, and prior repair breakdown (all <5%).

A triad of lesions specific to obstetrical trauma has been identified by endoanal US: right anterolateral external defects, right anterolateral internal defects, and disruption of perineal body *(4)* (Figs. 5 and 6).

Two prospective studies of anal US before and after vaginal delivery have been performed *(17,18)*. The first from London *(17)* studied 100 primiparous and 50 multiparous women 6 wk prior and 6 wk after delivery with symptom questionnaires, anal endosonography, and additional neurophysiologic testing. Predelivery, none of the primiparous women had anal sphincter defects on anal US. After delivery, 35% were found to have defects of one or both sphincters, though only 13% of the primiparous women complained of new bowel symptoms (fecal urgency and/or incontinence). Of the multiparous women, 40% had sphincter defects found by anal US prior to delivery (19% complained of bowel symptoms), and 6% had new symptoms after delivery (all three of these women had combined sphincter defects, and in two out of three, these were new). Sphincter defects developed in 8 out of 10 primiparous women that underwent forceps delivery.

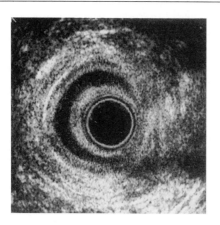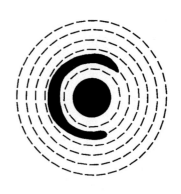

Fig. 5. Anterior defect secondary to traumatic forceps delivery. Reproduced with permission from ref. *4.*

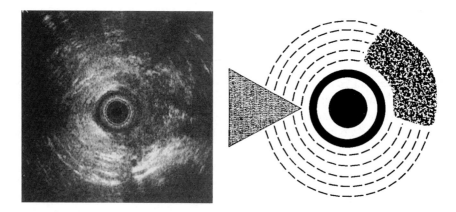

Fig. 6. Hypoechoic defect in the right anterolateral quadrant of external sphincter. Reproduced with permission from ref. *4.*

The second study from France *(18)* also studied women with questionnaires and anal US before and 6–8 wk after delivery. A total of 202 women delivering vaginally were studied, and new sphincter defects were found in 21.2% of primiparous women, 20.6% of secundiparous woman, and 1.9% of multiparous women. Independent risk factors for sphincter defects were forceps delivery, perineal tears, episiotomy, and low parity. Persistent anal incontinence occurred in 7% of patients after delivery, but only half of these were found to have anal sphincter defects.

Another study has been performed in 150 primiparous women immediately after delivery in whom there was no evidence of a third or fourth degree tear *(19)*. Thirty (20%) had a defect of the EAS alone, two (1.3%) had a defect of the IAS alone, and 10 (6.7%) had combined defects. Three to eleven months after delivery, 96% of women returned a survey on bowel habits. Twenty-two (15%) reported incontinence (five of whom reported this before delivery), and 15 out of 22 had defects found on anal US. The odds ratio for the association of anal sphincter defects and fecal incontinence 3 mo after delivery was 7.9. However, the positive

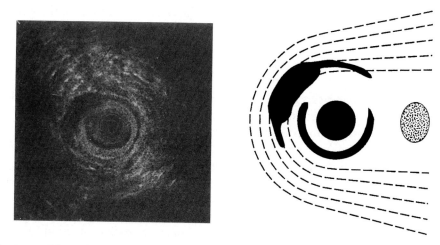

Fig. 7. An intersphincteric abscess is seen as hypoechoic area with horseshoe extensions running to the right and left. Reproduced with permission from ref. 4.

predictive value of finding an anal sphincter defect immediately after delivery for predicting incontinence 3 mo later was only 37%. Incontinence during pregnancy and birth weight >3500 g were other risk factors for incontinence 3 mos after delivery.

5.2. Peri Ano-Rectal Fistulas

Endoanorectal US can be useful to image clinically evident or suspected peri-anorectal fistulas. Dr. Bartram and colleagues at St. Mark's Hospital, London, have performed significant studies in this area. According to Dr. Bartram, the goals of a preoperative imaging exam are: (i) define the anatomy of any track and/or abscess within intersphincteric zone; (ii) determine if there is transphincteric extension; (iii) locate an internal opening; (iv) demonstrate any ischiorectal, supralevator, or infralevator abscess; and (v) assess the integrity of the sphincters (4).

Tracks appear as hypo-echoic bands within the intersphincteric zone and, if circumferential, are termed "horseshoe". If a track extends into the EAS, it is transphincteric (Fig. 7). Scars appear hypo-echoic, fairly homogenous, and have a regular outline. Abscesses are hypoechoic or of mixed echogenicity and have a less regular outline. Small echogenic areas may be found within an abscess and cause posterior shadowing. These may be due to foreign matter, calcified granulation tissue, or gas bubbles.

In the first 22 patients studied by endoanal US at 7 MHz followed by surgery at St. Mark's Hospital: two unsuspected foreign bodies were identified by US; four out of four horseshoe extensions were imaged correctly; 12 intersphincteric abscesses were identified by US, and 10 were found at surgery; 8 out of 12 internal openings were found by US; and zero out of four infra- or supralevator abscesses were identified by US (20).

Because of difficulty in always identifying an internal opening, Dr. Bartram revised his criteria for an internal opening to include one or more of the following features: (i) intersphincteric track contacts IAS; (ii) defect seen in IAS at point of contact with track; or (iii) actual break of subepithelial tissues (4). However, most subsequent studies have demonstrated continued difficulty in the assessment of an internal opening with conventional endoanal US (21,22). An exception to this was a study in which 122 of 130 internal openings were successfully identified by endoanal US (23). Criterion I was defined as a root-like budding formed by the intersphincteric tract that contacts the IAS (seen in 57 of 122). Criterion II was defined as root-like budding with an IAS defect (seen in 50 of 122). Criterion III was defined as subepithelial breach connecting to intersphincteric tract through IAS defect (seen in 15 of 122). Using a combination of these criteria, sensitivity and specificity for detecting internal opening with endoanal US was 94 and 87%, respectively.

Hydrogen peroxide has been used to enhance the assessment of peri-anal fistula with endoanal US. In a study of 21 patients assessed by endoanal US at 7 MHz with and without 3% hydrogen peroxide infusion into fistula prior to surgery, US alone was correct in fistula assessment in 62% cases, and hydrogen peroxide-enhanced scanning was correct in 95%. An internal opening was found with the hydrogen peroxide-enhanced imaging in 48% and during surgery in 90% (22). In a study comparing accuracy of physical exam, endoanal US at 10 MHz, and hydrogen peroxide-enhanced endoanal US with surgical findings in 26 patients, the following rates, respectively, were obtained: 65.4, 50, and 76.9% for primary tracts; 73.1, 65.4, and 88.8% for secondary tracts; 80.8, 80.8, and 92.3% for horseshoe extensions; and 23.1, 53.8, and 53.8% for internal openings (24).

Endoanal US was not found to be useful for mapping rectovaginal fistulas in a preoperative study of 25 women. The fistula was found with US in only 28% of these patients. However, 92% were correctly found to have an anterior sphincter defect on US, which guided the choice of surgical repair (25).

5.3. Anal Carcinoma

Endoanal US is well suited for loco-regional clinical staging of anal carcinoma because size, depth, and extension of the primary tumor can be determined, as well as the presence or absence of perirectal lymph nodes.

The tumor-node-metastasis (TNM) classification system for anal canal carcinoma was initially developed based on physical exam findings alone and is as follows:

- TX: primary tumor can not be assessed.
- T0: no evidence of primary tumor.
- Tis: carcinoma *in situ*.
- T1: tumor 2 cm or less in greatest dimension.
- T2: tumor >2 cm, <5 cm in greatest dimension.
- T3: tumor >5 cm in greatest dimension.
- T4: tumor of any size that involves adjacent organs (e.g., vagina, urethra, bladder).

- NX: regional lymph nodes can not be assessed.
- N0: no regional lymph node metastasis.
- N1: metastasis in perirectal lymph nodes.
- N2: metastasis in unilateral internal iliac and/or inguinal nodes.
- N3: metastasis in perirectal and inguinal nodes or bilateral internal iliac and/or inguinal nodes.

- MX: distant metastasis can not be assessed.
- M0: no distant metastasis.
- M1: distant metastasis (26).

Very few studies have specifically studied endoanal US as applied to anal carcinoma staging, but the studies published to date suggest information affecting treatment decisions can be obtained. Roseau et al. (27) studied 20 patients prior to therapy (18 radiotherapy and two combined chemoradiotherapy) and then subsequently following therapy at 2- to 5-mo intervals for 4–17 mo. Early follow-up showed a >50% reduction in tumor size in all cases. Early posttreatment abdominoperineal resection was done in two patients with persistent rectal or vaginal invasion and in one patient with persistent lymphadenopathy. In three patients (all originally T1 or T2 N0) tumor growth was found on consecutive follow-up US at 6, 10, and 12 mo, and these patients underwent surgery. The authors reported that there was "good correlation between ultrasonic images and operative findings" in the six patients that underwent surgery.

Magdeburg et al. *(28)* examined patients prior to therapy and patients after initial therapy for anal carcinoma utilizing an older staging system. The US results influenced therapeutic decisions in 27 of 30 patients (the other three patients refused treatment or were lost to follow-up). Of the 15 patients studied prior to therapy, four were referred for immediate surgery. Two patients (US stage T1 and T2) underwent local excision. The T1 lesion was found to actually be pathologic stage T2. Two patients (ultrasound stage T3) underwent rectal amputation. One of these was actually a pathologic T4 (invasion of vagina). Of the seven patients studied after primary surgical therapy, residual tumor was identified in five and confirmed by biopsy. These patients went on to receive radiation or chemoradiation. In four patients who had had either external beam radiation or combined surgery and radiation, US mapping of recurrent tumor was useful in guiding interstitial brachytherapy.

Giovannini et al. *(29)* recently proposed an EUS-based clinical staging system for anal carcinoma:

- usT1: involvement of mucosa and submucosa without infiltration of IAS.
- usT2: involvement of IAS with sparing of EAS.
- usT3: involvement of EAS.
- usT4: involvement of pelvic organ.

- N0: no suspicious perirectal lymph nodes.
- N+: perirectal lymph nodes having EUS criteria of malignancy (e.g., round, hypoechoic).

One hundred forty-six patients with anal carcinoma were staged by rectal exam (standard TN staging) and EUS (US TN stage). Treatment and follow-up data were available on 115 patients. Eighty percent of tumors clinically staged T1–T2N0 showed complete response to radiation therapy, while 94.5% of usT1–T2N0 tumors did. US T (usT1–2 vs usT3–4) ($p = 0.001$) and N (N0 vs N+) ($p = 0.03$) staging were both highly predictive of local recurrence, while clinical T and N staging were not predictive. In a multivariate analysis of factors correlated with survival, US T stage was the single significant ($p = 0.0001$) factor.

5.4. Rectal Carcinoma

Endorectal US is well suited to locoregional staging of rectal adenocarcinoma (Fig. 8). The results of preoperative staging can be used to guide treatment decisions, ranging from endoscopic mucosal resection or transanal excision to neoadjuvant chemoradiation, followed by anterior resection or abdominoperineal resection depending on location and stage of tumor. The TNM staging system for colorectal cancer is as follows:

- TX: primary tumor can not be assessed.
- T0: no evidence of primary tumor.
- Tis: carcinoma *in situ*.
- T1: tumor invades submucosa.
- T2: tumor invades muscularis propria.
- T3: tumor invades through the muscularis propria into subserosa or nonperitonealized perirectal tissues.
- T4: tumor directly invades other organs or structures.

- NX: regional lymph nodes can not be assessed.
- N0: no regional lymph node metastasis.
- N1: metastasis in one to three perirectal lymph nodes.
- N2: metastasis in four or more perirectal lymph nodes.

- MX: distant metastasis can not be assessed.
- M0: no distant metastasis.
- M1: distant metastasis *(26)*.

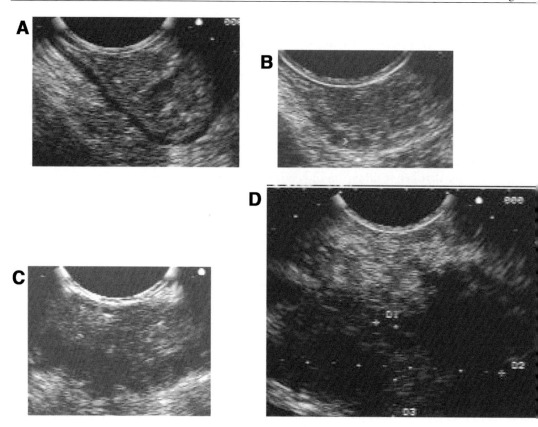

Fig. 8. Rectal cancers imaged with linear array echoendoscope at 7.5 MHz. (A) T1. (B) T2. (C) T3. (D) T4

Table 1
Accuracy of EUS in Rectal Cancer Staging as Compared to Histologic Findings

First author (yr) (reference)	No. of patients	Instrument	T stage accuracy	N stage accuracy
Boyce (1992) (31)	45	Olympus GF-UM2/3 scope	89%	79%
Nielsen (1996) (32)	100	7 MHz probe	85%	—
Massari (1998) (33)	75	Olympus GF-UM3 scope	90.7%	76%
Marone (2000) (34)	53	Olympus CF-UM-20 scope	81%	70%
Akahoshi (2000) (35)	39	Fuginon 7.5 MHz probe	82%	72%
Hunnerbein (2000) (36)	63	12.5 MHz probe	86%	85%

In a 1995 review, Hildebrandt and Feifel (30) reported the accuracy of rectal EUS assessment of tumor penetration (17 studies, 1985–1994) ranged from 60–94% and the accuracy for lymph node assessment (7 studies, 1986–1992) ranged from 73–81%.

Several more recent studies addressing the accuracy of EUS in staging rectal cancer as compared to histologic analysis are summarized in Table 1.

Two additional studies looked at more specific questions about tumor staging and subsequent treatment. The first study evaluated the accuracy of rectal EUS in determining earlier stage (<T3) vs T3 disease *(37)*. Among 70 patients who underwent immediate surgery, 18 of 19 pathologic T3 lesions were correctly identified by EUS. EUS correctly identified 44 of 51 patients as having <T3 disease. Forty-five patients who were initially staged as T3/4 underwent neoadjuvant chemoradiation. At operation, 56% had reduction in T stage, 31% had persistent nodal involvement, and 22% had a complete pathologic response. Five of seven who experienced recurrence at a median of 12 mo after diagnosis were in the subgroup of 10 patients who both failed to downstage T stage and had persistent nodal involvement *(37)*.

The second study utilized Olympus GF-UM2/3 echoendoscopes to examine 154 patients with early stage rectal cancer (T2) and compared EUS staging with pathologic staging *(38)*. T1 lesions were subclassified as T1-slight (invasion confined to superficial third of submucosa) or T1-massive (invasion extending to deeper mucosa). Overall accuracy rates for EUS detection of T1-slight, T1-massive, and T2 rectal carcinomas were 96, 97, and 96%, respectively. Overall accuracy for lymph node staging was 72%. No patients staged by EUS as T1-slight had positive lymph nodes. Based on their findings, the authors recommended consideration of endoscopic resection or local excision for lesions staged T1-slight, and radical operation for those staged T1-massive *(38)*.

Interobserver agreement of EUS staging of rectal cancers varies according to T stage *(39)*. Thirty-seven patients at two centers in France underwent videotaped EUS for rectal cancer staging. Six months later, four independent observers reviewed the tapes for both T and N staging, and interobserver agreement was estimated using the κ coefficient. Agreement was fair for usT1 ($\kappa = 0.40$), poor for usT2 ($\kappa = 0.20$), and good for usT3 ($\kappa = 0.58$) lesions. The agreement was also good for assessing metastatic involvement of lymph nodes ($\kappa = 0.54$).

EUS features of lymph nodes which suggest malignancy are size >1 cm, round shape, hypoechoic appearance, and well demarcated borders *(40)*. However, as seen in Table 1, EUS accuracy based on imaging alone is only in the 70–85% range. With a manual dissection technique, 45% of metastatic lymph nodes in 50 patients with rectal cancer were smaller than 5 mm *(41)*. In a study that examined EUS detection of metastatic lymph nodes as stratified by size, sensitivity of EUS was poor: 13.3% of lymph nodes <5 mm, 33.3% of lymph nodes 5–10 mm, and 20.4% of lymph nodes >10 mm *(42)*.

To improve the accuracy of lymph node staging, FNA has been employed. In a multicenter study of EUS-guided FNA, 192 lymph nodes (nine of which were perirectal) were aspirated *(43)*. The median number of passes required was two. The sensitivity–specificity–positive predictive value–negative predictive value–accuracy were as follows: 92, 93, 100, 86, and 92%, respectively. No complications from lymph node aspiration occurred. As compared to EUS imaging criteria of lymph node size >10 mm, EUS FNA had similar sensitivity, but significantly superior specificity (93 vs 24%) and accuracy (92 vs 69%).

The use of neoadjuvant chemoradiation therapy for advanced rectal cancers is becoming more common. Unfortunately, EUS staging accuracy is decreased after radiation treatment. Radiation has been found to cause thickening of the rectal wall, loss of normal wall layer appearance, increased echogenicity corresponding to fibrosis (leading to overstaging), and increased echogenicity of lymph nodes originally felt to be malignant (leading to understaging) *(44,45)*. In a few small studies, EUS T staging for rectal cancer after preoperative radiation therapy was accurate in 9 of 19 *(44)*, 15 of 17 *(45)*, and 24 of 56 patients *(46)*.

Rectal EUS can also be used to detect recurrence of rectal cancer after sphincter sparing surgery. In a 1995 review, Romano et al. reported that 110 local recurrences were identified by EUS in 600 patients (nine studies published between 1985 and 1993) and that 30 of 110 recurrences were found solely by EUS *(47)*. In a more recent prospective study, Lohnert et al. followed 338 patients after surgery for rectal cancer with either endorectal or endovaginal US

(48). In these patients, 721 exams were done, and 116 recurrences were found by US. In terms of detecting local recurrence in these 116 patients, digital rectal exam was not helpful in 91, flexible sigmoidoscopy was not helpful in 80, and tumor markers were not helpful in 25.

CONCLUSION

Endoanorectal US is an effective tool to assess anorectal pathology, both benign and malignant conditions, preoperatively. It is safe and relatively easy to perform. US-guided FNA can be used to confirm diagnoses, including suspected metastatic spread or cancer recurrences. The fact that the performance and interpretation of US examinations is operator-dependent is seen by some as a limitation of this tool. Also, the availability of EUS varies widely throughout this country. Future research directions in this field should include outcome studies of the impact of staging anorectal carcinomas, cost-effectiveness studies, and impact on quality of life.

REFERENCES

1. Wild JJ, Reid JM. *Ultrasound in Biology and Medicine.* Kelly-Fry E (ed.), American Institute of Biological Sciences, Washington, DC, 1957, pp. 30–45.
2. DiMagno EP, Regan PT, Wilson DA, et al. Ultrasonic endoscope. *Lancet,* **22** (1980) 629–631.
3. Kremkau FW. *Diagnostic Ultrasound: Principles and Instruments.* 5th ed., WB Saunders, Philadelphia, PA, 1998.
4. Bartram CI, Burnett SJD. *Atlas of Anal Endosonography.* Butterworth-Heinemann Ltd., Oxford, 1991.
5. Konerding MA, Dzemali O, Gaumann A, Malkusch W, Eckardt VF. Correlation of endoanal sonography with cross-sectional anatomy of the anal sphincter. *Gastrointest. Endosc.,* **50** (1999) 804–810.
6. Role of Endoscopic Ultrasonagraphy, *ASGE Guidelines for Clinical Application.* ASGE Publication No. 1043, 2000.
7. Rosch T, Dittler HJ, Fockens P, et al. Major complications of endoscopic ultrasonagraphy: results of a survey of 42,105 cases. *Gastrointest. Endosc.,* **39** (1993) 341.
8. Tjandra JJ, Milsom JW, Schroeder T, Fazio VW. Endoluminal ultrasound is preferable to electromyography in mapping anal sphincteric defects. *Dis. Colon Rectum,* **36** (1993) 689–692.
9. Burnett SJ, Speakman CT, Kamm MA, Bartram CI. Confirmation of endosonographic detection of external anal sphincter defects by simultaneous electromyographic mapping. *Br. J. Surg.,* **78** (1991) 448–450.
10. Law PJ, Kamm MA, Bartram CI. A comparison between electromyography and anal endosonography in mapping external anal defects. *Dis. Colon Rectum,* **33** (1990) 370–373.
11. Sentovich SM, Blatchford GJ, Rivela LJ, Lin K, Thorson AG, Christensen MA. Diagnosing anal sphincter injury with transanal ultrasound and manometry. *Dis. Colon Rectum,* (1997) **40** 1430–1434.
12. Romano G, Rotondano G, Esposito P, et al. External anal sphincter defects: correlation between pre-operative anal endosonography and intraoperative findings. *Br. J. Radiol.,* (1996) **69** 6–9.
13. Meyenberger C, Bertschinger P, Zala GF, Buchman P. Anal sphincter defects in fecal incontinence: correlation between endosonography and surgery. *Endoscopy,* **28** (1996) 217–224.
14. Sultan AH, Kamm MA, Talbot IC, Nichols RJ, Bartram CI. Anal endosonography for identifying external sphincter defects confirmed histologically. *Br. J. Surg.,* **81** (1994) 463–465.
15. Keating JP, Stewart PJ, Eyers AA, et al. Are special investigations of value in the management of patients with fecal incontinence? *Dis. Colon Rectum,* **40** (1997) 896–901.
16. Rieger NA, Sweeney JL, Hoffmann DC, Young, JF, Hunter A. Investigation of fecal incontinence with endoanal ultrasound. *Dis. Colon Rectum,* **39** (1996) 860–863.
17. Sultan AH, Kamm MA, Hudson CN, Thomas JM, Bartram CI. Anal-sphincter disruption during vaginal delivery. *N. Engl. J. Med.,* **329** (1993) 1905–1911.
18. Abramowitz L, Sobhani I, Ganansia R, et al. Are sphincter defects the cause of anal incontinence after vaginal delivery? *Dis. Colon Rectum* (2000) **43** 590–596.
19. Faltin DL, Boulivan M, Irion O, Bretones S, Stan C, Weil A. Diagnosis of anal sphincter tears by postpartum endosonography to predict fecal incontinence. *Obstet. Gynecol.,* **95** (2000) 643–647.
20. Law PJ, Talbot RW, Bartram CI, Northover JM. Anal endosonography in the evaluation of perianal sepsis and fistula in ano. *Br. J. Surg.,* **76** (1989) 752–755.
21. Deen KI, Williams JG, Hutchinson R, Keighley MR, Kumar D. Fistulas in ano: endoanal ultrasonographic assessment assists decision making for surgery. *Gut,* **35** (1994) 391–394.

22. Poen AC, Felt-Bersma RJ, Eijsbouts QA, Cuesta MA, Meuwissen SG. Hydrogen peroxide-enhanced transanal ultrasound in the assessment of fistula-in-ano. *Dis. Colon Rectum*, **41** (1998) 1147–1152.

23. Cho DY. Endosonographic criteria for an internal opening of fistula-in-ano. *Dis. Colon Rectum*, **42** (1999) 515–518.

24. Ratto C, Gentile E, Merico M, et al. How can the assessment of fistula-in-ano be improved? *Dis. Colon Rectum*, **43** (2000) 1375–1382.

25. Yee LF, Birnbaum EH, Read TE, Kodner IJ, Fleshman JW. Use of endoanal ultrasound in patients with rectovaginal fistulas. *Dis. Colon Rectum*, (1999) **42** 1057–1064.

26. Fleming ID, Cooper JS, Henson DE, et al. (eds.), *AJCC Cancer Staging Handbook*. Lippencott-Raven, Philadelphia, PA, 1998.

27. Roseau G, Palazzo L, Colardelle P, Chaussade S, Couturier D, Paolaggi JA. Endoscopic ultrasonography in the staging and follow-up of epidermoid carcinoma of the anal canal. *Gastrointest. Endosc.*, **40** (1994) 447–450.

28 Magdeburg B, Fried M, Meyenberger C. Endoscopic ultrasonography in the diagnosis, staging, and follow-up of anal carcinomas. *Endoscopy*, **31** (1999) 359–364.

29. Giovannini M, Bardou VJ, Barclay R, et al. Anal carcinoma: prognostic value of endorectal ultrasound-results of a prospective multicenter study. *Endoscopy*, **33** (2001) 231–236.

30. Hildebrandt U, Feifel G. Importance of endoscopic ultrasonography staging for treatment of rectal cancer. *Gastrointest. Endosc. Clin. N. Am.*, (1995) **5** 843–849.

31. Boyce GA, Sivak MV, Lavery IC, et al. Endoscopic ultrasound in the pre-operative staging of rectal carcinoma. *Gastrointest. Endosc.*, (1992) **38** 468–471.

32. Nielsen MB, Qvitzau S, Pedersen JF, Christiansen J. Endosonography for preoperative staging of rectal tumours. *Acta Radiol.*, **37** (1996) 799–803.

33. Massari M, De Simone M, Cioffi U, Rosso L, Chiarelli M, Gabrielli F. Value and limits of endorectal ultrasonography for preoperative staging of rectal carcinoma. *Surg. Laparosc. Endosc.* (1998) **8** 438–444.

34. Marone P, Petrulio F, de Bellis M, Battista Rossi G, Tempesta A. Role of endoscopic ultrasonography in the staging of rectal cancer: a retrospective study of 63 patients. *J. Clin. Gastroenterol.*, **30** (2000) 420–424.

35. Akahoshi K, Kondoh A, Nagaie T, et al. Preoperative staging of rectal cancer using a 7.5 MHz front-loading US probe. *Gastrointest. Endosc.*, (2000) **52** 529–534.

36. Hunerbein M, Totkas S, Ghadimi BM, Schlag PM. Preoperative evaluation of colorectal neoplasms by colonoscopic miniprobe ultrasonography. *Ann. Surg.*, (2000) **232** 46–50.

37. Adams DR, Blatchford GJ, Lin KM, Ternent CA, Thorson AG, Christensen MA. Use of preoperative ultrasound staging for treatment of rectal cancer. *Dis. Colon Rectum*, (1999) **42** 159–166.

38. Akasu T, Kondo H, Moriya Y, et al. Endorectal ultrasonography and treatment of early stage rectal cancer. *World J. Surg.*, (2000) **24** 1061–1068.

39. Burtin P, Rabot AF, Heresbach D, Carpentier S, Rousselet MC, Le Berre N, Boyer J. Interobserver agreement in the staging of rectal cancer using endoscopic ultrasonography. *Endoscopy*, **29** (1997) 620–625.

40. Tio TL, Tytgat GN. Endoscopic ultrasonagraphy in analyzing periintestinal lymph node abnormality. *Scand. J. Gastroenterol.*, **21(Suppl 123)** (1986) 158–163.

41. Andreola S. Leo E, Belli F, et al. Manual dissection of adenocarcinoma of the lower third of the rectum specimens for the detection of lymph node metastases smaller than 5 mm. *Cancer*, **77** (1996) 607–612.

42. Spinelli P, Schiavo M, Meroni E, et al. Results of EUS in detecting perirectal lymph node metastases of rectal cancer: the pathologist makes the difference. *Gastrointest. Endosc.*, **49** (1999) 754–758.

43. Wiersema MJ, Vilmann P, Giovannini M, Chang KJ, Wiersema LM. Endosonography-guided fine-needle aspiration biopsy:diagnostic accuracy and complication assessment. *Gastroenterology*, **112** (1997) 1087–1095.

44. Napoleon BN, Pujol BN, Berger F, et al. Accuracy of endosonography in staging of rectal cancer treated by radiotherapy. *Br. J. Surg.*, (1991) **78** 785–788.

45. Glaser F, Kuntz D, Schlag P, Herfarth C. Endorectal ultrasound for the control of preoperative radiotherapy of rectal cancer. *Ann. Surg.*, (1993) **217** 64–71.

46. Lin DE, Vanagunas A, Stryker S. Endoscopic ultrasound restaging of rectal cancer is inaccurate following neoadjuvant chemo-radiation therapy. *Gastrointest. Endosc.*, **51** (2000) AB171.

47. Romano G, Belli G, Rotondano G. Colorectal cancer diagnosis of recurrence. *Gastrointest. Endosc. Clin. N. Am.*, (1995) **5** 831–841.

48. Lohnert MS, Doniec JM, Henne-Bruns D. Effectiveness of endoluminal sonography in the identification of occult local rectal cancer recurrences. *Dis. Colon Rectum* (2000) **43** 483–491.

20 Colonic Transit and Motility

William J. Snape, Jr.

CONTENTS

1. INTRODUCTION: BASIC PRINCIPALS OF MOTILITY

1.1. General

The upper gastrointestinal tract transports food that has been eaten allowing digestion and ultimately absorption. The colon in humans has a storage and evacuation function and conserves fluid and electrolytes. In some mammals, i.e. the horse and the rabbit, the colon has a major function in the absorption of nutrients. The sphincters, placed at the junction between different parts of the gut, are specialized areas of smooth muscle, which regulate the forward and backward movement of intestinal contents. The ileocecal valve maintains a lower bacterial count in the small intestine by decreasing reflux of colonic contents into the ileum. The anal sphincter maintains contents in the colon until an appropriate time for expulsion.

In health, the movement of gastrointestinal contents is regulated strictly. This control of smooth muscle contraction is maintained by a complex interaction between excitatory and inhibitory neural stimuli exerted by myenteric nerves and circulating neuropeptides.

1.2. Electrophysiology

The rhythm and rate of contraction of the visceral smooth muscle of the stomach, small intestine, and colon is maintained by the intrinsic contractions of individual muscle cells. The rhythm of the cells is specific for each area of the gut, since each of the major sections of the gut has a different function. Electrical changes in the muscle membrane initiate intracellular biochemical reactions that result in muscle contraction. The intrinsic rate of spontaneous electrical depolarization of the muscle cell varies and is dependent on the location of muscle.

The esophagus has a slow wave rhythm that may be extensively modulated by the enteric nerves (1). In the stomach, the slow waves have a frequency of 3 cycles/min (2). Disturbance

From: *Colonic Diseases*
Edited by: T. R. Koch © Humana Press Inc., Totowa, NJ

in the generation of slow wave activity will lead to gastric retention *(3)*. The frequency increases in the duodenum to approx 11 cycles/min, with a decrease in the frequency seen in the distal small intestine *(4,5)*. The colon has an irregular slow wave rhythm of 3–6 cycles/min. The control of the slow wave rhythm appears to be set by the interstitial cells of Cajal (ICC) *(6,7)*. Migrating spike bursts may be the electrophysiologic event controlling long distance movement of colonic contents *(8,9)*.

1.3. Contractility

The electrical activity of the colonic smooth muscle initiates a contractile response in each of the layers of the muscular wall. Circular and longitudinal muscles have different functions. Throughout the gut, circular contractions segment the lumen, mixing the contents to expose the mucosa to continually different contents. The longitudinal muscle shortens the bowel, helping to move intraluminal contents forward.

The circular muscle contractions are phasic, which mixes the intraluminal contents and moves the bolus back and forth *(10–12)*. The longitudinal muscle has tonic contractions that shorten the colon causing net forward movement of the colonic intraluminal contents *(11–13)*. The differential contractions of the colonic smooth muscle layers is controlled by the enteric nervous system, as well as differences in the receptor subtypes for both stimulatory (e.g., substance P) or inhibitory (e.g., vasoactive intestinal peptide [VIP]) neurohormones *(14,15)*. The movement of intraluminal contents through the colon is dependent on both contraction and relaxation of the smooth muscle. In addition to phasic and tonic contractions, high amplitude propagating contractions are important for the propulsion of intraluminal contents through the colon *(16,17)*.

The motility patterns are normally coordinated to allow orderly transit of contents through the colon which "fine-tunes" the absorption of salt and water. Slow transit enhances the mucosal extraction of water, causing hard stools and constipation. Rapid transit causes frequent soft stools. Diarrhea associated with colonic motility disorders is low in volume (<400 mL/d), since most intestinal fluid has been absorbed in the small intestine. Table 1 lists the diseases or syndromes that cause disordered colonic motility. Many of the systemic diseases that affect gastric and small intestinal motility also alter colonic motility.

1.4. Sensation

Signals from the sensory afferent nerves help coordinate the colonic contractions through a series of neural reflexes *(18)*. Sensation from these sensory nerves helps the individual monitor and control their bowel function. The sensory system has been examined in detail, and numerous mediators have been identified that control afferent sensory recognition (Table 2) *(19)*. Changes in the tone of the colon will modify the sensory recognition. The increase in rectocolonic tone that occurs after eating increases sensory input that controls local and central nervous system-related reflexes *(20)*. Faulty function in the visceral afferent nerves may be, in part, responsible for many of the symptoms of functional bowel disease.

2. TECHNIQUES TO MEASURE MOTILITY

Clinical and research techniques allow measurement of the different parameters of colonic motility: (i) intraluminal pressure; (ii) tone; (iii) electrical signals; (iv) transit; and (v) visceral sensation. Computerized methods for data acquisition and analysis allow the clinical application of colonic motility measurements, which will hopefully improve our care of these patients.

Table 1
Pathogenesis of Colonic Motility Disorders

Slow transit

- Increased segmenting contraction
- Irritable bowel syndrome (spastic)
- Anal outlet obstruction
- Acquired anismus
- Irritable bowel syndrome (inertia)
- Ogilvie's syndrome
- Progressive systemic sclerosis

- Primary constipation
- Diverticular disease
- Congenital-Hirschsprung's disease
- Decreased segmenting contractions
- Primary colonic pseudo-obstruction
- Diabetes mellitus
- Spinal cord injury

Rapid transit

- Functional diarrhea
- Surreptitious abuse of laxatives

- Bile salt diarrhea

Table 2
Peripheral Pain Mediators

Agents acting indirectly on afferent nerves	*Agents acting directly on afferent nerves*
• Noradrenalin	• Prostaglandin E_2, I_2
• Interleukin-1, -8, -6	• diHETE
• TNF-α	• Adenosine, ATP
• Bradykinin	• Bradykinin
• Leukotriene B_4	• Serotonin
• Complement 5a	• CGRP, Substance P
• Substance P, VIP	

Abbreviations: diHETE, di-15(S)- or 15(R)-hydroxyeicosatetraenoic acid; ATP, adenosine triphosphate; CGRP, calcitonin gene-related peptide; TNF, tumor necrosis factor

2.1. Intraluminal Pressure Measurement

Intraluminal pressure remains the most widely used technique to define the colonic contractile state. As the smooth muscular wall of the colon contracts, intraluminal pressure is generated. Water-perfused catheters and solid state pressure catheters can be placed throughout the colon to measure phasic pressure changes. Pressure catheter can measure a tonic contraction, but changes in colonic wall tone are best measured with the barostat. Intraluminal pressure is analyzed for frequency of contraction, amplitude and duration of contractions (motility index), and pattern of contractions (16). Intraluminal pressure is a measure of a change in contraction of a large segment of the colon, encompassing many smooth muscle cells (21).

2.2. Measurement of Smooth Muscle Tone

Tone of the muscle wall of the colon can be measured with a computerized technique (barostat) that measures volume changes at a constant pressure (22–24). This technique provides complimentary information to intraluminal pressure measurements. The barostat allows measurement of colonic wall relaxation, also. A change in tone provides background upon which phasic contractions are superimposed.

2.3. Electrophysiologic Measurement

Changes in the membrane potential of the colonic smooth muscle membrane generate an electrical signal that can be measured. Research studies have used several techniques to measure this parameter. Electrodes placed in contact with the colonic mucosa by a clip or suction have recorded electrical responses of the colon that are similar to signals measured by sewing electrodes onto the serosal side of the bowel (25–27). The drop in electrical potential of the cell membrane leads to contraction of the smooth muscle.

Both slow waves and spike potentials can be measured using the electrodes that are in contact with the colonic mucosa. Measurement of the myoelectrical activity gives a specific measurement of the smooth muscle at that point of the colon. This avoids the potential difficulties of changes in luminal diameter that can affect the intraluminal pressure.

Preliminary studies suggest that electrical activity can be measured from the colon using surface skin electrodes much like the electrogastrogram (28,29). The surface electrodes are most effective at measuring the slow wave component of the electrical signal.

2.4. Measurement of Colonic Transit

In patients with constipation, assessment of colonic transit differentiates an abnormality in colonic motility from anal sphincter or pelvic floor disturbances. The characteristics of the patient's stool or the absolute number of bowel movements in a week correlates poorly with the measured transport of intraluminal contents through the colon. However, the form of the stool appears to differentiate between pseudodiarrhea and constipation (30,31). When measuring the colonic transit, the patient should maintain their usual diet and respond to the urge to move their bowels. Variations in the caloric content and fiber composition of the diet alter the transit of intraluminal material through the colon (32,33). The patient's response to an urge for a bowel movement also alters colonic transit. If healthy patients resist the urge to move their bowels, transit through the distal colon is greatly slowed; even transit through the proximal colon is decreased (34).

There are several methods that provide an objective and clinically useful measurement of colonic transit. The most widely used is a measurement of the transit of radio-opaque markers through the colon (35,36). Newer techniques have used radioisotopic markers to measure colonic transit (16,37–39). Both techniques allow estimation of the regional movement of intraluminal contents. However, the measurement of rapid flow through the colon may require use of the radionuclide markers and more frequent monitoring of the images (39–42). The total colonic and regional transit time can be quantified.

If the total transit time is >75 h, the patient has slow transit constipation caused by abnormal colonic motility or functional obstruction at the anal outlet. Therapy is directed toward improving the transit of intraluminal contents. Patients with normal transit constipation may require re-education about normal bowel habits and further discussion to understand the exact problem causing their symptoms (43). Some patients with outlet obstruction may feel that evacuation is incomplete and still have a normal frequency of stools. Patients with constipation associated with delayed transit exhibited greater psychological well-being compared to those with constipation and normal colonic transit (44).

2.5. Measurement of Sensation

The afferent sensation in the rectum provides a signal for needing to move the bowels. This sensation also provides a cue to the individual to contract their external anal sphincter, maintaining fecal continence. An intense sensory input leads to the feeling of urgency (45).

Balloon distention of the rectum and colon has been used to measure visceral sensitivity. Healthy patients first feel colorectal distention after infusion of 10–30 cc of air into the distending balloon. The maximum tolerable volume of distention in healthy subjects is greater than 100 cc of air. The development of computer-controlled balloon distention allows standardization of the sensory measurement. Phasic distention activates the splanchnic afferent nerves and is a better discriminator of disturbed sensory perception compared to a gradual ramp distention to the same volume (46).

Patients with functional bowel disease have increased visceral sensation leading to abdominal discomfort.

3. COLONIC MOTILITY IN HEALTHY SUBJECTS

There are few to no colonic contractions during sleep, but propagating contractions increase in frequency on awakening (47–49). Rapid eye movement sleep also is associated with an increased frequency of propagating contractions similar to arousal (50).

During the day, patients have minimal colonic motility during periods of fasting. Eating stimulates colonic contractions. The fat component of the meal is the major stimulus to colonic contractions (51), whereas protein ingestion inhibits colonic contraction (51,52). The major postprandial increase in motility occurs in the proximal descending colon. The movement of ileal contents into the proximal colon may initiate the increase in distal colonic contractions. This increased activity of segmenting contractions in the region of the splenic flexure moves colonic contents forward and backward, enhancing absorption of water and electrolytes (16). Eating also increases propagating contractions, which rapidly propel the colonic contents distally into the rectosigmoid junction. Stress also stimulates an increase colonic contractions (53,54). The altered bowel habits, especially diarrhea, that occur during stress may be related to the release of neurohormones (55,56). The mediator of the increased colonic motility is presently unknown.

Bisacodyl is a potent stimulant of colonic motility causing propagating contractions. Bisacodyl stimulates a propagating contraction that progresses through the distal half of the colon in healthy subjects (57,58). Bisacodyl appears to stimulate the colon through the myenteric plexus. Patients with defective myenteric plexus often have no response to the drug (57).

4. CLINICAL PRESENTATION OF COLONIC MOTILITY DISORDERS

Alterations in colonic motility can lead to abdominal pain and an alteration in bowel habit. These symptoms reflect abnormalities in either the motility of the colon or in the threshold for visceral sensory nerve activity. The pain can be localized anywhere over the anatomic location of the colon, but is generally in the lower abdomen (59). The link with altered colonic motility is suggested by increase in the cramping discomfort after eating and by improvement in the pain with a bowel movement. Motility disturbances of the colon can lead to either constipation or diarrhea. Anatomic lesions of the colon affecting the colonic mucosa (e.g., colitis) or obstructing the colonic lumen (e.g., carcinoma) must be excluded. Bloating and a feeling of abdominal distention commonly occur in colonic motility disorders due to changes in visceral sensitivity (60). There is no abnormality in the amount of colonic gas in bloated patients (61).

There are few signs of colonic motility disorders. The absence of abnormalities, such as rebound abdominal tenderness or rectal bleeding, support the presence of functional colonic disease. Some anatomic colonic diseases also have a disturbance in colonic motility (e.g., increased propagating contractions in ulcerative colitis), which may exacerbate the underlying disease.

5. COLONIC MOTILITY IN PATIENTS

In constipated patients, either increased or decreased segmenting contractions can slow transit through the colon. Functional partial obstruction results from increased segmenting contractions, since the segmentation impedes movement of colonic contents. In approx 50% of chronically constipated patients, there is an increase in post-prandial colonic motility. The other patients have an absent postprandial response (colonic inertia), which causes the slow movement of the colonic contents (62). The patients with inertia often have intermittent abdominal pain associated with nausea and vomiting in addition to their constipation (63). This may reflect either a generalized gastrointestinal motility disorder or a reflex proximal gut inhibition by a distended colon or rectum. Similar observations can be made in children (64).

Propagating contractions are invariably absent in patients with slow colonic transit and constipation, suggesting that these contractions are necessary for net forward movement of feces into the distal rectosigmoid (62,65,66). Bisacodyl, which stimulates propagating contractions, may function as a prokinetic in patients with constipation (57,58).

The absence of high amplitude propagation contractions in constipation is contrasted with the increased number of high amplitude propagating contractions occurring after eating and during the fasting phase in patients with functional diarrhea or ulcerative colitis (40,67). Patients with diarrhea and rapid colonic transit have decreased colonic segmenting contractions and increased numbers of contractions propagating into the rectum. As a result, intraluminal contents are rapidly transported distally. When these powerful contractions carry the colonic contents into the rectum, the patient experiences urgency. Increased intraluminal concentrations of bile salts may contribute to the diarrhea and the increase in propagating contractions (68–70)

A portion of the patients with constipation-associated irritable bowel syndrome and patients with diverticular disease have increased segmenting colonic contractions (17,63,71). The increased intraluminal pressure may reflect a defect of modulating colonic contractions.

Patients with diarrhea-associated irritable bowel syndrome and patients with ulcerative colitis have increased frequency of propagating contractions (40,67). An increase in propagating contractions can cause a faster transit through the colon, urgency, and even fecal incontinence.

6. FUTURE APPLICATIONS OF COLONIC MOTILITY MEASUREMENTS

There is a great deal of interest in correlating colonic symptoms to an actual motility pattern. This has proven difficult, since the symptoms of colonic dysfunction are often vague and nonspecific. In addition, specific symptoms, such as diarrhea, can be caused by diametrically opposing motility patterns, despite fulfilling careful clinical definition (Rome 2 criteria) (72). Diarrhea can be associated and presumably caused by rapid intestinal transit, by slow intestinal transit with bacterial overgrowth, or by increased colonic propagating contractions. Clinical therapy would be best directed by determining the motility that was causing the underlying symptom. However, motility testing is moderately invasive, requires a significant effort to perform the studies, and can be expensive.

Improvement in the clinical measurement of gastrointestinal motility should improve treatment of symptoms caused by colonic dysfunction. Radionuclide transit, cutaneous myoelectrical activity, magnetic resonance imaging (MRI) radiography, and ultrasound are being evaluated as methods to measure gastrointestinal function (39,62,73–75). The colon has not been as well studied as the stomach, gallbladder and upper gut, but should lend itself to further study.

The ultimate aim is to identify a pathophysiological abnormality in smooth muscle motility or afferent sensory system and provide treatment with a specific drug that will correct the defect. This will require increased understanding of colonic motility and the development of specific drugs to correct the abnormality.

REFERENCES

1. Preiksaitis HG, Diamant NE. Phasic contractions of the muscular components of human esophagus and gastroesophageal junction in vitro. *Can. J. Physiol. Pharmacol.*, **73** (1995) 356–363.
2. Becker JM, Kelly KA. Antral control of canine gastric emptying of solids. *Am. J. Physiol.*, **245** (1983) G334–G338
3. Telander RL, Morgan KG, Kreulen DL, Schmalz PF, Kelly KA, Szurszewski JH. Human gastric atony with tachygastria and gastric retention. *Gastroenterology*, **75** (1978) 497–501.
4. Christensen J, Schedl HP, Clifton JA. The basic electrical rhythm of the duodenum in normal human subjects and in patients with thyroid. *J. Clin. Invest.*, **43** (1964) 1659–1667.
5. Vantrappen G, Janssens J, Hellemans J, Ghoos Y. The interdigestive motor complex of normal subjects and patients with bacterial overgrowth of the small intestine. *J. Clin. Invest.*, **59** (1977) 1158–1166.
6. Sanders KM. A case for interstitial cells of Cajal as pacemakers and mediators of neurotransmission in the gastrointestinal tract. *Gastroenterology*, **111** (1996) 492–515.
7. Barajas-Lopez C, Berezin I, Daniel EE, Huizinga JD. Pacemaker activity recorded in interstitial cells of Cajal of the gastrointestinal tract. *Am. J. Physiol.*, **257** (1989) C830–C835.
8. Christensen J, Anuras S, Hauser RL. Migrating spike bursts and electrical slow waves in the cat colon: effect of sectioning. *Gastroenterology*, **66** (1974) 240–247.
9. Schang JC, Devroede G. Fasting and postprandial myoelectric spiiking activity in the human sigmoid colon. *Gastroenterology*, **85** (1983) 1048–1053.
10. Ritchie JA, Truelove SC, Ardran GM, Tuckey MS. Propulsion and retropulsion of normal colonic contents. *Dig. Dis. Sci.*, **16** (1971) 697–704.
11. Sarna SK. Physiology and pathophysiology of colonic motor activity. *Dig. Dis. Sci.*, **36** (1991) 998–1018.
12. Sarna SK. Physiology and pathophysiology of colonic motor activity. *Dig. Dis. Sci.*, **36** (1991) 827–862.
13. Prins NH, Akkermans LM, Lefebvre RA, Schuurkes JA. 5-HT(4) receptors on cholinergic nerves involved in contractility of canine and human large intestine longitudinal muscle. *Br. J. Pharmacol.*, **131** (2000) 927–932.
14. Warner FJ, Liu L, Lubowski DZ, Burcher E. Circular muscle contraction, messenger signalling and localization of binding sites for neurokinin A in human sigmoid colon. *Clin. Exp. Pharmacol. Physiol.*, **27** (2000) 928–933.
15. Burleigh DE. Motor responsiveness of proximal and distal human colonic muscle layers to acetylcholine, noradrenaline, and vasoactive intestinal peptide. *Dig. Dis. Sci.*, **35** (1990) 617–621.
16. Moreno-Osset E, Bazzocchi G, Lo S, et al. Association between post-prandial changes in colonic intraluminal pressure and transit. *Gastroenterology*, **96** (1989) 1265–1273.
17. Narducci F, Bassotti G, Granata MT, et al. Colonic motility and gastric emptying in patients with irritable bowel syndrome. Effect of pretreatment with octylonium bromide. *Dig. Dis. Sci.*, **31** (1986) 241–246.
18. Kreulen DL, Szurszewski JH. Reflex pathways in the abdominal prevertebral ganglia: evidence for a colo-colonic inhibitory reflex. *J. Physiol.*, **295** (1979) 21–32.
19. Bueno L, Fioramonti J, Delvaux M, Frexinos J. Mediators and pharmacology of visceral sensitivity: from basic to clinical investigations. *Gastroenterology*, **112** (1997) 1714–1743.
20. Malcolm A, Phillips SF, Camilleri M, Hanson RB. Pharmacological modulation of rectal tone alters perception of distention in humans. *Am. J. Gastroenterol.*, **92** (1997) 2073–2079.
21. Sasaki Y, Hada R, Nakajima H, Munakata A. Difficulty in estimating localized bowel contraction by colonic manometry: a simultaneous recording of intraluminal pressure and luminal calibre. *Neurogastroenterol. Motil.*, **8** (1996) 247–253.
22. Choi MG, Camilleri M, O'Brien MD, Kammer PP, Hanson RB. A pilot study of motility and tone of the left colon in patients with diarrhea due to functional disorders and dysautonomia. *Am. J. Gastroenterol.*, **92** (1997) 297–302.
23. Ford MJ, Camilleri M, Wiste JA, Hanson RB. Differences in colonic tone and phasic response to a meal in the transverse and sigmoid human colon. *Gut*, **37** (1995) 264–269.
24. O'Brien MD, Camilleri M, von der Ohe MR, et al. Motility and tone of the left colon in constipation: a role in clinical practice? *Am. J. Gastroenterol.* **91** (1996) 2532–2538.
25. Snape WJ Jr, Carlson GM, Cohen S. Human colonic myoelectric activity in response to prostigmin and the gastrointestinal hormones. *Am. J. Dig. Dis.*, **22** (1977) 881–887.
26. Bueno L, Fioramonti J, Ruckebusch Y, Frexinos J, Coulom P. Evaluation of colonic myoelectrical activity in health and functional disorders. *Gut*, **21** (1980) 480–485.

27. Schang JC, Devroede G, Hebert M, Hemond M, Pilote M, Devroede L. Effects of rest, stress, and food on myoelectric spiking activity of left and sigmoid colon in humans. *Dig. Dis. Sci.*, **33** (1988) 614–618.

28. Hamid SA, Reddy SN, Lagmay GL, Le T, Snape WJJ. Electrocolonography (EcG) in Children. *Gastroenterology*, **112** (1997) A743.

29. Reddy SN, Lagmay GL, Le T, DiLorenzo C, Hyman PE, Snape WJJ. Electrocolonography (EcG). *Gastroenterology*, **110** (1996) A743.

30. Heaton KW, O'Donnell LJ. An office guide to whole-gut transit time. Patients' recollection of their stool form. *J. Clin. Gastroenterol.*, **19** (1994) 28–30.

31. Probert CS, Emmett PM, Cripps HA, Heaton KW. Evidence for the ambiguity of the term constipation: the role of irritable bowel syndrome. *Gut*, **35** (1994) 1455–1458.

32. Burkitt DP, Walker A, Painter NS. Effect of dietary fibre on stools and transit-times, and its role in the causation of disease. *Lancet*, **2** (1972) 1408–1412.

33. Kaufman PN, Richter JE, Chilton HM, et al. Effects of liquid versus solid diet on colonic transit in humans. *Gastroenterology*, **98** (1990) 73–81.

34. Klauser AG, Voderholzer WA, Heinrich CA, Schindlbeck NE, Muller-Lissner SA. Behavioral modification of colonic function. *Dig. Dis. Sci.* **35** (1990) 1271–1275.

35. Hinton J, Lennard-Jones JE, Young AC. A new method for studying gut transit times using radioopaque markers. *Gut*, **10** (1969) 842–847.

36. Metcalf AM, Phillips SF, Zinsmeister AR, MacCarty RL, Beart RW, Wolff BG. Simplified assessment of segmental colonic transit. *Gastroenterology*, **92** (1987) 40–47.

37. Jian R, Najean Y, Bernier JJ. Measurement of intestinal progression of a meal and its residues in normal subjects and patients with functional diarrhoea by a dual isotope technique. *Gut*, **25** (1984) 728–731.

38. Krevsky B, Malmud LS, D'ercole F, Maurer AH, Fisher RS. Colonic transit scintigraphy: a physiologic approach to the quantitative measurement of colonic transit in humans. *Gastroenterology*, **91** (1986) 1102–1112.

39. Proano M, Camilleri M, Phillips SF, Brown ML, Thomforde GM. Transit of solids through the human colon: regional quantification in the unprepared bowel. *Am. J. Physiol.*, **258** (1990) G856–G862.

40. Bazzocchi G, Ellis J, Villanueva-Meyer J, Reddy SN, Mena I, Snape WJ, Jr. Effect of eating on colonic motility and transit in patients with functional diarrhea. Simultaneous scintigraphic and manometric evaluations [see comments]. *Gastroenterology*, **101** (1991) 1298–1306.

41. Camilleri M, Zinsmeister AR. Towards a relatively inexpensive, noninvasive, accurate test for colonic motility disorders. *Gastroenterology*, **103** (1992) 36–42.

42. von der Ohe MR, Camilleri M, Kvols LK, Thomforde GM. Motor dysfunction of the small bowel and colon in patients with the carcinoid syndrome and diarrhea. *N. Engl. J. Med.*, **329** (1993) 1073–1078.

43. Chaussade S, Khyari A, Roche H, Garret M, Gaudric M, Couturier D, Guerre J. Determination of total and segmental colonic transit time in constipated patients. *Dig. Dis. Sci.*, **34** (1989) 1168–1172.

44. Wald A. Colonic transit and anorectal manometry in chronic idiopathic constipation. *Arch. Intern. Med.*, **146** (1986) 1713–1716.

45. Salvioli B, Bharucha AE, Rath-Harvey D, Pemberton JH, Phillips SF. Rectal compliance, capacity, and rectoanal sensation in fecal incontinence. *Am. J. Gastroenterol.*, **96** (2001) 2158–2168.

46. Lembo T, Munakata J, Mertz H, et al. Evidence for the hypersensitivity of lumbar splanchnic afferents in irritable bowel syndrome [see comments]. *Gastroenterology*, **107** (1994) 1686–1696.

47. Narducci F, Bassotti G, Gaburri M, Morelli A. Twenty four hour manometric recording of colonic motor activity in healthy man. *Gut*, **28** (1987) 17–25.

48. Bassotti G, Gaburri M. Manometric investigation of high-amplitude propagated contractile activity of the human colon. *Am. J. Physiol.*, **255** (19880 G660–G664

49. Fioramonti J, Bueno L. Diurnal changes in colonic motor profile in conscious dogs. *Dig. Dis. Sci.*, **28** (1983) 257–264.

50. Furukawa Y, Cook IJ, Panagopoulos V, McEvoy RD, Sharp DJ, Simula M. Relationship between sleep patterns and human colonic motor patterns [see comments]. *Gastroenterology*, **107** (1994) 1372–1381.

51. Wright SH, Snape WJ Jr, Battle WM, Cohen S, London RL. Effect of dietary components on gastrocolonic response. *Am. J. Physiol.*, **238** (1980) G228–G232

52. Levinson S, Bhasker M, Gibson TR, Morin R, Snape WJ Jr. Comparison of intraluminal and intravenous mediators of colonic response to eating. *Dig. Dis. Sci.*, **30** (1985) 33–39.

53. Narducci F, Snape WJ J., Battle WM, London RL, Cohen S. Increased colonic motility during exposure to a stressful situation. *Dig. Dis. Sci.*, **30** (1985) 40–44.

54. Welgan P, Meshkinpour H, Beeler M. Effect of anger on colon motor and myoelectric activity in irritable bowel syndrome. *Gastroenterology*, **94** (1988) 1150–1156.

55. Williams CL, Peterson JM, Villar RG, Burks TF. Corticotropin-releasing factor directly mediates colonic responses to stress. *Am. J. Physiol.*, **253** (1987) G582–G586

56. Williams CL, Villar RG, Peterson JM, Burks TF. Stress-induced changes in intestinal transit in the rat: a model for irritable bowel syndrome. *Gastroenterology*, **94** (1988) 611–621.

57. Hamid SA, Di Lorenzo C, Reddy SN, Flores AF, Hyman PE. Bisacodyl and high-amplitude-propagating colonic contractions in children. *J. Pediatr. Gastroenterol. Nutr.*, **27** (1998) 398-402.

58. Preston DM, Lennard-Jones JE. Pelvic motility and response to intraluminal bisacodyl in slow-transit constipation. *Dig. Dis. Sci.*, **30** (1985) 289–294.

59. Waller SL, Misiewicz JJ. Prognosis in the irritable-bowel syndrome. *Lancet*, **2** (1969) 754–756.

60. Whitehead WE, Holtkotter B, Enck P, et al. Tolerance for rectosigmoid distention in irritable bowel syndrome. *Gastroenterology*, **98** (1990) 1187–1192.

61. Lasser RB, Bond JH, Levitt MD. The role of intestinal gas in functional abdominal pain. *N. Engl. J. Med.*, **293** (1975) 524–526.

62. Bazzocchi G, Ellis J, Villanueva-Meyer J, et al. Post-prandial colonic transit and motor activity in chronic constipation. *Gastroenterology*, **98** (1990) 686–693.

63. Bazzocchi G, Ellis J, Villanueva-Meyer J, et al. Postprandial colonic transit and motor activity in chronic constipation. *Gastroenterology*, **98** (1990) 686–693.

64. Di Lorenzo C, Flores AF, Reddy SN, Snape WJ Jr, Bazzocchi G, Hyman PE. Colonic manometry in children with chronic intestinal pseudo- obstruction. *Gut*, **34** (1993) 803–807.

65. Bassotti G, Chiarioni G, Vantini I, et al. Anorectal manometric abnormalities and colonic propulsive impairment in patients with severe chronic idiopathic constipation. *Dig. Dis. Sci.*, **39** (1994) 1558–1564.

66. Bassotti G, Imbimbo BP, Betti C, Dozzini G, Morelli A. Impaired colonic motor response to eating in patients with slow-transit constipation. *Am. J. Gastroenterol.*, **87** (1992) 504–508.

67. Reddy SN, Bazzocchi G, Chan S, et al. Colonic motility and transit in health and ulcerative colitis. *Gastroenterology*, **101** (1991) 1289–1297.

68. Flynn M, Darby C, Hyland J, Hammond P, Taylor I. The effect of bile acids on colonic myoelectrical activity. *Br. J. Surg.*, **66** (1979) 776–779.

69. Snape WJ Jr, Shiff S, Cohen S. Effect of deoxycholic acid on colonic motility in the rabbit. *Am. J. Physiol.*, **238** (1980) G321–G325.

70. Taylor I, Basu P, Hammond P, Darby C, Flynn M. Effect of bile acid perfusion on colonic motor function in patients with the irritable colon syndrome. *Gut*, **21** (1980) 843–847.

71. Trotman IF, Misiewicz JJ. Sigmoid motility in diverticular disease and the irritable bowel syndrome. *Gut*, **29** (1988) 218–222.

72. Mearin F, Badia X, Balboa A, et al. Irritable bowel syndrome prevalence varies enormously depending on the employed diagnostic criteria: comparison of Rome II versus previous criteria in a general population. *Scand. J. Gastroenterol.*, **36** (2001) 1155–1161.

73. Cucchiara S, Salvia G, Borrelli O, et al. Gastric electrical dysrhythmias and delayed gastric emptying in gastroesophageal reflux disease [see comments]. *Am. J. Gastroenterol.*, **92** (1997) 1103–1108.

74. Undeland KA, Hausken T, Svebak S, Aanderud S, Berstad A. Wide gastric antrum and low vagal tone in patients with diabetes mellitus type 1 compared to patients with functional dyspepsia and healthy individuals. *Dig. Dis. Sci.*, **41** (1996) 9–16.

75. Rentsch M, Paetzel C, Lenhart M, Feuerbach S, Jauch KW, Furst A. Dynamic magnetic resonance imaging defecography: a diagnostic alternative in the assessment of pelvic floor disorders in proctology. *Dis. Colon Rectum*, **44** (2001) 999–1007.

21

Defecography and Related Radiologic Imaging Techniques

Vincent H. S. Low

CONTENTS

1. INTRODUCTION

The patient with pelvic floor and anorectal dysfunction may present with a variety of symptoms such as urinary or defecatory dysfunction, urogenital or anorectal prolapse, pelvic or abdominal pain, and dyspareunia *(1–5)*. Occasionally, rectal bleeding may eventually be found to be due to rectal prolapse. Physical examination of these patients will frequently identify the underlying anatomical abnormality that results in these clinical presentations *(5–7)*. However, various radiological imaging techniques may be appropriately called upon to complement the workup of these patients to confirm the clinical suspicion as well as to identify unsuspected findings and defects that may impact upon the management decisions *(5,7–10)*. This chapter will review the current range of imaging techniques available to assess the pelvic floor either anatomically or functionally and discuss aspects of radiologic interpretation, strengths, and weaknesses of each modality.

2. DEFECOGRAPHY

Defecography (or evacuation proctography) is a fluoroscopic radiologic technique that assesses the function of the pelvic floor structures during the stresses imposed by the efforts of rectal evacuation. In its most basic form, opacification of the rectum is performed to provide an impetus for the patient to perform a forced evacuation, as well as to demonstrate the anatomical changes in this structure during this maneuver. Various modifications of this technique employ opacification of other pelvic floor structures to provide additional imaging

From: *Colonic Diseases*
Edited by: T. R. Koch © Humana Press Inc., Totowa, NJ

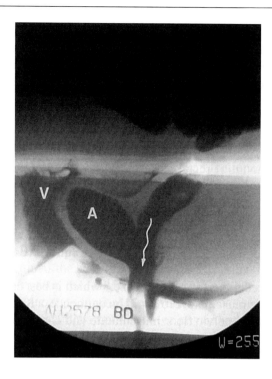

Fig. 1. Anterior Rectocele. A thirty-two-yr-old woman, G1P1 1 yr ago, with development of constipation (sensation of incomplete evacuation) relieved by digital splinting into her vagina and dyspareunia. Defecogram (late evacuation phase) shows a narrow necked 3 × 4 cm rectocele (A), extending anteriorly from the column of evacuating rectal contrast paste (curved arrow). It deforms the adjacent vaginal contour, the apex of the rectocele pushing up against the vaginal introitus (V).

considered pathological *(1,3,14)*. A rectocele greater than 4 cm in size is considered large and, if demonstrated to retain barium as well as contribute to feelings of incomplete evacuation, would then warrant surgical intervention as such patients may benefit from therapy *(3,10)*.

3.2. Rectal Prolapse

The inward invagination and downward migration of redundant rectal mucosa, occurring as the rectum evacuates, may take on a variety of forms. Milder degrees of such prolapse should be interpreted with caution and may indeed be a normal phenomenon *(3)*. Localized anterior rectal wall prolapse is a particularly common finding, reported to occur in 50% of female subjects without symptoms *(13)*. It may, however, represent a precursor to greater degrees of prolapse *(1,3,19)*. As the prolapse extends circumferentially to become a full intussusception formation, this may result in obstructive defecation as the prolapsed tissue prevents further evacuation of upper rectal content (Fig. 2). As the prolapse extends towards and eventually through the anal orifice, it may also be responsible for development for solitary rectal ulcer syndrome and result in rectal bleeding as well as become clinically overt resulting in rectal pain at the end of evacuation *(4)*.

3.3. Colorectal Inertia

Patients with these conditions are characterized typically by severe long-standing constipation, with very infrequent defecation (once every several days or weeks). As a result, they

21

Defecography and Related Radiologic Imaging Techniques

Vincent H. S. Low

CONTENTS

1. INTRODUCTION

The patient with pelvic floor and anorectal dysfunction may present with a variety of symptoms such as urinary or defecatory dysfunction, urogenital or anorectal prolapse, pelvic or abdominal pain, and dyspareunia *(1–5)*. Occasionally, rectal bleeding may eventually be found to be due to rectal prolapse. Physical examination of these patients will frequently identify the underlying anatomical abnormality that results in these clinical presentations *(5–7)*. However, various radiological imaging techniques may be appropriately called upon to complement the workup of these patients to confirm the clinical suspicion as well as to identify unsuspected findings and defects that may impact upon the management decisions *(5,7–10)*. This chapter will review the current range of imaging techniques available to assess the pelvic floor either anatomically or functionally and discuss aspects of radiologic interpretation, strengths, and weaknesses of each modality.

2. DEFECOGRAPHY

Defecography (or evacuation proctography) is a fluoroscopic radiologic technique that assesses the function of the pelvic floor structures during the stresses imposed by the efforts of rectal evacuation. In its most basic form, opacification of the rectum is performed to provide an impetus for the patient to perform a forced evacuation, as well as to demonstrate the anatomical changes in this structure during this maneuver. Various modifications of this technique employ opacification of other pelvic floor structures to provide additional imaging

From: *Colonic Diseases*
Edited by: T. R. Koch © Humana Press Inc., Totowa, NJ

and clinical information *(11)*. It should be noted that the commonly used clinical bony land-marks of the pelvis (pubic symphysis and coccygeal tip) are not readily visible on defecography, and the radiologist uses the ischial tuberosities as the standard bony landmark for interpretation *(12)*.

2.1. Technique

The defecographic procedure requires modification of standard radiologic fluoroscopic equipment with addition of a commode on which the patient is seated to allow observation of the pelvic floor structures during evacuation *(4,8)*. The examination is usually performed in the lateral projection, although the frontal projection has been described as useful in certain situations (lateral prolapse or enteroceles) *(1,3,13)*. Various structures in the pelvic floor will be opacified using appropriate contrast materials comprising the rectum (posterior compartment), vagina (middle compartment), and bladder (anterior compartment) *(11)*. The small bowel and external landmarks may also be opacified *(12)*.

Opacification of the rectum is the key component of this examination. This is accomplished with a commercial barium paste, this thick consistency is used to simulate stool *(1,3)*. The precise consistency is not crucial, as normal feces varies in consistency *(14)*. Liquid contrast should not be used, because this does not allow for physiologic rectal function, the liquid imposes abnormal stresses on the continence mechanism and produces abnormal responses of anal canal closure and pelvic floor musculature contractions *(4,13)*. The volume of paste is also not crucial, sufficient should be introduced to produce the sensation of slight urgency of evacuation, but should not result in painful stress to the patient. Excess paste is not a problem, as this would reflux into the sigmoid segment above the rectum *(4,10,13)*. A volume of 300 mL is usually sufficient.

In my practice, the vagina is opacified with 20 mL of high density barium. Demonstration of the vagina has been proven of value to allow visualization of the rectal vaginal gap, as separation would indicate the presence of prolapsing viscera into this space. Deformity of the vagina has also been found useful to identify the predominant pelvic floor deformity either from the anterior compartment (cystocele), causing posterior vaginal displacement, vs posterior compartment (rectocele), causing anterior vaginal displacement. The use of a contrast soaked tampon to opacify the vagina should be avoided, as the stiffness of this structure result in splinting and prevents development of pelvic floor prolapse during the fluoroscopic procedure *(3,4,10,13,15)*. I have found placement of a folded gauze square into the introitus useful, as it reduces the leakage of contrast from the vagina, as well as demonstrates the position of the urogenital hiatus in relation to the rest of the pelvic floor, and also allows visualization of vaginal migration in relation to the hiatus *(16,17)*.

Small bowel opacification is also a useful routine maneuver and is accomplished with the patient ingesting 500 mL of low density barium 1 h before the fluoroscopic procedure *(10)*. This will allow visualization of any potential small bowel segment that may herniate or prolapse into the pelvic floor (enterocele). The external soft tissue landmarks, which are obvious on clinical observation, are not routinely visible fluoroscopically. The urogenital hiatus will usually be rendered visible by normal leakage of contrast from the vagina. The anal dimple may be easily demonstrated by leaving a small smear of rectal paste at the orifice as the rectal catheter is removed. If assessment of the position and mobility of the perineal body is required, this surface landmark could be rendered visible by placement of an opaque marker prior to the fluoroscopic examination *(4,13)*. Opacification of the bladder (accomplished per urethral catheter with 50–200 mL of sterile urographic contrast) allows simultaneous demonstration of bladder deformities during evacuation (dynamic cystoproctography) *(6,10,11)*.

The patient sits on the defecographic commode and fluoroscopy and images are obtained initially at rest, followed by a "squeeze," which attempts to demonstrate the patient's effective continence mechanism. Finally, the patient is asked to strain, and then proceed to evacuate the rectal contents as completely as possible. It is usually during this final maneuver that deformities of the pelvic floor are most manifest *(12)*.

2.2. The Normal Defecogram

The examination begins with the patient at rest. A subjective assessment of the rectal volume is made based on the amount of rectal paste introduced. Objective measurements of rectal diameter, anal canal length, anorectal angle, and position of the anorectal junction in relation to bony landmarks (ischial tuberosities) can be made. The anorectal angle is usually measured between the axis of the anal canal against the posterior rectal margin *(1)*. This is normally 90° with a range of 60–120°. The anorectal junction is situated usually 5 mm above the ischial tuberosities reference level, with a normal range from 20 mm above to 10 mm below this level *(3,13,14)*.

The patient is then asked to perform a "squeeze," which is best explained as an attempt to actively contract the pelvic musculature to avoid incontinence, a Kegel maneuver. The resultant increase in tension of the pelvic floor musculature and contraction of the voluntary anal sphincter results in anterior and superior displacement of the anorectal junction. The actual impression by the puborectalis muscle sling may be actually visualized as an indentation upon the posterior rectal contour just above the anorectal junction *(13)*. Elevation of the pelvic floor by 10–15 mm should be expected. The anorectal angle should reduce by 15–25° *(3,4,13,14)*.

With strain, these effects of the pelvic floor muscular activity should reverse with resultant descent of the pelvic floor to a resting level and increase of the anorectal angle by 10–30°. Upon actual defecation, the anal canal should open to at least 1.5 cm in diameter *(3)*. Further pelvic floor descent should occur, usually by 20 mm, but up to 40 mm has been reported as considered normal. The anorectal angle should increase, to at least >90° and as much as 140° *(13,14)*. The posterior rectal impression, due to the puborectalis sling, should disappear. Rectal evacuation should proceed from the upper segment progressively through into the lower rectal segment and should be complete after a few attempts and within 60 s. Observation of the development of structural and functional abnormalities is most likely to occur in this final phase of the examination. Because of the chronicity of their problems, many patients have learned to perform a variety of splinting maneuvers (with vaginal, perineal, or rectal digital pressure). They should be encouraged to demonstrate these maneuvers, during the radiographic exercise, to identify the mechanism of their actions as an aid to understanding their symptoms *(1,4,12)*.

3. ABNORMAL FINDINGS

3.1. Rectocele

A rectocele is a focal outpouching of the rectal wall beyond its expectant line *(4,13)*. Rectoceles usually extend anteriorly and appear most prominently during the evacuation phase of the defecogram (Fig. 1). Occasionally occurring laterally and rarely posteriorly, these deformities are usually evident clinically by digital rectal examination. Defecography is of value in the evaluation of these deformities to differentiate a narrow necked rectocele, which suggests a focal defect in the rectal fascia, vs a broadly capacious akinetic rectum, which may be similar in perception to rectal examination *(10,18)*. Furthermore, a rectocele may be transient during evacuation, as it may empty with further effort of evacuation. Rectoceles when small (<2 cm) may be seen in normal individuals and should not always be

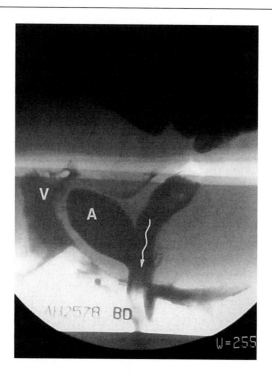

Fig. 1. Anterior Rectocele. A thirty-two-yr-old woman, G1P1 1 yr ago, with development of constipation (sensation of incomplete evacuation) relieved by digital splinting into her vagina and dyspareunia. Defecogram (late evacuation phase) shows a narrow necked 3 × 4 cm rectocele (A), extending anteriorly from the column of evacuating rectal contrast paste (curved arrow). It deforms the adjacent vaginal contour, the apex of the rectocele pushing up against the vaginal introitus (V).

considered pathological *(1,3,14)*. A rectocele greater than 4 cm in size is considered large and, if demonstrated to retain barium as well as contribute to feelings of incomplete evacuation, would then warrant surgical intervention as such patients may benefit from therapy *(3,10)*.

3.2. Rectal Prolapse

The inward invagination and downward migration of redundant rectal mucosa, occurring as the rectum evacuates, may take on a variety of forms. Milder degrees of such prolapse should be interpreted with caution and may indeed be a normal phenomenon *(3)*. Localized anterior rectal wall prolapse is a particularly common finding, reported to occur in 50% of female subjects without symptoms *(13)*. It may, however, represent a precursor to greater degrees of prolapse *(1,3,19)*. As the prolapse extends circumferentially to become a full intussusception formation, this may result in obstructive defecation as the prolapsed tissue prevents further evacuation of upper rectal content (Fig. 2). As the prolapse extends towards and eventually through the anal orifice, it may also be responsible for development for solitary rectal ulcer syndrome and result in rectal bleeding as well as become clinically overt resulting in rectal pain at the end of evacuation *(4)*.

3.3. Colorectal Inertia

Patients with these conditions are characterized typically by severe long-standing constipation, with very infrequent defecation (once every several days or weeks). As a result, they

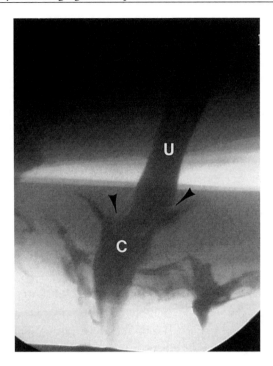

Fig. 2. Internal Rectal Prolapse. A thirty-nine-yr-old woman with long-standing constipation (sensation of incomplete evacuation) relieved by digital rectal pressure. Defecogram (mid evacuation phase) shows good lower rectal segment emptying but development of circumferential internal rectal mucosal prolapse (arrow heads), with more pronounced involvement of the anterior wall, protruding to the level of the anal canal (C). This mass of redundant rectal tissue then cuts-off the rectal column preventing evacuation of further content from the upper rectal segment (U). The internal mass effect of the prolapsed tissue is also contributing to the sensation of incomplete evacuation.

manifest considerable retention of feces with associated symptoms of abdominal distention and bloating. Imaging of these patients demonstrate no physical obstructive process, instead, colonic inertia is characterized by diffuse failure of the colon to evacuate. The value of defecography in these patients is to demonstrate if the rectum is similarly involved, usually in preparation for colonic shortening surgery. Patients who exhibit normal rectal evacuation would be expected to do well with colonic resection. If the inertia appears to involve the rectum as well (characterized at defecography by a patulous rectum which fails to evacuate), surgical management would be less likely to be successful and efforts should remain initially with medical therapy including stool softening agents and stimulatory laxatives.

3.4. Pelvic Floor Dyskinesia

Defecatory symptoms may also be due to abnormal contractile activity of the pelvic floor musculature. These result in constipation with a variety of names given to this syndrome including dyskinetic (nonrelaxing), puborectalis muscle, spastic pelvic floor syndrome, paradoxical sphincter contraction, and rectal dyschezia *(12)*. During attempted evacuation, there is failure of the pelvic floor to descend due to persistent contractile activity of the pelvic floor muscles. The normal effacement of the anorectal angle does not occur and there may indeed be paradoxical increased and acute angulation. During defecography, these features will be observed, and there will be incomplete evacuation despite repeated attempts by the patient *(1,3,4,10,20)*. The chronic staining by the patient usually results in the development of associated other rectal pelvic floor deformities, such as rectoceles and prolapse. The diagnosis of this syndrome as the underlying etiology for constipation will avoid inappropriate surgery of the observed rectal and pelvic deformities. Instead, management should begin with a retraining regime to develop appropriate relaxation of the pelvic floor musculature during evacuation *(10)*.

Conversely, excessive pelvic floor laxity may also produce symptoms. This is recognized as the descending perineum syndrome where the pelvic floor landmarks are located more than 3 to 4 cm below the ischial tuberosities *(21,22)*. Further pelvic floor descent may occur during evacuation. Patient may perceive constipation due to impaired ability of the rectum to empty, as well as prolapse of various viscera into the pelvic space. The patient may also suffer synchronous incontinence due to failure of the voluntary sphincter mechanism to perform adequately *(10,23)*. During defecography, low lying pelvic floor with obtuse anorectal angulation is observed, and assessment can be made of adequate or otherwise rectal evacuation as well as other pelvic organ abnormalities *(7)*.

3.5. *Enteroceles and Other Rectovaginal Gap Hernias*

The rectovaginal gap is a potential space between the posterior surface of the vagina and the anterior margin of the rectum, usually supported by a fascia. This supportive tissue may become deficient either due to previous obstetric or other trauma. Herniation of various viscera into this space may then occur, usually as a consequence of chronic and repeated straining. Detection and identification of these hernias may escape clinical evaluation because these hernias may not develop until the patient exerts maximal straining effort, such as occurs during defecation *(24)*. In addition, the beginnings of such herniations may occur above the reach of the digital pelvic examination. Defecography has been found most useful in the detection of these herniations, especially in the patient proceeding towards pelvic floor repair for the management of other obvious deformities, such as rectoceles and rectal prolapses *(6,7)*. The identification of this group of lesions allows simultaneous repair of the rectovaginal septum, as well as management of the pelvic floor diaphragm defect. Without the benefit of this information, the presence of the persistent herniation will result in prompt redevelopment of pelvic floor symptoms and, therefore, an unsatisfactory surgical result *(6,8,10)*. The importance of detecting these lesions also highlights the importance of the defecography technique to include opacification of the vagina and small bowel *(4,12,17)*.

The space of the widened rectovaginal gap is most commonly filled with herniating loops of small bowel (enterocele) (Fig. 3). The full extent of the defect and herniation may not become apparent unless the patient exerts the maximal effort of straining *(6,7)*. Enteroceles are considered small if <4 cm in size and large if >6 cm in depth *(10)*. Enteroceles are easily identified if the small bowel has been opacified with oral contrast *(12)*. The observation of rectovaginal gap widening without small bowel herniation suggest the presence of herniation of some other viscera. The sigmoid colon may be responsible, and this can usually be deduced by the observation of bowel without contrast, but with gas and feces within the widened rectovaginal space. Less commonly, a posteriorly prolapsing uterus, herniation of mesentery or omentum may fall into this space *(7,10,13)*. Regardless of the content of the widened rectovaginal space, symptoms may be produced as a consequence of the mass effect upon the adjacent structures. If the herniation causes external mass effect upon the middle rectal segment, this may cause interruption of rectal evacuation, resulting in constipation due to retained rectosigmoid feces. The mass effect of the enterocele or other hernia within the posterior perineal space may leave the patient with the sensation of incomplete rectal evacuation despite

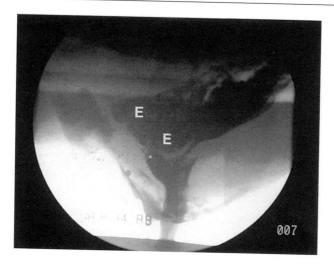

Fig. 3. Enterocele. A seventy-two-yr-old woman with constipation (feeling of incomplete evacuation). Physical examination revealed a capacious rectum with anterior rectocele. Defecogram demonstrates complete rectal evacuation. A broad anterior rectocele was observed during evacuation, but is also completely evacuated. A large enterocele (E) develops as the rectum empties, the true source of the patient's symptom of persistent perineal fullness (perceived as rectal fullness and hence incomplete evacuation).

adequate rectal emptying. Extension of the hernia towards the perineal body will result in an overt perineal bulge with associated local discomfort and symptoms. Extension anteriorly into the posterior vaginal wall may result in vaginal prolapse and dyspareunia (12).

3.6. Cystocele

A cystocele is recognized by descent of the bladder base below the inferior margin of the pubic symphysis, usually observed only at maximal straining. It is usually evident clinically and may be confirmed with specific bladder imaging studies such as cystometry or cystography. Bladder opacification during defecography may be useful to assess the global involvement of abnormal bladder migration in the context of other pelvic floor deformities (6,10). Without bladder opacification, cystocele may still be recognized as a concave impression on the superior aspect of the bladder and resultant posterior and inferior migration of the vagina during defecation (17). If bladder opacification is performed, additional information can be observed, such as rotation of the bladder neck into the vagina indicating hypermobility of the bladder neck (Fig. 4). The bladder neck configuration itself can also be observed during straining to assess for intrinsic urethral sphincter efficiency, or otherwise, and resultant urinary continence (10,11,21,25).

4. OTHER RADIOGRAPHIC TECHNIQUES

The plain abdominal radiograph has very little value in the assessment of the patient with defecatory dysfunction. Gross amounts of fecal constipation may be evident in the severely constipated patient, but the plain radiograph remains notoriously inaccurate in its ability to assess less severe but still symptomatic degrees of constipation. The plain radiograph is of value when taken in conjunction with ingestion of a Sitzmarks capsule (Konsyl Pharmaceuticals, Fort Worth, TX). This is a commercially available dissolvable capsule, which contains

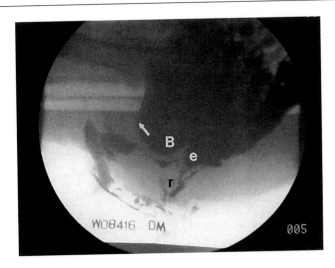

Fig. 4. Cystocele. A forty-eight-yr-old woman with variable inability to control urinary emptying and occasional fecal incontinence. Defecogram (including bladder [B] opacification) shows rapid downward prolapse of the bladder by 5 cm onto the vaginal contour. As a result, the vesicourethral junction (arrow) is angulated upwards. As she evacuates there is prolapse of rectal mucosa (r) to the anal verge and observation of a small enterocele (e).

24 small opaque markers. A plain abdominal radiograph is obtained 5 d after ingestion of the capsule. In the presence of normal colonic function, 80% or more of the markers should have been evacuated. The presence of 6 or more retained markers suggest impaired colonic evacuatory function and may provide an understanding of the cause of patients constipation. A widespread distribution of retained markers suggests diffuse colonic inertia. A localized distribution of the retained markers suggests an obstructive phenomenon just distal to the location of the residual markers *(26,27)*.

Barium enema is the radiological investigation of choice to diagnose or exclude structural obstructive lesions (strictures), in the context of obstruction or constipation, or mucosal lesions (polyps, masses, or ulcers), in the context of rectal bleeding *(28)*. It is also useful to define the colorectal anatomy prior to proposed colonic surgery. It will not, however, substitute for defecography in the assessment of functional disorders of the rectum or pelvic floor. Only the most gross of rectal anatomical deformities will be evident on the distended barium enema. Most of the abnormalities as described above, which become evident during the evacuation phase of a defecogram, will not be visible during an enema *(12)*.

5. ULTRASOUND

Endoanal ultrasonography uses a high frequency (greater than 7 Mhz) circumferential transducer, which will produce a 360° circular image *(29,30)*. This technique is optimal for the direct visualization of the internal anal sphincter. This structure is consistently visible as a concentric homogenous hypoechoic ring a few millimeters peripheral to the margin of the transducer and external to a hyperechoic submucosal layer *(30)*. This modality is most useful to assess the structural integrity of the internal anal sphincter seen normally as a symmetrical and circumferential ring. A focal gap in the ring would indicate a sphincter tear *(31,32)*. Conversely, the demonstration of sphincter thickening may indicate hypertrophy as an etiology for obstructed defecation *(33)*. It may also detect associated fistulas, abscesses, or tumors. It should be noted that the function of these transducers requires the presence of a surrounding water bath or hard plastic sheath to allow good sonographic contact between the device and the anal canal surface. As a consequence, there is distention of the anal canal. This, in turn, leads to considerable variation in reported normal and abnormal thickness of the internal anal sphincter (reports range from 1.3–2.7 mm) *(29,30)*. Each individual ultrasound laboratory would have its own range of normal values depending on the size of the transducer package, because the larger the diameter of the probe, would result in greater distention of the anal canal and normal thinning of the muscle layer.

The high frequency of the endoanal ultrasound probe prevents examination of further distant perianal structures, and even the external anal sphincter is not reliably demonstrated. Alternative means of examination, such as by an abdominal, transvaginal, or perineal approach may be used to examine the remainder of the pelvic viscera *(34–38)*. In the assessments of the pelvic floor, examination of the bladder and its neck may by of relevance. Abdominal and vaginal approaches are suitable for detection of masses or cysts. Transperineal scanning is a reliable means to visualize the bladder and the urethra without the acoustic shadowing artifact from the pubic bone. This technique has been used to assess residual post-void bladder volume and to visualize bladder neck mobility *(39)*.

6. MAGNETIC RESONANCE IMAGING

Magnetic resonance imaging (MRI) is an established diagnostic imaging modality that has the potential to provide exquisite soft tissue definition. This modality also allows imaging of the patient in multiple planes directly and allows the soft tissues of the pelvis to be visualized without the assistance of special contrast material. Despite the apparent advantages of MRI, there are drawbacks and limitations. The preparation for imaging requires selection of a variety of technical variables, which will impact upon the resulted image quality. Some of the sequences may take several minutes, requiring considerable patient cooperation, otherwise motion artifact will degrade the image. The choice of the field-of-view examined would also effect the ability to identify normal structures or pathology, a smaller chosen field-of-view would allow resolution of smaller structures, but will prevent detection of potential abnormalities at the edge the examination field. The direction of imaging needs to be chosen, and the slice plane should be parallel or perpendicular to the structure of interest to allow it to be optimally displayed. Errors in the selection of any or some of these criteria for MRI may degrade the quality of the examination, and this, in turn, may lead to errors in diagnosis.

MRI in the evaluation of the patient with incontinent defecatory difficulty is usually used to assess the morphology of the anal sphincters. This is optimally performed with a dedicated endoanal coil, which places the imaging technology at closest proximity to the area of interest *(40,41)*. This technique sacrifices the ability to visualize the other structures of the pelvic floor and may require additional imaging with external body coils. Anal sphincter studies usually combine sagittal or coronal scans with axial series perpendicular to the axis of the anal canal. The use of a small field-of-view allows sufficient spatial resolution (0.5 mm) to discriminate the various muscle layers. As with endoanal ultrasound, the size and configuration of the endoanal coil (which is used specific to the manufacturer of the MRI scanner) will result in different degrees of distention of the anal canal (ranging from 7–19 mm). These coils results in stretching of the anal canal lumen and the various layers of the anal canal, including the internal and external sphincter muscles, which would be displayed as concentric circles *(40–43)*. Imaging laboratories, which use a body coil to examine the anal canal as well as the pelvic floor globally, should insert a soft catheter in the anal canal to produce a similar distention, otherwise the superficial layers of the anus will crumple together and will not be differentiated from each other *(30,44,45)*.

The internal anal sphincter is the structure of most interest in the MRI of the incontinent patient, and the aim is to detect integrity or otherwise of this structure *(1)*. It appears as a low signal (dark) ring, which should be intact circumferentially just deep to the mucosa and submucosa of the anal canal. Depending on the technology used for imaging, the sphincter muscle has been reported to range in thickness from 0.5–4 mm *(40,41)*. It is, therefore, important that each imaging laboratory establish its independent normal values for interpretation of its diagnostic imaging studies rather than refer to publications based on imaging with different equipment *(30,42,45)*.

Techniques that allow a more global pelvic floor examination (using a body or an endovaginal coil) allows visualization of the other pelvic floor muscles and groups, including the external anal sphincter, puborectalis sling, pubococcygeus, and the levator plate *(46,47)*. Apart from demonstration of these normal structures, MRI permits the visualization of pelvic pathology in relationship to these normal structures. Masses, fluid collections, infection, fistula tracts, and scars are well recognized *(42–45,48)*.

Recent advances in MRI have been directed towards modifications in dynamic scanning as an alternative to radiographic defecography *(49–55)*. These techniques have the potential advantage over radiographic defecography of being able to image in a variety of planes, without ionizing radiation, and with the ability to visualize all the pelvic luminal and muscular structures without special contrast opacification. Major disadvantages of these techniques are the inability to image in a seated (physiological) position and to ensure an adequate straining effort as can be achieved with forced rectal evacuation. These currently remain evolving technologies.

7. CONCLUSION

The use of imaging techniques is optimized by close cooperation between the referring clinician and the imaging radiologist. This is especially true of the patient with pelvic floor dysfunction. It should be recognized that there is a wide overlap of defecographic findings between normal subjects and the symptomatic patient *(3,12,13,56)*. The abnormal findings at defecography should not be the only criteria for decision making. A totally normal defecogram will indicate that anorectal dysfunction is not the etiology in a patient with constipation. Otherwise, the result of defecography should be combined with other anatomical and functional evaluations to formulate a plan of management *(12,56)*.

REFERENCES

1. Hiltunen KM, Kolehmainen H, Matikainen M. Does defecography help in diagnosis and clinical decision-making in defecation disorders? *Abdom. Imaging*, **19** (1994) 355–358.
2. Karasick S, Ehrlich S. Evacuation proctography (defecography): Roentgenographic findings in 274 consecutive patients. In *Programs and Abstracts of the 94th Annual Meeting of the American Roentgen Ray Society*. New Orleans, LA, 1994, p. 71.
3. Ott DJ, Donati DL, Kerr RM, Chen MYM. Defecography: results in 55 patients and impact on clinical management. *Abdom. Imaging*, **19** (1994) 349–354.
4. Shorvon PJ, Stevenson GW. Defecography: setting up a service. *Br. J. Hosp. Med.*, **41** (1989) 460–466.
5. Harvey CJ, Halligan S, Bartram CI, Hollings N, Sahdev A, Kingston K. Evacuation proctography: A prospective study of diagnostic and therapeutic effects. *Radiology*, **211** (1999) 223–227.
6. Kelvin FM, Maglinte DDT, Hornback JA, Benson JT. Pelvic prolapse: Assessment with evacuation proctography (defecography). *Radiology*, **184** (1992) 547–551.
7. Kelvin FM, Hale DS, Maglinte DDT, Patten BJ, Benson JT. Female pelvic organ prolapse: Diagnostic contribution of dynamic cystoproctography and comparison with physical examination. *Am. J. Roentgenol.*, **173** (1999) 31–37.

8. Brubaker L, Retzky S, Smith C, Saclarides T. Pelvic floor evaluation with dynamic fluoroscopy. *Obstet. Gynecol.*, **82** (1993) 863–868.

9. Fenner DE. Diagnosis and assessment of sigmoidoceles. *Am. J. Obstet. Gynecol.*, **175** (1996) 1438–1442.

10. Maglinte DDT, Kelvin FM, Hale DS, Benson JT. Dynamic cystoproctography: a unifying diagnostic approach to pelvic floor and anorectal dysfunction. *Am. J. Roentgenol.*, **169** (1997) 759–767.

11. Kelvin FM, Maglinte DDT, Benson JT, Brubaker LP, Smith C. Dynamic cystoproctography: A technique for assessing disorders of the pelvic floor in women. *Am. J. Roentgenol.*, **163** (1994) 368–370.

12. Weidner AC, Low VHS. Imaging studies of the pelvic floor. *Obstet. Gynecol. Clin. N. Am.*, **25** (1998) 825–848.

13. Shorvon PJ, McHugh S, Diamant NE, Somers S, Stevenson GW. Defecography in normal volunteers: results and implications. *Gut*, **30** (1989) 1737–1749.

14. Ikenberry S, Lappas JC, Hana MP, Rex DK. Defecography in healthy subjects: comparison of three contrast media. *Radiology*, **201** (1996) 233–238.

15. Archer BD, Somers S, Stevenson GW. Contrast medium gel for marking vaginal position during defecography. *Radiology*, **182** (1992) 278–279.

16. Ho LM, Low VHS, Freed KS. Vaginal opacification during defecography: utility of placing a folded gauze square at the introitus. *Abdom. Imaging*, **24** (1999) 562–564.

17. Low VHS, Ho LM, Freed KS. Vaginal opacification during defecography: direction of vaginal migration aids in diagnosis of pelvic floor pathology. *Abdom. Imaging*, **24** (1999) 565–568.

18. Cundiff GW, Weidner AC, Visco AG, Addison WA, Bump RC. An anatomical and functional assessment of the discrete defect posterior colporrhaphy. In *Abstract of the 24th Scientific Meeting of the Society of Gynecologic Surgeons*. Orlando, FL, 1997.

19. McGee SG, Bartram CI. Intra-anal intussusception: Diagnosis by posteroanterior stress proctography. *Abdom. Imaging*, **18** (1993) 136–140.

20. Halligan S, Bartram CI, Park HJ, Kamm HA. Proctographic features of anismus. *Radiology*, **197** (1995) 679–682.

21. Oettle GJ, Roe AM, Bartolo DCC, Mortensen NJ. What is the best way of measuring perineal descent? A comparison of radiographic and clinical methods. *Br. J. Surg.*, **72** (1985) 999–1001.

22. Parks AG, Porter NH, Hardcastle J. The syndrome of the descending perineum. *Proc. R. Soc. Med.*, **59** (1966) 477–450.

23. Henry MM, Parks AG, Swash M. The pelvic floor musculature in the descending perineum syndrome. *Br. J. Surg.*, **69** (1982) 470–472.

24. Altringer WE, Saclarides TJ, Dominguez JM, Brubaker LP, Smith CS. Four-contrast defecography: pelvic "floor-oscopy." *Dis. Colon Rectum*, **38** (1995) 695–699.

25. Versi E, Cardozo L, Studd J, et al. Distal urethral compensatory mechanisms in women with an incompetent bladder neck who remain continent, and the effect of the menopause. *Neurourol. Urodyn.*, **9** (1990) 579–590.

26. Ahmed M. Anorectal manometry, EMG, defecography and colonic transit studies to evaluate constipation. *Pract. Gastroenterol.*, **23** (1999) 52–62.

27. Mertz H, Naliboff B, Mayer E. Physiology of refractory chronic constipation. *Am. J. Gastroenterol.*, **94** (1999) 609–615.

28. Karasick S. Does barium enema predict defecographic abnormalities? In *Programs and Abstracts of the 96th Annual Meeting of the American Roentgen Ray Society*. San Diego, CA, 1996, p. 83.

29. Gantke B, Schafer A, Enck P, Lubke H. Morphology and function: sonographic, manometric, and myographic evaluation of the anal sphincters. *Dis. Colon Rectum*, **36** (1993) 1037–1041.

30. Schafer A, Enck P, Furst G, Kahn TH, Frieling T, Lubke HJ. Anatomy of the anal sphincters: comparison of anal endosonography to magnetic resonance imaging. *Dis. Colon Rectum*, **37** (1994) 777–781.

31. Law PJ, Kamm MA, Bartram CI. A comparison between electromyography and anal endosongraphy in mapping external anal sphincter defects. *Dis. Colon Rectum*, **33** (1990) 370–373.

32. Meyenberger C, Bertschinger P, Zala GF, Buchmann P. Anal sphincter defects in fecal incontinence: correlation between endosonography and surgery. *Endoscopy*, **28** (1996) 217–224.

33. Nielsen MB, Rasmussen OO, Pedersen JF, Christiansen J. Anal endosonographic findings in patients with obstructed defecation. *Acta Radiol.*, **34** (1993) 35–38.

34. Frudinger A, Bartram CI, Kamm MA. Transvaginal versus anal endosonography for detecting damage to the anal sphincter. *Am. J. Roentgenol.*, **168** (1997) 1435–1438.

35. Kohorn EL, Scioscia AL, Jeanty P, Hobbins JC. Ultrasound cystourethrography by perineal scanning for the assessment of female stress urinary incontinence. *Obstet. Gynecol.*, **68** (1986) 269–272.

36. Peschers U, Schaer G, Anthuber C, DeLancey JO, Schuessler B. Changes in vesical neck mobility following vaginal delivery. *Obstet. Gynecol.*, **88** (1996) 1001–1006.

37. Stewart LK, Wilson SR. Transvaginal sonography of the anal sphincter: reliable, or not? *Am. J. Roentgenol.*, **173** (1999) 179–185.

38. Rubens DJ, Strang JG, Bogineni-Misra S, Wexler IE. Transperineal sonography of the rectum: anatomy and pathology revealed by sonography compared with CT and MR imaging. *Am. J. Roentgenol.*, **170** (1998) 637–640.

39. Roehrborn CG, Peters PC. Can transabdominal ultrasound estimation of postvoiding residual replace catheterization? *Urology*, **16** (1988) 445–449.

40. deSouza NM, Puni R, Zbar A, Gilderdale DJ, Coutts GA, Krausz T. MR imaging of the anal sphincter in multiparous women using an endoanal coil: Correlation with in vitro anatomy and appearances in fecal incontinence. *Am. J. Roentgenol.*, **167** (1996) 1465–1471.

41. Hussain SM, Stoker J, Lameris JS. Anal sphincter complex: Endoanal MR imaging of normal anatomy. *Radiology*, **197** (1995) 671–677.

42. deSouza NM, Gilderdale DJ, MacIver DK, Ward HC. High-resolution MR imaging of the anal sphincter in children: a pilot study using endoanal receiver coils. *Am. J. Roentgenol.*, **169** (1997) 201–206.

43. Stoker J, Hussain SM, van Kempen D, Elevelt AJ, Lameris JS. Endoanal coil in MR imaging of anal fistulas. *Am. J. Roentgenol.*, **166** (1996) 360–362.

44. Hussain SM, Stoker J, Schouten WR, Hop WC, Lameris JS. Fistula in ano: Endoanal sonography versus endoanal MR imaging in classification. *Radiology*, **200** (1996) 475–481.

45. Schaer GN, Koechli OR, Schuessler B, Haller U. Improvement of perineal sonographic bladder neck imaging with ultrasound contrast medium. *Obstet. Gynecol.*, **86** (1995) 950–954.

46. Fielding JR, Dumanli H, Schreyer AG, et al. MR-based three-dimensional modeling of the normal pelvic floor in women: Quantification of muscle mass. *Am. J. Roentgenol.*, **174** (2000) 657–660.

47. Tan IL, Stoker J, Zwaborn AW, Entius KAC, Calame JJ, Lameris JS. Female pelvic floor: Endovaginal MR imaging of normal anatomy. *Radiology*, **206** (1998) 777–783.

48. Sultan AH, Kamm MA, Hudson CN, Thomas JM, Bartram CI. Anal-sphincter disruption during vaginal delivery. *N. Engl. J. Med.*, **329** (1993) 1905–1911.

49. Delemarre JBVM, Kruyt RH, Doornbos J, et al. Anterior rectocele: assessment with radiographic defecography, dynamic magnetic resonance imaging, and physical examination. *Dis. Colon Rectum*, **37** (1994) 249–259.

50. Goodrich MA, Webb MJ, King BF, Bampton AEH, Campeau NG, Riedener SJ. Magnetic resonance imaging of pelvic floor relaxation: dynamic analysis and evaluation of patients before and after surgical repair. *Obstet. Gynecol.*, **82** (1993) 883–891.

51. Healy JC, Halligan S, Reznek RH, et al. Dynamic MR imaging compared with evacuation proctography when evaluating anorectal configuration and pelvic floor movement. *Am. J. Roentgenol.*, **169** (1997) 775–779.

52. Goh V, Halligan S, Kaplan G, Healy JC, Bartram CI. Dynamic MR imaging of the pelvic floor in asymptomatic subjects. *Am. J. Roentgenol.*, **174** (2000) 661–666.

53. Schoenenberger AW, Debatin JF, Guldenschuh I, Hany TF, Steiner P, Krestin GP. Dynamic MR defecography with a superconducting, open-configuration MR system. *Radiology*, **206** (1998) 641–646.

54. Kelvin FM, Maglinte DDT, Hale DS, Benson JT. Female pelvic organ prolapse: a comparison of triphasic dynamic MR imaging and triphasic fluoroscopic cystocolpoproctography. *Am. J. Roentgenol.*, **174** (2000) 81–88.

55. Yang A, Mostwin JL, Rosenshein NB, Zerhouni EA. Pelvic floor descent in women: dynamic evaluation with fast MR imaging and cinematic display. *Radiology*, **179** (1991) 25–33.

56. Freimanis MG, Wald A, Caruana B, Bauman DH. Evacuation proctography in normal volunteers. *Invest. Radiol.*, **26** (1991) 581–585.

22 Cross-Sectional Imaging of the Large Bowel

Diego R. Martin, Ming Yang, and Paul Hamilton

CONTENTS

1. INTRODUCTION

There has been considerable evolution of imaging techniques applied to visualization of pathology related to the large bowel. As recently as 10–15 yr ago, the predominant technique for colon imaging depended on plain film radiography. More recently, technological developments have facilitated use of computed tomography (CT), magnetic resonance imaging (MRI), and ultrasound. Plain radiography is now considered to be of limited relative value, and generally, a test having low diagnostic yield. Radiography in combination with rectally administered contrast agents has been found useful for assessing mucosal and structural abnormalities. Optimal technique uses double-contrast barium enema, where a combination of a positive contrast, barium, thinly coats the intestinal mucosal surface, while the lumen is distended with a negative contrast, air, which is insufflated transrectally. In order to achieve effective coating of the entire colon, the patient is required to perform a variety of maneuvers while on the imaging table. There is exhaustive review of plain film and double-contrast radiography techniques in the literature, and this chapter will instead concentrate on newer state-of-the-art imaging based on CT and MR.

2. CROSS-SECTIONAL IMAGING TECHNIQUES

2.1. CT: Technology and Methodology

CT uses ionizing X-ray radiation, similar to that used for plain film radiography. However, where the plain film image is generated using a system that has a radiation source, patient, and film remaining in static relative position, the CT scanner uses a radiation source and detector

From: *Colonic Diseases*
Edited by: T. R. Koch © Humana Press Inc., Totowa, NJ

system that rotates around the patient. In the past 15 yr there has been marked improvement in this technology (1–3). Improvements have been based on better reconstruction programs, using backscatter image reconstruction algorithms, faster computers, and significant innovations in the design of the rotating radiation-detection devices. Initially, there was development of the slip-ring technology, allowing maintenance of high voltage power supply to the X-ray tube, while this tube is rotating around the patient. More recently, there has been development of solid-state detectors that are built to dimensions of 1.25 mm squares, and then assembled into multirow detector arrays, allowing high-resolution imaging (1–3). This has been combined with spiral scanning, where the radiation source and detector array revolve rapidly around the patient during imaging, while the patient table slides continually through the gantry. This allows more rapid imaging, and constructs an image data set that can be treated as a volume (4–8). Initially, imaging relied on generating a two-dimensional slice, one slice at a time, then moving the patient to the next increment, and performing the next slice while the patient remains immobile during image acquisition. This creates a tremendous problem with misregistration, particularly in imaging mobile structures such as bowel (9–11). Misregistration is caused by having two contiguous slices performed with the soft tissue structures moving and not lining up exactly with the prior image slice due to even slight movements occurring between imaging of the two neighboring slices. Spiral imaging, performed rapidly during a single breath-hold, can reduce or eliminate misregistration by decreasing the time to acquire the image data set and by creating data that is mathematically treated as a volume covering the entire scanned part of the patient, rather than generating a scan by combining individually scanned slices. The volumetric data acquired from a spiral scanner can then be retrospectively sliced into thickness as desired and prescribed by the operator, with slicing occurring mathematically. The volumetric data also has the potential to be reconstructed in slices oriented in planes different from the primary transverse plane in which the imaging was performed. Volumetric data can also be used to construct three-dimensional images, using specially adapted software. Volume rendering allows depiction of tubular structures, such as large bowel, using fly-through software that produces images with the perspective from within the bowel lumen, appearing similar to the view from a colonoscope (Fig. 1). The imager can then use the computer to move along the length of the bowel, changing directions and angle of view as desired. However, despite the undeniable sophistication and complexity of these developments in image data post-processing, it is still felt that the most important images are the source images from which the three-dimensional views are generated. The source images can be viewed using computer workstations, typically as part of a picture archival computer system (PACS) that have the capability of rapidly scrolling through a stacked set of two-dimensional images (12,13). Considering the number of individual images generated in an optimal spiral CT of the abdomen and pelvis, typically over 220 and sometimes greater than 500–600 images, hard copy filming is no longer practical. Furthermore, soft copy reading on a PACS is known to lead to superior visual interpretation of images, as compared to reading from sheets of film (12,13). Rapid scrolling through a set of stacked two-dimensional images facilitates interpretation by the visual system of the reader, creating the illusion of looking at a three-dimensional

---

Fig. 1. *(opposite page)* Colonographic imaging using CT (A and B) and MRI (C–E). Three-dimensional reconstruction obtained from axial two-dimensional source images allows depiction of large bowel mucosal contours with a view from inside the lumen (A). This study showed a 1.5-cm polypoid mass (A, arrowheads). However, these findings are nonspecific, and although identical in appearance to an adenoma or adenocarcinoma, require correlation with the two-dimenstional source images (B). Corresponding focus (B, arrow) demonstrates features typical of retained stool demonstrating mottled lower

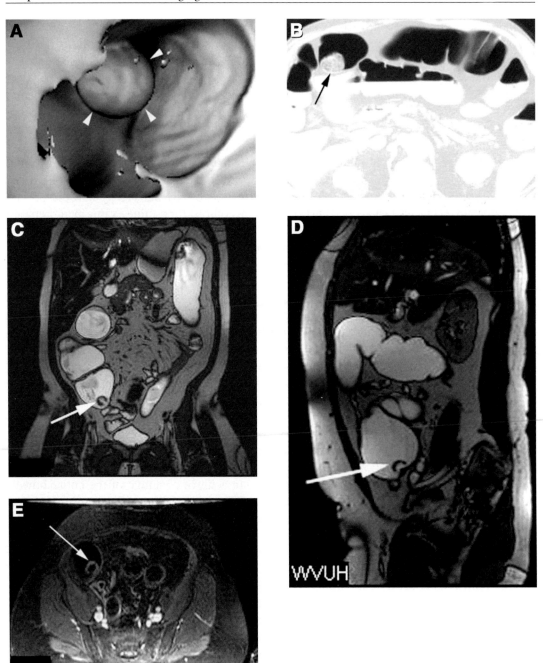

density gas within the structure. Note that the source images are viewed using lung window-level settings to improve contrast between intraluminal gas and bowel wall. MR colonography is shown on T-FISP coronal (C) and sagittal (D) images using water enema contrast and on 3D-VIBE axial image (E) after intravenous gadolinium enhancement. Superb contrast and motion-insensitive delineation of bowel wall is obtained on T-FISP images, showing a benign linear polypoid defect arising from the base of the cecum (C and D, arrow). Similarly, this defect is seen on 3D-VIBE (E, arrow). Although 3D-VIBE produces less contrast relative to T-FISP and has greater bowel motion sensitivity, it provides excellent visualization of the extra-enteric structures, including retroperitoneum (note bright iliac arteries and veins seen just below the iliac bifurcation) and liver (not shown).

picture. The phenomenon particularly is applicable to tubular structures, such as bowel. Usual protocols for imaging of the abdomen and pelvis can include oral and rectal administration of radiodense iodinated contrast agent, to opacify the large and small bowel lumen. This approach can facilitate visualization of most of the important large bowel disease processes. Protocols for specific evaluation of the large bowel mucosa, especially designed for detection of premalignant polyps and small tumors, are currently undergoing intense evaluation. These techniques can generally be referred to as CT colonography (14–31). The technique showing greatest promise involves insufflating air into the large bowel per rectum, to yield a fully distended bowel. The patient requires preparation using a bowel cleansing protocol starting the evening prior to imaging. Polyps, either solitary, metachronous, or multiple polyps associated with polyposis syndromes, can be diagnosed on CT and MRI. Sensitivity can be improved using oral and rectal contrast agents. On CT imaging, contrast for routine exams in unprepared bowel usually consists of dilute water-soluble iodinated solution, yielding radiodense positive contrast, within the bowel lumen. The contrast can be administered orally, and can be supplemented by per-rectal administration. However, more dedicated techniques are evolving in order to maximize sensitivity for small mucosal lesions, particularly for detecting premalignant polyps. CT colonography is a technique that is analogous to double-contrast barium enema, dependent on preparing the bowel with a cleansing protocol, and subsequently distending the large bowel with a contrast agent at the time of imaging. The contrast agent showing greatest favor is gas, either air or CO^2, administered rectally while the patient is on the CT table. The patient bowel is distended to tolerance, the patient then placed prone on the imaging table, and imaging performed using thin slice protocols, such as 2.5 mm thickness on a multirow detector scanner. The gas produces a dark or negative contrast within the lumen. In order to visualize all bowel wall surfaces, the patient is rotated to the supine position and imaging repeated to minimize the risk of missing lesions on the dependent aspect that may be obscured by layering residual fluid or stool. The patient must breath-hold in order to reduce motion degradation and misregistration. Scans performed on single row detector CT require multiple breath-hold scans, typically two to three, in order to achieve coverage of the entire bowel. Scans using current generation multidetector row CT can scan through the entire abdomen during a single breath-hold period. This increased speed has been shown to reduce motion and misregistration artifacts and reduce the problem of bowel gas leakage with loss of bowel lumen distension (24). Both the source two-dimensional images and reconstruction three-dimensional volume-rendered images are then viewed on a workstation, with three-dimensional volume-rendered images used for colonoscopy-like depiction and fly-through visualization. It is found that the volume-rendered images are useful as a supplement to findings made on the two-dimensional slices, to confirm or reevaluate questionable findings, and that this approach is more reliable and time-efficient as compared to relying only on three-dimensional reconstruction images using current generation software. Early studies show that polyp size resolution is possible to the range of 1.0 cm, below which the sensitivity and negative predictive value of the exam begins to diminish to levels well below that of conventional colonoscopy (14–31). As experience continues, it is hoped that CT colonography will improve further.

2.2. MR Technology and Methodology

MRI has evolved to become a major imaging method for detection and characterization of most of the important diseases of the abdomen and pelvis (32–37). Despite considerable evolution in the techniques used to generate MR images over the past 15 yr, abdominal imaging is still based upon obtaining some form of T1-weighted and T2-weighted images. A T1-weighted image, regardless of method, generates characteristic patterns of signal intensity, where structures having higher water content, such as the central spinal fluid (CSF) surrounding the spinal cord, generally are depicted as having lower signal. T2-weighted images, regardless of method, will show structures with high water content as having high signal. On gray scale image display, high signal is depicted as white, and low signal as black, with signal between these two extremes depicted on a gradient gray scale. Fat can appear as high signal on most types of fast T1- and T2-weighted sequences. At times, the high fat signal can interfere with visualization of structures. Fat-suppressed imaging uses certain methods to selectively suppress or eliminate signal derived from fat-containing tissues and can facilitate visualization of certain pathologies, especially those related to the retroperitoneum and peritoneum (32). Conspicuity of bowel pathology can be improved with fat suppression imaging, as reduction of the surrounding fat signal can sometimes improve the contrast between bowel serosa and adjacent fat (32). Intravenously administered contrast, gadolinium chelate, has become a critical additional tool in MRI. Gadolinium is a intravascular agent that can increase the signal generated on T1-weighted images by up to 10,000-fold. Administered intravenously, gadolinium will lead to enhanced contrast of vascular tissues. Enhancing vascular tissues include abnormal tissues, such as areas of inflammation or infection or vascular tumors (32–36). Enhanced imaging is particularly critical for evaluation of solid organs, including the liver, and must be utilized for optimal detection of both diffuse as well as focal diseases, such as metastases. Historically, MRI of the abdomen has depended upon a combination of standard spin echo and fast spin echo T1- and T2-weighted sequences, which required respiratory gating in order to reduce respiratory motion image degradation. Acquisition times typically extend up to 7 to 8 min, and respiratory gating may be difficult or impossible in patients who have irregular respiratory patterns, as can be seen in patients with abdominal pain. In our experience, total scan times would extend to between 45 and 90 min using these longer sequence techniques, particularly with patients having irregular or tachypnic respiratory patterns typically requiring longer time in the scanner due to failure of respiratory gating and image degradation, frequently requiring repetition of imaging sequences. More recently, the movement towards development of abdominal MRI protocols that are dependent on rapid breath-hold T1- and T2-weighted sequences has led to the ability to shorten overall exam times.

In fact, using these techniques, we have demonstrated that MR abdominal imaging can be performed even in the acute setting with total scan times similar to those of CT imaging, and less than that required for ultrasound scanning. Rapid imaging is generally dependent on obtaining T1-weighted images using a so-called spoiled gradient echo technique, and T2-weighted images utilizing a single shot echo train technique. Using these newer sequences, a series of images covering most of the abdomen can be obtained typically between 19–25 s scan time. This typically is within the patients' ability to suspend respiration, which is important to reduce motion-related deterioration and motion-related misregistration between slices. Most of the motion that leads to image deterioration is related to low frequency and high amplitude motion, resulting from respiration and gastrointestinal tract motility. By making sequences faster, the degree of motion sensitivity can be reduced. Certain sequences are inherently less sensitive to motion deterioration. For example, a typical single shot fast spin echo technique images one slice at a time at a rate of around one slice/s, but acquires most of the critical contrast data within 200 ms, and results in relative motion insensitivity. Such sequences can yield diagnostic quality images even if the patient is moving and breathing during the examination. Another feature of MRI is the ability to acquire data sets volumetrically, using a three-dimensional acquisition. This permits reconstruction of two-dimensional slices for viewing tissues in any desired plane. Alternatively, the same data set can be used to create three-dimensional images using volume rendering, shaded surface display, or maximum intensity projection techniques, using dedicated software. Such images can be displayed on a computer workstation and moved to allow the viewer to see selected tissues from any perspective. Advantages of MRI over CT include the ability to generate significantly greater soft tissue contrast resolution, in the order of 10- to 10,000-fold greater than in CT imaging. Typically, CT imaging has superior spatial resolution. However, this difference is diminishing as newer sequences being developed for soft tissue imaging are approaching levels associated with state of the art CT scanning, with the ability to dice tissue into images resolving in the order of 2.0-mm-sided cubes, called voxels. Another advantage of MRI over CT scanning is related to the temporal resolution obtained after administration of intravenous contrast. This results from various factors, including the fact that the volume of gadolinium contrast required for adequate enhancement in a patient is typically less than 20% the volume of contrast required in CT imaging. This results in a tighter peak contrast bolus, which allows improved imaging resolution between arterial, capillary, and venous phases of enhancement. Furthermore, MRI is routinely performed dynamically. That is, immediately following administration of intravenous contrast, a series of MR images are repeated through the abdomen, one after the other, in order to temporally resolve and capture the bolus of contrast within the different vascular phases. Although, in theory, the same approach could be performed with CT, this is not done routinely due to the increase in radiation dosage. CT imaging can only be performed in the transverse plane. Any imaging obtained in the alternate sagittal or coronal planes requires reconstruction of the primary images. However, MRI can be performed in any plane as prescribed by the operator. This includes oblique planes that can be useful for imaging of irregularly oriented structures. For example, imaging of the rectum in the sagittal plane can be very useful for assessing the presacral space, normally a space oriented obliquely relative to the true transverse plane of the patient. On CT, neighboring structures with oblique orientation to the transverse plane are susceptible to volume averaging, which results in blurring tissue margins together, and potential obscuring of important detail such as posterior rectal tumor. MRI in the sagittal plane can provide excellent visualization of the posterior rectal wall and presacral space (38–40).

Another critical development in MRI has been the development of multiple-element surface coils (41, 42). Such coils have the capability of being placed directly on the patient and as close as possible to the tissues from which the signal is generated. As signal will diminish as a square of the distance from the source, surface coils can yield significant improvement in image quality. Furthermore, there is development currently permitting utilization of multiple surface coils concurrently, which can facilitate imaging of large fields of view. In combination with co-processing techniques, this can facilitate significant reduction in acquisition time for any given sequence. It is predicted that this technology will allow scanning through the abdomen using volumetric acquisitions in the order of 4 to 5 s.

More recently, dedicated methodology for assessing colon mucosal surface to improve detection for small irregularities including premalignant polyps is being developed. The general approach can be referred to as MR colonography (Fig. 1). As with CT or plain film imaging, the patient undergoes a bowel preparation protocol starting the evening prior to scanning. The bowel must be distended with intralumenal contrast at the time of examination. One of the strengths of MRI is the numerous sequences available, each producing specific different patterns of contrast between different tissues and substances, based on characteristic molecular environments. The authors (43) have compared a variety of combinations of different intralumenal contrast agents, namely water, gas, or dilute gadolinium, and different sequences, including half-fourier single shot echo-train spin echo T2 (HASTE), true free induction with steady-state precession (T-FISP), and three-dimensional gradient echo (3D-VIBE). Each of these sequences have attributes particularly well suited for bowel imaging. Early data has shown that optimal combinations include T-FISP with water, and 3D VIBE with water or air supplemented with intravenously administered gadolinium to achieve enhanced contrast of the bowel mucosa. There has been early investigation of alternative strategies where bowel preparation would not be required. Experimentation with an approach not even requiring bowel distension has been proposed. However, to date, the images are suboptimal. In contrast, early data using optimized techniques are extremely encouraging, and visualization of bowel mucosa appears significantly improved compared to CT. Furthermore, MRI permits scanning in any plane. Acquisition of images in two or three orthogonal planes ensures that primary image slices will always be available to show bowel wall in optimal cross-sectional view, regardless of how convoluted the bowel may be. This feature diminishes the reliance on time-consuming post-processing volume-rendered analysis and ensures that all lesions will be visualized with minimal risk for misregistration or reconstruction artifacts, improving detection sensitivity and reducing false positive detection rates for small lesions, as compared to CT.

3. DISEASES OF THE LARGE BOWEL:
A CROSS-SECTIONAL IMAGING PERSPECTIVE

In the following section, the most important large bowel disease entities that can be well depicted by MR and CT cross-sectional imaging will be discussed.

3.1. Congenital Malformations

Malrotation and malposition, micro-colon, Hirschprung's disease, imperforate anus, and duplications are all congenital abnormalities where imaging is critical for diagnostic assessment (38,40,44–48). In most cases, plain radiography or fluoroscopy utilizing water-soluble intraluminal contrast is the basis for imaging examination. However, anorectal abnormality, including imperforate anus, is an exception, as MRI is the technique of choice for determination of the extent of atresia and for determination of the optimal surgical approach (38,40). Generally, MRI has been found most useful for delineation of cloacal abnormalities.

3.2. Infection and Inflammation

3.2.1. Ulcerative Colitis and Crohn's Disease

Both CT and MR have proven to be valuable in the diagnosis of inflammatory bowel disease (34,35,49–55). Diagnosis using either modality is dependent on identification of certain patterns. In particular, ulcerative colitis is identified as an abnormality of the large bowel extending from the rectum proximally as contiguous disease (Fig. 2). Abnormality can be identified in the form of colorectal wall thickening associated with either abnormal dilatation or narrowing. The transition between residual normal colon and diseased bowel wall can usually be identified. Ulcerative colitis, a mucosal disease, develops mucosal ulcers resulting from coalescence of micoabscesses in the crypts of Lieberkuhn. In chronic cases, the colon shortens, the walls thicken, and there is loss of huastral markings, leading to a so-called lead pipe appearance. Pan-colitis with backwash ileitis can be identified as disease involving the entire colon, with evidence of wall thickening involving the terminal ileum, and associated with a patulous ileocecal valve. There is significant risk for development of colonic adenocarcinoma, which becomes significant after 10 yr of disease, and if the entire colon is involved. Although colonoscopy and/or double contrast barium enema examination has been used to assess for tumor development, the role for MR colonography may become a method of choice, given that there is no ionizing radiation risk and that patients are relatively young. Mucosal dysplasia is a premalignant finding and is used to determine indication for prophylactic colectomy. Diagnosis is made by colonoscopic random biopsy. To date, dysplasia has not been diagnosed on imaging. For a diagnosis of ulcerative colitis, important negative findings on imaging include absence of any disease involving the serosal aspect of the bowel. Namely, there should be no evidence of involvement of mesenteric fat and no evidence of fistulization or perforation. In contradistinction, diagnosis of Crohn's Disease is dependent upon identification of bowel wall thickening with associated involvement of serosa and adjacent mesenteric fat, evidence of fistulization, abscess formation or mesenteric fibrosis with bowel tethering, or by evidence of skip lesions with intervening relatively normal bowel interposed between diseased segments (Fig. 3). Sensitivity for diagnosis of colorectal disease is improved by administration of perrectal intraluminal contrast. Toxic megacolon is a process that can be associated with multiple etiologies, but most commonly is associated with ulcerative colitis. Unlike ulcerative colitis, toxic megacolon is a transmural process. Imaging shows marked abnormal dilatation of the entire large bowel, and the entire bowel wall enhances after intravenous contrast administration. However, diagnosis requires characteristic clinical presentation with debilitating bloody diarrhea, fever, leukocytosis, and abdominal pain.

3.2.2. INFECTIOUS COLITIS AND PSEUDOMEMBRANOUS COLITIS

Based solely on imaging, the differential diagnosis for large bowel wall thickening visualized on CT or MR studies would include infectious etiologies resulting in infectious colitis or from pseudomembranous colitis. Pan-colitis, resulting in an appearance comparable to ulcerative colitis, has been described with pseudomembranous colitis (56–63). Serosal and pericolic fat (Fig. 4) involvement is considered rare with pseudomembranous colitis, but can occur in up to 20–25% of cases. In such cases, pericolic fat may be edematous and inflamed on CT or MR, and free fluid may develop within the peritoneum. Disease may be segmental and can selectively involve either proximal or distal colon. Interestingly, the severity of imaging findings does not always correlate with clinical severity. Imaging findings on CT have included descriptions such as the halo sign and the accordion sign. These findings are nonspecific in that it is a description of images showing mucosal and submucosal edema, visualized in short or long axis relative to the bowel.

3.2.3. DIVERTICULITIS

Diverticulitis is another inflammatory infectious etiology that is well imaged by CT or MRI (32,52,58,64–71). Typically, the culprit diverticulum can be identified, with surrounding inflammatory changes identified in the pericolic fat. The sigmoid colon is most commonly involved. In more advanced disease, a long segment of several centimeters of large bowel is usually involved, and can be identified as a region of abnormal bowel wall thickening, luminal narrowing, and pericolic stranding involving the adjacent fat. More advanced disease with perforation is associated with extravasation of intralumenal contrast, extralumenal fluid, and abscess formation. Extralumenal intraperitoneal gas may be identified, but it typically is small in volume and located in the region adjacent to the perforation. Large quantities of free intraperitoneal gas are required for identification by plain film radiography, which is far less sensitive for detection of bowel perforation as compared to CT examination. CT and MRI, compared to other imaging modalities, are considered most sensitive for even very mild or early diverticulitis. CT and MRI are useful for determination of other acute and chronic complications of perforation. Acute abscess may form. Chronically, there may develop strictures or fistulas to neighboring bowel segments, to bladder, or vagina (72–75).

3.2.4. Epiploic Appendagitis

This disease entity likely results from a thrombosis of a draining vein, or possibly due to torsion and secondary thrombophlebitis involving a colonic epiploic appendage *(58,70,76–79)*. This entity is benign and self-limiting. However, it can be clinically confused with other inflammatory or infectious conditions such as diverticulitis, appendicitis, or inflammatory bowel disease. CT or MRI findings can be pathognomonic (Fig. 5), and critical to clinical management and avoidance of unnecessary surgical intervention.

3.2.5. Radiation Colitis

This process is always associated with an appropriate history and has a distribution of disease that coincides with the radiation portal. CT and MRI will demonstrate wall thickening, luminal narrowing, serosal involvement with stranding extending into the pericolic or omental fat, fistula formation, and perforation with abscess, depending on severity *(58)*.

3.3. Vascular

Ischemic injury of the large bowel *(32,80–83)*can result from either large vessel proximal disease involving the superior mesenteric artery or inferior mesenteric artery or from distal small vessel disease. In most cases of arterial insufficiency, critical proximal disease is not demonstrated, as it appears most cases result from small vessel disease, most commonly due to atherosclerosis. However, approx one-third of cases will show proximal disease that can be demonstrated on either CT angiography or MR angiography. Imaging can be used in order to screen for cases that should go on to percutaneous angiographically guided angioplasty or stent procedure. Inflammatory etiologies typically involve the end organ vessels and are beyond resolution of imaging by CT or MR. Venous thrombosis is also well diagnosed by either CT or MR angiography and can result in similar changes in the bowel. Findings on either CT or MRI include large bowel abnormal dilatation with thinning of the wall in the acute phase. This can be followed by development of abnormal wall thickening and narrowing of the lumen (Fig. 6). This evolution can occur over a period of hours to days, following an acute episode of ischemia. In subsequent days to weeks, the bowel can be seen to either recover and return to a more normal appearance or, alternatively, may develop fibrosis with fixed narrowing and stricture. In severe cases, there may also be perforation, and abscess formation in the acute phase (Fig. 7). Distribution of disease can be helpful for diagnosis as the initial appearance of ischemic bowel may be nonspecific. The most common area of ischemic injury, secondary to athersclerotic disease or hypoperfusion states involves the splenic flexure, or so-called watershed region (Fig. 6).

3.4. Appendix

Appendicitis is a common indication for CT or MRI *(32,58,84–93)*. It is generally shown that CT has higher sensitivity and less interobserver variation than ultrasound in diagnosis of acute appendicitis. More recently, there is growing evidence to show that MRI of the abdomen and pelvis can have sensitivity and specificity for diagnosis of appendicitis comparable to CT imaging. The advantage of MRI over CT is the ability to avoid ionizing radiation, which is particularly a factor in younger patients. Diagnosis is based on identification of thickening of the wall of the appendix and associated peri-appendicial inflammation within the adjacent fat (Fig. 8). In more advanced disease, there may be perforation, abscess formation, and fistulization to the cecum. Identification of an appendicolith can be supportive of the diagnosis, but is not essential. Only because of improved and more frequently used CT and MRI, it has been noted that there is a subset of appendicitis, associated with very mild inflammation, that may

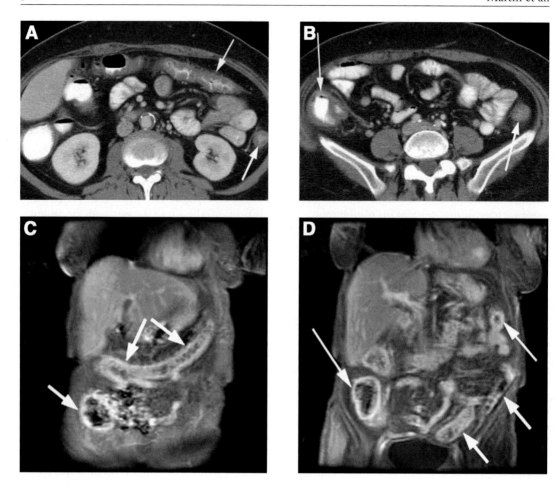

Fig. 2. Pan-colitis of ulcerative colitis, on CT (A and B) and MR (C and D) images. CT scan performed with oral, rectal, and intravenous contrast shows thickening of the bowel wall with selected images showing transverse and descending colon (A, arrows), and ascending and descending colon (B, arrows). In another patient, MR coronal T1-weighted gradient echo imaging with fat suppression and gadolinium enhancement shows diffuse abnormal enhancement of the large bowel, indicative of inflammation, with no uninvolved segments (C and D-, arrows). Although the second patient shown here had less wall thickening, MRI is much more sensitive for detection of inflammation, compared to CT, and, therefore, less dependent on the need to detect wall thickening, which is a variable finding and at least partly dependent on severity of disease.

Fig. 3. *(opposite page)* Crohn's disease shown on CT (A–E) and MR (F) images. Axial CT images with oral and intravenous contrast show concentric abnormal thickening of the terminal ileum (A, arrow on left side of image), descending colon (A, arrow on right side of image), and distal transverse colon (B, arrow). Bowel wall thickening is associated with transmural inflammation in this case. The intervening large bowel is relatively spared. Scan through the lower abdomen (C) shows sigmoid (C, arrowheads) to be diffusely thickened and irregular with narrowing, tethering, and possible fistula to an adjacent small bowel loop, with formation of a small abscess (C, above arrowheads). Other associated complications related to inflammatory bowel disease are shown on coronal reconstruction images (C and D), including gallstone formation (d, superior arrow), avascular necrosis of the femoral head (D, inferior arrow), and ankylosing spondylitis (E, arrows). A 10-yr-old male presented with nonspecific right lower quadrant abdominal pain and was studied with nonionizing MRI performed with oral and per-rectal water contrast. A transverse T-FISP image through the lower abdomen shows diffuse thickening of the terminal ileum (F, arrow), but complete sparing of the large bowel and cecum (F, arrowhead). Findings were confirmed by large bowel endoscopy.

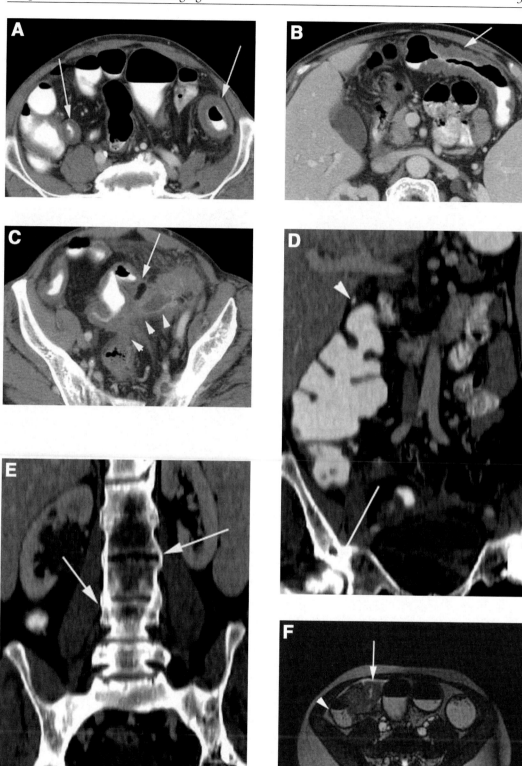

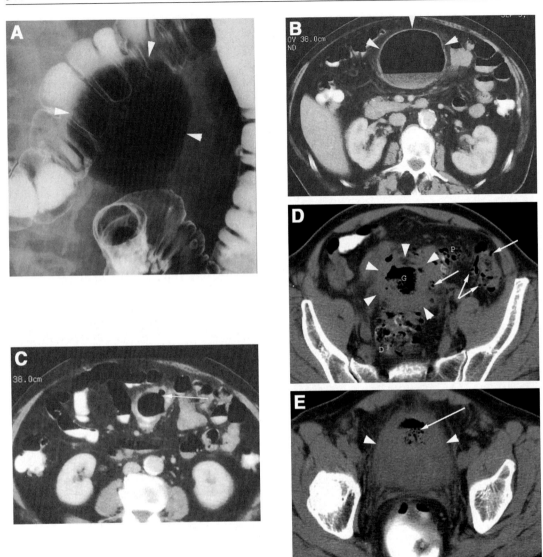

Fig. 4. Diverticular disease examples, simple and complex. Plain radiography (A) and CT examinations (B and C) on a patient with a sigmoid giant diverticulum. A large gas-containing structure is identified on plain radiographs (A, arrowheads) located immediately adjacent and above the sigmoid colon. Uncomplicated small diverticula are identified adjacent to the gas-containing mass in the sigmoid and large bowel. CT examination through the gas-containing mass (B, arrowheads) shows a giant diverticulum filled with gas and fluid, with very mild hazy opacity in the adjacent fat indicating edema and/or inflammation. The neck of the diverticulum is shown arising from the mid-sigmoid colon (C, arrow), confirming the diagnosis. Another patient, who presented with lower abdominal pain, loose bowel movements, dysuria with cloudy urine, borderline elevated body temperature and mild leukocytosis, is shown with diverticulitis complicated by abscess formation and fistulization to urinary bladder (D and E). This patient has innumerable diverticula scattered throughout the distal colon and sigmoid (a few examples are shown: D, arrows). The proximal (D, "P") and distal (D, "D") sigmoid colon is shown with a thick-walled abscess (D, arrowheads) arising from the anterior–superior surface. The abscess has central low attenuation gas (D, "G") consistent with bowel perforation. The urinary bladder (E, arrowheads) has a mottled gas-fluid level (E, arrow) demonstrated within the lumen, indicative of fistulous communication with the abscess and sigmoid colon.

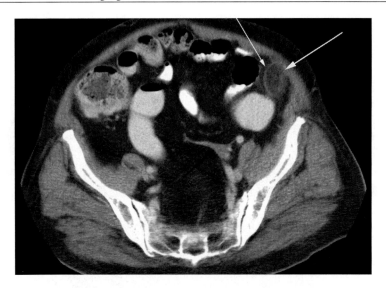

Fig. 5. Appendagitis epiploica. Transverse oral and intravenous contrast-enhanced CT imaging through the lower abdomen shows fatty lobule with well-circumscribed thin soft tissue density boundary (arrows). Inflammation can be inferred from the slightly elevated fuzzy density within and immediately adjacent to the lobule, indicating fat with slightly increased water content. A small amount of dependent free fluid is identified (black arrow). These are characteristic features.

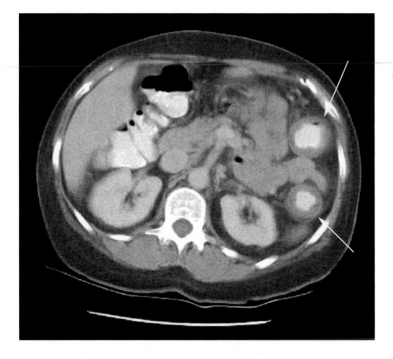

Fig. 6. Colonic ischemia. CT scan through the mid-abdomen after administration of rectal and intravenous contrast shows concentric wall thickening of the splenic flexure (arrows). The remainder of the large bowel had normal configuration (not shown).

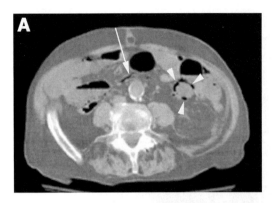

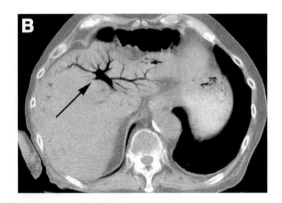

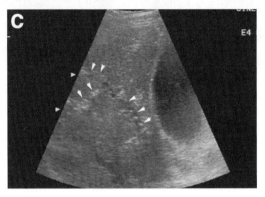

Fig. 7. Bowel infarction with pneumatosis coli and portal venous gas. CT imaging with oral and without intravenous contrast shows tiny gas pocket collections within the walls of large bowel (A, arrowheads) and gas extending into the draining small portal venous branches (A, arrow). Gas has further been carried into the liver intraparenchymal portal venous system (B, arrow). Intrahepatic portal venous gas can also be demonstrated on ultrasound imaging of the liver (C, arrowheads), as demonstrated by linear segments of brightly echogenic tiny foci that are highly mobile or flowing during the real-time examination.

Fig. 8. *(opposite page)* Images from six different patients with acute appendicitis showing a range of characteristic features on CT (A–E), and on MR (F and G). CT examination shows diffuse concentric wall thickening with evidence of an appendicolith (A, arrow) as indicated by a central intraluminal focal density surrounded by a lower attenuation band of fluid. Mild appendicitis (B) is demonstrated by mild wall thickening of the appendix (B, arrow head) and adjacent edema or thickening of the lateral conal and anterior pararenal fascia (B, arrows). In 2 other cases with mild appendicitis (C and D) concentric appendix wall thickening with a small pocket of fluid accumulated in the tip of the appendix (C, arrow) and tenting of the root of the appendix to form the shape of an arrow head (D, arrow), is demonstrated. More severe appendicitis (E) has resulted in abscess formation (E, arrows) adjacent to the cecum, with extravasation of intraluminal contrast (E, arrow head). The appendix is no longer identifiable within the abscess. Selected MRI through the cecum and terminal ileum of another patient with acute appendicitis, perforation, and abscess formation (F–H) is shown with coronal (F) and axial (G) breath-hold T2-weighted fat-suppressed and postgadolinium-enhanced breath-hold T1-weighted fat-suppressed (H) images. Water-sensitive T2-weighted images show central fluid with the abscess (F, straight arrow) with cecal tip and fluid lateral to the cecum draped around the lateral aspect of the abscess (F and G, curved arrow). The terminal ileum is displaced superior and medial to the abscess (F–H, arrowheads). An appendicolith is identified as a round low signal focus sitting on the dependent aspect of the abscess cavity (G, straight arrow). Abnormal gadolinium enhancement involving the terminal ileum (H, central arrowhead) indicates inflammation. Inflammation of the pericecal (H, anterior arrowhead) and retro-peritoneal fat (H, posterior arrowhead) also is demonstrated.

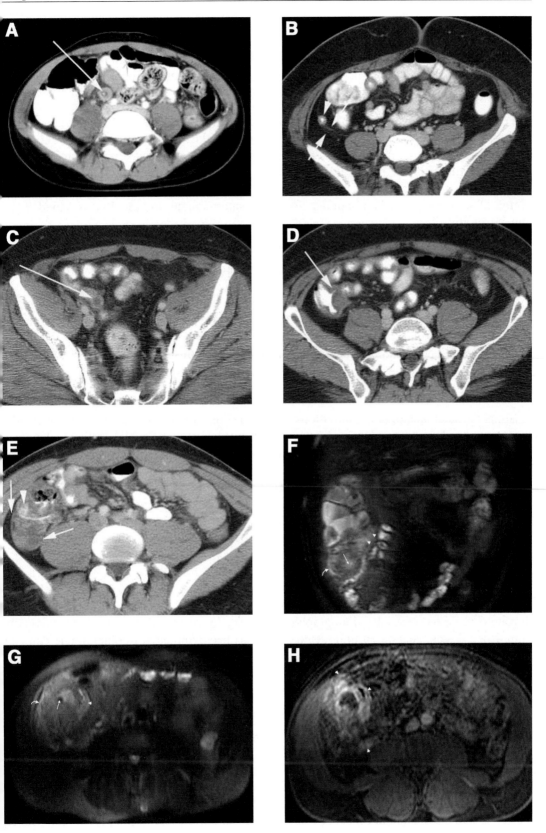

be self-limiting or may respond to medical management using antibiotics. Prior to availability of high-quality CT, either these patients were taken to surgery, or had an uncertain clinical diagnosis followed by resolution of symptoms. The natural history of nonsurgical resolving appendicitis is a topic of current research, to determine incidence of recurrent disease.

3.4.1. Focal Mesenteritis

Focal mesenteritis is a condition seen in postappendectomy patients. This condition occurs at the appendectomy site and results from inflammation of the mesenteric fat immediately adjacent to the appendectomy site. Presentation may occur yr after surgery and can clinically appear indistinguishable from acute appendicitis. Treatment is supportive, as this is an entirely benign and self-limiting process. CT or MRI is diagnostic and is based on identification of a region of well-circumscribed high density, high water content, inflamed fat, situated at the appendectomy site.

3.4.2. Pseudomyxoma Peritonei

Pseudomyxoma peritonei (94–101) is a neoplastic process usually associated with the appendix or ovary. This disease entity is associated with a low-grade mucinous tumor that can lead to extensive mucin production and deposition throughout the peritoneal free-space. This develops a characteristic appearance on CT and MRI with low-density material collections within the peritoneum and around solid organs. In particular, mucin deposition around the liver and spleen results in a scalloped contour irregularity characteristic for this entity.

3.5. Polyps

3.5.1. Adenomatous

Simple tubular adenoma, tubulovillous adenoma (Fig. 9), and villous adenoma represent a spectrum of polyps both in size and in degree of dysplasia (33,102–104). Villous adenomas typically are the largest polyps at presentation and are associated with the highest degree of malignancy pathologically. Imaging signs related to malignancy include size (approx malignancy risk: >2.0 cm, 50%; 1.0–2.0 cm, 10%; 0.5–1.0 cm, 1%; <0.5 cm, 0%), sessile appearance (polyp is broader at the base than at the tip), puckering of the colonic wall at the polyp base, and irregularity of the polyp surface. Sensitivity for detection of polyps on routine CT or MR scans performed on patients with no bowel preparation, using oral and intravenous contrast, is poor for solitary small, <0.5-cm polyps, and moderate for polyps >1 to 2 cm in size. Using CT colonography, (see Subheading 2.1.) sensitivity for detection of polyps down to 1.0 cm is significantly improved, with results reported indicating up to 90% sensitivity, which is approaching that of colonoscopy. To this point in development there appears to be a detection threshold based on size, and colonographic sensitivity for polyps <1.0 cm in size is markedly diminished. Latest generation multidetector CT has been compared to older single detector array scanning, but there so far is no evidence to show that polyp detection sensitivity is improved, although there is less artifact from motion and less problem with loss of bowel distension in multidetector CT due to faster scanning with shorter exam times.

Familial Polyposis Coli and Gardner's Syndrome

It may be that both entities may represent a spectrum of the same disease, with both showing an autosomal-dominant inheritance pattern (33,104). Diagnosis is dependent on identification of innumerable polyps, usually >100, and usually more numerous in the distal colon and rectum. Colon adenocarcinoma develops in 30% of patients by 10 yr, and 100% by 20 yr, with multifocal carcinoma identified in 50%. Extracolonic intra-abdominal manifestations on imaging include gastric hamartomas, gastric or duodenal adenomas, periampullary carcinoma,

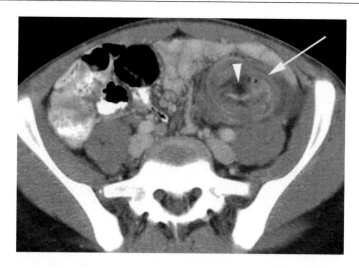

Fig. 9. Colocolic intussusception. Intussuceptum carries vessels and mesenteric fat, seen as low density on this transverse CT image through the descending colon (arrowhead), centrally within the expanded lumen of the intussuscipiens (arrow). Findings shown here are pathognomonic. A lead point mass is not identified in this study, and only rarely is identifiable in the unreduced intussusception.

and jejunal and ileal polyps. In theory, MR using dedicated bowel imaging techniques should be more sensitive than CT for detection of subtle mucosal abnormalities. Mesenteric and subcutaneous fibromatosis is another association that can appear as a nonspecific soft tissue mass on CT, and as soft tissue with late enhancement on MR. This process is particularly associated with prior surgical procedures or even minor trauma, presumably due to a propensity to excessive desmoid reaction to tissue injury. Associations with dental abnormalities, skull outer table osteomas, epidermoid cysts, ocular fundal pigmental lesions, and thyroid carcinoma have been described. Other polyposis syndromes include autosomal recessive Turcot's syndrome *(105)*, associated with central nervous system malignancy and nonhereditary Canada-Cronkhite syndrome, which mostly involves the colon and stomach with increased risk for colon adenocarcinoma.

3.5.3. HAMARTOMATOUS

Juvenile polyposis *(33)* may have a familial component, and usually presents in children <10 yr of age, and can commonly present as a solitary rectal polyp. Peutz-Jeghers syndrome *(33)* is autosomal dominant and can affect the colon in up to 30% of patients, although the small bowel is usually involved and appears as a carpet of submucosal polyps causing mucosal surface lobulation. Gastric, duodenal, and ovarian carcinoma occurs with increased incidence.

3.5.4. INFLAMMATORY

Ulcerative colitis can cause pseudopolyps in the acute phase due to mucosal hyperplasia interposed with eroded mucosa, which appear as branching linear surface polyps. Larger sessile polyps can develop in disease that is more chronic.

3.5.5. HYPERPLASTIC

These form as solitary or multiple polyps most commonly in the distal colon and rectum. Nodular lymphoid hyperplasia is most common in children, resulting is small submucosal lobulation, and is difficult to visualize on conventional CT or MRI.

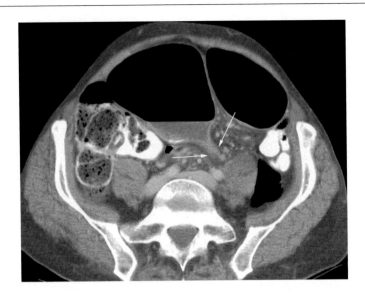

Fig. 10. Sigmoid volvulus shown on transverse CT image through the lower abdomen and pelvis. The sigmoid mesenteric root is acting as a pedicle around which the sigmoid colon has rotated, creating a "pinched" appearance of the colon at the level of the volvulus (arrows). The colon proximal to the volvulus is markedly dilated.

3.5.6. MISCELLANEOUS

Other causes of lower abdominal pain includes intussusception (Fig. 9) and volvulus (Fig. 10). Both conditions can be diagnosed on cross-sectional imaging. Intussusception in children is most commonly benign, but in adults is more likely a result of a mass found at the intussusception lead point.

3.6. Neoplasms

3.6.1. ADENOCARCINOMA

By far the most clinically important primary neoplasm of the colon is adenocarcinoma *(32,106,107)*. Diagnosis can be made of larger tumors on standard CT or MRI (Fig. 11), but dedicated colonography can yield very high sensitivity. Furthermore, unlike barium enema studies, CT or MRI can simultaneous stage the tumor, assessing metastatic involvement, particularly of lymph nodes and liver. MRI for local staging and assessment of direct extension is the method of choice, with the ability to detect submucosal periserosal direct invasion in rectal tumors. Perirectal involvement can be critical in determining treatment strategy, with disease confined to within the perirectal fascia treated surgically, possibly after radiation. MRI techniques have included use of local rectal coils *(108)*, but surface coil systems have been found to yield good results and also permit good visualization of the remainder of the pelvis. In other tumors, size criteria has been used to diagnose metastatically involved lymph nodes, with nodes >1.0 cm in size considered abnormal. Unfortunately, it has been found that this criteria is insensitive in metastatic rectal adenocarcinoma, where perirectal metastatic lymph nodes are commonly <1.0 cm at presentation. Use of superparamagnetic iron oxide particles has been shown on MRI to have the ability to discriminate normal from diseased nodes. The principle is that intravenously administered iron oxide particles are taken up by normal lymph nodes by reticuloendothelial cells, which results in decrease in signal on T2-weighted imaging.

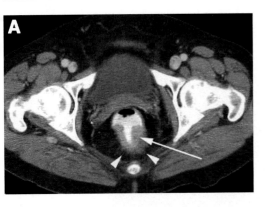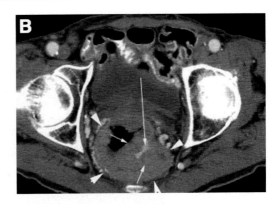

Fig. 11. Rectal polyp and adenocarcinoma. CT imaging through the rectum after rectal and intravenous contrast administration shown eccentric wall thickening along the posterior rectum (A, arrow), subsequently determined to be adenocarcinoma. Ill-defined stranding along the posterior margins corresponds to local tumor infiltration into the perirectal space in this patient, although this finding has been shown to be nonspecific for tumor invasion. In another patient, intravenous contrast enhanced CT through the pelvis shows a large polypoid mass (B, arrows) with a central enhancing vascular core (B, long arrow). Outer margins of the mass, expanding the thickened walls of the rectum, are also shown (B, arrowheads). The polyp was found to represent a fibrovascular polyp with malignant transformation.

Diseased nodes cannot take up the agent, and are distinguishable as high signal nodes. Positron emission tomography (PET) imaging using radioactive fluorodeoxyglucose (FDG) has also been shown to have promise for detecting local nodal metastases *(109,110)*, and can be used for whole body scans to detect remote lymphatic and hematogenously spread metastatic disease. Ultrasound, using a rectal probe, has shown promise for determining depth of rectal wall invasion and assessing involvement of the submucosa and serosa *(108)*, but lacks in ability to assess local or remote lymphatic disease and is not able to assess the remainder of the large bowel or sigmoid. MRI of the liver has been shown to be superior to CT for detection sensitivity and specificity of focal lesions. MRI and CT portography have comparable sensitivity, but MR has better specificity and is noninvasive. In summary, the best imaging tools available for detection and staging of adenocarcinoma, either the initial presentation or recurrent disease, are the combination MRI and PET. The cost-effectiveness of using these two imaging tools in combination as routine protocol has not yet been determined. However, it can be predicted that cost of these tests will diminish as demand and availability increases.

3.6.2. Other Tumors

These include benign lipoma (Fig. 12) and relatively rare leiomyoma, fibroma, hemangioma, and neurofibroma. Lipoma usually occurs in the cecum adjacent to the ileocecal valve, and can be specifically diagnosed based on demonstrating a smoothly marginated mass with fat density on CT, and fat signal on MR *(32)*, confirmed on fat-suppressed spoiled gradient echo images.

Other malignant neoplasms, far less common than adenocarcinoma, include lymphoma, carcinoid, leimyosarcoma, melanoma, squamous cell carcinoma of the anal canal, and metastases, usually due to direct extension to rectum or sigmoid from pelvic tumors (ovary, cervix, prostate, or bladder) or extension to involve the transverse colon via the transverse mesocolon (pancreas or stomach) *(32,107,111–117)*. Based on the pattern of tumor growth, these tumors can usually be diagnosed on imaging, with MR generally superior, particularly for assessment

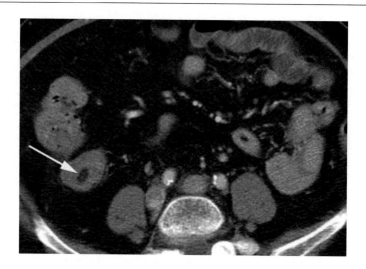

Fig. 12. Lipoma. Transverse CT image shows a low density fat-containing well-circumscribed mass protruding into the cecal lumen just above the ileocecal valve. These are almost always benign lesions and are most commonly found in the region of the ileocecal valve.

of the pelvic soft tissues. Carcinoid can have characteristic features diagnosed on MRI, with evidence of elevated signal on T2-weighted images, and intense contrast enhancement. Fibrosis with tethering of the bowel in a stellate configuration is commonly seen with mesenteric carcinoid metastases, and can be identified on CT and MRI. Carcinoid often metastasizes to the liver, appearing as hypervascular metastases. Carcinoid is the most common cause of hypervascular liver metastases (32,52,118). MR is the most specific imaging modality in determining carcinoid liver metastases, again with the finding of elevated signal on T2-weighted images and the demonstration of hypervascularity on dynamically acquired post-gadolinium images.

4. SUMMARY

This is a most exciting time for application of the latest imaging techniques for assessment of important colon diseases. It is expected that MRI will play an increasing role to supplement or replace CT and ultrasound for numerous conditions, with the advantages of being able to produce a comprehensive examination that has no serious associated health hazards, avoiding both the risks of ionizing radiation and iodinated contrast agents. It is expected that colon screening for premalignant lesions will become increasingly supported in the healthcare systems of economically developed nations, and that cross-sectional imaging, and quite likely MRI, could supplement or replace conventional double-contrast barium enema radiography.

REFERENCES

1. Berland LL, & Smith JK. Multidetector-array CT: once again, technology creates new opportunities. *Radiology*, **209** (1998) 327–329.
2. Hu H, He HD, Foley WD, Fox SH. Four multidetector-row helical CT: image quality and volume coverage speed. *Radiology*, **215** (2000) 55–62.
3. Rubin GD. Data explosion: the challenge of multidetector-row CT. *Eur. J. Radiol.*, **36** (2000) 74–80.
4. Stoll E, Stern C, Stucki P, Wildermuth S. A new filtering algorithm for medical magnetic resonance and computer tomography images. *J. Digit. Imaging*, **12** (1999) 23–28.

5. McFarland EG, Brink JA, Loh J, et al. Visualization of colorectal polyps with spiral CT colography: evaluation of processing parameters with perspective volume rendering. *Radiology*, **205** (1997) 701–707.

6. Hopper KD, Iyriboz AT, Wise SW, Neuman JD, Mauger DT, Kasales CJ. Mucosal detail at CT virtual reality: surface versus volume rendering. *Radiology*, **214** (2000) 517–522.

7. Fishman EK, Horton KM, Urban BA. Multidetector CT angiography in the evaluation of pancreatic carcinoma: preliminary observations. *J. Comput. Assist. Tomogr.*, **24** (2000) 849–853.

8. Reed JE, Johnson CD. Automatic segmentation, tissue characterization, and rapid diagnosis enhancements to the computed tomographic colonography analysis workstation. *J. Digit. Imaging*, **10** (1997) 70–73.

9. Brown SJ, Hayball MP, Coulden RA. Impact of motion artefact on the measurement of coronary calcium score. *Br. J. Radiol.*, **73** (2000) 956–962.

10. Thoeni RF. Colorectal cancer. Radiologic staging. *Radiol. Clin. N. Am.*, **35** (1997) 457–485.

11. Lupetin AR, Cammisa BA, Beckman I, et al. Spiral CT during arterial portography. *Radiographics*, **16** (1996) 723–743.

12. D'Asseler Y, Koole M, Van Laere K, et al. PACS and multimodality in medical imaging. *Technol. Health Care*, **8** (2000) 35–52.

13. Foord KD. PACS workstation respecification: display, data flow, system integration, and environmental issues, derived from analysis of the Conquest Hospital pre-DICOM PACS experience. *Eur. Radiol.*, **9** (1999) 1161–1169.

14. Rex DK, Vining D, Kopecky KK. An initial experience with screening for colon polyps using spiral CT with and without CT colography (virtual colonoscopy). *Gastrointest. Endosc.*, **50** (1999) 309–313.

15. Rogalla P, Bender A, Bick U, Huitema A, Terwissscha van Scheltinga J, Hamm B. Tissue transition projection (TTP) of the intestines. *Eur. Radiol.*, **10** (2000) 806–810.

16. Ahlquist DA, Johnson CD. Screening by CT colonography: too early to pass judgment on a nascent technology. *Gastrointest. Endosc.*, **50** (1999) 437–440.

17. Bauerfeind P, Luboldt W, Debatin JF. Virtual colonography. *Baillieres Best Pract. Res. Clin. Gastroenterol.*, **13** (1999) 59–65.

18. Callstrom MR, Johnson CD, Fletcher JG, et al. Ct colonography without cathartic preparation: feasibility study. *Radiology*, **219** (2001) 693–698.

19. Chen SC, Lu DS, Hecht JR, Kadell BM. CT colonography: value of scanning in both the supine and prone positions. *Am. J. Roentgenol.*, **172** (1999) 595–599.

20. Dachman AH, Kuniyoshi JK, Boyle CM, et al. CT colonography with three-dimensional problem solving for detection of colonic polyps. *Am. J. Roentgenol.*, **171** (1998) 989–995.

21. Dave SB, Wang G, Brown BP, McFarland EG, Zhang Z, Vannier MW. Straightening the colon with curved cross sections: an approach to CT colonography. *Acad. Radiol.*, **6** (1999) 398–410.

22. Fletcher JG, Johnson CD, Welch T.J, et al. Optimization of CT colonography technique: prospective trial in 180 patients. *Radiology*, **216** (2000) 704–711.

23. Hara AK, Johnson CD, Reed JE, et al. Reducing data size and radiation dose for CT colonography. *Am. J. Roentgenol.*, **168** (1997) 1181–1184.

24. Hara AK, Johnson CD, MacCarty RL, Welch TJ, McCollough CH, Harmsen WS. CT colonography: single- versus multi-detector row imaging. *Radiology*, **219** (2001) 461–465.

25. Johnson CD, Hara AK, Reed JE. Computed tomographic colonography (Virtual colonoscopy): a new method for detecting colorectal neoplasms. *Endoscopy*, **29** (1997) 454–461.

26. Johnson CD, Dachman AH. CT colonography: the next colon screening examination? *Radiology*, **216** (2000) 331–341.

27. Macari M, Berman P, Dicker M, Milano A, Megibow AJ. Usefulness of CT colonography in patients with incomplete colonoscopy. *Am. J. Roentgenol.*, **173** (1999) 561–564.

28. Rogalla P, Meiri N, Ruckert JC, Hamm B. Colonography using multislice CT. *Eur. J. Radiol.*, **36** (2000) 81–85.

29. Rubin DT, Dachman AH. Virtual colonoscopy: a novel imaging modality for colorectal cancer. *Curr. Oncol. Rep.*, **3** (2001) 88–93.

30. Tafazoli F, Taylor J, McFarland EG, Gianfelice D, Lepanto L, Reinhold C. New imaging techniques for the evaluation of gastrointestinal diseases. *Can. J. Gastroenterol.*, **14(Suppl D)** (2000) 163D–180D.

31. Valev V, Wang G, Vannier MW. Techniques of CT colonography (virtual colonoscopy). *Crit. Rev. Biomed. Eng.*, **27** (1999) 1–25.

32. Chung JJ, Semelka RC, Martin DR, Marcos HB. Colon diseases: MR evaluation using combined T2-weighted single-shot echo train spin-echo and gadolinium-enhanced spoiled gradient-echo sequences. *J. Magn. Reson. Imaging*, **12** (2000) 297–305.

33. Semelka RC, Marcos HB. Polyposis syndromes of the gastrointestinal tract: MR findings. *J. Magn. Reson. Imaging*, **11** (2000) 51–55.

34. Shoenut JP, Semelka RC, Silverman R, Yaffe CS, Micflikier AB. Magnetic resonance imaging in inflammatory bowel disease. *J. Clin. Gastroenterol.*, **17** (1993) 73–78.

35. Shoenut JP, Semelka RC, Magro CM, Silverman R, Yaffe CS, Micflikier AB. Comparison of magnetic resonance imaging and endoscopy in distinguishing the type and severity of inflammatory bowel disease. *J. Clin. Gastroenterol.*, **19** (1994) 31–35.

36. Marcos HB, Semelka RC. Evaluation of Crohn's disease using half-fourier RARE and gadolinium- enhanced SGE sequences: initial results. *Magn. Reson. Imaging*, **18** (2000) 263–268.

37. Martin DR, Semelka RC. MR imaging of pancreatic masses. *Magn. Reson. Imaging Clin. N. Am.*, **8** (2000) 787–812.

38. Sachs TM, Applebaum H, Touran T, Taber P, Darakjian A, Colleti P. Use of MRI in evaluation of anorectal anomalies. *J. Pediatr. Surg.*, **25** (1990) 817–821.

39. O'Donovan AN, Somers S, Farrow R, Mernagh JR, Sridhar S. MR imaging of anorectal Crohn disease: a pictorial essay. *Radiographics*, **17** (1997) 101–107.

40. Paley MR, Ros PR. MRI of the rectum: non-neoplastic disease. *Eur. Radiol.*, **8** (1998) 3–8.

41. Rivera M, Vaquero JJ, Santos A, Ruiz-Cabello J, del Pozo F. MRI visualization of small structures using improved surface coils. *Magn. Reson. Imaging*, **16** (1998) 157–166.

42. Schenck JF, Hart HR, Jr, Foster TH, Edelstein WA, Hussain MA. High resolution magnetic resonance imaging using surface coils. *Magn. Reson. Annu.*, (1986) 123–160.

43. Martin DR, Yang M, Thomasson D, Acheson C. MR colonography development of optimized method with ex vivo and in vivo systems. *Radiology*, **225** (2002) 597–602.

44. Cianfarani S, Vitale S, Stanhope R, Boscherini B. Imperforate anus, bilateral hydronephrosis, bilateral undescended testes and pituitary hypoplasia: a variant of Hall-Pallister syndrome or a new syndrome. *Acta. Paediatr.*, **84** (1995) 1322–1324.

45. Estrada RL, Mindelzun RE. The retropancreatic colon: a congenital anomaly. *Abdom. Imaging.*, **22** (1997) 426–428.

46. Herman TE, Coplen D, Skinner M. Congenital short colon with imperforate anus (pouch colon). Report of a case. *Pediatr. Radiol.*, **30** (2000) 243–246.

47. Inoue Y, Nakamura H. Adenocarcinoma arising in colonic duplication cysts with calcification: CT findings of two cases. *Abdom. Imaging*, **23** (1998) 135–137.

48. Pfluger T, Czekalla R, Koletzko S, Munsterer O, Willemsen UF, Hahn K. MRI and radiographic findings in Currarino's triad. *Pediatr. Radiol.*, **26** (1996) 524–527.

49. Freeman AH. CT and bowel disease. *Br. J. Radiol.*, **74** (2001) 4–14.

50. Tarjan Z, Zagoni T, Gyorke T, Mester A, Karlinger K, Mako EK. Spiral CT colonography in inflammatory bowel disease. *Eur. J. Radiol.*, **35** (2000) 193–198.

51. Durno CA, Sherman P, Williams T, Shuckett B, Dupuis A, Griffiths AM. Magnetic resonance imaging to distinguish the type and severity of pediatric inflammatory bowel diseases. *J. Pediatr. Gastroenterol. Nutr.*, **30** (2000) 170–174.

52. Kettritz U, Shoenut JP, Semelka RC. MR imaging of the gastrointestinal tract. *Magn. Reson. Imaging Clin. N. Am.*, **3** (1995) 87–98.

53. Semelka RC, Shoenut JP, Silverman R, Kroeker MA, Yaffe CS, Micflikier AB. Bowel disease: prospective comparison of CT and 1.5–T pre- and postcontrast MR imaging with T1-weighted fat-suppressed and breath-hold FLASH sequences. *J. Magn. Reson. Imaging*, **1** (1991) 625–632.

54. Rieber A, Wruk D, Potthast S, et al. Diagnostic imaging in Crohn's disease: comparison of magnetic resonance imaging and conventional imaging methods. *Int. J. Colorectal. Dis.*, **15** (2000) 176–181.

55. Sabir N, Sungurtekin U, Erdem E, Nessar M. Magnetic resonance imaging with rectal Gd-DTPA: new tool for the diagnosis of perianal fistula. *Int. J. Colorectal. Dis.*, **15** (2000) 317–322.

56. Fishman EK, Kavuru M, Jones B, et al. Pseudomembranous colitis: CT evaluation of 26 cases. *Radiology*, **180** (1991) 57–60.

57. Hamrick KM, Tishler JM, Schwartz ML, Koslin DB, Han SY. The CT findings in pseudomembranous colitis. *Comput. Med. Imaging Graph.*, **13** (1989) 343–346.

58. Horton KM, Corl FM, Fishman EK. CT evaluation of the colon: inflammatory disease. *Radiographics*, **20** (2000) 399–418.

59. Kawamoto S, Horton KM, Fishman EK. Pseudomembranous colitis: can CT predict which patients will need surgical intervention? *J. Comput. Assist. Tomogr.*, **23** (1999) 79–85.

60. Kawamoto S, Horton KM, Fishman EK. Pseudomembranous colitis: spectrum of imaging findings with clinical and pathologic correlation. *Radiographics*, **19** (1999) 887–897.

61. Megibow AJ, Streiter ML, Balthazar EJ, Bosniak, MA. Pseudomembranous colitis: diagnosis by computed tomography. *J. Comput. Assist. Tomogr.*, **8** (1984) 281–283.
62. Wilcox CM, Gryboski D, Fernandez M, Stahl W. Computed tomographic findings in pseudomembranous colitis: an important clue to the diagnosis. *South. Med. J.*, **88** (1995) 929–933.
63. Yankes JR, Baker ME, Cooper C, Garbutt J. CT appearance of focal pseudomembranous colitis. *J. Comput. Assist. Tomogr.*, **12** (1988) 394–396.
64. Chintapalli KN, Chopra S, Ghiatas AA, Escola CC, Fields SF, Dodd GD, 3rd. Diverticulitis versus colon cancer: differentiation with helical CT findings. *Radiology*, **210** (1999) 429–435.
65. Jang HJ, Lim HK, Lee SJ, Choi SH, Lee MH, Choi MH. Acute diverticulitis of the cecum and ascending colon: thin-section helical CT findings. *Am. J. Roentgenol.*, **172** (1999) 601–604.
66. Luboldt W, Luz O, Vonthein R, et al. Three-dimensional double-contrast MR colonography: a display method simulating double-contrast barium enema. *Am. J. Roentgenol.*, **176** (2001) 930–932.
67. Marinella MA, Mustafa M. Acute diverticulitis in patients 40 years of age and younger. *Am. J. Emerg. Med.*, **18** (2000) 140–142.
68. Minardi AJ, Jr, Johnson LW, Sehon JK, Zibari GB, McDonald JC. Diverticulitis in the young patient. *Am. Surg.*, **67** (2001) 458–461.
69. Rao PM, Rhea JT. Colonic diverticulitis: evaluation of the arrowhead sign and the inflamed diverticulum for CT diagnosis. *Radiology*, **209** (1998) 775–779.
70. Rao PM. CT of diverticulitis and alternative conditions. *Semin. Ultrasound CT MR*, **20** (1999) 86–93.
71. Urban BA, Fishman EK. Targeted helical CT of the acute abdomen: appendicitis, diverticulitis, and small bowel obstruction. *Semin. Ultrasound CT MR*, **21** (2000) 20–39.
72. Liu CH, Chuang CK, Chu SH, et al. Enterovesical fistula: experiences with 41 cases in 12 years. *Changgeng Yi Xue Za Zhi*, **22** (1999) 598–603.
73. Netri G, Verbo A, Coco C, et al. The role of surgical treatment in colon diverticulitis: indications and results. *Ann. Ital. Chir.*, **71** (2000) 209–214.
74. White TB, Allen HA, 3rd, Ives CE. Portal and mesenteric vein gas in diverticulitis: CT findings. *Am. J. Roentgenol.*, **171** (1998) 525–526.
75. Kawamura YJ, Sugamata Y, Yoshino K, et al. Appendico-ileo-vesical fistula. *J. Gastroenterol.*, **33** (1998) 868–871.
76. Birjawi GA, Haddad MC, Zantout HM, Uthman SZ. Primary epiploic appendagitis: a report of two cases. *Clin. Imaging*, **24** (2000) 207–209.
77. Hiller N, Berelowitz D, Hadas-Halpern I. Primary epiploic appendagitis: clinical and radiological manifestations. *Isr. Med. Assoc. J.*, **2** (2000) 896–898.
78. Rao PM, Wittenberg J, Lawrason JN. Primary epiploic appendagitis: evolutionary changes in CT appearance. *Radiology*, **204** (1997) 713–717.
79. Sirvanci M, Tekelioglu MH, Duran C, Yardimci H, Onat L, Ozer K. Primary epiploic appendagitis: CT manifestations. *Clin. Imaging*, **24** (2000) 357–361.
80. Simon AM, Birnbaum BA, Jacobs JE. Isolated infarction of the cecum: CT findings in two patients. *Radiology*, **214** (2000) 513–516.
81. Ha HK, Rha SE, Kim AY, Auh YH. CT and MR diagnoses of intestinal ischemia. *Semin. Ultrasound CT MR* **21** (2000) 40–55.
82. Rademaker J. Veno-occlusive disease of the colon—CT findings. *Eur. Radiol.*, **8** (1998) 1420–1421.
83. Rha SE, Ha HK, Lee SH, et al. CT and MR imaging findings of bowel ischemia from various primary causes. *Radiographics*, **20** (2000) 29–42.
84. Applegate KE, Sivit CJ, Myers MT, Pschesang B. Using helical CT to diagnosis acute appendicitis in children: spectrum of findings. *Am. J. Roentgenol.*, **176** (2001) 501–505.
85. Birnbaum BA, Wilson SR. Appendicitis at the millennium. *Radiology*, **215** (2000) 337–348.
86. Brice J. What should CT's role be in pediatric appendicitis? *Diagn. Imaging (San Franc)*, **Suppl** (2000) 21–23.
87. Daniels IR, Chisholm EM. Suspected acute appendicitis: is ultrasonography or computed tomography the preferred imaging technique? *Eur. J. Surg.*, **166** (2000) 910.
88. Funaki B. Nonenhanced CT for suspected appendicitis. *Radiology*, **216** (2000) 916–918.
89. Hardin DM, Jr. Acute appendicitis: review and update. *Am. Fam. Physician*, **60** (1999) 2027–2034.
90. Karakas SP, Guelfguat M, Leonidas JC, Springer S, Singh SP. Acute appendicitis in children: comparison of clinical diagnosis with ultrasound and CT imaging. *Pediatr. Radiol.*, **30** (2000) 94–98.
91. Lane MJ, Mindelzun RE. Appendicitis and its mimickers. *Semin. Ultrasound CT MR*, **20** (1999) 77–85.
92. Styrud J, Josephson T, Eriksson S. Reducing negative appendectomy: evaluation of ultrasonography and computer tomography in acute appendicitis. *Int. J. Qual. Health Care*, **12** (2000) 65–68.

93. Wise SW, Labuski MR, Kasales CJ, et al. Comparative assessment of CT and sonographic techniques for appendiceal imaging. *Am. J. Roentgenol.*, **176** (2001) 933–941.

94. Geusens E, Vanhoenacker P, De Man R, Van Oost J, Verbanck J. Mucocele of the appendix. *J. Belge Radiol.*, **77** (1994) 17–18.

95. Hinson FL, Ambrose NS. Pseudomyxoma peritonei. *Br. J. Surg.*, **85** (1998) 1332–1339.

96. Low RN, Barone RM, Lacey C, Sigeti JS, Alzate GD, Sebrechts CP. Peritoneal tumor: MR imaging with dilute oral barium and intravenous gadolinium-containing contrast agents compared with unenhanced MR imaging and CT. *Radiology*, **204** (1997) 513–520.

97. Matsuoka, Y., Masumoto, T., Suzuki, K., et al. Pseudomyxoma retroperitonei. *Eur. Radiol.*, **9** (1999) 457–459.

98. Sugarbaker, P.H., Ronnett, B.M., Archer, A., et al. Pseudomyxoma peritonei syndrome. *Adv. Surg.*, **30** (1996) 233–280.

99. Yasar A, De Keulenaer B, Opdenakker G, Malbrain M. Pseudomyxoma peritonei in association with primary malignant tumor of the ovary and colon. *J. Belge Radiol.*, **80** (1997) 233–234.

100. Zissin R, Gayer G, Kots E, Apter S, Peri M, Shapiro-Feinberg M. Imaging of mucocoele of the appendix with emphasis on the CT findings: a report of 10 cases. *Clin. Radiol.*, **54** (1999) 826–832.

101. Zissin R, Gayer G, Fishman A, Edelstein E, Shapiro-Feinberg M. Synchronous mucinous tumors of the ovary and the appendix associated with pseudomyxoma peritonei: CT findings. *Abdom. Imaging*, **25** (2000) 311–316.

102. Beaulieu CF, Napel S, Daniel BL, et al. Detection of colonic polyps in a phantom model: implications for virtual colonoscopy data acquisition. *J. Comput. Assist. Tomogr.*, **22** (1998) 656–663.

103. Hara AK, Johnson CD, Reed JE. Colorectal lesions: evaluation with CT colography. *Radiographics*, **17** (1997) 1157–1167.

104. Williams SC, Peller PJ. Gardner's syndrome. Case report and discussion of the manifestations of the disorder. *Clin. Nucl. Med.*, **19** (1994) 668–670.

105. Scribano E, Loria G, Ascenti G, Cardia E, Molina D, Gaeta M. Turcot's syndrome: a new case in the first decade of life. *Abdom. Imaging*, **20** (1995) 155–156.

106. Wimmer AP, Bouffard JP, Storms PR, Pilcher JA, Liang CY, DeGuide JJ. Primary colon cancer without gross mucosal tumor: unusual presentation of a common malignancy. *South. Med. J.*, **91** (1998) 1173–1176.

107. Yeung KW, Kuo YT, Huang CL, Wu DK, Liu GC. Inflammatory/infectious diseases and neoplasms of colon. Evaluation with CT. *Clin. Imaging*, **22** (1998) 246–251.

108. Joosten FB, Jansen JB, Joosten HJ, Rosenbusch G. Staging of rectal carcinoma using MR double surface coil, MR endorectal coil, and intrarectal ultrasound: correlation with histopathologic findings. *J. Comput. Assist. Tomogr.*, **19** (1995) 752–758.

109. Goldberg MA, Lee MJ, Fischman AJ, Mueller PR, Alpert NM, Thrall JH. Fluorodeoxyglucose PET of abdominal and pelvic neoplasms: potential role in oncologic imaging. *Radiographics*, **13** (1993) 1047–1062.

110. Yoshioka, T., Fukuda, H., Fujiwara, T., et al. FDG PET evaluation of residual masses and regrowth of abdominal lymph node metastases from colon cancer compared with CT during chemotherapy. *Clin. Nucl. Med.*, **24** (1999) 261–263.

111. Ahn, M.J., Park, Y.W., Han, D., et al. A case of primary intestinal T-cell lymphoma involving entire gastrointestinal tract: esophagus to rectum. *Korean J. Intern. Med.*, **15** (2000) 245–249.

112. Frick MP, Salomonowitz E, Hanto DW, Gedgaudas-McClees K. CT of abdominal lymphoma after renal transplantation. *Am. J. Roentgenol.*, **142** (1984) 97–99.

113. Martin DR, Semelka RC, Chung JJ, Balci NC, Wilber K. Sequential use of gadolinium chelate and mangafodipir trisodium for the assessment of focal liver lesions: initial observations. *Magn. Reson. Imaging*, **18** (2000) 955–963.

114. Parker LA, Vincent LM, Ryan FP, Mittelstaedt CA. Primary lymphoma of the ascending colon: sonographic demonstration. *J. Clin. Ultrasound*, **14** (1986) 221–223.

115. Schmid C, Vazquez JJ, Diss TC, Isaacson PG. Primary B-cell mucosa-associated lymphoid tissue lymphoma presenting as a solitary colorectal polyp. *Histopathology*, **24** (1994) 357–362.

116. Wyatt SH, Fishman EK, Hruban RH, Siegelman SS. CT of primary colonic lymphoma. *Clin. Imaging*, **18** (1994) 131–141.

117. Pelage JP, Soyer P, Boudiaf M, et al. Carcinoid tumors of the abdomen: CT features. *Abdom. Imaging*, **24** (1999) 240–245.

118. Semelka RC, Martin DR, Balci C, Lance T. Focal liver lesions: Comparison of dual-phase CT and multisequence multiplanar MR imaging including dynamic gadolinium enhancement. *J. Magn. Reson. Imaging*, **13** (2001) 397–401.

III COLORECTAL DISEASE

23   Hirschsprung's Disease and Neonatal Disorders

Carol Lynn Berseth

Contents

1. INTRODUCTION

Hirschsprung's disease, or congenital aganglionic megacolon, accounts for 20–25% of cases of neonatal obstruction. It occurs in approximately one of 5000 births *(1)*, may occur in families *(2,3)*, and occurs more commonly in males than females *(1,3,4)*. Approximately 20% of infants with Hirschsprung's disease will have other associated anomalies *(1,3)*, most notably Down's syndrome *(1,3)*. The first curative surgery was introduced in 1948 *(5)*; however, this procedure has been refined and altered, as described in Subheading 5.

2. GENETICS

Histologically Hirschsprung's disease is described to consist of the absence of ganglia cells in the distal intestinal tract. The anus is always involved with variable lengths of distal intestine. A number of cases of Hirschsprung's disease among families have been reported, and there is an increased incidence of Hirschsprung's disease among patients with Down's syndrome, Waardensburg syndrome, and central hypoventilation syndrome. In turn, patients with Hirschsprung's disease are more likely to have additional anomalies of the cardiovascular or genitourinary systems *(6–8)*.

There is increasing evidence that Hirschsprung's disease may result from mutations in any one of several genes singly or in combination. Mutations of these genes may give dominant, recessesive or polygenic patterns of inheritance *(9,10)*. Numerous genetic mutations have been identified to result in the common phenotype of mutations associated with Hirschsprung's

From: *Colonic Diseases*
Edited by: T. R. Koch © Humana Press Inc., Totowa, NJ

disease. Two groupings of genes, *RET/GDNF/NTN* and *EDNRB/EDN3/ECE-1*, are involved in two different signaling pathways while another, *SOX10*, is a transcription factor. All of these genes, which have been identified in humans, are present in murine models, and recent advances in the use of molecular probes and immunohistochemical probes have permitted investigators to gain a better understanding of the development of the enteric nervous system (ENS) and, thus, the underlying pathology in Hirschsprung's disease. The neural and glial cells that form the ganglia of the gastrointestinal tract originate in the vagal and sacral neural crest populations. Vagal enteric neural crest cells arise from the cranial portion of the neural tube and migrate throughout the gastrointestinal tract in a cranial to caudal manner. Sacral neural crest cells arise from the caudal neural tube and migrate for a distance distally. For normal innervation of the gut to occur, neural crest cells must migrate to the gut, differentiate, and survive. All three aspects of this process have been studied in this disease.

A truncating mutation of *SOX10*, a transcription factor, has been identified in individuals who have Hirschsprung's disease associated with Waardenberg syndrome *(11)*. In *SOX10*-deficient mice, mutant neural crest cells appear to have excessive cell death early in their migratory pathway *(12)*.

One signaling pathway in Hirschsprung's disease involves *RET*, a gene in cells of neural crest origin that encodes a receptor tyrosine kinase and binds the two ligands, glial cell line-derived neurotrophic factor (GDNF) and neurturin (NTN). *RET*-expressing cells are multipotential progenitors of the mammalian ENS.

RET signaling promotes survival, proliferation, and differentiation of ENS progentors in the fetus. Thirty to fifty percent of individuals with familial Hirschsprung's disease carry *RET* mutations. In mice homozygotic for null mutations of *RET* and the ligand GDNF, the ENS fails to develop in the distal esophagus and gastric cardia, and the mice die shortly after birth.

Mutations of the ligand NTN result in more subtle abnormalities. Mice with null mutations of NTN have reduced innervation in the myenteric plexus and abnormal intestinal motility. NTN-deficient mice have a reduced number of fine acetyl cholinesterase-positive fibers in the small intestine and a reduction in substance P-expressing fibers *(13)*.

The second signaling pathway involved in Hirschsprung's disease is EDNRB/EDN3/ECE-1. Endothelin-B-receptor (EDNRB) is one of 2 G protein-coupled membrane receptors for endothelin. This receptor binds to the ligand EDN3. Endothelin-converting enzyme (ECE-1) cleaves the inactive precursor of EDN to produce the active EDN3 ligand.

Megacolon appears in two strains of mice, the homozygous lethal spotted strain (which has mutations in EDRB) and the piebald lethal strain (which has mutations of EDN3). The latter strain is also characterized by a decrease in skin pigmentation due to the absence of cutaneous melanocytes that also migrate from neural crest cells. The embryonic guts in this strain do not contain cells with neurogenic potential, providing support to the theory that Hirschsprung's disease may be due to failure of neural crest cells to migrate to the gut *(14)*. This apparent migration defect also may be caused by an alteration in the microenvironment of the intestinal wall of the affected area that inhibits the colonization by neuroblasts *(15)*. Other investigators have studied wild-type–lethal spotted chimeric mice, in which a genetic marker for neuroblasts was present. In these animals, the primary defect for megacolon is not the lack of neural migration, but rather a defect in the surrounding mesenchymal interactions with neural cells in the gut wall *(16)*.

In another series of studies, Hirschsprung's disease appears to be associated with yet another developmental abnormality in neural differentiation. Mutations in neurotrophic factors also inhibit normal development and survival of gut neurons *(17,18)*. These include nerve growth factor, which functions as a trophic and chemotactic agent and promotes outgrowth of axons to establish synapses (17), and neurotrophic factor-3, which promotes development of enteric neurons and glia (18). Kuroda et al. has shown the signal for mRNA for neural growth factor is less intense in mice with congenital megacolon than is seen in controls (19).

Chakravarti has estimated that *RET* mutations account for approximately half of cases of Hirschsprung's disease and mutations in EDNRB for 5% (20). Fujimoto et al. has studied the distribution of extracellular matrix proteins and cell matrix interactions in the gut of the human embryo. His observations suggest that enteric neurogenesis is dependent upon extracellular matrices, fibronectin, and hyaluronic acid for provision of a migration pathway and laminin and collagen type IV to promote outgrowth of neurites from neurons that have "settled" in the gut wall (21). Thus, the microenvironment of the smooth muscle cells may inhibit the ingrowth of neural crest cells (22).

3. CLINICAL PRESENTATION

Although Hirschsprung's Disease is congenital in etiology, only 15% of patients are actually diagnosed during the first month of life. Rather, the majority is diagnosed by 4 mo, with some diagnoses delayed until early preschool age. During the newborn period, infants with Hirschsprung's disease may pass their first meconeum stool beyond 48 h, have infrequent stooling, reluctance to feed, abdominal distention, or bilious vomiting. The non-neonate often presents with decreased stool frequency and abdominal distention, which may be accompanied by recurrent fecal impaction or a history of the parents using rectal suppositories and/or frequent enemas to stimulate stool production, which may be described to be "ribbon-like". Some infants will present with diarrhea or fulminent enterocolitis. On digital exam, the rectal tone may be normal, but the rectal vault may be empty and explosive expulsion of stool may occur on removal of the finger.

The abdominal radiographs of the newborn may demonstrate dilated gas or fluid-filled loops of intestine (Fig. 1). In the non-neonate, intestinal loops may be distended and filled with fecal material. Although the barium enema is considered to be diagnostic, it may not be definitive during the first 2 wk of life, as sufficient time may not have elapsed for the classic transition zone to develop. In the non-neonate, the classic radiographic findings include: (i) dilated loops of bowel proximal to the site of aganglionosis; (ii) a transition zone, a funnel-shaped area that lies between the distended proximal bowel and the narrowed distal bowel; and (iii), narrowed bowel distal to the transition zone (Fig. 2). In addition, there may be large quantities of inspissated fecal material at the upper border of the aganglionic segment. The dilatation of the proximal bowel is due to the functional obstruction created by the presence of the aganglionic bowel and hypertrophy of the normal bowel above the site of the functional obstruction. Films taken approx 24–48 h after the instillation of barium may permit the identification of delays in colonic emptying. Lateral views of the pelvis while contrast material is still in place may help to better visualize transition zones that are low in the pelvis (see Fig. 2, right panel). It should be noted that the barium enema is nondiagnostic in patients with total colon Hirschsprung's Disease (23). Anorectal manometry may be performed in older children. Typically, the resting pressure of the internal anal sphincter is normal or high, the rectosphincteric reflex is absent when the rectal balloon is inflated, and the rectal wall may be resistant to stretch.

4. DIAGNOSIS

The definitive diagnosis of Hirschsprung's disease is made by rectal biopsy. In most cases suction biopsies performed at the bedside yield adequate specimens (24). However, in a small number of infants, a full thickness biopsy at laparoscopy may be necessary. Alternatively,

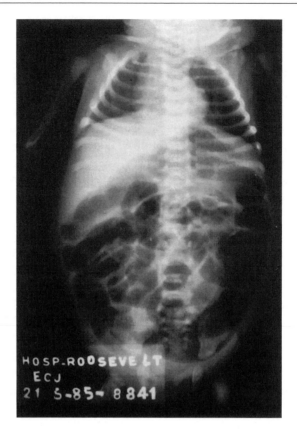

Fig. 1. A newborn with Hirschsprung's disease. On the third day of life this infant developed abdominal distension and vomiting. An abdominal radiograph of this infant showed the presence of loops of small and large bowel distended by air with a paucity of gas in the rectum. Kindly provided by Dr. Gerardo Cabrera-Meza, Texas Children's Hospital.

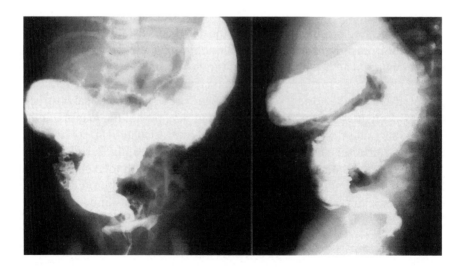

Fig. 2. A newborn with Hirschsprung's disease. When a barium enema was administered to this infant, the colon was distended (left panel), and a funnel-like narrowing was present in the distal segment (right panel). Kindly provided by Dr. Gerardo Cabrera-Meza, Texas Children's Hospital.

serial specimens to delineate the extent of the aganglionic segment may be done when a colostomy is performed as part of a two-stage repair. Once a diagnosis has been made, the extent of the disease must be determined. This identification is usually done when a colostomy is created for a two-stage repair or during the preliminary definitive repair when a one-stage repair is used. The most common lesion extends to the rectosigmoid area (75% of cases), while less commonly to the descending colon (11%), the splenic flexure (4%), the transverse colon (2%), the ascending colon (1%), and the entire colon (8%) (4). Two variants of this latter diagnosis may occur. One is called zonal aganglionosis, wherein segments of aganglionic colon lie adjacent to proximal and distal normal ganglionic areas. In another variant, the myenteric plexus is deficient, but the submucosal plexus is normal (25).

Hirschsprung's disease results as the absence of the intrinsic innervation of the distal colon and both the myenteric and submucosal plexuses are absent. The extrinsic innervation (i.e., the sympathetic and parasympathetic nerves derived from the spinal cord) is preserved and, at times, increased, perhaps due to the lack of feedback inhibition by ingrowth of the intrinsic nerves. As a result, enlarged bundles of sympathetic and parasympathetic nerves are seen between the circular and longitudinal muscles. Because these trunks contain acetyl cholinesterase, staining for acetyl cholinesterase has aided the accuracy of diagnosis, especially beyond 3 wk postnatal age when the acetyl cholinesterase positive fibers have proliferated into the lamina propria. For the most accurate diagnosis, it is recommended that some diagnostic biopsy sections be stained with hematoxylin and eosin (H & E) and some with acetyl cholinesterase. Hirschsprung's disease is diagnosed if neurons are absent in the H & E sections and the acetyl cholinesterase stain is positive.

Other stains using antibodies to neural and glial-cell markers have been recently introduced. For example an S-100 antibody may show hypertrophied submucosal nerve trunks to be present in the aganglionic colon (26). Staining for nitric oxide synthase for Hirschsprung's disease has also been described in six patients (27).

5. TREATMENT

Although the definitive treatment is surgical repair, there are three alternatives for initial treatment, including rectal irrigation (28), colostomy, or primary repair (29). Rectal irrigation may be used several times/d in patients whose aganglionic segments do not extend above the sigmoid. These irrigations decompress the intestine until further evaluation and growth are achieved in preparation for a definitive surgical repair (1). Alternatively, a colostomy is created proximal to the aganglionic segment, which is identified by performing serial biopsies. This procedure also permits decompression of the bowel and permits the infant to grow larger until a definitive repair can be done approx 12 mo later. As anesthetic techniques have improved, there has been a recent shift to attempt primary repair in the neonatal period, reserving the use of the colostomy for those patients who present with enterocolitis. In these latter patients, the colostomy permits the decompression of the bowel and permits time for the inflammatory events of the enterocolitis to resolve.

Regardless, whether repair is done using two operations (i.e, the colostomy followed by a definitive repair) or one (i.e., primary repair), the classic operation for Hirschsprung's disease consists of removal of the aganglionic segment and pulling the normally innervated bowel down to the anus. The major procedures are those of Swenson (30), Duhamel (31), Soave-Boley (32,33) and Georgeson (34). The Swenson procedure includes the dissection of the rectum to a point just proximal of the dentate line posteriorly, leaving a 2-cm segment of abnormal bowel anteriorly. The bowel is then divided at the transition zone, and the distal aganglionic segment is pulled down and everted out the anus. The aganglionic segment is then amputated just proximal to the dentate line, and the proximal ganglionic bowel is pulled down and sewn to this level. During the Duhamel procedure, the aganglionic segment remains in place, and the ganglionic segment is brought posterior to it. These two portions of bowel are anastomosed to create an opening between the two. The Soave-Boley procedure involves dissection of the outer wall of the rectum (as does the Swenson) with dissection of the inner wall of the bowel or an endorectal mucosal protectomy with the rectal muscle layer left in place. The Georgeson procedure uses laparoscopic instruments to mobilize the intra-abdominal rectum. The mucosal sleeve is then removed from the aganglionic segment via a transanal dissection, using an anastomosis that is identical to that of the Soave-Boley procedure.

For patients who have total colonic aganglionsis, total colectomy and ileostomy with or without a pouch has been done in adults. The two procedures suggested for infants are those proposed by Martin *(35)* and Boley *(36)*. Martin's procedure consists of an extended Duhamel with a long side-to-side anastomosis of retained sigmoid and left colon to the normal small bowel, which is then passed retrorectally and placed near the dentate line. The Boley procedure consists of anatomizing the cecum and ascending colon as an on-lay patch graft to the most distal normal small bowel. This is then pulled through the amputated rectum that has been stripped of its mucosa, and a primary anastomosis is done. Regardless of the surgical technique used, these patients often lose significant amounts of water and electrolytes postoperatively and have difficulties with stool continence. Care should also be taken to examine whether the patient has associated anomalies, as total aganglionosis may be associated with Waardenburg's syndrome, the Smith-Lemli-Opitz syndrome, and congenital failure of automatic control of ventilation or central hypoventilation syndrome *(6–8)*.

6. OUTCOME

Postoperatively, as many as 15–20% of patients develop enterocolitis (Fig. 3). Enterocolitis can occur within days or years following surgery *(37)*, and it is the most common cause of mortality and postoperative morbidity *(38)*. The cause of this complication has not been elucidated, and it is thought to be multifactorial. The lack of relaxation of the distal bowel permits stool to stagnate, which, in turn, permits an increased number of fecal breakdown products to accumulate. As the bowel distends and intraluminal pressure rises, the resulting decreases in intramural capillary blood flow inhibit the function of the protective mucosal barrier. Finally, fecal breakdown products, bacteria, and toxin cause inflammation of the bowel wall and gain access to the blood stream. Patients develop abdominal distention, foul-smelling diarrhea, fever, and sepsis. Often the colon shows mucosal ulcers, bacterial proliferation (most typically of the *Clostridium* type), and occasionally perforation. Treatment includes rectal irrigations using warm saline, nasogastric suction, and intravenous antibiotics. In the event that enterocolitis is present prior to the confirmation of a diagnosis of Hirschsprung's disease, a colostomy is performed when the patient has clinically recovered, and definitive surgery delayed for about 12 mo. A second pull-through may be required for those patients who have already had a previous definitive repair.

Regardless of the surgical technique used for definitive repair, a few patients develop severe complications, including dehiscence of the pull-through bowel, severe rectal strictures, pelvic abscess, and chronic perineal fistulas. These complications are treated secondarily with a posterior sagittal approach that permits the resection of the stricture areas, mobilization of the proximal normal agaganglionic bowel, and anastomosis with the anal canal.

Other complications that may occur are anal stricture, incontinence, constipation, and cuff abscess. In spite of these complications, it is estimated that 90% of patients undergoing surgery have a satisfactory outcome *(1)*. A recent report of eight adult patients who had operations as

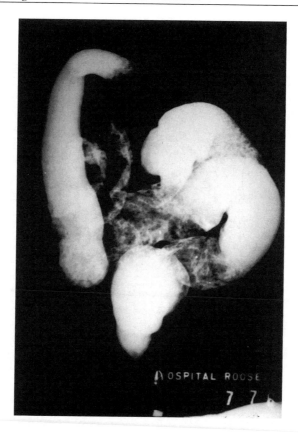

Fig. 3. An infant with Hirschsprung's disease who presented with enterocolitis. Note the presence of the typical radiographic findings for Hirschsprung's disease in the colon accompanied by the presence of pneumatosis intestinalis in the distal small intestine. Kindly provided by Dr. Gerardo Cabrera-Meza, Texas Children's Hospital.

adults reports similar outcomes *(39)*. The most commonly reported adverse outcomes are incontinence and constipation *(1)*. Unfortunately, no prospective trial has compared the outcomes from the various procedures. One study has shown similar outcomes for infants managed using primary repairs compared to those with two-stage repairs up to 17 mo postoperatively *(40)*.

Among 48 adults who had repair as infants, approx 60% were found to have complete fecal control, 31% had occasional staining and/or gas incontinence, 8% had constant fecal soiling, and 10% had constipation *(41)*. A recent study has described that functional outcome was significantly poorer among patients who had had repairs involving the creation of extended lengths of aganglionic–aganglionic common channels done in an attempt to maximize fluid reabsorption postoperatively *(42)*. Other investigators developed a scoring system to assess stool evacuation, abdominal distention, fecal soiling, and severe incontinence. Using this scoring system to evaluate 53 patients up to 23 yr postoperatively, they demonstrated that patients who had short segment disease had progressive improvement in outcome throughout childhood and adolescence *(38)*. In one study among 178 adults, 16 had symptoms of obstruction. Although the results of manometric evaluation of these patients were similar to others who were assymptomatic, 14 of these 16 patients had abnormal histologic features, including neuronal dysplasia *(9)*, aganglionosis *(4)*, and gaglioneuromatosis of the colon *(1)*. In yet

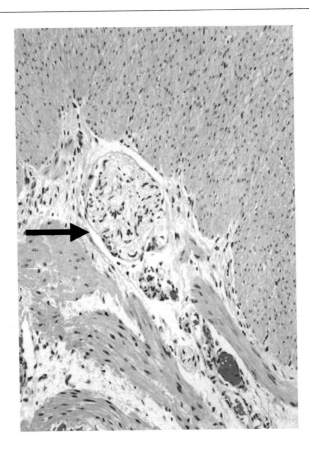

Fig. 4. High power view of the muscularis propria shows an abnormally thick nerve fascicle (arrow) associated with a paucity of myenteric ganglion cells. Figure kindly provided by Dr. Hannes Vogel, Texas Children's Hospital.

another study, there was a positive correlation between functional outcome for fecal incontinence and lower anal resting pressure. Di Lorenzo et al. has found colonic manometry useful for identifying the pathophysiology and to direct treatment in symptomatic children *(43)*. Aggressive intervention to improve fecal continence appears to be warranted, as psychosocial development is impaired among those who have ongoing problems *(44–46)*. Sijmons has recently observed that adults with Hirschsprung's disease associated with *RET* mutations are at greater risk for tumor formation in early adulthood *(47)*.

Outcome for total colonic aganglionosis is poor. Tsuji et al. reported a series of 48 patients over 17 yr *(48)*. Most of these patients had had more than one operation, 82% had fecal incontinence, and 63% had weights below the 2nd percentile for age at age 15 yr *(48)*.

7. INTESTINAL NEURONAL DYSPLASIA AND MATURATIONAL ARREST

Intestinal neuronal dysplasia refers to a variety of histological abnormalities seen in children who have symptoms similar to those seen in Hirschsprung's disease *(49)*. Histologically, these diseases are characterized by hyperplasia of the enteric nerve plexuses, an abnormal distribution of neural elements (Fig. 4), the presence of giant ganglia (Fig. 5) or ectopic ganglia, and increased acetyl cholinesterase activity *(49–52)*. The presence of ganglioneuromas is almost always associated with type IIb multiple endocrine neoplasia syndrome. Intestinal neuronal

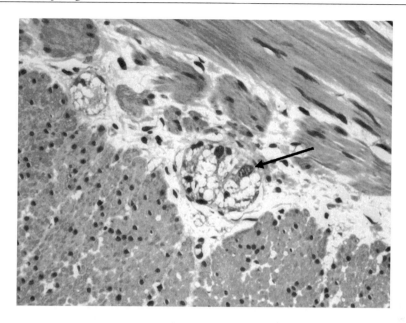

Fig. 5. An isolated giant ganglion cell (arrow) within the myenteric plexus, which normally would contain groups of smaller ganglion cells. Figure kindly provided by Dr. Hannes Vogel, Texas Children's Hospital.

dysplasia may be localized to the colon or disseminated throughout the small and large intestines. It may occur in association with Hirschsprung's disease *(53)*, causing clinical symptoms after surgical repair for Hirschsprung's disease, or in isolation. Most patients can be managed with laxatives and enemas. However, internal sphincter myectomy may be necessary for patients in whom symptoms persist *(50)*. Because there is little correlation of the clinical course with histology, it is recommended that decisions concerning surgery be made on the clinical course rather than the histological findings.

Maturational arrest, or hypoganglionosis, may present histologically in a variety forms, including deficiency of all neural and glial cell elements to deficiency of argyrophilic neurons *(54,55)*. Specific standardized histological criteria for this entity have not been established. As for patients with intestinal neuronal dysplasia, there is an inconsistency of histologic findings, clinical manifestation, treatments, and outcomes. Some patients have benefited from a Soave procedure for severe symptoms *(50)*.

REFERENCES

1. Skinner M. Hirschsprungs's disease. *Curr. Prob. Surg.*, **33** (1996) 389.
2. Carter CO, Evans K, Kickmam VJ. Children of those treated surgically for Hirschsprungs'disease. *J. Med. Genet.*, **18** (1981) 87.
3. Passarge E. The genetics of Hirschsprung's disease. Evidence for heteogeneious etiology and a study of sixty-three families. *N. Engl. J. Med.*, **276** (1967) 138.
4. Kleinhaus S, Boley SJ, Sheran M, Sieber WK. Hirschsprung's disease, a survey of the members of the Surgical Section of the American Academy of Pediatrics. *J. Pediatr. Surg.*, **14** (1979) 588–597.
5. Swenson O, Bill AH. Resection of rectum and rectosigmoind with preservation of the sphincter for benign spastic lesions producing megacolon, an experimental study. *Surgery*, **24** (1948) 212–216.
6. Farndon P, Bianchi A. Waardenburg's syndrome associated with total aganglioniosis. *Arch. Dis. Child.*, **58** (1983) 932–933.

7. Zizka J, Maresova J, Kerekes Z, Juttnerova V, Balicek P. Intestinal aganglionosis in the Smith-Lemli-Opitz syndrome. *Acta Paediatr. Scand.*, **72** (1983) 141–143.

8. Stern M, Hellwege H, Gravinghoff L, Lambrecht W. Total aganglionosis of the colon (Hirschsprung's diseases) and congenital failure of automatic control of ventilation (Ondine's curse). *Acta Paediatr. Scand.*, **70** (1981) 121–124.

9. Hofstra RMW, Osinga J, Buys, CHCM. Mutations in Hirschsprung's disease, when does a mutation contribute to the phenotype? *Eur. J. Hum. Genet.*, **5** (1997) 180–185.

10. Badner JA, Sieber WK, Garver KL. A genetic study of Hirschsprung's Disease. *Am. J. Hum. Genet.*, **46** (1990) 568–580.

11. Touraine RL, Attie-Bitach T, Manceau E. Neurologic phenotype in Waardenberg and syndrome type 4 correlates with novel SOX10 truncating mutations and expression in developing brain. *Am. J. Hum. Genet.*, **66** (2000) 1496–1503.

12. Kapur RP. Early death of neural crest cells is responsible for total aganglionosis in SOX10 (Dom)/SOX10 (Dom) mouse embryos. *Pediatr. Dev. Pathol.*, **2** (1999) 559–569.

13. Pattyn A, MorinX, Cremer H, Gordis C, Brunet JF. The homobox gene phox 26 is essential for the development of autonomic neural crest derivatives. *Nature*, **399** (1999) 366–70.

14. Rothman TP, Gershon MD. Regionally defective colonization of the terminal bowel by precursors of enteric neurons in lethal spotted mutant mice. *Neuroscience*, **12** (1984) 1293–1311.

15. Jacobs-Cohen RJ, Payette RF, Gershon MD, Rothman TP. Inability of neural crest cells to colonize the presumptive aganglionic bowel of ls/ls mice, requirement for a permissive microenvironment. *J. Comp. Neurol.*, **255** (1987) 425–438.

16. Kapur RP, Yost C, Palmiter RD. Aggregation chimeras demonstrate that the primary defect responsible for aganglionic megacolon in lethal spotted mice is not neuroblast autonomous. *Development*, **117** (1993) 993–999.

17. Thoenen H, Edgar D. Neurotrophic factors. *Science*, **229** (1985) 238–342.

18. Chalazonitis A, Rothman TP, Chen JX, Lanballe F, Barbacid M, Gershon M. Neurotrophin-3 induces neural crest-derived cell from fetal rat to develop in vitro as neurons or glia. *J. Neurosci.*, **14** (1994) 6571–6584.

19. Kuroda T, Ueda M, Nakano M, Saeki M. Altered production of nerve growth factor in agtagnlionic intestines. *J. Pediatr. Surg.*, **29** (1994) 288–293.

20. Chakravarti A. Endothelin receptor-mediated signaling in Hirschsprung's disease. *Hum. Molec. Genet.*, **5** (1996) 303–307.

21. Fujimoto T, Hata J, Yokoyama S, Mitomi T. A study of the extracellular matrix protein as the migration pathway of neural crest cell for the gut. Analysis in human embryos with special reference to the pathogenesis of Hirschsprung's disease. *J. Pediatr. Surg.*, **24** (1989) 550–556.

22. Parikh D, Tam P, Lloyd D, Van Velzen D, Edgar D. Quantitative and qualitative analysis of the extracellular matrix protein, laminin, in Hirschsprung's disease. *J. Pediatr. Surg.*, **27** (1992) 991–996.

23. De Campo J, Mayne V, Boldt D, de Campo M. Radiological findings in total aganglionosis coli. *Pediatr. Radiol.*, **14** (1984) 205.

24. Andrassy R, Issacs H, Weitzman J. Rectal suction biopsy for the diagnosis of Hirschsprung's disease. *Ann. Surg.*, **193** (1981) 419.

25. McMahon RA, Moore CCM, Cussen LJ. Hirschsprung's-like syndromes in patients with normal ganglion cells on suction rectal biopsy. *J. Pediatr. Surg.*, **16** (1981) 835–839.

26. Robey S, Kuhajda F, Yardley J. Immunoperoxidase stains of ganglion cells and abnormal mucosal nerve proliferations in Hirschsprung's disease. *Hum. Pathol.*, **19** (1988) 432–437.

27. Vanderwinden J, DeLaet M, Schiffmann S, et al. Nitric oxide synthase distribution in the enteric nervous system of Hirschsprung's disease. *Gastroenterology*, **105** (1993) 969–973.

28. Carcassonne M, Morrisson-Lacombe G, Letourneau JN. Primary corrective operation without decompression in infants less than three months of age with Hirschsprung's disease. *J. Pediatr. Surg.*, **17** (1982) 241–243.

29. So HB, Schwartz DL, Becker JM, Daum F, Schneider KM. Endorectal "pull-through" without preliminary colostomy in neonates with Hirschsprung's disease. *J. Pediatr. Surg.*, **15** (1980) 470–471.

30. Swenson L, Bill A. Resection of the rectum and rectosigmoid with preservation of the sphincter for benign spastic lesions producing magacolon. *Surgery*, **24** (1948) 212–216.

31. Duhamel B. Rectrorectal and transanal pull-through procedure for the treatment of Hirschsprung's disease. *Dis. Colon Rectum*, **7** (1964) 455–460.

32. Soave F. A new surgical technique for the treatment of Hirschsprung's disease. *Surgery*, **56** (1964) 1007.

33. Boley S. New modification of the surgical treatment of Hirschsprung's disease. *Surgery*, **56** (1964) 1015.

34. Georgeson K, Fuenfer M, Hardin W. Primary laparoscopic pull through for Hirschsprung's disease in infants and children. *J. Pediatr. Surg.*, **30** (1995) 1017.

35. Martin LW. Surgical management of total colonic aganglionosis. *Ann. Surg.*, **176** (1972) 343–350.

36. Boley SJ. A new operative approach to total colonic aganglionosis. *Surg. Gynecol. Obstet.*, **159** (1984) 481–484.
37. Blane C, Elhalaby E, Coran A. Enterocolitis following endorectal pull-through in children with Hirschsprung's disease. *Pediatr. Radiol.*, **24** (1994) 164.
38. Reding R, de Ville de Goyet J, Gosseye S, et al. Hirschsprung's disease, a 20-year experience. *J. Pediatr. Surg.*, **32** (1997) 1221–1225.
39. Pheikkinen M, Huikuri K, Jarvinen H. Adult Hirschsprung's disease. Clinical features and functional outcome after surgery. *Dis. Colon Rectum*, **33** (1990) 65–69.
40. Langer JC, Fitzgerald PG, Winthrop AL, et al. One versus two stage Soave pull-through for Hirschsprung's disease in the first year of life. *J. Pediatr. Surg.*, **31** (1996) 33–37.
41. Bjornland K, Diseth TH, Emblem R. Long-term functional, manometric and endosonographic evaluation of patients operated upon with the Duhamel technique. *Pediatr. Surg. Int.*, **13** (1998) 24–28.
42. Hoehner JC, Ein SH, Shankdling B, Kim PC. Long-term morbidity in total colonic aganglionosis. *J. Pediatr. Surg.*, **33** (1998) 961–965.
43. Di Lorenzo C, Solzi GF, Flores AF, Schwankovsky L, Hyman PE. Colonic motility after surgery for Hirschsprung's disease. *Am. J. Gastroenterol.*, **95** (2000) 1759–1764.
44. Yanchar NL, Soucy P. Long-term outcome after Hirschsprung's disease: patients' perspectives. *J. Pediatr. Surg.*, **34** (1999) 1152–1160.
45. Diseth TH, Egeland T, Emblem R. Effects of anal invasive treatment and incontinence on mental health and psychosocial functioning of adolescents with Hirschsprung's disease and low anorectal anomalies. *J. Pediatr. Surg.*, **33** (1998) 468–475.
46. Van Kuyk EM, Brugman-Boezeman AT, Wissink-Essink M, Severjnen RS, Festen C, Bleijenberg G. Defecation problems in children with Hirschsprung's disease: a biopsychosocial approach. *Pediatr. Surg. Int.*, **16** (2000) 312–316.
47. Sijmons RH, Hofstra RMW, Wijburg FA, et al. Oncological implications of *RET* gene mutations in Hirschsprung's disease. *Gut*, **43** (1998) 542–547.
48. Tsuji H, Spitz L, Kiely EM, Drake DP, Pierro A. Mangagement and long-term follow-up of infants with total colonic aganglionosis. *J. Pediatr. Surg.*, **34** (1999) 158–161.
49. Puri P, Wester T. Intestinal neuronal dysplasia. *Sem. Pediatr. Surg.*, **7** (1998) 181–186.
50. Dickson JAS, Variend S. Colinic neuronal dysplasia. *Acta Pediatr. Scand.*, **72** (1983) 635–637.
51. Munakata K, Morita K, Okabe, I, Sueoka H. Clinical and histologic studies of neuronal intestinal dysplasia. *J. Pediatr. Surg.*, **20** (1985) 231–235.
52. Koletzko S, Jesch I, Faus-Kessler T, et al. Rectal biopsy for diagnosis of intestinal neuronal dysplasia in children: a prospective multicenter study on interobserver variation and clinical outcome. *Gut*, **44** (1999) 853–861.
53. Fadda B, Pistor G, Meier-Ruge W. Symptoms, diagnosis, and therapy of neuronal intestinal dysplasia masked by Hirschsprung's disease. *Pediatr. Surg. Int.*, **2** (1987) 76–80.
54. Sacher P, Briner J, Stauffer UG. Unusual cases of neuronal intestinal dysplasia. *Pediatr. Surg. Int.*, **6** (1991) 225–226.
55. Meier-Ruge WA, Brunner LA, Engert J. A correlative morphometric and clinical investigation of hypoganglionosis of the colon in children. *Eur. J. Pediatr. Surg.*, **9** (1999) 67–74.

24 Acute Megacolon, Acquired Megacolon, and Volvulus

Marc Stauffer and Timothy R. Koch

Contents

1. INTRODUCTION: ACUTE MEGACOLON

1.1. Historical Overview

Marked dilation of the colon to a threshold diameter above which there is risk of colonic perforation is termed megacolon. In this chapter, we will not be considering "toxic megacolon," which is an acute dilation of the colon associated with colitis. Acute megacolon can occur either secondary to an acute obstructive process or with no evidence for a mechanical origin. Different studies have described the risk of perforation of the cecum in acute megacolon. During acute dilation, the risk of ischemic changes with subsequent cecal perforation rises with diameter of the cecum ranging from >9 cm to >12 cm. Colonic ischemia has been reported in up to 10% of patients with acute colonic distention.

In 1948, Ogilvie (1) first described two cases of large intestine colic due to sympathetic deprivation. He presented two patients who exhibited signs and symptoms compatible with bowel obstruction. Barium studies failed to reveal any evidence for a mechanical obstruction. In both cases, exploratory surgery was performed to confirm these results. The operative findings were that of extensive malignant disease involving the celiac axis and semilunar ganglion with a normal nonobstructed colon. He postulated that retroperitoneal infiltration resulted in sympathetic deprivation with unopposed parasympathetic stimulation causing excessive and uncoordinated contraction. Since that time, the term Ogilvie's syndrome has been applied to patients with rapid dilation of the colon without an identifiable mechanical cause. Dudley, in 1958, coined the term pseudo-obstruction, which has become synonymous with Ogilvie's syndrome (2).

1.2. Pathophysiology

The exact mechanism for development of acute colonic pseudo-obstruction remains uncertain. It is hypothesized that colonic pseudo-obstruction results from an imbalance in the regu-

From: *Colonic Diseases*
Edited by: T. R. Koch © Humana Press Inc., Totowa, NJ

Table 1
Conditions Associated with the Development of Acute Megacolon

Post-surgical	Acute medical disorders	Neurological disorders
Total hip arthroplasty	Metastatic cancer	Muscular dystrophy
Spinal surgery	Congestive heart failure	Cerebral infarction
Lumbar laminectomy	Myocardial infarction	Parkinson's disease
Renal transplantation	Appendicitis	Guillain-Barré syndrome
Hysterectomy	Cholecystitis	
Cesarean section	Pancreatitis	
Cystectomy	Pneumonitis	
Coronary artery bypass graft		

Medications	Metabolic disorders	Miscellaneous disorders
Imipramine	Hypothyroidism	Varicella zoster infection
Interleukin-2	Diabetes mellitus	Mechanical ventilation
Clonidine	Pheochromocytoma	Hypoxia
Lactulose	Electrolyte imbalance	Hip fracture
Amphetamines	(Hypokalemia, hypercalcemia,	Trauma
Opiate agonists	Hypomagnesemia)	Burn patient
Anticholinergics	Uremia	Alcoholism
Tricyclic antidepressant		Lead poisoning
Calcium channel antagonist		Idiopathic

lation of colonic motor activity due to a disruption of the autonomic nervous system. Sympathetic fibers innervating the colon are classically considered to be inhibitory, while parasympathetic fibers are classically considered to be stimulatory. Parasympathetic innervation could increase colonic contractility, while sympathetic innervation could decrease colonic motility. It has been theorized that extrinsic factors could cause a disruption of this autonomic regulation leading to excessive parasympathetic suppression, sympathetic stimulation, or both, resulting in acute colonic pseudo-obstruction. In this model, colonic dilation occurs as the result of muscle atony. In support of this model, interruption of parasympathetic outflow to the gut, rendering the descending colon and rectosigmoid immobile and excessively compliant, may occur in lumbosacral trauma, therefore promoting the development of megacolon. In addition, patients with lumbar spinal surgery and lumbar spinal stenosis are more susceptible to the development of megacolon (3).

1.3. Potential Causes of Acute Megacolon

As many as 95% of patients with acute megacolon have been reported to have an associated medical or surgical condition (see Table 1). Conditions associated with the development of acute megacolon include postsurgical conditions (4,5), acute medical disorders, metabolic and endocrine disorders, neurological disorders, medications (6–10), and miscellaneous disorders including infections (11).

1.4. Signs and Symptoms of Acute Megacolon

Symptoms in patients who have developed acute megacolon can include those of obstruction: mainly crampy, spasmodic abdominal pain, vomiting, borborygmi (audible rumbling or gurgling of the intestine), abdominal distention, and obstipation. On physical examination,

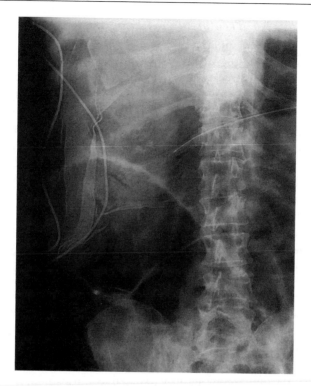

Fig. 1. Patient with acute abdominal distension following an orthopedic surgical procedure. An abdominal flat plate X-ray reveals dilation of the colon with marked cecal dilation in the right lower quadrant. These findings are consistent with the diagnosis of acute megacolon or Ogilvie's syndrome.

percussion may reveal resonance or tympany due to trapped air. Auscultation may intermittently demonstrate loud, high pitched, and hyperactive bowel sounds.

Signs of peritonitis including abdominal guarding, rigidity, and rebound tenderness, often associated with leukocytosis support both a diagnosis of colonic perforation and the need for surgical intervention under emergency circumstances. Surgical intervention in these circumstances would include consideration of performing a colectomy or tube cecostomy.

1.5. Diagnosis of Acute Megacolon

The diagnosis of acute megacolon is made when patients who present with rapid development of abdominal distention have an abdominal X-ray showing colonic gaseous distention with cecal or transverse colonic diameter greater than 9–12 cm, with a predominance of right colon dilation (see Fig. 1). It has been suggested that following plain abdominal radiographs, 2 additional films consisting of a right lateral decubitus abdominal view followed by a prone lateral view of the pelvis should be obtained *(12)*. It has been demonstrated that gaseous distension of the rectum occurs in 75% of patients examined with pseudo-obstruction, but this finding is not consistent in patients with a structural obstruction of the colon *(12)*.

Additional evaluation by lower endoscopy or exploratory laporotomy should reveal no evidence for mechanical obstruction. A radiocontrast enema using a water soluble contrast media without gaseous distension has also been demonstrated to be effective and safe in excluding a mechanical obstruction in these patients.

1.6. Treatment of Acute Megacolon

The treatment of acute megacolon is based on the prevention of colonic perforation induced by ischemia due to prolonged colonic distension. Proper treatment is an extensively debated topic. The literature is also somewhat difficult to read, since some authors consider colonoscopy to be a "conservative method". While all patients and their risks must be individualized, in general, cecal dilation to greater than 12 cm or acute dilation lasting greater than 24 h would suggest the need for early intervention without a trial of conservative measures.

Initial management of patients with acute megacolon may, therefore, involve conservative measures *(13)*: (i) correction of an underlying cause; (ii) evaluation for immediate discontinuation of medications that can alter colonic motility (such as narcotics, anticholinergic medications, or calcium channel antagonists) (see Table 1); (iii) correction of electrolyte abnormalities and metabolic disturbances; (iv) permit nothing to eat or drink by mouth; (v) nasogastric suction; (vi) intravenous fluid replacement; and (vii) consideration of placement of a soft rectal tube (one must consider the risk of perforation) while periodically repositioning the patient side-to-side. It has been reported that cancer patients with acute megacolon respond well and safely to conservative measures *(13)*.

These patients require repeated reevaluation. In those patients who have failed to correct their acute megacolon within 24 h of conservative management, further treatment options include the use of erythromycin *(14)*, neostigmine *(15–18)*, colonoscopy with decompression *(19–23)*, or cecostomy *(24–25)*.

The use of erythromycin in Ogilvie's syndrome is limited to case reports *(14)*. It is based on the increase in gastrointestinal motor activity induced by intravenous erythromycin. The suggested dose is 250 mg of erythromycin in 250 mL of saline (0.9%) given intravenously every 8 h for 3 d. A rapid response should not be expected and this regimen should not be utilized if a rapid response appears necessary.

Since the original report by Dr. William Snape, Jr. et al. on the effect of anticholinesterases on colonic motor activity *(15)*, the use of these pharmacological drugs to induce flatus passage has been examined. Neostigmine increases cholinergic activity and its use in this condition supports the theory that this colonic disorder is due to decreased parasympathetic activity.

With the use of neostigmine methylsulfate, a test dose of 0.5 mg should be considered; it is given slowly by intravenous injection with potentially simultaneous cardiac monitoring owing to a potential for cardiac disrhythmia. A main concern is the development of cholinergic crisis as manifested by increasing muscle weakness and difficulty with respirations. This requires immediate treatment with intravenous atropine sulfate (0.6–1.2 mg). For colonic decompression, protocols have utilized neostigmine methylsulfate with 2.0 mg given intravenously over 3–5 min. An immediate clinical response to treatment is defined as the passage of flatus or stool with a reduction in abdominal distention on physical examination within 30 min of administration. It is not yet certain whether increasing colonic contractile activity increases pressure in the right colon to a level that might be dangerous in the presence of colonic ischemia.

In clinical studies *(16–18)*, it has been reported that up to 90% of patients who receive neostigmine have an immediate clinical response. However, this treatment may fail in up to 20% of patients who have a recurrence of megacolon requiring colonoscopic decompression of the colon. Further work is required to determine whether neostigmine therapy is appropriate for patients with more severe colonic distention or prolonged colonic distention.

Patients who have had a poor response to conservative management or neostigmine may be candidates for colonic decompression by colonoscopy with or without placement of a decompression tube *(19–24)*. This technique was originally described in 1977 by Kukora and associates *(19)*. Recurrence rates in these patient have been reported to range from 40–58%, with improved results described in patients who also had decompression tubes placed during lower endoscopy *(20)*. Placement of decompression tubes during colonoscopy may however be technically difficult. Reports suggest that colonoscopic decompression can be safely performed in those patients who have progressed to colonic ischemia *(21)*. Placement of the patient on their left lateral side after colonoscopic decompression may reduce the risk of recurrent colonic distention *(24)*.

Surgical intervention is generally recommended for patients with signs of peritonitis or persistent or worsening distention despite colonic decompression. In selected patients, surgeons with the proper experience and training may be able to perform a cecostomy using laparoscopic techniques as demonstrated by case reports *(25,26)*. However, surgery does present risk to the patient since even in the absence of perforation, the mortality rate for an open surgical procedure ranges up to 26% in those patients believed to have viable bowel at the time of surgery.

1.7. Morbidity and Mortality

Colonic perforation and colonic ischemia are uncommon unless the diameter of the cecum is >12 cm. However, some authors have suggested that the duration of colonic dilation may be as important as a risk factor. The approximate risk of spontaneous colonic perforation is 3% with a related mortality of up to 50% in those patients with a colonic perforation and peritonitis.

2. ACQUIRED MEGACOLON

2.1. Background and Definition

Chronic acquired megacolon may be the result of a congenital disorder such as Hirschsprung's disease, or it may be the result of a chronic colonic disorder. Acquired megacolon can be defined by radiological techniques as a distal sigmoid colon >6.5 cm in diameter (see Fig. 2) *(27)*. Constipation is a common symptom in acquired megacolon since 77% of patients with megacolon have constipation *(28)*. Most reports of acquired megacolon have focused on dilation of the distal colon. However, chronic acquired megacolon involving the right colon has been reported in conjunction with impaired colonic muscle tone *(29)*.

2.2. Associated Conditions

Despite the multiple causes of acquired megacolon, alteration of enteric nerves appears to be a common risk factor for development of acquired megacolon. Megacolon is a clinical feature of chronic spinal cord injury *(3)*, Chagas' disease, Von Recklinghausen's disease, myotonic dystrophy, and intestinal ganglioneuromatosis *(30)*. The association between acquired megacolon and chronic neurological and psychiatric disorders has been examined by epidemiologic methods *(31)*. The conditions associated with development of acquired megacolon are summarized in Table 2.

2.3. Pathophysiology

The pathophysiological process involved in development of acquired megacolon is incompletely understood. Based on the morphological alteration of enteric nerves in acquired megacolon, studies of colonic neurochemicals identified a decrease in colonic nerves containing the inhibitory neurochemical, vasoactive intestinal peptide (VIP) *(32)*. Further work revealed a decrease in the tissue antioxidant, glutathione, in colonic muscularis externa from patients with acquired megacolon *(33)*. These patients with chronic acquired megacolon had multiple underlying neurological disorders: dementia, cerebral infarction, quadriplegia, cerebral palsy,

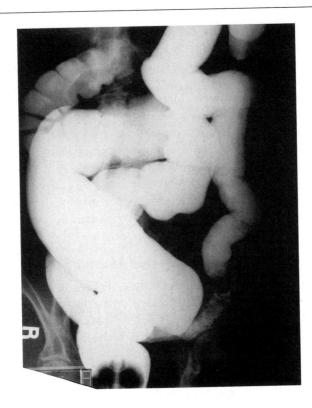

Fig. 2. A barium colon X-ray in a patient with chronic constipation revealed elongation and dilation of the sigmoid colon consistent with the diagnosis of acquired megacolon.

Table 2
Conditions Associated with the Development of Chronic Megacolon

Neurological disorders

Presenile dementia	Alzheimer's disease
Parkinson's disease	Multiple sclerosis
Quadriplegia or chronic spinal cord injury	Neurofibromatosis (Von Recklinghausen's disease)
Multiple endocrine neoplasia, Type 2b	Hirschsprung's disease
(intestinal ganglioneuromatosis)	

Miscellaneous disorders

Infections: Chagas' disease	Schizophrenia
(South American trypanosomiasis)	Idiopathic
Myotonic dystrophy	

and schizophrenia. The results suggest that loss of the potentially neuroprotective antioxidant, glutathione, may lead to changes in intrinsic colonic nerves. An interesting recent manuscript described a decrease in the density of interstitial cells of Cajal in Chagasic megacolon *(34)*. Since interstitial cells of Cajal may function as pacemakers, by regulating the activation of intrinsic colonic nerves, their absence could lead to a relative atony of the colon.

As physiological correlates, an in vitro physiological study has demonstrated diminished nitric oxide production in colonic circular smooth muscle obtained from patients with acquired megacolon *(35)*. Potential explanations could include depletion of tissue levels of L-arginine (the substrate for nitric oxide), decreased capacity to recycle citrulline to arginine, or decreased release of VIP from the circular smooth muscle of the colon. Decreased nitric oxide production as a colonic inhibitory neurochemical could increase the occurrence of nonpropagating contractions (previously termed "spastic constipation").

In a related in vivo physiological study of sigmoid megacolon, both nonadrenergic relaxation induced by balloon distention and relaxation induced by superfusion of VIP were decreased compared to sigmoid colon in normal controls *(36)*. Altered inhibitory nerve input to colonic smooth muscle could induce constipation by reducing the magnitude of smooth muscle relaxation regulated by intrinsic inhibitory nerves and by diminished inhibition of colonic phasic contractions. This potential mechanism would be consistent with the development of constipation in individuals receiving opiates who have been found to have both an increase in nonpropagating contractions of the rectum with slowed colonic transit in the right colon. Progression to colonic hypertrophy and elongation could be the result of prolonged cholinergic nerve-mediated contractions of circular smooth muscle (work hypertrophy). An additional proposed mechanism is the loss of inhibition of smooth muscle proliferation. Indeed, VIP has been shown to inhibit DNA synthesis in cultured smooth muscle cells.

2.4. Clinical Presentation

In the usual clinical presentation, the patient with acquired megacolon will be seen for increasing constipation as manifested by difficulty initiating defecation or infrequent defecation. Patients may also present with a new or recurrent fecal impaction. Less commonly, the patient presents with signs of peritonitis due to a colonic perforation induced by a stercoral (pressure) ulcer of the rectum or sigmoid colon.

The patients generally note lower abdominal distension and discomfort. In severe cases, nausea, emesis, anorexia, and weight loss may be present. Physical examination generally reveals a distended abdomen with palpable masses in the right and left lower quadrants of the abdomen and a fecal impaction on digital rectal examination. In severe cases, evidence for protein–calorie malnutrition may be evidenced by muscle mass wasting. Plain abdominal radiographs will often show colonic distention with impaction of feces diffusely throughout the colon. The differential diagnosis and evaluation of patients with constipation is presented more fully in Chapter 27 in this text.

Remarkably, patients with acquired megacolon do not generally present with colon cancer. Indeed, investigators have reported that colon cancer is quite rare in those individuals with Chagasic megacolon. In an interesting rat study, rats with megacolon induced by the use of neuropathic chemicals were resistant to the development of colon cancer induced by the carcinogen dimethylhydrazine despite the high rate of colon cancer in littermates without megacolon *(37)*.

2.5. Treatment

Clinical studies to examine the treatment of acquired megacolon are required. Our medical treatment strategy has been dictated by three elements. First, studies have shown that the magnitude of colonic contractions required to induce propagation is lower with liquid in the colon compared to solid material in the colon. Second, since acquired megacolon is a risk factor for the development of colonic volvulus, we try to prevent recurrent fecal impaction. Third, a chronic strategy appears to be required. Although there are reports in the pediatric gastrointestinal literature that colonic megacolon may reverse with chronic colonic disimpaction, there is minimal evidence that this is true in adult patients. With our typical patient, we will ask the patient to be instructed on a low-fiber low-residue diet. The second line of therapy is the addition of a stool softener or osmotic agent to increase the water content of the stool. This is described in more detail in Chapter 27. As a third line of therapy, we will ask the patient to use a suppository per rectum at least three times weekly after a warm breakfast to try to induce rectal evacuation. Especially in spinal cord patients, the use of suppositories containing a mixture of sodium bicarbonate with potassium bitartrate in a water soluble polyethylene glycol base may be effective. In the presence of megarectum, strategies to induce colorectal evacuation are often unrewarding.

Surgical intervention to treat acquired megacolon is reserved for patients with a chronic symptom that includes persistent weight loss, recurrent fecal impaction, a history of sigmoid volvulus, or abdominal symptoms that are intractable to medical and dietary therapy and greatly compromise the patient's lifestyle. Some surgical studies have reported that a majority of patients who have developed refractory acquired megacolon will require surgical intervention. Prior to surgical consideration, we evaluate the patient's gastric and small intestinal motility to try to avoid suggesting surgery to patients with evidence for a diffuse pseudo-obstruction. This is generally not possible, however, in patients who present with an acute colonic volvulus. Surgical intervention could include subtotal colectomy with formation of a Hartmann's pouch and ileostomy, or subtotal colectomy with ileorectal anastomosis in younger patients and in those patients with manometric evidence supporting good anal sphincter function. Surgical reports suggest that greater than 80% of patients with acquired megacolon are improved by surgical intervention (38). Complications have been reported in up to 20% of patients and include small bowel obstruction, anastomotic stricture, anastomotic hemorrhage, wound infection, hemorrhagic gastritis, and pancreatitis. As in all surgical procedures, there is a risk of mortality, although the mortality rate is not well defined due to the small patient numbers in surgical reports.

2.6. Future Work

Future studies in this area would benefit from longitudinal examination of individuals with chronic constipation who have evidence for slow transit constipation, a rectal outlet disorder, or a primary neurological disorder. At this time, evaluation of patients for potential surgical intervention for acquired megacolon provides no certainty of the original cause for developing acquired megacolon. An improved approach would include long-term follow-up of patients who have had complete evaluation of chronic constipation. Additional biochemical studies that might provide information about nitric oxide production in patients with acquired megacolon could include determination of tissue levels of L-arginine (the precursor of nitric oxide), determination of the capacity to recycle citrulline to arginine, and determination of VIP release from circular smooth muscle.

3. VOLVULUS

3.1. Background and Definition

In simplest terms, a volvulus is a twisting or folding of the colon on its mesentary. Volvulus of the colon can induce an acute intestinal obstruction. The most frequent volvulus is a sigmoid volvulus followed by cecal volvulus. Transverse colon volvulus makes up only an estimated 2% of cases of volvulus. Four issues that make volvulus important and interesting include its description in ancient literature, its apparent age-related rise in incidence, its potential relationship to a high dietary fiber intake, and the potential risk of development of volvulus in patients with megacolon.

3.2. Etiology

The world-wide incidence of volvulus as a cause of bowel obstruction varies widely *(39)*. Although volvulus is a rare cause of intestinal obstruction in the United States, there are two international populations that require special mention. It has been reported that the incidence of sigmoid volvulus is high in West African populations utilizing a very high fiber diet *(40)*. Factors that predispose to the development of a sigmoid volvulus include a long mobile sigmoid loop and a short basis of mesentary around which the volvulus occurs *(40)*. The implication of the study is that a high fiber diet induces colonic lengthening, perhaps due to incomplete colonic evacuation. The frequent use of enemas was also suggested to be a potential risk factor for the development of volvulus *(40)*. A second noteworthy patient population is the development of sigmoid volvulus in the Andes Mountains *(41)*. It is hypothesized that due to low atmospheric pressure, gases (carbon dioxide, methane, and hydrogen) produced in the colon are present in higher relative gas volume, thus inducing a chronic distention of redundant colon *(41)*. This interesting theory could be linked with individuals chronically eating a high fiber diet if it could be shown that flatus production in the colon is directly related to the average dietary fiber intake.

A major risk factor for the development of sigmoid volvulus is the presence of megacolon. Conditions in which acquired megacolon is common, including Hirschsprung's disease and spinal cord injury, are associated with the development of sigmoid volvulus *(42,43)*. It has been suggested that chronic distention will produce a differential elongation with greater lengthening of the antimesenteric border of colon *(44)*. In this model, elongation of the mesenteric border is restricted by the mesentery and its vessels *(44)*. As lengthening of the colon progresses, the mesenteric border could induce progressive curvature of the colon due to fixation along the length of the mesentery. This increasing curvature could, therefore, place the colon in the configuration of a volvulus.

Other unusual reported associations with volvulus include development of transverse colon volvulus in the presence of *Clostridium difficile* colitis *(45)*, cecal volvulus in the presence of Celiac sprue *(46)*, and transverse colon volvulus in the presence of Chilaiditi's syndrome (interposition of the hepatic flexure of the colon between the liver and the right hemidiaphragm) *(47)*.

Cecal volvulus comprises 25–40% of all cases of colonic volvulus, and on average patients with cecal volvulus are 10–20 yr younger than patients with sigmoid volvulus. The incidence of volvulus during pregnancy is reported at 1/1500 to 1/66,000 deliveries with up to 44% of the diagnoses being cecal volvulus. It is proposed that as uterine enlargement occurs during pregnancy, it can raise redundant or abnormally mobile cecum out of the pelvis, most commonly during the third trimester of pregnancy *(48,49)*. Other risk factors for the development of cecal volvulus include prior abdominal surgery with internal adhesions, unpressurized air travel, coughing, pelvis mass, atony of the colon, and extreme exertion *(49)*.

3.3. Presentation

In the United States, volvulus is an uncommon cause of intestinal obstruction. Patients may present with complaints of abdominal distention, crampy lower abdominal pain, obstipation, and emesis. On physical examination, common findings include abdominal distension, tender and/or palpable abdominal mass, and an empty rectum on digital rectal examination.

In clinical presentation, volvulus of the cecum may be misdiagnosed as a chronic or recurrent appendicitis. Proper diagnosis requires a high index of suspicion.

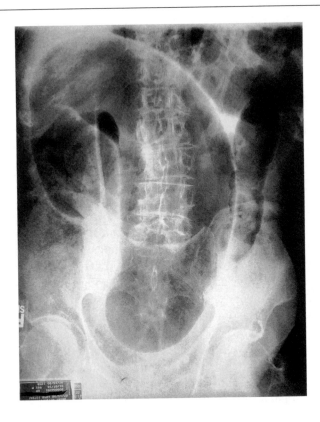

Fig, 3. Patient with acute abdominal distension and obstipation. On an abdominal flat plate X-ray, dilation of the sigmoid colon was identified. Features of distended sigmoid colon arising from the pelvis and a point of apparent termination are consistent with the diagnosis of sigmoid volvulus.

3.4. Diagnosis

The diagnosis of volvulus is often confirmed by plain abdominal radiography. As shown in Fig. 3, the diagnosis of a sigmoid volvulus is suggested by features of distended sigmoid colon arising from the pelvis and a point of apparent termination. Specific and sensitive radiologic signs of sigmoid volvulus on plain abdominal radiographs include: (i) apex of the loop under the left hemidiaphragm; (ii) inferior convergence on the left; and (iii) a left flank overlap sign (50). An additional radiologic sign of sigmoid volvulus that has been suggested from review of plain abdominal radiographs is identification of dilated sigmoid colon that ascends cephalad to the transverse colon (51).

The presence of a sigmoid volvulus can be confirmed and temporarily treated by performance of lower endoscopy. Caution should be taken in attempting to reduce a sigmoid volvulus by advancement of the endoscope if ischemic appearing colon is identified, since the risk of perforation of the colon may be increased. Since reduction of a sigmoid volvulus by performance of lower endoscopy can produce a very rapid release of a mixture of liquid stool and gases during colonic decompression, the endoscopist must take proper care to protect against potential contamination of the room and nearby health care personnel. The recurrence rate of sigmoid volvulus is reported to be >80% in patients at a mean of 3 mo follow-up following colonoscopic reduction and decompression without surgical intervention.

A radiocontrast enema without gaseous distention has been demonstrated to be effective for the diagnosis of cecal volvulus. The use of colonoscopy for confirmation and temporary treatment of a cecal volvulus is not as clear as in the case of sigmoid volvulus. It is thought that the risk of colonic perforation is increased by performing colonoscopy on patients with cecal volvulus. Available clinical studies also suggest a high failure rate during attempted colonoscopic decompression in patients with cecal volvulus.

3.5. Treatment

Definitive treatment of colonic volvulus requires surgical intervention (52–57). Surgical treatment of sigmoid volvulus generally involves performance of a sigmoid colectomy. There is a high recurrence rate reported following simple detorsion of the colon for treatment of sigmoid volvulus. It has been known for at least 20 yr that the recurrence rate following sigmoid colectomy is high in patients with megacolon at the time of surgery (53). It has been suggested that in patients with sigmoid volvulus and megacolon, subtotal colectomy should be considered (56). Perioperative mortality following sigmoid colectomy for sigmoid volvulus is up to 14% in multiple surgical series.

Suggested surgical therapies for cecal volvulus include tube cecostomy, simple detorsion, cecopexy, and performance of a right hemicolectomy. Due to high recurrence rates, most individuals with cecal volvulus are presently treated by performance of a right hemicolectomy. The mortality rates for surgical treatment of cecal volvulus are higher than in surgical treatment of sigmoid volvulus. The mortality rate is higher for those patients with necrotic colon at the time of surgery and patients who require emergency surgical intervention. If necrotic or gangrenous colon is present, a right hemicolectomy is required and consideration must be given for formation of a temporary ileostomy and distal mucous fistula.

REFERENCES

1. Ogilvie WH. Large intestine colic due to sympathetic deprivation: a new clinical syndrome. *BMJ*, **2** (1948) 671–673.
2. Dudley HA, Sinclair IS, McLaren IF, McNair TJ, Newsam JE. Intestinal pseudo-obstruction. *J. R. Coll. Surg. Edinb.*, **3** (1958) 206–217.
3. Harari D, Minaker KL. Megacolon in patients with chronic spinal cord injury. *Spinal Cord*, **38** (2000) 331–339.
4. O'Malley KJ, Flechner SM, Kapoor A, et al. Acute colonic pseudo-obstruction (Ogilvie's syndrome) after renal transplantation. *Am. J. Surg.*, **177** (1999) 492–496.
5. Ballaro, A, Gibbons CLM, Murray DM, Kettlewell MGW, Benson MK. Acute colonic pseudo-obstruction after total hip replacement. *J. Bone Joint Surg.*, **79** (1997) 621–623.
6. Wright, R. Lactulose-induced megacolon. *Gastrointest. Endosc.*, **34** (1988) 489–490.
7. Stieger DS, Cantieni R, Frutiger A. Acute colonic pseudo-obstruction (Ogilvie's syndrome) in two patients receiving high dose clonidine for delirium tremens. *Intensive Care Med.* **23** (1997) 780–782.
8. Sood A, Kumar R. Imipramine induced acute colonic pseudo-obstruction (Ogilvie's syndrome): a report of two cases. *Indian J. Gastroenterol.*, **15** (1996) 70–71.
9. Ohri SK, Patel T, Desa CBL, Spencer J. Drug-induced colonic pseudo-obstruction. *Dis. Colon Rectum*, **34** (1991) 346–350.
10. Post AB, Falk GW, Bukowski RM. Acute colonic pseudo-obstruction associated with interleukin-2 therapy. *Am. J. Gastroenterol.*, **86** (1991) 1539–1541.
11. Walsh TN and Lane D. Pseudo-obstruction of the colon associated with varicella-zoster infection. *Ir. J. Med. Sci.*, **151** (1982) 318–319.
12. Low VHS. Colonic pseudo-obstruction: Value of prone lateral view of the rectum. *Abdom. Imaging*, **20** (1995) 531–533.
13. Sloyer AF, Panella VS, Demas BE, et al. Ogilvie's syndrome: Successful management without colonoscopy. *Dig. Dis. Sci.*, **33** (1988) 1391–1396.
14. Bonacini M, Smith OJ, Pritchard T. Erythromycin as therapy for acute colonic pseudo-obstruction (Ogilvie's syndrome). *J. Clin. Gastroenterol.*, **13** (1991) 475–487.

15. Snape WJ Jr, Carlson GM, Cohen S. Human colonic myoelectric activity in response to prostigmin and the gastrointestinal hormones. *Dig. Dis.*, **22** (1977) 881–887.

16. Stephenson BM, Morgan AR, Salaman JR, Wheeler MH. Ogilvie's syndrome: A new approach to an old problem. *Dis. Colon Rectum*, **38** (1995) 424–427.

17. Turegano-Fuentes F, Munoz-Jimenez F, DelValle-Hernandez E, et al. Early resolution of Ogilvie's syndrome with intravenous neostigmine. *Dis. Colon Rectum*, **40** (1997) 1353–1357.

18. Ponec RJ, Saunders MD, Kimmey MB. Neostigmine for the treatment of acute colonic pseudo-obstruction. *N. Eng. J. Med.*, **341** (1999) 137–141.

19. Kukora JS, Dent TL, Thomas L. Colonoscopic decompression of massive nonobstructive cecal dilation. *Arch. Surg.*, **112** (1977) 512–517.

20. Harig JM, Fumo DE, Loo FD, et al. Treatment of acute nontoxic megacolon during colonoscopy: tube placement verses simple decompression. *Gastrointest. Endosc.*, **34** (1987) 23–27.

21. Fiorito JJ, Schoen RE, Brandt LJ. Pseudo-obstruction associated with colonic ischemia: successful management with colonoscopic decompression. *Am. J. Gastroenterol..*, **86** (1991) 1472–1476.

22. Jetmore AB, Timmcke AE, Gathright JB, Hicks TC, Ray JE, Baker JW. Ogilvie's syndrome: colonoscopic decompression and analysis of predisposing factors. *Dis. Colon Rectum*, **35** (1992) 1135–1142.

23. Geller A, Petersen BT, Gostout C. Endoscopic decompression for acute colonic pseudo-obstruction. *Gastrointest. Endosc.*, **44** (1996) 144–150.

24. Estela CM, Burd DAR. Conservative management of acute pseudo-obstruction in a major burn. *Burns*, **25** (1999) 523–525.

25. Duh QY, Way LW. Diagnostic laparoscopy and laparoscopic cecostomy for colonic pseudo-obstruction. *Dis. Colon Rectum*, **36** (1993) 65–70.

26. Vaughn P, Schlinkert RT. Management of cecal perforation secondary to Ogilvie's syndrome by laparoscopic tube cecostomy. *J. Laparoendosc. Surg.*, **5** (1995) 339–341.

27. Preston DM, Lennard-Jones JE, Thomas BM. Towards a radiologic definition of idiopathic megacolon. *Gastrointest. Radiol.*, **10** (1985) 167–169.

28. Kantor JL. A clinical study of some common anatomical abnormalities of the colon. I. The redundant colon. *Am. J. Roentenol.*, **12** (1924) 414–430.

29. von der Ohe MR, Camilleri M, Carryer PW. A patient with localized megacolon and intractable constipation: Evidence for impairment of colonic muscle tone. *Am. J. Gastroenterol.*, **89** (1994) 1867–1870.

30. Feinstat T, Tesluk H, Schuffler MD, et al. Megacolon and neurofibromatosis: A neuronal intestinal dysplasia. *Gastroenterology*, **86** (1984) 1573–1579.

31. Sonnenberg A, Tsou VT, Muller AD. The "institutional colon": a frequent colonic dysmotility in psychiatric and neurologic disease. *Am. J. Gastroenterol.*, **89** (1994) 62–66.

32. Koch TR, Schulte-Bockholt A, Telford GL, Otterson MF, Murad TM, Stryker SJ. Acquired megacolon is associated with alteration of vasoactive intestinal peptide levels and acetylcholinesterase activity. *Regul. Pept.*, **48** (1993) 309–319.

33. Koch TR, Schulte-Bockholt A, Otterson MF, et al. Decreased vasoactive intestinal peptide levels and glutathione depletion in acquired megacolon. *Dig. Dis. Sci.*, **41** (1996) 1409–1416.

34. Hagger R, Finlayson C, Kahn F, DeOliveira R, Chimelli L, Kumar D. A deficiency of interstitial cells of Cajal in Chagasic megacolon. *J. Auton. Nerv. Syst.*, **80** (2000) 108–111.

35. Koch TR, Otterson MF, Telford GL. Nitric oxide production is diminished in colonic circular muscle from acquired megacolon. *Dis. Colon Rectum*, **43** (2000) 821–828.

36. Aoki N, Tomita R, Nogai N, Munekata K, Kurose Y, Morita K. Peristaltic reflex and peptidergic nerve control in megacolon. *Nippon Heikatsukin Gakkai Zasshi*, **25** (1989) 233–235.

37. Barcia SB, Oliveira JSM, Pinto LZ, Mucillo G, Zucoloto S. The relationship between megacolon and carcinoma of the colon: an experimental approach. *Carcinogenesis*, **17** (1996) 1777–1779.

38. Belliveau P, Goldberg SM, Rothenberger DA, Nivatvongs S. Idiopathic acquired megacolon: the value of subtotal colectomy. *Dis. Colon Rectum*, **25** (1982) 118–121.

39. Ballantyne G. Review of sigmoid volvulus-Clinical patterns and pathogenesis. *Dis. Colon Rectum*, **25** (1982) 823–830.

40. Schagen Van Leeuwen JH. Sigmoid volvulus in a West African population. *Dis. Colon Rectum*, **28** (1985) 712–716.

41. Asbun HJ, Castellanos H, Balderrama B, et al. Sigmoid volvulus in the high altitude of the Andes: review of 230 cases. *Dis. Colon Rectum*, **35** (1992) 350–353.

42. Fenton-Lee D, Ywo BW, Jones RF, Engel S. Colonic volvulus in the spinal cord injured patient. *Paraplegia*, **31** (1993) 393–397.

43. Sarioglu A, Tanyel CH, Buyukpamukcu N, Hisconmez A. Colonic volvulus: a rare presentation of Hirschsprung's disease. *J. Pediatr. Surg.*, (1997) **32** 117–118.
44. Perry EG. Intestinal volvulus: a new concept. *Aust. NZ J. Surg.*, **53** (1983) 483–486.
45. Yaseen ZH, Watson RE, Hean HA, Wilson ME. Case report: transverse colon volvulus in a patient with Clostridium difficile pseudomembranous colitis. *Am. J. Med. Sci.*, **308** (1994) 147–150.
46. Riobo P, Turbi C, Banet R, et al. Colonic volvulus and ulcerative jejunoileitis due to occult Celiac sprue. *Am. J. Med. Sci.* (1998) **315** 317–318.
47. Plorde JJ, Raker EJ. Transverse colon volvulus and associated Chilaiditi's syndrome: case report and literature review. *Am. J. Gastroenterol.*, **91** (1996) 2613–2616.
48. John H, Gyr T, Giudici G, Martinol S, Marx A. Cecal volvulus in pregnancy. Case report and review of literature. *Arch. Gynecol. Obstet.*, **258** (1996) 161–164.
49. Montes H, Wolf J. Cecal volvulus in pregnancy. *Am. J. Gastroenterol.*, **94** (1999) 2554–2555.
50. Burrell HC, Baker DM, Wardrop P, Evans AJ. Significant plain film findings in sigmoid volvulus. *Clin. Radiol.*, **49** (1994) 317–319.
51. Javors BR, Baker SR, Miller JA. The northern exposure sign: A newly described finding in sigmoid volvulus. *Am. J. Roentgenol.*, **173** (1999) 571–574.
52. Ballantyne GH, Brandner MD, Beart RW, Ilstrup DM. Volvulus of the colon. *Ann. Surg.*, **202** (1985) 83–92.
53. Ryan P. Sigmoid volvulus with and without megacolon. *Dis. Colon Rectum*, **25** (1982) 673–679.
54. Friedman JD, Odland MD, Bubrick MP. Experience with colonic volvulus. *Dis. Colon Rectum*, **32** (1989) 409–416.
55. O'Mara CS, Wilson TH Jr, Stonesifer GL, Cameron JL. Cecal volvulus: analysis of 50 patients with long-term follow-up. *Curr. Surg.*, (1980) **37** 132–136.
56. Chung YF, Eu KW, Nyam DC, Leong AF, Ho YH, Seow-Choen F. Minimizing recurrence after sigmoid volvulus. *Br. J. Surg.*, **86** (1999) 966–967.
57. Grossmann EM, Longo WE, Stratton MD, Virgo KS, Johnson FE. Sigmoid volvulus in department of veterans medical centers. *Dis. Colon Rectum*, **43** (2000) 414–418.

25 Diverticular Disease

Gordon L. Telford, Susan W. Telford, and Mary F. Otterson

CONTENTS

1. INTRODUCTION

Colonic diverticular disease can manifest as either diverticulosis or diverticulitis. With diverticulosis, noninflamed diverticula are present with or without symptoms. Although most patients with diverticulosis have no or only mild symptoms, complications of hemorrhage or infection occur in 15–30% of affected patients; about 30% of these patients require operative treatment. When diverticulitis develops, one or more diverticula become infected. This can lead to perforation of a diverticulum with pericolic infection (peridiverticulitis), abscess formation, or free perforation with peritonitis. As a result, patients can develop fistulas, hemorrhage, colonic obstruction, or other complications. Henchey et al. *(1)* devised a classification for the inflammatory conditions encountered with colonic diverticulitis. Stage I is a small confined pericolonic abscess, Stage II is a larger abscess, Stage III is suppurative peritonitis, and Stage IV is fecal peritonitis.

Diverticulosis occurs more commonly in Western countries. The incidence depends on the age of the population studied, varying from <2% in patients younger than 30 yr old to 30–50% in patients older than 50 yr of age *(2)*. Colonic diverticular disease is a major public health problem in the United States and a continuing challenge for general surgeons.

2. PATHOLOGIC ANATOMY

The majority of colonic diverticula are false diverticula. True diverticula are rare and occur more frequently in the right colon. True diverticula involve all layers of the bowel wall:

From: *Colonic Diseases*
Edited by: T. R. Koch © Humana Press Inc., Totowa, NJ

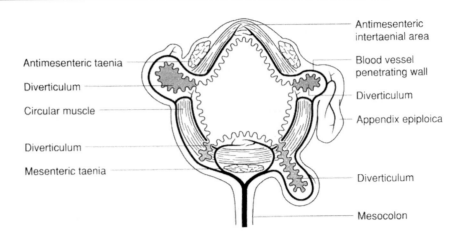

Fig. 1. Cross-section of the colon illustrating the relation of diverticula to blood vessels penetrating the circular muscle layer, the taeniae, and the appendices epiploicae. [Reprinted with permission from: ref. 27.]

mucosa, submucosa, and muscularis externa. With false diverticula, the mucosa and submucosa herniate through the muscularis externa. The vast majority of false diverticula emanate from weak points in the colonic wall where mesenteric blood vessels penetrate the circular muscle layer (Fig. 1). False diverticula also can occur along the antimesenteric border in the intertaenial area *(3)*.

The sigmoid colon contains the majority of colonic diverticula, although they can be present throughout the intra-abdominal colon *(2,4)*. Diverticulosis is limited to the sigmoid colon in up to 65% of patients. In about 35% of patients, at least one other area of the colon is involved. In only 1–4% of patients is the sigmoid colon not involved with diverticula. Diverticula do not occur in the rectum.

3. PATHOPHYSIOLOGY

Decreased dietary fiber is the most consistent factor associated with the high incidence of diverticulosis in Western populations *(5)*. Although called a disease of Western industrialized civilization, diverticulosis may better be described as a disease of affluence and refined food products. As people in some Western nations have decreased their intake of dietary fiber, the incidence of diverticulosis has increased. In contrast, diverticulosis is rare in less affluent nonindustrialized countries. Diverticulosis is also unusual in Japan, however, where the population continues to eat a diet high in fiber.

The mechanism of development of diverticula in response to a diet low in fiber is unknown. One hypothesis states that when circular muscular contractions occur in patients with small amounts of stool in their colons, which occurs in patients with diets low in fiber, the colonic lumen can be totally occluded. When two such occluding contractions occur close together, the lumen of the intervening segment of colon is isolated, and high pressure is generated in that segment. Theoretically, increased pressure results in the formation of diverticula by placing increased tension on the colonic wall. In some patients, there also appears to be a decrease in tensile strength of the colon wall. Pressure–volume curves in patients with diverticulosis demonstrate decreased colon wall tension compared with controls. The combination of colonic segmentation and decreased wall tension may be more important than either factor in isolation.

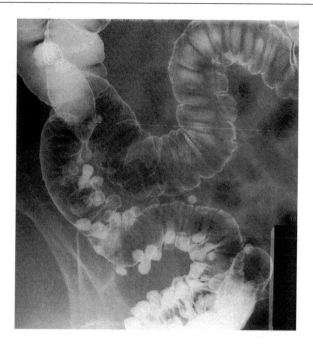

Fig. 2. Barium enema demonstrating multiple colonic diverticula.

4. CLINICAL PRESENTATION AND DIFFERENTIAL DIAGNOSES

4.1. Diverticulosis

Noninflamed colonic diverticula are not well accepted as a cause of abdominal pain or discomfort. In patients with abdominal pain and evidence of noninflamed diverticula on barium enema, the diverticula are not usually the cause of symptoms (Fig. 2). A more plausible explanation for the pain that occurs in patients with diverticula is the excessive pressure exerted by segmentation of the colon. Although diverticulosis should be considered in the differential diagnosis of a patient with intermittent mild to moderate lower abdominal pain, other diagnoses that should be eliminated include chronic constipation, diverticulitis, irritable bowel syndrome, and adenocarcinoma of the colon. Irritable bowel syndrome is thought, by some, to be a prediverticular condition and is a diagnosis made by exclusion.

4.2. Diverticulitis

Symptoms of diverticulitis are fever, bloating, obstipation, lower abdominal pain, and lower abdominal tenderness. A lower abdominal mass, tachycardia, and an elevated white blood cell count with a left shift are frequently seen. Depending on the precise location of the inflammation and whether there is free abdominal perforation, abdominal pain and tenderness can vary markedly. With free perforation and generalized peritonitis, it is often difficult to differentiate diverticulitis from other causes of perforated viscus. Suspicion of diverticulitis is heightened when the process is localized to the left lower quadrant and there is a palpable, tender mass. The differential diagnosis for diverticulitis includes perforated colon cancer, acute appendicitis, perforated peptic ulcer, acute-onset ulcerative colitis, acute-onset Crohn's colitis, and ischemic colitis

Perforated sigmoid colon cancer is often difficult to differentiate from diverticulitis. Patient histories are frequently similar with vague poorly defined lower abdominal pain and a tender left lower quadrant mass. Although helpful, colonoscopy is not always diagnostic. The inflammation that results from the perforation can make it difficult to pass a colonoscope through the involved area, and it may be impossible to visualize the mucosa. Therefore, if carcinoma cannot be eliminated preoperatively, a thorough examination must be performed intraoperatively. If adenocarcinoma of the colon can not be absolutely eliminated as a possible diagnosis, then a cancer operation must be performed. Computed tomography (CT) evidence of pericolic lymph nodes in patients suspected of having diverticulitis should raise the suspicion of underlying colonic cancer (6). The patient's history is usually helpful in differentiating appendicitis from diverticulitis, unless the diverticula are right sided in origin, and then a CT scan can be very helpful in differentiating between the two diagnoses. Inflammatory bowel disease and ischemic colitis can be diagnosed by flexible sigmoidoscopy. For ulcerative colitis or Crohn's disease, the patient's history usually includes a history of inflammatory bowel disease, but when the onset is acute, diverticulitis may be difficult to distinguish from inflammatory bowel disease. Caution should be exercised in diagnosing Crohn's disease in the presence of diverticular disease (7).

4.3. Hemorrhage

Hemorrhage can occur with either diverticulosis or diverticulitis, although massive bleeding is more typically associated with diverticulosis (Fig. 3A, B). It is important to distinguish hemorrhage as a complication of diverticulosis from colonic angiodysplasia (8). Patients who bleed from angiodysplasia and diverticulosis are usually asymptomatic before the hemorrhage, and in both cases, the blood loss can be massive. Patients who develop massive bleeding secondary to inflammatory bowel disease usually have a history of colitis. Occasionally, a patient with colitis presents with a fulminant course and no history of the disease. Ischemic colitis is usually accompanied by a history of abdominal pain, diarrhea, and vascular occlusive disease in other areas. The differential diagnosis of lower gastrointestinal bleeding must always include the various causes of massive upper gastrointestinal bleeding.

4.4. Obstruction

Diverticulitis and its complications account for about 13% of all cases of large bowel obstruction. The relatively high incidence (7%) of adenocarcinoma in patients with sigmoid diverticular disease, and the relative difficulty of making the diagnosis of adenocarcinoma of the colon when a large phlegmonous mass is present, is a significant problem in evaluating patients with sigmoid colon obstruction (6). Colonoscopy is helpful only when the endoscope can pass beyond the area of obstruction and biopsy specimens can be obtained.

5. DIAGNOSIS AND THERAPY

5.1. Diverticulosis

Patients who present with a combination of chronic intermittent lower abdominal pain and diverticula on barium enema should initially be treated nonoperatively. The diverticula are not considered to be the cause of the pain, and surgical therapy is not indicated. Colectomy is generally reserved for treatment of complications of diverticular disease.

Population studies have demonstrated that diverticula can be prevented by consuming a diet high in fiber, and such a diet has been widely prescribed for the treatment of symptomatic diverticulosis. Vegetarians have a lower incidence of diverticulosis than nonvegetarians. No study, however, has shown that a diet high in fiber prevents the complications of diverticulosis. Likewise, the efficacy of fiber supplements or bulk laxatives to treat the pain associated with

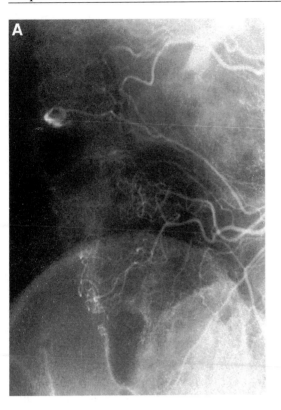
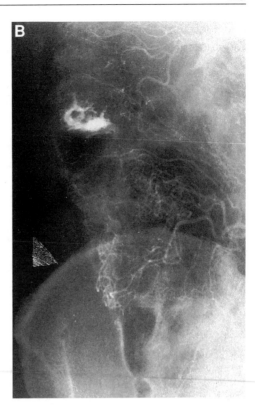

Fig. 3. Superior mesenteric arteriogram in a patient with bleeding from a right colon diverticulum. (A) Early roentgenogram with contrast material outlining the diverticulum (arrow). (B) Late roentgenogram demonstrating overflow of contrast material into the colonic lumen. [Reprinted with permission from ref. *27*.]

diverticula is controversial. Studies have demonstrated that an increase in dietary fiber can improve symptoms related to constipation and that may explain the improvement in pain with a diet high in fiber.

Diverticular hemorrhage should be treated surgically depending on its risk of recurrence. In over 70% of patients with diverticular hemorrhage, bleeding stops spontaneously, and 75% of these patients do not have recurrent bleeding. In the 25% of patients whose bleeding recurs, even if the bleeding is managed successfully by nonoperative means, segmental colectomy should be performed, because most of these patients have subsequent hemorrhage.

Angiodysplasia of the right colon is a more common cause of massive lower gastrointestinal bleeding than previously appreciated. In one study, half the patients with angiodysplasia had diverticula, which is not surprising, because both diseases occur predominately in the elderly. All of the bleeding angiodysplastic lesions were in the right colon, which may explain why massive colonic hemorrhage tends to be right-sided in origin.

Before an operative resection is undertaken it is important that the precise source of the bleeding be identified since it may not be a left colon diverticula and instead be a right colon angiodysplasia. In that circumstance a left colectomy would not resect the area of hemorrhage. Colonoscopy and tagged red blood cell scans may not be routinely helpful in identifying the precise source of the hemorrhage. The best study is an arteriogram. Once the area of hemorrhage is identified, an appropriate resection can be performed. If the area of hemorrhage can not be identified, an abdominal colectomy and ileostomy should be performed. When the patient has completely recovered, the ileostomy can be taken down and ileorectostomy performed.

5.2. Diverticulitis

Diverticulitis is a complication of diverticulosis, but the exact progression from one entity to the other is not entirely clear. One theory is that diverticulitis occurs when feces are impacted in a diverticulum causing obstruction of the neck of the diverticulum or abrasion of the thin-walled diverticulum. This can progress to infection. Another theory states that microperforation occurs as a result of increased intraluminal pressure, leading to spillage of colonic contents. Either event could result in infection of the surrounding pericolic tissues or free perforation. The process, once initiated, can result in a self-limiting infection with no or minimal clinical symptoms or cause progression to clinically significant infection, requiring hospitalization and surgical intervention. When the infection is progressive, other complications can occur.

If a clinical diagnosis of mild diverticulitis is made, therapy should be initiated immediately. Treatment for mild distress in a patient tolerating oral hydration should include 7–10 d of outpatient oral broad-spectrum antimicrobral therapy, which includes anaerobic coverage (e.g., trimethoprim–sulfamethoxazole or ciprofloxacin and metronidazole) (9,10). Most patients with an acute episode of diverticulitis severe enough to require hospitalization can be initially treated with intravenous fluids, bowel rest, broad-spectrum antibiotics, and analgesics. Older studies suggest that morphine sulfate should be avoided, since it increases intracolonic pressure (11). Meperidine may be more appropriate, since it does not increase intracolonic pressure (12). Signs and symptoms of severe diverticulitis include fever, tachycardia, leukocytosis with increased percentage of neutrophils, abdominal pain (usually in the left lower quadrant) severe enough to require analgesics, abdominal tenderness, and a lower abdominal fullness or mass.

If nausea, vomiting, or abdominal distention develops, nasogastric suction should be instituted. The patient should be reexamined frequently for progression of disease. If, despite therapy, the patient does not improve within 24 h or he or she gets worse, complications of diverticulitis probably exist, and further therapy is necessary. There is some controversy regarding patients under the age of 35 yr with diverticulitis. Some authors have suggested that these patients should undergo elective surgical resection because of the recurrent nature and frequency of serious complications. Others suggest that the increased frequency of complications and surgery is secondary to delay or inaccurate diagnosis, and not because of an increased severity of disease in younger patients (9,13).

Only about 20% of patients develop complications with their first episode of diverticulitis; this rises to 60% with recurrent episodes. Although a water-soluble contrast enema radiograph frequently provides the diagnosis of diverticulitis (Fig. 4), CT has become the preferred diagnostic test in patients who do not improve within 24 h, who are assumed to have a complication of diverticulitis (Fig. 5). CT scanning is the safest and most cost-effective method and has the additional potential benefit of allowing percutaneous drainage for the treatment of an abscess (9).

Radiologically guided percutaneous drainage has been recommended as the initial therapeutic maneuver in patients with diverticular abscesses greater than 5 cm in diameter. Most small abscesses will regress with antibiotics and do not require radiologic drainage unless the patient does not improve or deteriorates. After CT drainage of an abscess, more than 50% of patients undergo a successful one-stage procedure of segmental colectomy and primary anastomosis at a later date (14). If percutaneous drainage is not feasible, or an abscess is not identified, surgical intervention is recommended.

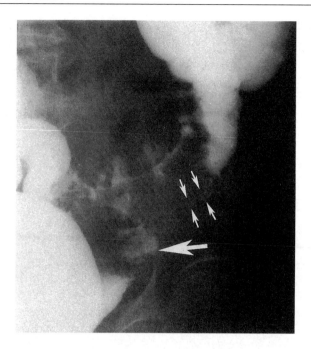

Fig. 4. Barium enema examination of the sigmoid colon with signs of diverticulitis. There is colonic narrowing, intramural tracking (small arrows), and an abscess inferior to the sigmoid colon (large arrow). [Reprinted with permission from ref. *27*.]

At the time of exploratory laparotomy, if the disease is localized, a segmental colectomy should be performed. The distal extent of the resection should always extend to the proximal rectum to decrease the chance of recurrence. The proximal extent of resection should include the segment involved with the acute disease plus any additional colon with signs of chronic disease as manifested by colonic thickening. With this approach, the recurrence rate after surgical resection is less than 10%. The only absolute contraindications to primary anastomosis are free perforation with generalized peritonitis, obstruction with unprepared bowel, and intraoperative conditions that do not warrant primary anastomosis, such as septic shock, ureteral injury, and other medical conditions that make a prolonged operation inadvisable. If resection is thought to be unsafe in the presence of a massive phlegmon or the patient is too unstable to undergo a resection, a diverting end colostomy with mucous fistula and drainage may be appropriate, with planned colonic resection at a later date after inflammation subsides. This approach is seldom necessary, however, and most patients can undergo resection of the diseased segment of bowel at the initial operation. Patients who do not have the involved segment resected do not do as well and have increased complications and mortality. Current trends suggest that laparoscopic resection of the diseased sigmoid colon may be possible (*15–18*). The laparoscopic approach has primarily been utilized for elective operations, however the conversion rate to an open procedure is high (ranging from 10–53%).

Most patients improve on a regimen of intravenous fluids, bowel rest, and broad-spectrum antibiotics, and emergency surgery is not necessary. Intravenous antibiotics should be continued for 7–10 d, and intravenous fluids and bowel rest should be continued until colonic function has normalized. A contrast enema should be performed subsequently to confirm the presumed diagnosis and to evaluate the extent of disease. If there is minimal disease and no sign of

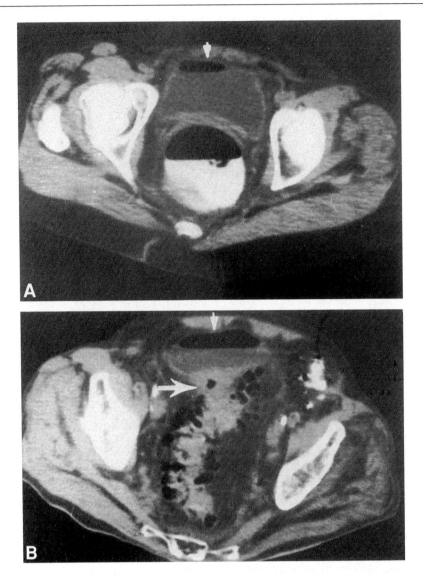

Fig. 5. (A) CT scan demonstrating air in the urinary bladder (arrow) in the presence of a colovesical fistula secondary to diverticulitis. (B) Air in the urinary bladder (small arrow) in association with a paravesical inflammatory mass (large arrow). [Reprinted with permission from ref. *28.*]

obstruction, fistula formation, or abscess, the patient can be discharged and followed as an outpatient. If any of these complications are present, a segmental resection should be performed before discharging the patient. After a second episode of diverticulitis, a resection should be performed, because the risk of further episodes of diverticulitis increases with each episode.

5.3. Obstruction

Patients who have experienced one or more episodes of diverticulitis can develop a fibrotic colonic stricture and partial large bowel obstruction. As stated earlier, when obstruction is diagnosed, it is important to differentiate between diverticulitis and colon carcinoma. Water-soluble contrast radiographs of the colon should be obtained to define completeness of obstruction. All patients should undergo sigmoidoscopy or colonoscopy to attempt biopsy of any masses. The extent of the workup depends on the condition of the patient and the completeness of the obstruction. Patients with an incomplete obstruction should be given a thorough but rapid preoperative evaluation in an attempt to secure a diagnosis. Because patients with complete obstructions require urgent operation, it is not always feasible to complete all tests before surgery.

If the obstruction is partial, complete preoperative bowel preparation should be carried out, including oral antibiotics. Patients with high-grade colonic obstruction do not tolerate rapid bowel preparation with laxatives or polyethylene glycol. Such patients should be prepared slowly, with extra time allowed for completion of the bowel cleansing. Once bowel preparation is complete, the patient with incomplete obstruction can undergo one-stage resection and primary anastomosis. Some authors have suggested that intraoperative colonic lavage may be a safe method for accomplishing single stage resection of the colon in selected patients with diverticulitis who require an urgent operation (19). This technique involves occlusion of the bowel lumen proximal to the pathologic process. Sterile corrugated plastic tubing is inserted through a colotomy proximal to the occlusion and secured. The distal end of the tubing is passed off the field. The cecum is cannulated through the stump of the appendix and the colon is lavaged with warm saline until the effluent is clear. The rectum is irrigated through a proctoscope to clear the remaining fecal material. Following resection of the pathologic process, a primary anastomosis is performed (20,21). This technique is most safely utilized for patients with bleeding or obstruction, rather than infectious complications of diverticulitis. Only 35–75% of patients who undergo colostomy for diverticular disease go on to have colostomy closure, because of the morbidity or the debilitated condition of many of these patients (9). In spite of this, a staged procedure is virtually mandated in the presence of generalized peritonitis. Unless colon carcinoma has been eliminated as a possible diagnosis, a cancer operation should be performed under all circumstances.

A diverting colostomy should be performed to relieve the obstruction in the patient with complete obstruction who cannot undergo bowel preparation. Resection of the diseased, obstructed segment of bowel can be performed during this operation or can be delayed until additional workup is complete. The evaluation to differentiate between carcinoma and diverticular diseases should be completed after the patient has recovered from the initial surgery.

When the patient has recovered from the first operation, which usually takes at least 1 mo, the next procedure may be performed. The second operation can be resection of the colostomy and the diseased segment of colon and reestablishment of bowel continuity by colorectostomy. When the diseased segment of bowel was removed during the first operation, the second procedure is a colostomy closure.

5.4. Fistula Formation

The development of fistulas from the diseased colon to other viscera or to skin may complicate diverticular disease. Colovesical fistulas account for about half of fistulas secondary to diverticulitis. Most patients with colovesical fistulas present with urinary tract symptoms, including urgency, dysuria, pneumaturia, and fecaluria. Despite what in retrospect often appear to be obvious symptoms, the diagnosis of colovesical fistula can be difficult to establish conclusively. Recurrent urinary tract infections in an elderly man should increase suspicion. Barium enema usually demonstrates diverticula and occasionally shows sigmoid narrowing. Only rarely does the fistulous tract actually fill. Cystoscopy demonstrates hyperemia and inflammation consistent with chronic cystitis, but the fistulous opening is seldom seen. CT scan with rectal contrast material has emerged as the most sensitive test for the presence of a colovesical fistula. In over 90% of patients, air is in the urinary bladder, and an indurated segment of sigmoid colon is observed adjacent to a locally thickened bladder wall *(22)*. In addition, after the rectal administration of barium, the patient's urine sediment should be checked for barium by radiograph of a spun urine sample. The presence of barium in the urine is further confirmation of a colovesical fistula.

Most patients with colovesical fistulas are treated effectively with a one-stage procedure consisting of segmental colectomy and closure of the fistulous opening in the bladder, although closure is not routinely necessary. The proximal margin of resection should include the segment of thickened, contracted colon, and any additional colon that is involved in the acute inflammation. As stated earlier, although it is not necessary to resect all the colon involved with diverticulosis, the resection should include sufficient colon to allow the anastomosis to be performed in an area of colon relatively free of diverticula. The distal resection margin should be the proximal rectum. If the fistulous opening is not identifiable, indicating that it is small in diameter, nothing needs to be done to identify the bladder opening. Urinary catheter drainage for 7–10 d, followed by cystographic verification of closure of the fistula, is sufficient therapy. Depending on the severity of the related complications of diverticulitis (obstruction, inflammation, abscess, sepsis, other fistulas), it may occasionally be necessary to perform a two-stage procedure, the first stage being segmental colectomy and colostomy formation, and the second stage consisting of closure of the colostomy. Either the one- or two-stage procedure can be done with low morbidity and mortality and with less than a 5% recurrence rate. The three-stage approach of diverting colostomy, then resection, and finally colostomy closure is not recommended, because the inflammatory process and the fistula are not removed at the first operation, leaving potential sources of sepsis.

Although rare in the past, recent reports indicate an increase in the occurrence of colovaginal fistulas. Almost all women with colovaginal fistulas have previously undergone a hysterectomy. The only consistent symptom is feculent vaginal discharge. About 40% of patients have intermittent abdominal pain and distention. A mass may be felt on pelvic examination; on vaginal speculum examination, the fistula opening is visible in 85% of cases. The diagnosis is confirmed in 50% of cases by barium enema. Vaginal contrast studies may also be helpful.

Unless other complications of diverticulitis are present, a one-stage procedure is appropriate. The involved colon is resected and a primary anastomosis performed. The vaginal defect is closed if this can be easily accomplished, but such a defect usually closes spontaneously.

Diarrhea, abdominal pain, and constitutional symptoms are frequently observed in patients with diverticular coloenteric fistulas. The usual signs of coloenteric fistula are abdominal tenderness, abdominal distention, and pelvic mass. Barium enema is diagnostic in 40–100% of patients. The preferred operative management of an uncomplicated coloenteric fistula is en bloc resection of the involved segment of small intestine, the fistula, and the diseased segment of colon. Primary anastomoses of both the small intestine and colon are then performed. If there are complicating factors, such as other fistulas, intra-abdominal abscess, or inadequate bowel preparation secondary to obstruction, primary anastomosis of the small intestine, combined with colostomy formation, is performed as the first stage of a two-stage procedure.

6. DIVERTICULITIS OF THE CECUM AND ASCENDING COLON

The actual incidence of right-sided diverticula is not known; estimates based on barium enema examinations are between 5 and 10% *(2)*. The incidence of true diverticula is higher in the cecum and ascending colon than in the remainder of the colon, but false diverticula still predominate. True diverticula tend to be solitary and to originate in the anterior cecum close to the ileocecal valve. They occur in only 1–2% of the population. Most are asymptomatic, and the diagnosis is usually made by pathologic examination. Of people with left-sided diverticulosis, 7–30% of them will also have right-sided diverticula (23). In a study of over 250 patients with right colonic diverticulitis, 81% had a solitary diverticulum, while 19% had multiple diverticula (24). There is an increased incidence of right colonic diverticula and diverticulitis and a lower than expected incidence of left-sided diverticulitis in the Asian population (25).

When patients with right-sided diverticula develop diverticulitis, the symptom complex is similar to that in acute appendicitis, and misdiagnosis is frequent (24,26). Patients with right-sided diverticulitis are generally younger than patients with left-sided disease and are older than most patients with appendicitis (26). Patients with right-sided diverticulitis are usually in their late 30s or 40s, whereas patients with left-sided diverticulitis are usually more than 50 yr of age (26). Patients with right-sided diverticulitis have a longer duration of illness than patients with appendicitis, infrequently vomit, and feel pain initially in the right lower quadrant rather than the middle abdomen. Despite these dissimilarities, misdiagnosis of acute appendicitis is made in over 60% of patients who are later found to have right-sided diverticulitis (24,26). In only 20% of cases is the correct diagnosis made preoperatively. CT scanning may improve diagnosis of right-sided diverticulitis. CT findings include thickening of the colonic wall, extraluminal mass involving the cecum or ascending colon, and signs of pericolic inflammation. CT scanning is recommended in patients with atypical appendicitis who are elderly and in whom right-sided diverticulitis is being considered as a diagnosis. Barium enema examination is seldom helpful because many patients have a single diverticulum that is not visible on barium examination. Associated findings, such as compression of the colon, are nonspecific and usually nondiagnostic.

At the time of surgical intervention, it may be difficult to establish a diagnosis of diverticulitis of the cecum or ascending colon. Most series report a correct intraoperative diagnosis in fewer than 60% of cases (26). The presence of an intact, normal appendix eliminates appendicitis as the diagnosis in almost all circumstances. Usually, a large inflammatory mass involves the cecum and ascending colon. In many cases, however, it is difficult to distinguish the mass from a perforated carcinoma, and a right hemicolectomy should be performed. If the resection can be accomplished without contamination of the peritoneal cavity, and a mechanical bowel preparation had been accomplished preoperatively, a primary anastomosis is acceptable. If there is spillage of abscess contents or bowel preparation was not feasible, an end ileostomy and mucous fistula can be performed. When the only abnormality noted at laparotomy is an inflamed diverticulum, a few authors propose leaving the diverticulum in situ and treating the patient with broad-spectrum antibiotics. If this therapy is undertaken, an appendectomy should be performed to avoid confusion if right lower quadrant symptoms recur. Most patients treated in this manner do well and do not develop recurrent diverticulitis.

If the diagnosis of right-sided diverticulitis is made before operation, the patient should be treated as with sigmoid diverticulitis. If improvement is noted with intravenous fluids, broad-spectrum antibiotics, bowel rest, and analgesics, therapy should be continued, and further testing performed when the patient recovers. If the patient does not improve or deteriorates, laparotomy is performed.

7. GIANT COLONIC DIVERTICULUM

Giant diverticula usually occur in the sigmoid colon, although they have been described in other areas of the left colon. Giant diverticula almost always arise from the antimesenteric border of the colon, unlike most left-sided diverticula, which develop where the vascular supply passes through the muscularis externa. Most are gas filled, and therefore, visible on plain abdominal radiographs. They range in size from 3–35 cm.

The pathogenesis of giant diverticula is not understood; they are assumed to be a complication of diverticulosis and not a separate entity. The most widely accepted explanation is that inflammation of a diverticulum causes narrowing of its neck and results in a ball-valve mechanism that entraps gases.

The predominant symptoms are abdominal pain, bloating, nausea, vomiting, and diarrhea. Physical findings include abdominal tenderness and a movable lower abdominal mass. Perforation causes diffuse abdominal pain, leukocytosis, fever, and signs of localized or generalized peritonitis. Although the diagnosis can be suspected based on plain radiographs of the abdomen, barium enema or CT scanning confirms the diagnosis. On barium enema, diverticula fill with barium in 50–70% of cases, and frequently, other diverticula are demonstrated. CT scanning of giant diverticula performed with intraluminal contrast usually demonstrates apposition of the colon and the giant diverticulum, as well as the presence of barium in the diverticulum. On CT scan, wall thickness is variable and has not proved to be diagnostic.

Giant colonic diverticula are managed surgically. The patient should undergo standard mechanical bowel preparation, including oral antibiotics. The diverticulum, along with the adjacent colon, should be resected in continuity. Bowel continuity can usually be restored by end-to-end primary anastomosis.

REFERENCES

1. Hinchey EJ, Schaal PGH, Richards GK. Treatment of perforated diverticular disease of the colon. *Adv. Surg.*, **12** (1978) 85–109.
2. Hughes LE. Postmortem survey of diverticular disease of the colon. *Gut*, **10** (1969) 336–344.
3. Slack WW. The anatomy, pathology and some clinical features of diverticulitis of the colon. *Br. J. Surg.*, **50** (1962) 185–190.
4. Spriggs EI, Marxer OA. Intestinal diverticula. *Q. J. Med.*, **19** (1925) 1.
5. Mendeloff AI. Thoughts on the epidemiology of diverticular disease. *Clin. Gastroenterol.*, **15** (1986) 855–877.
6. Chintapalli KN, Esola CC, Chopra S, Ghiatas AA, Dodd GC, 3rd. Pericolic mesenteric lymph nodes: An aid in distinguishing diverticulitis from cancer of the colon. *Am. J. Roentgenol.*, **169** (1997) 1253–1255.
7. Gledhill A, Dixon MF. Crohn's-like reaction in diverticular disease. *Gut*, **42** (1998) 392–395.
8. Welch CE, Athanasoulis CA, Galdabini JJ. Hemorrhage from the large bowel with special reference to angiodysplasia and diverticular disease. *World J. Surg.*, **2** (1978) 73–83.
9. Ferzoco LB, Raptopoulos V, Silen W. Acute Diverticulitis. *N. Engl. J. Med.*, **338** (1998) 1521–1526.
10. Freeman SR, McNally PR. Diverticulitis. *Med. Clin. N. Am.*, **77** (1993) 1149–1167.
11. Painter NS, Truelove SC. The intraluminal pressure in diverticulosis of the colon. *Gut*, **5** (1964) 201–213.
12. Arfwidsson S. Pathogenesis of multiple diverticula of the sigmoid colon in diverticular disease. *Acta Chir. Scand. Suppl.*, **342** (1964) 1–68.
13. Spivak H, Weinrauch S, Harvey JC, Surick B, Ferstenberg H, Friedman I. Acute colonic diverticulitis in the young. *Dis. Colon Rectum*, **49** (1997) 570–574.
14. Stabile BE, Puccio E, Van Sonnenberg E, Neff CC. Preoperative percutaneous drainage of diverticular abscesses. *Am. J. Surg.*, **159** (1990) 99–104.
15. Memon MA, Fitztgibbons RJ. The role of minimal access surgery in the acute abdomen. *Surg. Clin. N. Am.*, **77** (1997) 1333–1353.
16. Bruce CJ, Coller JA, Murray JJ, Schoetz DJ, JR, Roberts PL, Rusin, LC. Laparoscopic resection for diverticular disease. *Dis. Colon Rectum*, **39(Suppl)** (1996) S1–6.
17. Eijsbouts QA, Cuesta MA, deBrauw LM, Siestses C. Elective laparoscopic-assisted sigmoid resection for diverticular disease. *Surg. Endosc.*, **11** (1997) 750–753.
18. Sher ME, Agachan F, Bortul M, Nogueras JJ, Weiss EG, Wexner SD. Laparoscopic surgery for diverticulitis. *Surg. Endosc.*, **11** (1997) 264–267.
19. Lee EC, Murray JJ, Coller JA, Roberts PL, Schoetz DJ, Jr. Intraoperative colonic lavage in nonelective surgery for diverticular disease. *Dis. Colon Rectum*, **40** (1997) 669–674.
20. Murray JJ, Schoetz DJ, Coller JA, Roberts PL, Veidenheimer MC. Intraoperative colonic lavage and primary anastomosis in nonelective colon resection. *Dis. Colon Rectum*, **34** (1991) 527–531.
21. Scott HJ, Lane IF, Glynn MJ. Colonic hemorrhage: a technique for rapid intraoperative bowel preparation and colonoscopy. *Br. J. Surg.*, **73** (1986) 390–391.

22. Woods RJ, Lavery IC, Fazio VW, jagelman DG, Weakley FL. Internal fistulas in diverticular disease. *Dis. Colon Rectum*, **31** (1988) 591–596.

23. Beranbaum SL, Zausner J, Lane B. Diverticular disease of the right colon. *Radiology*, **115** (1972) 334–348.

24. Graham SM, Ballantyne GH. Cecal diverticulitis: a review of the American experience. *Dis. Colon Rectum*, **30** (1987) 821–826.

25. Katz DS, Lane MJ, Ross BA, Gold BM, Jeffrey RB, Jr, Mindelzun RE. Diverticulitis of the right colon revisited. *Am. J. Roentgenol.*, **171** (1998) 151–156.

26. Gouge TH, Coppa GF, Eng K, Ranson JH, Localio SA. Management of diverticulitis of the ascending colon: 10 years' experience. *Am. J. Surg.*, **145** (1983) 387–391.

27. Otterson MF, Telford GT. Diverticular Disease. In *Surgery: Scientific Principles and Practice*. 3rd ed., Greenfield LJ, Mulholland MW, Oldham KT, Zelenock GB,Lillemoe KD (eds.), Lippincott-Raven, Philadelphia, PA, 2001, pp. 1137–1140.

28. Sarr MG, Fishman EK, Goldman SM. Enterovesical fistula. *Surg. Gynecol. Obstet.*, **164** (1987) 41–48.

26 Current Understanding of Colorectal Neoplasia

Melanie B. Thomas and Robert A. Wolff

CONTENTS

1. INTRODUCTION

Colorectal cancer is the second most common cause of cancer-related death in the United States. For the year 2000, an estimated 130,200 new cases will be diagnosed (93,800 colon cancers and 36,400 rectal cancers) with 56,300 deaths expected in that year. Colorectal cancer accounts for 11% of all cancer deaths in the United States (Surveillance, Epidemiology, and End Results [SEER] 2000 data, see Website: www.seer.cancer.gov). Of note, incidence rates declined by 2.1% between 1992 and 1996, and recent data suggest that mortality rates for colorectal cancer may also be declining. These trends may be attributable to increased screening efforts, "prophylactic polypectomy," and improved adjuvant therapies and should bolster even greater efforts in detection, prevention, and treatment.

Over the past several years, investigators have made important discoveries in genetics and carcinogenesis, in screening and prevention, and in anticancer therapy, which may reduce the overall incidence and mortality of this disease. This chapter reviews our current understanding of colorectal cancer, describing the known genetic mutations and risk factors, as well as the available and emerging screening, prevention, and therapeutic strategies.

2. EPIDEMIOLOGY AND ETIOLOGY OF COLORECTAL NEOPLASIA

2.1. Geographic Distribution

Colorectal cancer is more common in Western industrialized countries (i.e., United States, Canada, Scandinavia, northern and western Europe, New Zealand) than in Asia, most of South

From: *Colonic Diseases*
Edited by: T. R. Koch © Humana Press Inc., Totowa, NJ

America, and in the black populations of Africa. Since 1978, the mortality rate for colon cancer has declined in some western European countries and in the United States, while the incidence and mortality rates for colorectal cancer have increased in Japan and China. Individuals who migrate from low-incidence regions assume the colon cancer risk of their adopted country, implicating interplay of environmental and genetic factors in the development of this disease. The age-specific incidence of colorectal cancer in the United States rises steadily, with more than 90% of cases diagnosed in patients 50 yr or older. The male:female ratio for colon cancer is 1.34 and 1.73 for rectal carcinoma (1).

2.2. Carcinogenesis

Results from Vogelstein's group (2), which were clinically verified by the National Polyp Study (3), suggest that colorectal neoplasia begins with an accumulation of genetic mutations ultimately leading to transformation of normal epithelium to dysplastic and malignant epithelium. Early mutations have included deletions in the tumor suppressor gene, APC, (which may be inherited or acquired) located on the long arm chromosome 5, and mutations in the K-ras oncogene. Later genetic events include deletions in a gene on 18q, the deleted in colon cancer mutation (DCC), and mutation of the tumor suppressor gene p53, on chromosome 17. The latter two events have been implicated in malignant transformation of colonic epithelium. Genetic mutations that occur in inherited colon cancer include those of the APC gene, and a variety of DNA mismatch repair enzymes. These genetic mutations eventually lead to phenotypic alterations in the colonic epithelium and are associated with the development of early, intermediate, and late adenomas that progress to invasive carcinoma with eventual metastases (4).

2.3. Risk Factors

General risk factors for the development of colorectal cancer include genetic predisposition, acquired risks, and environmental factors. These factors are involved in a complex interplay that leads to a stepwise progression from normal colonic mucosa to adenomatous polyps to invasive cancer. The neoplastic process often develops in individuals who have acquired or inherited genetic mutations and may be further promoted by environmental, dietary, or other factors.

A personal or family history of colorectal cancer or polyps, older age, and inflammatory bowel disease (IBD) have all been associated with an increased risk of colorectal cancer. Other possible risk factors include a sedentary lifestyle and a diet high in fat, low in dietary fiber, or deficient in specific micronutrients. Cigarette smoking has been implicated in the formation of colonic adenomas and carcinomas, with the relative risk correlating with total exposure and duration of smoking (5).

2.3.1. DIET

Some studies have shown that a "Western" diet rich in saturated fat is associated with an increased risk of colon cancer, whereas a diet that includes a high proportion of fruit and vegetables seems to protect against colorectal cancer (6). Dietary fat has been shown to promote tumors in animal models of colorectal cancer. A high-fat diet may alter the colonic flora, leading to a predominance of anaerobic species. Certain enzymes capable of metabolizing procarcinogens to overt carcinogens are present in higher concentrations in the large bowel. It should be noted that the role of dietary fat has not been firmly established, and some studies have failed to demonstrate that a high-fat diet is associated with an increased risk nor that a high-fiber diet offers a protective benefit (7).

Fiber may provide a protective effect by decreasing the concentration of fecal carcinogens and decreasing their transit time, thus reducing the period of exposure to colonic mucosa. Some

Table 1
Lifetime Risks of Colorectal Cancer

Characteristic	Incidence
General population	5%
Personal history of colorectal cancer	15–20%
IBD	15–40%
Adenomatous polyps: personal	Variable[a]
HNPCC	70–80%
FAP	>95%

[a]Adapted from ref.8.

studies have suggested that fresh fruits and vegetables are protective, although whether this effect is due to the fiber content or to the presence of other micronutrients and antioxidants remains unclear. Moreover, the protective benefit of fiber, micronutrients, or antioxidants has not been consistently demonstrated. A recent prospective study of 88,757 women, aged 34–59 yr, who participated in the Nurses Health Study begun in 1976 found no association between fiber intake (measured in g/d) and the risk of colorectal cancer during 16 yr of follow-up.

2.3.2. ADENOMATOUS POLYPS

Colorectal tumors occur more often among patients with adenomatous polyps than among patients without polyps. Carcinoma is present in 5% of adenomas, and in general, the risk correlates with the histology and the size of the polyp. The potential for malignant transformation is 8–10 times higher for villous and tubulovillous adenomas than for tubular adenomas. Just over 1% of adenomatous polyps <1 cm are malignant, whereas up to 40% of adenomas >2 cm are malignant (1).

Whether the presence of simple hyperplastic polyps represents a risk for development of colorectal cancer has recently been disputed. Historically, researchers believed that the presence of these benign lesions did not represent any added risk for developing colorectal cancer. However, a recent study in which proximal adenomas were found in patients with distal hyperplastic polyps questions this assumption (8).

2.3.3. INFLAMMATORY BOWEL DISEASE

Patients with IBD (ulcerative colitis or Crohn's disease) are at increased risk of developing colorectal carcinoma. For patients with ulcerative colitis, the risk of colorectal cancer correlates with the duration of active disease, extent of colitis, development of mucosal dysplasia, and duration of symptoms. The risk for colon cancer is also higher among patients with Crohn's disease than among the general population, although to a lesser extent than among those with ulcerative colitis.

2.3.4. FAMILIAL SYNDROMES

Table 1 lists the estimated risk of developing colorectal cancer attributable to various hereditary syndromes. Most of the genetic abnormalities associated with the development of colorectal cancer involve deletion of fragments of chromosomes, a phenomenon known as allelic loss or loss of heterozygosity (LOH), or errors in DNA mismatch repair. The following molecular markers are associated with particularly aggressive colorectal cancer: loss of expression of the *DCC* gene, *p11*, *p27*, or *p53*, or overexpression of thymidylate synthase (TS), *ki67*, or *bcl-2*. Researchers are actively investigating the effectiveness and practical value of incorporating these markers into screening for groups at high risk for colorectal cancer.

Sporadic colon cancers comprise approx 80% of all cases, with the remainder attributed to inherited syndromes. Familial adenomatous polyposis (FAP), Gardner's syndrome, and hereditary nonpolyposis colon cancer (HNPCC) are all inherited in an autosomal-dominant pattern; FAP and Gardner's syndrome represent <1% of familial colorectal cancer, while HNPCC accounts for 6–15% of cases *(4,9,10)*.

2.3.5. FAP

FAP results in a high penetrance of disease, whereby patients who inherit the genetic disorder are very likely to develop colon cancer. In individuals with FAP, thousands of adenomatous polyps grow throughout the colon and rectum, and some of these polyps invariably progress to cancer. Prophylactic resection of the entire colon and rectum should be performed, as the adenomatous polyps in patients with FAP are too numerous for endoscopic removal. The syndrome is caused by a mutation of *APC*, a tumor suppressor gene located at 5q21. When *APC* is mutated, the function of both *APC* alleles is lost: one defective allele is inherited as a mutated gene from a parent, and the other is mutated in individual colon cells in early childhood. The onset of malignancy in untreated patients occurs at an average age of 42 yr, therefore, invasive cancer develops 20–30 yr after the initiation of the polyposis. The polyps accumulate other mutations in oncogenes and tumor suppressor genes that convert benign adenomas to malignant tumors *(11)*. In cases of FAP, mutations in other tumor suppressor genes, such as *p53* and *DCC*, combined with the activation of protooncogenes, especially K-*ras*, occur sequentially in the neoplastic transformation of the bowel epithelium *(2)*.

2.3.6. HNPCC

The genetic penetrance of HNPCC, also known as Lynch's syndrome, is lower than that of FAP, but remains significant, ranging from 30–70% *(11)*. HNPCC consists of two clinical subgroups: Lynch I, which involves tumors of the large bowel only, and Lynch II, which includes carcinomas of the large bowel, endometrium, and ovaries *(12)*. Adenomas develop in persons with HNPCC at roughly the same rate as in the general population. However, an adenoma that develops in the colon or rectum of a patient with HNPCC rapidly progresses to carcinoma.

Patients with HNPCC do not have the *APC* gene mutation that characterizes FAP. Rather, HNPCC is caused by defects in DNA mismatch repair. DNA replication is often imperfect, and correct transmission of the genetic code relies on the ability of the cells' DNA mismatch repair system to correct the sequence. Several proteins participate in the repair process and are encoded by various genes, at least four of which are mutated in the germ line of patients with HNPCC, thereby causing the HNPCC syndromes *(11)*. Additional mutations involving tumor suppressor genes and oncogenes rapidly accumulate in these DNA repair-deficient cells, and as a result, a benign adenoma progresses to a malignant one in only 3–5 yr. Recently, mutations in the human homologues of the bacterial *muy*HLS gene complex (hMSH2, hMLH1, hPMS1, and hPMS2) were found to predispose to the development of HNPCC. Such mutations lead to genetic instability, which is reflected in errors in DNA replication (also known as replication errors or microsatellite instability) *(13,14)*.

3. SCREENING FOR COLORECTAL NEOPLASIA

3.1. General Considerations

As with screening tests for all types of diseases, the presence of such risk factors as genetic predisposition or such epidemiological factors as disease prevalence in a geographic area increases the sensitivity of a test. Researchers have, therefore, attempted to stratify populations in order to identify individuals who are at the greatest risk of developing colorectal cancer and

Table 2

Current Recommendations for Colorectal Cancer Screening[a]

Patient populations	Screening tests
General population and patient with any distant relative with colorectal cancer (CRC) or polyps.	FOBT annually and sigmoidoscopy every 3–5 yr or colonoscopy every 10 yr, beginning at age 50.
Patient with first-degree relative with CRC.	FOBT annually and sigmoidoscopy every 3–5 yr or colonoscopy every 10 yr. Begin at age 40.
Moderate risk patients[b].	Polyp removal; repeat colonsocopy at 3 yr; if normal, extend interval to 5 yr.
Patient with two first-degree relatives with CRC or patient with one first-degree relative with colorectal cancer diagnosed at 50 yr of age or younger.	Colonoscopy every 3–5 yr. Begin screening at age 40 or 10 yr younger than youngest affected relative.
Patient with HNPCC risk[c].	Colonoscopy every 2 yr, then yearly after age 40. Begin screening at age 25 or 10 yr younger than the youngest affected relative. Consider genetic counseling and testing.
Patient with FAP risk[c].	Sigmoidsocopy every 1 to 2 yr. Begin screening at age 12 yr. Genetic counseling and testing.
Patient with personal history of CRC.	Total colon examination (TCE) (ACBE or colonoscopy) within 1 yr after resection. Repeat at 3 yr if normal. Repeat at 5 yr if normal.
Patient with personal history of adenoma.	Polyp removal. Repeat at 3 yr. Repeat at 5 yr if normal.

[a]Adapted from refs. *19* and *60*.

[b]Moderate-risk patients are defined as those found to have adenomatous polyps, either villous or nonvillous, patients with a first-degree relative <60 yr of age, with a history of colorectal cancer or adenomas, or colorectal cancer in more than one first-degree relative of any age *(19)*. Individuals who have been previously diagnosed with early-stage colorectal cancer, that is those who underwent surgery with curative intent, should undergo follow-up colonoscopy or ACBE within 1 yr of diagnosis, then at 3 yr and if normal, every 5 yr thereafter.

[c]High-risk patients include those with a personal or family history of FAP, HNPCC, juvenile *Polyposis coli*, Peutz-Jeghers syndrome, or IBD of at least 8 yr duration.

who would benefit most from screening and surveillance. Numerous tests have been developed over the years to screen individuals at risk for colorectal cancer, and the subject of screening various populations continues to be studied and debated. The 5-yr survival rate of patients diagnosed with early-stage colorectal cancer is 90%, compared with less than 5% for patients diagnosed with stage IV disease. Presently, less than 40% of cases of colorectal cancer are discovered early *(15)*. It is, therefore, believed that increased detection of premalignant lesions and early-stage tumors will improve overall survival for patients with colorectal cancer. Current recommendations for colorectal cancer screening are listed in Table 2.

3.2. Detection Methods

3.2.1. FECAL OCCULT BLOOD TESTING

Of all of the screening modalities for colorectal cancer, fecal occult blood testing (FOBT) may be the most controversial. Although several large trials *(16–18)* have shown an increase in the percentage of early-stage colorectal cancers discovered, only one large, randomized trial has conclusively demonstrated that the use of FOBT decreased mortality *(17)*. The use of rehydrated slides resulted in a high percentage of patients undergoing unnecessary colonoscopy. In addition, workers have questioned the statistical ability of FOBT to detect colorectal cancers in a cost-effective manner. Nevertheless, the current recommendation of the American College of Physicians is that all individuals over age 40 yr undergo annual FOBT *(19)*.

3.2.2. SIGMOIDOSCOPY

The 60-cm flexible sigmoidoscope can be inserted as far as the descending colon. This instrument can visualize more of the colon than can be reached by the rigid sigmoidoscope or by digital rectal examination. Sigmoidoscopy does not require sedation and is relatively inexpensive. Since it is a very safe procedure, it can be performed by primary care physicians and may be suitable for screening large populations at low risk. However, this method is not appropriate for screening patients suspected to have HNPCC, in which approximately two-thirds of the lesions are right-sided. For patients in whom flexible sigmoidoscopy has detected adenomas in the distal colon, current practice dictates full colonoscopy. Importantly, recent studies show that the presence or absence of adenomas in the distal colon is not necessarily indicative of the presence of proximal lesions, and sigmoidoscopy may miss nearly 50% of all colonic lesions *(20)*. Most oncologists would agree that any adenomatous lesion in the distal colon or rectum warrants evaluation of the entire colon. Methods to assess the entire colon include air-contrast barium enemas (ACBE), colonoscopy, and the newer "virtual" radiographic colonoscopy.

3.2.3. ACBE

In some settings, high-quality ACBE plus flexible sigmoidoscopy may be substituted for full colonoscopy. The technique is limited by its lack of sensitivity for small polyps (<1 cm in diameter) and for areas within the rectosigmoid, hepatic, and splenic flexures, where large bowel loops may overlap making a single lumen difficult to identify. In addition, ACBE is unsuitable as a screening or surveillance technique for HNPCC, ulcerative colitis, or flat adenoma syndrome *(21)*.

3.2.4. COLONOSCOPY

Full visual examination of the rectum and colon to the level of the cecum is considered the gold standard for evaluating the colon for lesions, but the optimal surveillance interval for the general population or for patients with risk factors for colorectal cancer has not been established. Colonoscopy not only enables full visualization of the entire colon, but also allows for biopsy or removal of any suspicious lesions. Several recent studies suggest the increasing importance of colonoscopy in colorectal cancer screening. One study showed that more than half of all the advanced proximal neoplasms found in colonoscopic screening of a series of asymptomatic men aged 50–75 yr would have been missed if only the distal colon had been evaluated *(20)*. In another retrospective study, 1994 patients were examined to determine whether the size and histologic features of distal lesions are predictive of proximal lesions, as the identification of these factors would help determine who should undergo full colonoscopy after sigmoidoscopic screening *(8)*. The findings in the distal and proximal colon are shown in Table 3.

Of the 50 patients with advanced proximal neoplasia, no polyps were found in 23 patients (46%). Thus, the proximal neoplasms of these patients would not have been detected under the current practice of conducting full colon evaluation only in patients with distal findings. The

Table 3
Findings in the Distal and Proximal Colon in Cohort of 1994 Patients[a]

Finding	Distal colon		Proximal colon	
	No.	%	No.	%
No polyp	1564	78.4	1686	84.6
Hyperplastic polyp	201	10.1	72	3.6
Tubular adenoma	168	8.4	186	9.3
Advanced neoplasm	61	3.1	50	2.5

[a]Adapted from ref. 8.

study also found that a polyp of any size or type was associated with an increased risk of histologically advanced proximal neoplasia and that the magnitude of risk was proportional to the histologic features of the distal lesion.

3.2.5. GENETIC TESTING

DNA analysis of stool samples for mutations of K-*ras* and other genes is becoming more readily available, but its usefulness in the clinic has yet to be determined. Genetic testing for *APC* mutation and for HNPCC is being employed to identify carriers of FAP and HNPCC, respectively. However, as yet unidentified mutations are likely to be present in some families, and a negative test at one time does not assure that an individual is not at risk for colorectal cancer. Thus, whenever genetic testing is being considered for an individual, genetic counseling prior to and after testing is strongly recommended.

4. DIAGNOSTIC EVALUATION AND STAGING

4.1. Clinical Presentation

Among the malignancies that occur in the colon itself, 60–70% of sporadic colorectal cancers are left-sided, whereas inherited colon cancer syndromes occur mainly in the right colon (12,22). Commonly, left-sided colorectal cancer may lead to a change in bowel habits, with constipation, small caliber stool, fecal impaction, or obstructive symptoms. Right-sided lesions are often associated with vague abdominal pain and bloating, acute or chronic gastrointestinal blood loss, or bowel obstruction. Colonic lesions of any location can cause bleeding, as evidenced by melena, hematochezia, positive hemoccult testing, or iron-deficiency anemia. Of particular concern are weight loss, anorexia, and other constitutional symptoms, which may reflect the presence of metastatic disease. Any unexplained iron deficiency anemia should prompt an evaluation of the gastrointestinal tract.

4.2. Pathology

More than 95% of all colorectal malignancies are adenocarcinomas. The other small percentage consists of mucinous and signet-ring cell subtypes, which generally display atypical patterns of spread and confer a poorer prognosis. Tumors with neuroendocrine and carcinoid differentiation are uncommon, and their treatment differs from that of adenocarcinoma. Adenocarcinomas have been classified on the basis of histology as well-differentiated, moderately differentiated, poorly differentiated, and undifferentiated. However, while tumor grade may provide additional prognostic information, it is not typically used in treatment planning (1).

4.3. Preoperative Staging

In cases of colorectal cancer, it is important to conduct a thorough staging evaluation before any surgical intervention, as treatment options are guided largely by staging information. However, preoperative evaluation is not always possible, particularly in the setting of acute bowel obstruction. A complete history and physical examination should be performed in conjunction with full colonoscopy with biopsies. Laboratory evaluation should include a complete blood count with differential, electrolytes, liver function studies, a carcinoembryonic antigen (CEA) level, and blood urea nitrogen (BUN) and creatinine. Imaging studies should include routine posteroanterior and lateral chest radiographs, abdominal ultrasound, or preferably, computed tomography (CT) scans of the abdomen and pelvis. For patients undergoing flexible sigmoidoscopy with biopsy as their initial diagnostic procedure, full colonoscopy to the cecum is recommended to exclude synchronous primary tumors that may occur in 3 to 4% of patients with colorectal neoplasms. If full colonoscopy is precluded by the presence of an obstructing lesion or the need for emergent surgery, a total colon evaluation should be undertaken soon after surgical intervention.

Anatomic differences between the rectum and colon produce different patterns of spread and often prompt different treatment strategies. Rectal cancers have been variably defined as those tumors occurring below the sacral promontory, below the peritoneal reflection, or situated <12–15 cm from the anal verge (23). The rectum resides in a funnel below the pelvic brim and is circumscribed posteriorly by the sacrum, laterally by the pelvic sidewalls, and anteriorly by either the prostate gland or the posterior wall of the vagina. The rectum also rests below the peritoneal reflection. Therefore, while the proximal and distal margins of resection can be ascertained with some certainty, the anatomy creates challenges in establishing the radial margin of resection. Thus, rectal cancers recur locally more often than do colonic neoplasms. Complete clinical staging of rectal cancer is particularly important when patients are being considered for preoperative therapy.

Importantly, rectal carcinomas more commonly metastasize to the lungs by venous and lymphatic drainage via the retroperitoneum, whereas colon cancers typically spread hematogenously to the liver through the portal circulation. Both colon and rectal cancers typically invade in a stepwise fashion, first through the mucosa, submucosa, and muscularis propria, then to the perirectal or pericolonic lymph nodes, and subsequently to the more distant lymph node groups, the liver, and the lungs.

4.4. Pathologic Staging

In colorectal cancer, the tumor-node-metastasis (TNM) classification system (Table 4) has replaced the Dukes classification system. Staging is used to provide prognostic information and to guide recommendations for treatment, particularly the use of adjuvant chemotherapy and radiation.

5. THERAPEUTIC OPTIONS

5.1. Local and Regional Control

Most patients with colorectal cancer present at a stage at which all gross tumor can be resected. Nevertheless, almost half of all patients with colorectal adenocarcinoma die of metastatic disease, as a result of residual microscopic disease not evident at the time of surgery. If complete resection of all gross disease is achieved, risk for relapse can be estimated based on pathological staging. Patients identified to be at relatively high risk for relapse may then be considered for additional local therapy in the form of radiotherapy, systemic adjuvant chemotherapy, or both.

Table 4
TNM Staging of Colorectal Cancer[a]

TNM stage	Primary tumor	Lymph node metastasis	Distant metastasis
0	Tis[b]	N0	M0
I	T1	N0	M0
	T2	N0	M0
II	T3	N0	M0
	T4	N0	M0
IIIA	Any T	N1	M0
IIIB	Any T	N2, N3	M0
IV	Any T	Any M	N1

[a] Adapted from (61).
[b] Tis: T1, tumor invades submucosa; T2, tumor invades muscularis propria; T3, tumor invades through muscularis mucosa to subserosa or pericolic or perirectal tissues; T4, tumor perforates the visceral peritoneum or directly invades other organs. N1, metastases to 1–3 regional lymph nodes; N2, metastases in four or more regional lymph nodes; N3, metastases to any lymph node along a named vascular trunk.

5.1.1. Surgical Management of Colon Cancer

The primary management of localized colon cancer is surgery to remove the affected segment of bowel, the adjacent mesentery, and the draining lymph nodes. Right, left, or transverse hemicolectomy is performed for tumors located in these respective areas. Pathologic staging can be completed once the surgical specimen has been removed. Patients with stage IV disease detected on initial evaluation do not necessarily require resection unless there is a risk of bowel obstruction, bleeding, or other complications. Compared with laparotomy, laparoscopic colectomy may be associated with lower morbidity but disadvantages include the potential for inadequate nodal resection, longer operative time, inability to palpate intra-abdominal organs, and increased risk of tumor seeding of the abdomen during specimen removal (24).

5.1.2. Local Therapy for Rectal Cancer

Owing to the confined nature of the pelvis and difficulties in achieving clear tumor margins (proximal, distal, and radial) while preserving sphincter function, resection of rectal tumors is generally more challenging than that of colon primaries. An abdominoperineal resection (APR) involves removal of the anus and sphincter muscle and creation of a permanent colostomy; this procedure may be necessary if the tumor is located in the distal rectum or if other tumor characteristics preclude obtaining an adequate surgical margin. A low anterior resection (LAR) is performed with sphincter-sparing techniques, often using an intraluminal circular stapler. A surgical margin of at least 2 cm is generally recommended. Patients who have localized, nontransmural cancer or who receive preoperative chemotherapy and radiation therapy may be resected with lesser distal margins (1). For patients with metastatic cancer at presentation, external-beam radiation therapy rather than surgical resection can be used to achieve local control in selected patients (25).

5.1.3. Preoperative Therapy for Rectal Cancer

For almost two decades, there has been increasing interest in the use of preoperative chemotherapy and radiation prior to surgical resection of primary rectal cancer. This modality had previously been reserved for patients with unresectable tumors. The rationale for preoperative chemoradiation is supported by several factors. First, preoperative therapy appears to be better tolerated. After an APR or LAR, the small bowel tends to sag into the pelvis and is therefore more likely to be exposed to radiation in the postoperative setting. Radiation of the small bowel leads to enteritis characterized by nausea, vomiting, and diarrhea (26). Second, patients are typically in better physiologic condition in the preoperative state. Third, preoperative therapy also offers a theoretic biological advantage. Prior to surgery, the tumor has an intact blood supply, which allows for greater cytotoxic delivery of both radiation therapy and chemotherapy, whereas in the postoperative setting, the pelvis is comparatively fibrotic and hypoxic. Fourth, some authorities have suggested that preoperative treatment allows for immediate treatment of micrometastatic disease and may also prevent the soiling of tumor cells locally at the time of resection. Although there is little data from randomized clinical trials, there is evidence to suggest preoperative therapy leads to tumor downstaging, thus enhancing the resectability of the primary rectal lesions, which may result in sphincter preservation. Surgeons in particular have argued that preoperative chemoradiation may allow for a sphincter-sparing procedure that would have been impossible without prior treatment of the primary tumor. This is supported by single-institution trials of preoperative therapy that report complete pathologic responses in about 20–25% of patients (27).

On a cautionary note, the decision to provide preoperative therapy relies on clinical staging, which may be imprecise. Therefore, patients with superficial lesions may undergo unnecessary chemoradiotherapy preoperatively. The reliance on clinical staging is a serious drawback making comparisons of preoperative therapy with postoperative therapy difficult. However, endorectal ultrasound provides useful information about primary tumor penetrance and perirectal nodal involvement–two areas in which CT scan is relatively insensitive–and is becoming widely accepted as a part of preoperative staging.

5.1.4. RADIOTHERAPY

External-beam radiotherapy for primary tumors of the colon is used occasionally, either in patients with locally advanced disease to decrease the chance for local recurrence or in patients with established local recurrence following surgical resection.

5.2. Adjuvant Therapy

5.2.1. ADJUVANT THERAPY FOR COLON CANCER

The rationale for adjuvant chemotherapy is straightforward. Patients with stage II and stage III colon cancer are at risk for microscopic metastases after surgical resection. Systemic therapy, usually in the form of chemotherapy has been employed in an attempt to irradicate these micrometastases. Numerous trials conducted in the 1970s and 1980s did not show a clear survival benefit to postoperative chemotherapy. However in 1988 the National Surgical Adjuvant Breast and Bowel Project (NSABP) published results of a large prospective trial comparing observation alone to immunotherapy with bacille Calmette-Guerin (BCG), and to chemotherapy consisting of 5-fluorouracil (5-FU), semustine, and vincristine (28–31). There was a small, but statistically significant survival advantage for patients receiving chemotherapy compared to surgery alone. Subsequently, numerous studies assessed 5-FU in combination with other modulators, such as levamisole and leucovorin (folinic acid) (32,33). Currently, for patients with stage III colon cancer (node-positive without clinically detectable metastases), adjuvant therapy with 5-FU and leucovorin for a total of 6 mo is the standard of care (34). This therapy can be delivered according to either the Roswell Park regimen of 5-FU and leucovorin or the Mayo Clinic regimen (Table 5). Adjuvant therapy should begin within 3–6 wk after surgery, unless surgical complications or medical co-morbidities warrant

Table 5
Summary of Common Chemotherapy Regimens for Colorectal Cancer

Adjuvant chemotherapy

Mayo Clinic Bolus: 5-FU 425 mg/m^2 + leucovorin 20 mg/m^2 on days 1–5 every 4 wk.
Roswell Park: 5-FU 500 mg/m^2 + leucovorin 500 mg/m^2 weekly for 6 wk with 2 wk rest.

Therapy for advanced disease

Mayo Clinic Bolus: 5-FU 425 mg/m^2 + leucovorin 20 mg/m^2 on days 1–5 every 4 wk.
Roswell Park: 5-FU 500 mg/m^2 + leucovorin 500 mg/m^2 weekly for 6 wk with 2 wk rest.
Saltz Regimen (Triple Therapy): irinotecan (CPT-11) 15 mg/m^2, 5-FU 500 mg/m^2, and leucovorin 20 mg/m^2, all given weekly for 4 wk with 2 wk rest.

Rectal (preoperatively or as adjuvant therapy)

Continuous infusion 5-FU 250–300 mg/m^2 M–F concurrent with external-beam radiation therapy for 5–5.5 wk.

a delay. The 5-yr rate of recurrence is 60% among untreated patients, compared with 40% in patients who receive 6 mo of adjuvant chemotherapy.

The decision of whether to use adjuvant 5-FU in patients with stage II colon cancer remains controversial and should be made on a case-by-case basis. Patients with stage II colon cancer have a 75% chance of long-term disease-free survival with surgical resection alone. At best, the use of adjuvant therapy increases this rate to approx 80%. However, certain clinical features, such as presentation with bowel obstruction or perforation, confer a worse prognosis and generally warrant adjuvant therapy for stage II colon cancer. Adjuvant therapy has also been recommended for patients with tumors with specific pathologic or molecular characteristics that confer a worse prognosis (e.g., poorly differentiated tumors, aneuploidy, high TS levels, loss of *dcc* expression, and certain *p53* gene mutations) *(33)*.

5.2.2. Adjuvant Therapy for Rectal Cancer

Since the mid-1970s, studies have shown that combined modality therapy offers a clear benefit for patients with stage II or III rectal cancer. The Gastrointestinal Tumor Study Group (GTSG) performed a randomized trial among patients with rectal cancer undergoing surgery for cure. Patients were randomized to four arms: observation, chemotherapy alone, radiation therapy alone, or combined-modality chemoradiotherapy. The rates of disease-free survival and overall survival were higher in the combined-modality therapy group than in the other arms *(35)*.

A subsequent trial comparing chemoradiotherapy with radiation therapy alone also showed that combined-modality treatment conferred an advantage for both disease-free and overall survival. In addition, a phase III intergroup trial demonstrated that, compared with bolus 5-FU delivered during radiation therapy, prolonged infusional 5-FU delivered with radiation therapy resulted in higher overall survival rates ($p = 0.005$) and a trend towards improved local control of disease. This study suggested that infusional 5-FU during the course of radiation therapy is a better radiosensitizer and provides superior protection from distant metastatic disease compared with bolus 5-FU *(36)*.

Currently, standard adjuvant therapy for patients with stage II or III rectal cancer should include combined-modality therapy consisting of 5-FU-based chemotherapy and external-beam radiation of the pelvis. Clinicians should strongly consider infusional 5-FU during the course of radiation therapy. Adjuvant treatment for stage II or III rectal cancer also involves the use of bolus 5-FU or 5-FU plus leucovorin for 4 mo. Whether chemoradiotherapy should be given first or should follow two cycles of bolus 5-FU has not been established.

6. PATTERNS OF SPREAD AND RECURRENCE AFTER PRIMARY THERAPY

6.1. General Considerations

As noted previously, 70% of patients presenting with colon cancer have disease that is resectable with curative intent, and the remaining 30% have advanced disease. However, among those who undergo surgical resection, 25% will recur; the approximate distribution of sites of relapse is as follows: 60%, multiple sites; 15%, liver metastases only, 4% pulmonary metastases only; 21%, local recurrence (15).

Patients with a history of early colorectal cancer have approx a 3 to 4% risk of local recurrence at the anastomotic site. These patients should undergo surveillance colonoscopy 6–12 mo after diagnosis and, if normal, at 3-yr intervals thereafter. In many cases, patients in whom the tumor recurs at the anastomotic site may undergo resection for cure. The same pathologic staging and associated prognosis as those used for the primary neoplasm apply to recurrence. As discussed previously, 3 to 4% of patients have synchronous primary tumors elsewhere in the colon at the time of initial diagnosis. Thus, full colonoscopy to the cecum must be performed shortly after surgery, if this not performed as part of the preoperative evaluation. Colon cancer tends to recur in the peritoneum, liver, and other distant sites, with a low rate of local recurrence. In contrast, rectal cancer more commonly recurs locally, by direct submucosal extension, or via intramural lymphatic spread. The spread of disease may be continuous or discontinuous. Owing to the venous drainage from the rectum, these rectal tumors more commonly produce pulmonary metastases which may be isolated or multifocal (37).

6.2. Management of Metastatic Disease

Although surgical resection of limited liver and lung metastases has led to long-term survival for some patients, surgical candidacy is a subject of ongoing debate. For patients with hepatic metastases not amenable to resection, newer ablative techniques, such as radiofrequency ablation and cryoablation, are under investigation. In addition, for patients with metastatic disease confined to the liver, regional delivery of chemotherapy via hepatic artery infusions (HAI) has been utilized with some success (38,39). In addition, for patients undergoing hepatic resection with curative intent, HAI chemotherapy combined with systemic chemotherapy has recently been shown to increase survival at 2 yr, compared to the delivery of systemic therapy alone (40). Placement of the HAI catheter is a surgical procedure with occasional life-threatening morbidity, including chemical hepatitis, irreversible biliary sclerosis, and gastrointestinal bleeding.

For patients with metastatic disease not amenable to surgical intervention, systemic chemotherapy with 5-FU has been the mainstay of palliative treatment since the late 1950s when the drug was first synthesized. A variety of schedules have been employed including bolus injection either weekly or daily for 5 d, or as continuous infusion given via central catheter and portable infusion pump. Objective response rates to 5-FU range from 15–25%. When 5-FU is administered as a bolus injection, it has been common to add leucovorin to enhance binding of 5-FU to its target, TS. Currently there is no consensus regarding the optimal dose and schedule of 5-FU with leucovorin, however two dosing schedules have been approved by the United States Food and Drug Administration (see Table 5).

The role of palliative chemotherapy has been questioned in asymptomatic patients with metastatic disease. An interesting study from the Nordic Gastrointestinal Tumor Adjuvant

Therapy Group sought to resolve this and showed that treatment with 5-FU, methotrexate, and leucovorin resulted in prolongation of symptom-free survival, progression-free survival, and overall survival, compared to patients who received treatment only when they became symptomatic (41). Despite this finding, 5-FU-based regimens provide only a modest survival advantage for patients with stage IV disease. However, with the advent of newer agents, such as irinotecan, survival times of patients with metastatic disease may be improving. Irinotecan, a potent inhibitor of topisomerase I, was originally given as second-line chemotherapy for patients in whom 5-FU was ineffective (42). Recently, two large randomized trials in the United States and Europe compared 5-FU plus leucovorin with 5-FU plus leucovorin plus irinotecan as first-line treatment of metastatic colorectal cancer. Both studies demonstrated that the response and overall survival rates for the group treated with triple-drug therapy were superior to those of the group treated with 5-FU plus leucovorin alone (43–45). The response rates for the triple-drug combination ranged from 35–40%, and the median time to disease progression was around 7 mo (43). These results prompted the United States Food and Drug Administration in the year 2000 to approve the use of this combination as first-line treatment of colorectal cancer; this treatment is the first new regimen approved for this disease in many years. Common chemotherapy regimens for both colon and rectal carcinoma are listed in Table 5.

7. THERAPEUTIC MODALITIES UNDER INVESTIGATION

Numerous agents are under investigation in the treatment of colorectal cancer. Two oral fluoropyrimidines: capecitabine and UFT, (a combination of tegafur and uracil) are being used in place of intravenous 5-FU. These agents avoid the need for central venous catheters and ambulatory pumps and are being studied in both the adjuvant and metastatic setting. To date, these drugs appear to result in objective response rates similar to those reported for intravenous 5-FU, but with more acceptable toxicity profiles.

Oxaliplatin, a third-generation platinum agent, has been shown to be effective against 5FU-resistant tumors, and synergistic with 5-FU (46,47). Oxaliplatin has been investigated extensively in Europe, where it has shown excellent response rates in clinical trials, notably in combination with 5-FU plus leucovorin (48–51). In Europe, oxaliplatin plus 5-FU plus leucovorin has been showed to improve response rates and progression-free survival compared to 5-FU plus leucovorin alone. Recently, oxaliplatin, along with infusional 5-FU, was approved by the United States FDA for use as second-line chemotherapy in patients who have failed treatment with 5-FU, leucovorin, and irinotecan (IFL).

In addition to investigation of new cytotoxic agents, new molecular targets have been identified that may prove to have clinical relevance. For example, colonic neoplasms appear to overexpress a variety of angiogenic factors crucial to the growth of metastatic deposits. Specifically, intratumoral overexpression of the endogenous factor, vascular endothelial growth factor (VEGF), has been implicated in tumor angiogenesis, and is associated with a worse prognosis. A number of small molecules and monoclonal antibodies have been developed that abrogate binding to, or function of the VEGF receptor. These agents are currently under clinical investigation. A variety of other receptor tyrosine kinases, including members of the epidermal growth factor receptor (EGF-R) family, HER2/neu, and EGF-R, have been implicated in tumor cell proliferation and metastases. Blocking intracellular signaling from these receptors using monoclonal antibodies to the EGF-R and HER2/neu (C225, or trastuzumab, and Herceptin™, respectively) have demonstrated promising clinical activity. These molecular targets continue to be the focus of intense study.

8. PREVENTION OF COLORECTAL CANCER

The goal of chemoprevention is to interfere with the cell-damaging effects of carcinogens before cancer develops. The agents most commonly studied in the prevention of colorectal cancer are the antioxidants B-carotene, vitamin C, and vitamin E, calcium, estrogen, and nonsteroidal antiinflammatory drugs (NSAIDS), such as aspirin, sulindac, and celocoxib (Celebrex ™).

Researchers believe that calcium works by binding bile and fatty acids and by directly inhibiting epithelial cell proliferation (52). Estrogen decreases the synthesis of secondary bile acids and decreases the production of insulin-like growth factor and may also have direct effects on colonic epithelium. Some epidemiologic studies suggest a higher incidence of colorectal cancer among individuals with a higher dietary intake of total calories and protein (53), whereas those with diets low in folate (and often with high alcohol intake) appear to be at increased risk of colorectal adenomas and carcinomas (54–56). Diets rich in β-carotene may provide some protective effect (57).

NSAIDs are the most widely studied agents for the prevention of colon cancer. These agents inhibit colorectal carcinogenesis, possibly by reducing endogenous prostaglandin production through cyclooxygenase (COX) inhibition. COX-1 is naturally expressed in many tissues, whereas COX-2 is induced by cytokines, growth factors, and mitogens (52). COX-2 expression is elevated in up to 90% of sporadic colon cancers and in up to 40% of colonic adenomas, but is not elevated normal colonic epithelium (58).

Sulindac, which is a nonselective inhibitor of both COX-1 and COX-2, has induced regression of large-bowel polyps in both animal models and patients with FAP. Controlled studies have shown a correlation between regular long-term use of aspirin and a reduced incidence of colorectal cancer. More recently, the COX-2-specific inhibitor celecoxib was shown to reduce the size and number of adenomatous polyps in patients with FAP (59). This agent is currently being studied in large, randomized chemoprevention trials.

REFERENCES

1. Cohen AM, Minsky B, Schilsky RL. Cancer of the colon. *Cancer Principles and Practice of Oncology.* 5th ed., DeVita VT, Hellman S, Rosenberg S. (eds.), Lippincott-Raven, Philadelphia, PA, 1997.
2. Vogelstein B, Fearon ER, Hamilton SR, et al. Genetic alterations during colorectal-tumor development. *N. Engl. J. Med.,* **319** (1988) 525–532.
3. Winawer SJ, Zauber AG, O'Brien MJ, et al. Randomized comparison of surveillance intervals after colonoscopic removal of newly diagnosed adenomatous polyps. The National Polyp Study Workgroup. *N. Engl. J. Med.,* **328** (1993) 901–906.
4. Houlston RS, Collins A, Slack J, et al. Dominant genes for colorectal cancer are not rare. *Ann. Hum. Genet.,* **56** (1992) 99–103.
5. Giovannucci E, Colditz GA, Stampfer MJ, et al., A prospective study of cigarette smoking and risk of colorectal adenoma and colorectal cancer in U.S. men. *J. Natl. Cancer Inst.,* **86** (1994) 183–191.
6. Slattery ML, Edwards SL, Boucher KM, Anderson K, Caan BJ, et al. Lifestyle and colon cancer: an assessment of factors associated with risk. *Am. J. Epidemiol.,* **150** (1999) 869–877.
7. Fuchs CS, Giovannucci EL, Colditz GA, et al. Dietary fiber and the risk of colorectal cancer and adenoma in women. *N. Engl. J. Med.,* **340** (1999) 169–176.
8. Imperiali G, Minoli G. Colonic neoplasm in asymptomatic patients with family history of colon cancer: results of a colonoscopic prospective and controlled study. Results of a pilot study of endoscopic screening of first degree relatives of colorectal cancer patients in Italy. *Gastrointest. Endosc.,* **49** (1999) 132–133.
9. Lynch HT, Lynch J. Genetics, natural history, tumor spectrum, and pathology of hereditary nonpolyposis colorectal cancer: an updated review. *Gastroenterology,* **104** (1993) 1535–1549.
10. Lynch HT, Smyrk TC, Lanspa SJ, et al. Upper gastrointestinal manifestations in families with hereditary flat adenoma syndrome. *Cancer,* **71** (1993) 2709–2714.

11. Vogelstein B. Genetic testings for cancer: the surgeon's critical role. In *26th Annula Meeting of the American College of Surgeons.* Elsevier Science, Baltimore, MD, 1998.

12. Lynch PM, Wargovich MJ, Lynch HT, et al. A follow-up study of colonic epithelial proliferation as a biomarker ina Native-American family with hereditary nonpolyposis colon cancer. *J. Natl. Cancer Inst.,* **83** (1991) 951–954.

13. Leach FS, Nicolaides NC, Papadopoulas N, et al. Mutations of a mutS homolog in hereditary nonpolyposis colorectal cancer. *Cell,* **75** (1993) 1215–1225.

14. Bronner CE, Baker SM, Morrison PT, et al. Mutation in the DNA mismatch repair gene homologue hMLH1 is associated with hereditary non-polyposis colon cancer. *Nature,* **368** (1994) 258–261.

15. August DA, Ottow RT, Sugarbaker PH. Clinical perspective of human colorectal cancer metastasis. *Cancer Metastasis Rev.,* **3** (1984) 303–324.

16. Mandel JS, Bond JH, Bradley M, et al. Sensitivity, specificity, and positive predictivity of the Hemoccult test in screening for colorectal cancers. The University of Minnesota's Colon Cancer Control Study. *Gastroenterology,* **97** (1989) 597–600.

17. Mandel JS, Bond JH, Church TR, et al. Reducing mortality from colorectal cancer by screening for fecal occult blood. Minnesota Colon Cancer Control Study. *N. Engl. J. Med.,* **328** (1993) 1365–1371.

18. Kewenter J. [Does screening influence mortality of colorectal cancer?]. *Lakartidningen,* **88** (1991) 601–602.

19. Ransohoff DF, Lang CA. Screening for colorectal cancer with the fecal occult blood test: a background paper. American College of Physicians. *Ann. Intern. Med.,* **126** (1997) 811–822.

20. Lieberman DA, Weiss DG, Bond JH, Ahnen DJ, Garewall H, Chejfec G. Use of colonoscopy to screen asymptomatic adults for colorectal cancer. Veterans Affairs Cooperative Study Group 380. *N. Engl. J. Med.,* **343** (2000) 162–168.

21. Toribara NW, Sleisenger MH. Screening for colorectal cancer. *N. Engl. J. Med.,* **332** (1995) 861–867.

22. Lynch HT, Lynch JF. Hereditary nonpolyposis colorectal cancer (Lynch syndromes I & II). Genetics, pathology, natural history, and cancer control, Part I. *Cancer Genet. Cytogenet.,* **53** (1991) 143–160.

23. Bruckner HW, Pitrelli J, Merrick M. *Cancer Medicine.* 5th ed., Bast R. (ed.), B.C. Decker, Hamilton, Ontario, Canada, 2000.

24. Wexner SD, Cohen SM, Johansen OB, Nogueras JJ, Jagelman DG. Laparoscopic colorectal surgery: a prospective assessment and current perspective. *Br. J. Surg.,* **80** (1993) 1602–1605.

25. Crane CH, Janjan NA, Abbruzzese JL, et al. Effective pelvic symptom control using initial chemoradiation without colostomy in metastatic rectal cancer. *Int. J. Radiat. Oncol. Biol. Phys.,* **49** (2001) 107–116.

26. Minsky BD, Cohen AM, Kemeny M, et al. Combined modality therapy of rectal cancer: decreased acute toxicity with the preoperative approach. *J. Clin. Oncol.,* **10** (1992) 1218–1224.

27. Janjan NA, Crane CN, Feig BW, et al. Prospective trial of preoperative concomitant boost radiotherapy with continuous infusion 5-fluorouracil for locally advanced rectal cancer. *Int. J. Radiat. Oncol. Biol. Phys.,* **47** (2000) 713–718.

28. Wolmark N, Wieand S, Rockette HE, et al., The prognostic significance of tumor location and bowel obstruction in Dukes B and C colorectal cancer. Findings from the NSABP clinical trials. *Ann. Surg.,* **198** (1983) 743–752.

29. Wolmark N, Rockette H, Wickerham DL, et al. Adjuvant therapy of Dukes' A, B, and C adenocarcinoma of the colon with portal-vein fluorouracil hepatic infusion: preliminary results of National Surgical Adjuvant Breast and Bowel Project Protocol C-02. *J. Clin. Oncol.,* **8** (1990) 1466–1475.

30. Mamounas E, Wieand S, Wolmark N, et al. Comparative efficacy of adjuvant chemotherapy in patients with Dukes' B versus Dukes' C colon cancer: results from four National Surgical Adjuvant Breast and Bowel Project adjuvant studies (C-01, C-02, C-03, and C-04). *J. Clin. Oncol.,* **17** (1999) 1349–1355.

31. Wolmark N, Rockette H, Mamanas E, et al. Clinical trial to assess the relative efficacy of fluorouracil and leucovorin, fluorouracil and levamisole, and fluorouracil, leucovorin, and levamisole in patients with Dukes' B and C carcinoma of the colon: results from National Surgical Adjuvant Breast and Bowel Project C-04. *J. Clin. Oncol.,* **17** (1999) 3553–3559.

32. Poon MA, O'Connell MJ, Wienad HS, et al. Biochemical modulation of fluorouracil with leucovorin: confirmatory evidence of improved therapeutic efficacy in advanced colorectal cancer. *J. Clin. Oncol.,* (1991) **9** 1967–1972.

33. Moore HC, Haller DG. Adjuvant therapy of colon cancer. *Semin. Oncol.,* **26** (1999) 545–555.

34. NIH. NIH consensus conference. Adjuvant therapy for patients with colon and rectal cancer. *JAMA,* **264** (1990) 1444–1450.

35. GTSG. Prolongation of the disease-free interval in surgically treated rectal carcinoma. Gastrointestinal Tumor Study Group. *N. Engl. J. Med.,* **312** (1985) 1465–1472.

36. O'Connell MJ, martenson JA, Wieand HS, et al. Improving adjuvant therapy for rectal cancer by combining protracted- infusion fluorouracil with radiation therapy after curative surgery. *N. Engl. J. Med.*, **331** (1994) 502–507.

37. Weiss L, Grundmann E, Torhorst J, et al. Haematogenous metastatic patterns in colonic carcinoma: an analysis of 1541 necropsies. *J. Pathol.*, **150** (1986) 195–203.

38. Lorenz M, Muller HH. Randomized, multicenter trial of fluorouracil plus leucovorin administered either via hepatic arterial or intravenous infusion versus fluorodeoxyuridine administered via hepatic arterial infusion in patients with nonresectable liver metastases from colorectal carcinoma. *J. Clin. Oncol.*, **18** (2000) 243–254.

39. Ambiru S, Miyazaki M, Ito H, Nakagawa K, Shimizu H, Nakajima N. Adjuvant regional chemotherapy after hepatic resection for colorectal metastases. *Br. J. Surg.*, **86** (1999) 1025–1031.

40. Kemeny N, Huang Y, Cohen AM, et al. Hepatic arterial infusion of chemotherapy after resection of hepatic metastases from colorectal cancer. *N. Engl. J. Med.*, **341** (1999) 2039–2048.

41. NGTATG. Expectancy or primary chemotherapy in patients with advanced asymptomatic colorectal cancer: a randomized trial. Nordic Gastrointestinal Tumor Adjuvant Therapy Group. *J. Clin. Oncol.*, **10** (1992) 904–911.

42. Conti JA, Kemeny NE, Saltz LB, et al. Irinotecan is an active agent in untreated patients with metastatic colorectal cancer. *J. Clin. Oncol.*, **14** (1996) 709–715.

43. Saltz LB, Cox JV, Blanke C, et al. Irinotecan plus fluorouracil and leucovorin for metastatic colorectal cancer. Irinotecan Study Group. *N. Engl. J. Med.*, **343** (2000) 905–914.

44. Cunningham D, Pyrhonen S, James RD, et al. Randomised trial of irinotecan plus supportive care versus supportive care alone after fluorouracil failure for patients with metastatic colorectal cancer. *Lancet*, **352** (1998) 1413–1418.

45. Ducreux M, Gil-Delgado M, Andre T, Ychou M, de Gramond A, Khayat D. [Irinotecan in combination for colon cancer]. *Bull. Cancer*, **Spec No** (1998) 43–46.

46. Mathe G, Kidani Y, Segiguchi M, et al. Oxalato-platinum or 1-OHP, a third-generation platinum complex: an experimental and clinical appraisal and preliminary comparison with cis- platinum and carboplatinum. *Biomed. Pharmacother.*, **43** (1989) 237–250.

47. Tashiro T, Kawada Y, Sakurai Y, Kidani Y. Antitumor activity of a new platinum complex, oxalato (trans-l-1,2- diaminocyclohexane)platinum (II): new experimental data. *Biomed. Pharmacother.*, **43** (1989) 251–260.

48. Andre T, Bensmaine MA, Louvet C, et al. Multicenter phase II study of bimonthly high-dose leucovorin, fluorouracil infusion, and oxaliplatin for metastatic colorectal cancer resistant to the same leucovorin and fluorouracil regimen. *J. Clin. Oncol.*, **17** (1999) 3560–3568.

49. Giacchetti S, Perpoint B, Zidani R, et al. Phase III multicenter randomized trial of oxaliplatin added to chronomodulated fluorouracil-leucovorin as first-line treatment of metastatic colorectal cancer. *J. Clin. Oncol.*, **18** (2000) 136–147.

50. Levi F, Giachetti S, Adam R, Zidani R, Metzger G, Misset JL. Chronomodulation of chemotherapy against metastatic colorectal cancer. International Organization for Cancer Chronotherapy. *Eur. J. Cancer*, **31A** (1995) 1264–1270.

51. de Gramont A, Figer A, Seymour M, et al. Leucovorin and fluorouracil with or without oxaliplatin as first-line treatment in advanced colorectal cancer. *J. Clin. Oncol.*, **18** (2000) 2938–2947.

52. Janne PA, Mayer RJ. Chemoprevention of colorectal cancer. *N. Engl. J. Med.*, **342** (2000) 1960–1968.

53. Benito E, Stiggelbout A, Boxch FX, et al. Nutritional factors in colorectal cancer risk: a case-control study in Majorca. *Int. J. Cancer*, **49** (1991) 161–167.

54. Giovannucci E, Stampfer MJ, Colditz GA, et al. Folate, methionine, and alcohol intake and risk of colorectal adenoma. *J. Natl. Cancer Inst.*, **85** (1993) 875–884.

55. Giovannucci E, Rimm EB, Ascherio A, Stampfer MJ, Colditz GA, Willett WC. Alcohol, low-methionine— low-folate diets, and risk of colon cancer in men. *J. Natl. Cancer Inst.*, **87** (1995) 265–273.

56. Baron JA, Sandler RS, Haile RW, Mandel JS, Mott LA, Greenberg ER. Folate intake, alcohol consumption, cigarette smoking, and risk of colorectal adenomas. *J. Natl. Cancer Inst.*, **90** (1998) 57–62.

57. Ferraroni M, LaVecchia C, D'Avanzo B, Negri E, Franceschi S, Decarli A. Selected micronutrient intake and the risk of colorectal cancer. *Br. J. Cancer*, **70** (1994) 1150–1155.

58. Eberhart CE, Coffey RJ, Radhika A, Giardiello FM, Ferrenbach S, DuBois RN. Up-regulation of cyclooxygenase 2 gene expression in human colorectal adenomas and adenocarcinomas. *Gastroenterology*, **107** (1994) 1183–1188.

59. Steinbach G, Lynch PM, Phillips RK, et al. The effect of celecoxib, a cyclooxygenase-2 inhibitor, in familial adenomatous polyposis. *N. Engl. J. Med.*, **342** (2000) 1946–1952.

60. Winawer SJ, Fletcher RH, Miller L, et al. Colorectal cancer screening: clinical guidelines and rationale. *Gastroenterology,* **112** (1997) 594–642.

61. Fleming ID, Cooper JS, Henson DE, American Joint Committee on Cancer, *Cancer Staging Manual.* 5th ed., Lippincott-Raven, Philadelphia, PA, 1997.

27 Constipation

Anne Lutz-Vorderbruegge and Arnd Schulte-Bockholt

Contents

1. INTRODUCTION

Constipation is a common problem in general practice as well as in specialized gastro-enterological care. The definition of this term however, remains difficult; patients and their physicians often do not agree on the exact meaning of the term. Patients who complain of constipation may describe infrequent defecation, pain or straining with defecation, passage of firm or small volume material, increased difficulty initiating evacuation, or a feeling of incomplete evacuation. According to the revised "Rome criteria" *(1)*, chronic constipation is defined if two or more of the following symptoms occur for at least 12 wk (not necessarily consecutively) within 12 mos: (i) straining in more than 25% of bowel motions; (ii) hard or pellet stools in more than 25% of bowel motions; (iii) a feeling of incomplete evacuation in more than 25 % of bowel motions; (iv) manual support of defecation in more than 25% of bowel motions; and (v) fewer than three bowel movements per week.

These criteria include subjective complaints. Bowel frequency has been used as an objective criterion, and the range between 3 and 21 bowel movements weekly has been proposed to be a normal defecation frequency. We define chronic constipation as a disorder lasting 6 mo or longer, in which individuals have two or fewer bowel movements per week. We consider a diagnosis of acute constipation in those individuals who have recently (<6 mo) had either decreased frequency of bowel movements or increased difficulty initiating evacuation.

2. EPIDEMIOLOGY

Constipation affects nearly 5 million people in the United States, corresponding to a prevalence rate of 2%, and 2.5 million people consult a physician yearly for constipation. In a meta-

From: *Colonic Diseases*
Edited by: T. R. Koch © Humana Press Inc., Totowa, NJ

analysis of 30 epidemiological studies, prevalence rates varied from 1.4–16.9 %, depending on the definition of constipation. The occurrence of constipation increases with advancing age, rising exponentially in prevalence after the age of 65. This disorder is three times more common in women than in men. According to older epidemiological studies, constipation is less common in caucasians than in other groups, however this was not confirmed by a recent study. It is more common in people with low income or lack of formal education. Recent epidemiological studies in the U.S. showed a clear geographical distribution; there are more frequent hospital discharges for constipation in rural than in urban states and in poorer and northern states (2). This suggests the potential influence of rural living and colder temperature as potential environmental factors.

In the U.S., laxatives are prescribed to more than 3 million people yearly, with 15% of women and 2% of men using laxatives on a regular basis. An estimated $250 million are spent yearly on laxatives purchased without a prescription, and the total amount spent on laxatives including prescriptions is at least $500 million yearly. These numbers are similar to those reported in European studies, and it has been noted that laxative use increases with patient age.

3. COMMON CAUSES

Constipation is a symptom that may be present in patients with many underlying medical disorders. Therefore, before beginning medical treatment, it is important to evaluate individuals for known origins of constipation (see Table 1). In general, we are more aggressive in the immediate evaluation of constipation in those patients presenting with acute constipation (present <6 mo).

In about 70% of individuals seen for a complaint of constipation, it is not possible to find a specific cause. These patients are classified as having idiopathic constipation. With regards to the type of constipation, these patients can be classified into two groups: those with a normal colon transit time (70–80% of all patients studied; for method, see Subheading 4.) and those with a pathological colon transit time (20–30% of all patients studied). This latter group can be divided into patients with slow transit constipation (30% of patients with pathological transit time, i.e., a colonic motility disorder) and those with outlet obstruction (70% of patients with pathological transit time, i.e., a rectal evacuation disorder) (3).

There are many theories and widespread beliefs concerning the cause of idiopathic constipation (4). Lack of dietary fiber, inadequately low fluid intake, lack of physical exercise, raised progesterone levels, suppression of the defecatory urge, and damage to the enteric nervous system by stimulant laxatives have all been suggested as reasons for constipation (5). Although some of these factors may play a partial role, there is little scientific evidence in recent studies to support these notions (6).

Morphological studies point to the possibility of degeneration of the enteric nerve system as a cause of idiopathic constipation. In these individuals, age might be a factor. A reduced number of argyrophilic neurons has been shown in some but not all surgical specimens of patients with slow transit constipation. Furthermore a decreased number of neurofilaments in enteric ganglia has been reported. Recently, decreased volume of interstitial cells of Cajal in patients with slow transit constipation was shown. Interstitial cells of Cajal play a central role in the autonomic regulation of gastrointestinal motility, especially in the colon.

In children, cows milk intolerance was identified in a high percentage of constipated patients. This apparent paradox can be explained by perianal lesions due to an allergy that led to painful defecation and subsequent constipation. It is unknown whether other food allergies play a similar role and how often this mechanism is of relevance in adults.

Table 1
Causes of Constipation

Mechanical obstruction	Neurogenic disorders	Systemic disease
Neoplasia and strictures	Hirschsprung's disease	Systemic sclerosis
Rectocele	Central nervous system diseases	Amyloidosis
Rectal prolapse	Heavy metal poisoning	
Endometriosis	(e.g., lead/mercury)	
Intussusception		

Medication-induced	Metabolic–endocrine disorders	Idiopathic constipation
Opiate analgesics	Hypothyroidism	Outlet obstruction
Anticholinergic agents	Diabetes mellitus with	Slow transit–colonic inertia
Calcium channel antagonists	autonomic neuropathy	Normal transit–irritable
Calcium-containing supplements	Uremia	bowel syndrome
Aluminum-containing antacids	Hypercalcemia–hypokalemia	
Vinca alkaloids		
Polystyrene binding resins		
Oral iron supplements		
Antidepressants		
Neuroleptic agents		
Anticonvulsants		

The complex course and mechanism of defecation can be seen in Fig. 1. In many cases, the cause of so-called idiopathic constipation will be a disturbance in the complex interactive mechanism of colon motility and rectosigmoidal evacuation, which, to date, still remains incompletely understood *(7)*.

4. DIAGNOSTIC EVALUATION OF THE PATIENT

Figure 2 presents our algorithm for the laboratory investigation and treatment at the initial presentation of a patient with constipation. In the first visit, we complete a history and physical examination including a rectal examination. Our goal is to try to differentiate between complaints of acute constipation (<6 mo) with progressive symptoms or chronic constipation (>6 mo).

A lifelong complaint suggests a congenital disorder. Associated symptoms such as weight loss, urinary symptoms, neurological complaints, or symptoms suggestive of hypothyroidism should be elicited to encourage specific investigation of a possible underlying disease *(8)*. The past history should include previous surgery in the pelvis, including colonic resection or prostate operations, an obstetric history (resulting in possible damage to the pelvic floor), and any illness that might have led to constipation (see Table 1), including illnesses that led to prolonged immobilization. A careful drug history will point to medications as a cause of constipation (Table 1).

The physical examination may uncover signs of neurological disease such as Parkinson's disease, endocrine disease, e.g., hypothyroidism, or psychiatric illness, such as depression. Abdominal palpation can reveal distension, coprostasis, or an inflammatory or neoplastic mass. Digital rectal examination can reveal stenosis (e.g., neoplastic), functional disorders of the anus, and whether a fecal impaction is present.

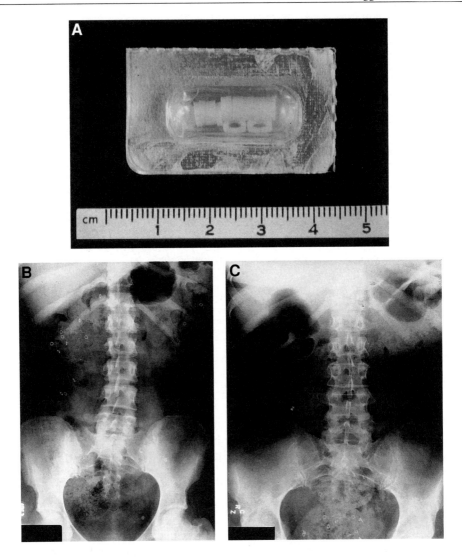

Fig. 1. (A) Sitzmark capsule to study colonic transit time. (B) Patient with slow transit constipation, i.e., colonic inertia (left). (C) Patient with outlet obstruction (right).

In patients with acute constipation or progressive symptoms (especially those patients older than 40 yr), exclusion of neoplastic, metabolic, or endocrine disorders associated with constipation is critical. Laboratory measurements should include hemoglobin level and erythrocyte sedimentation rate (ESR), potassium, calcium, glucose, creatinine, and thyroid stimulating hormone. We also perform a complete colonoscopy (or a proctosigmoidoscopy and barium colon X-ray) in order to exclude mechanical obstruction due to neoplasia, diverticular stricture, or endometriosis. If this evaluation provides a specific diagnosis, we treat the underlying disease. If no specific diagnosis is made, we recommend a high fiber intake as described below.

In patients with chronic constipation, the first step is to encourage a high dietary fiber intake and/or prescribe fiber supplements (9). In those patients who have not improved with a high fiber intake, we perform a laboratory evaluation and endoscopy, as described earlier. If this is normal, we then proceed to a colonic transit study. These patients, by definition,

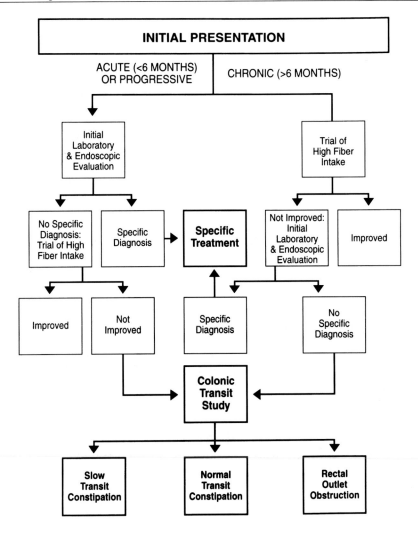

Fig. 2. Algorithm for the evaluation and management of constipation.

have idiopathic constipation, and this test is performed to determine the subtype of constipation. Because of improved patient compliance and ease of interpretation, we use the Hinton method for examination of colonic transit (see Fig. 3) *(10)*. After fecal disimpaction (if present), the patient ingests a single gelatine capsule containing 20 nonabsorbable markers. These are commercially available (Sitzmarks, Konsyl Pharmaceuticals, Fort Worth, TX; or Mauch, Münchenstein, Switzerland), but can also be manufactured inexpensively using gelatine capsules and radio-opaque particles (available at Eduard Plazotta, München, Germany; or, e.g., catheters cut into small pieces). During the study, the patient remains off all laxatives, suppositories, enemas, and constipation-associated medications. An abdominal flat plate X-ray is taken after 5 d. In multiple published studies, normal individuals pass at least 80% or 16 out of 20 markers at 5 d. If the study is abnormal, markers may be retained in the rectosigmoid region (consistent with a diagnosis of rectal outlet obstruction) or more diffusely throughout the colon (consistent with a diagnosis of slow transit constipation).

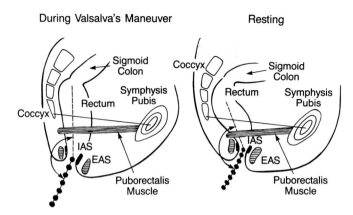

Fig. 3. The process of normal defecation includes the following mechanisms: (i). colorectal motility (fast propulsive contractions of high amplitude); (ii) anorectal sensation, i.e., defecatory urge; (iii) reflectory relaxation of the internal anal sphincter; (iv) voluntary relaxation of the external anal sphincter; and (v) increase in intra-abdominal pressure (Valsalva's maneuver) leading to initiation of defecation after relaxation of the puborectal muscle with straightening of the rectoanal angle and increase in intraluminal pressure.

In patients with rectal outlet obstruction, stenosis (e.g., carcinoma or Hirschsprung's disease), neurological causes, and functional causes must be differentiated. After endoscopy has been performed (with deep rectal biopsies 2 to 3 cm proximal to the dentate line in those patients younger than 30 yr if Hirschsprung's disease is suspected), further evaluation may include anorectal manometry with measurement of rectal compliance. Specialized centers may further evaluate outlet obstruction with electromyographic studies of the external anal sphincter, and defecography (conventional fluoroscopic monitoring of defecation of thickened barium). Patients with paradoxical contraction of the external anal sphincter during defecation (anismus) can be identified by manometry, electromyogram (EMG), and defecography *(11)*. Motivated patients with anismus are candidates for biofeedback therapy to relearn relaxation of the external anal sphincter.

In future studies, functional magnetic resonance tomography (MRT) may replace conventional defecography. After instillation of 200–300 mL of ultrasound gel into the rectum, MRT of the minor pelvis is performed at rest, while squeezing the anal sphincter, and during straining. The nonphysiologic position does not appear to reduce the diagnostic value of this method, as comparative studies between conventional defecography and functional MRT have shown. The limited availability of the method and the costs at present restrict the use of this diagnostic tool to specialized centers *(12)*.

There are further diagnostic methods that have not yet been evaluated in large patient numbers and whose value in the diagnostic workup of constipated patients still has to be elucidated. These include colonic manometry, scintigraphic colonic transit studies, positron emission tomography, and anal endosonography.

5. THERAPY

5.1. Dietary Fiber

In patients with chronic constipation, we initially recommend high fiber intake. The average American diet is estimated to include 15–20 g of fiber daily. To utilize fiber in therapy of

Table 2
Agents Used in Treatment of Constipation

Group	Comments
1. Bulk–fiber	• Least side effects but may cause obstruction.
a. Soluble: psyllium, guar, pectin	• Fermentation increases flatus.
b. Insoluble–Inorganic:	• Not fermented.
Cellulose, Polycarbophil salts	
2. Osmotic	• May impair fluid and electrolyte balance.
a. Salts:	• Inexpensive.
magnesium salts,	• Magnesium accumulation if renal insufficiency.
sodium phosphate	• Phosphate accumulation if renal insufficiency.
b. Sugars or sugar alcohols: lactulose,	• Increases flatus.
lactose, mannitol	
sorbitol, glycerol, PEG solutions	• Expensive.
3. Stimulants/irritants	• Tachyphylaxis occurs.
Bisacodyl and phenolpthalein (diphenols)	• Active only if bile salts and bacteria present.
Cascara–senna–aloe–casanthranol	• Require bacterial cleavage.
(anthraquinones)	
Castor oil (rizinoleic acid)	• Not routinely used, poor taste.
Docusate salts	• Poorly effective.
Chenocholic acid	• Expensive.
4. Prokinetic agents	• Abdominal cramping, avoid in outlet obstruction.
Cisapride, Bethanecol chloride	• Not available at present.
Neostigmine bromide	• May induce cholinergic crisis.
Naloxone HCl	• Requires parenteral delivery.
5. Enema and suppository	• Self administered enema may produce perforation.
Sodium phosphates, glycerol, sorbitol,	
lactulose, mineral oil, bisacodyl,	
CO_2-producing suppository	

constipation, we recommend 25–30 g of total fiber intake daily. Specifically, patients can utilize bran (8 g fiber/30 g serving), shredded wheat (3 g fiber/30 g serving), corn meal (5 g fiber/120 g serving), brown rice (5.5 g fiber/120 g serving), whole wheat or rye bread (2 g fiber/30 g serving), brown, Navy, or red beans (8 g fiber/120 g serving), corn, broccoli, or peas (4 g fiber/120 g serving), prunes (5.5 g fiber/120 g serving), and an apple or pear (5 g fiber/medium fruit).

When we instruct patients on a high fiber intake, we also discuss the initiation of the gastrocolonic response. In most individuals, gastric distension can increase phasic contractions of the rectosigmoid region. Due to the normal circadian rhythm of colonic motility, this response may be more pronounced in the morning. We recommend that patients eat a warm meal or drink a warm fluid after arising in the morning.

5.2. Drug Treatment of Constipation

There are five major groups of agents that have been used in the medical treatment of constipation (see Table 2) (13).

5.2.1. BULK AGENTS

Since most individuals seem unable on a daily basis to reach 30 g of total fiber intake, they will likely require fiber supplements. These supplements should be used with a meal and adequate fluid intake. These bulk agents include soluble and insoluble fiber supplements. Fiber and fiber supplements are a diverse group of nonstarch cabohydrates that are not digestible by humans. Cellulose and lignin are fibrous and insoluble, and have their greatest effect on fecal bulk. Noncellulose polysaccarides include hemicellulose pectin, gums, algal polysaccarides, such as guar, and the synthetic resin polycarbophil. These substances are viscous, soluble, have a high water binding capacity, and appear to influence colonic motility. Most soluble fibers are digested by bacteria and may contribute to a laxative action by increasing osmotic pressure of stool and by increasing fecal mass. Colonic bacterial fermentation of soluble fibers may also produce metabolites that directly influence fluid transport and motility. Water soluble fiber supplements may, however, slow nutrient absorption and decrease transit through the upper gastrointestinal tract.

Colonic gas formation is a common side effect, but often subsides after a week, due to adaptation of intestinal flora. It occurs especially after consumption of soluble fiber, therefore these substances can be avoided. Patients who have excessive flatulence may benefit by prescribing a polycarbophil salt, 1 g up to four times daily. Among the commonly used supplements, psyllium obtained from plantago seeds has few side effects. It is taken as a dose of 3 to 4 g of fiber in at least 250 mL of fluid, such as fruit juice (as a taste corrector) up to three times daily.

Patients with gastrointestinal stenosis or intestinal pseudo-obstruction should avoid fiber. Cellulose may bind cardiac glycosides and other drugs; therefore, ingestion of drugs and laxatives should be separated in time as much as possible. Intestinal obstruction and bezoar formation are unusual complications of the use of fiber supplements. Allergic reactions have also been described, especially with plant gums, but fiber supplements generally have the fewest side effects among laxatives.

5.2.2. Osmotic Agents

The second major class of laxatives are osmotic agents. These compounds increase the water content of fecal material. This effect may be beneficial in patients with constipation, because the transit of liquid fecal material in human colon is more rapid than transit of solid material. Magnesium salts, such as sulfate or citrate of magnesia, have been extensively used and are relatively safe if used as directed. These substances are available as an over-the-counter laxative at every drugstore in the U.S.A. They are contraindicated for long-term use in patients with congestive heart failure or renal insufficiency. Patients receiving these agents for a prolonged time should periodically have screening of their serum magnesium and creatinine level. Sodium phosphate is another salt often used as an osmotic laxative. It is more pleasant tasting than the magnesium salts, but phosphate and sodium accumulation can occur in patients with diminished renal function.

Poorly absorbed mono- or disaccharides or alcohol derivatives (such as lactulose, sorbitol, or glycerol) may also be beneficial in treatment of constipation. These substances increase osmotic pressure in the colon and are metabolized by colonic bacteria to increase intraluminal bacterial mass. Sorbitol 70% syrup or glycerol are less expensive alternatives to lactulose. Most patients receive benefit from 30 mL of these substances once or twice daily, although the therapeutic dose has to be determined empirically. One to three days may be required before a laxative effect begins. Common side effects include gas formation, due to fermentation by colonic bacteria.

Polyethyleneglycol (PEG; molecular weight [MW] 3350 D) electrolyte solutions are non-absorbable polyalcohols in a saline isotonic solution containing 60 g PEG/L. These solutions are commonly used in preparation for colonoscopy, since there is no net ion absorption or loss,

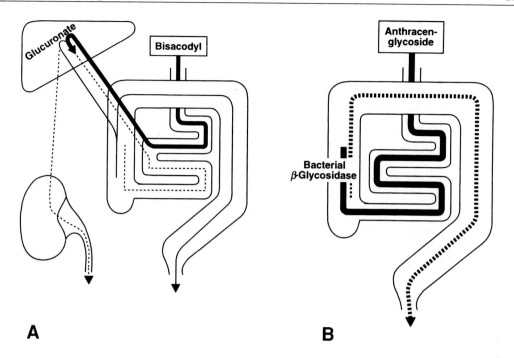

Fig. 4. Pharmacokinetic mechanisms for diphenols (hepatic glucuronidation is necessary) and anthraquinones (bacterial cleavage is necessary).

and dehydration does not occur because of their isotonicity. In patients with constipation, PEG electrolyte solutions can be given regularly in smaller doses (in Europe, commercially available preparations contain 13.81 g), one to five times daily *(14)*. This leads to regular bowel motions in most patients with less gas formation than lactulose *(15)*. Two randomized placebo-controlled study studies proved the effectiveness of this medication (evidence level Ib or grade A) *(16)*. A relative disadvantage of PEG solutions is their higher price.

5.2.3. STIMULANT LAXATIVES

The third major class of laxatives includes irritant or stimulant laxatives. These agents may be beneficial in short term usage. This class contains anthraquinone compounds, such as the extracts of senna, aloe, cascara, or rhubarb, and diphenylmethane derivatives, including phenolphthalein and bisacodyl. These substances have a prokinetic action, increase intestinal secretion, and diminish intestinal absorption. The active ingredients in the anthraquinone group are glycoside derivatives of danthron. Danthron itself has been withdrawn from the market because of its association with hepatic and intestinal tumors. Anthraquinones are nonabsorbable, and the active component, rheinanthrone, is formed by bacterial cleavage. By contrast, bisacodyl and phenolphtalein are absorbed by the small intestine, undergo glucuronidation in the liver, and then are excreted into the bile. Glucuronidated derivatives are not absorbable and will pass into the colon where deconjugation by bacteria forms the active diphenol compound. These substances have a laxative effect only if bile flow is not obstructed and bacteria are present in the colon (see Fig. 4). Due to enterohepatic circulation, their laxative effect is delayed until 6–10 hours after ingestion.

The dose for using anthraquinones in constipation is variable, because most commercial preparations are not standardized. The adult dose for the proprietary preparation, cascara

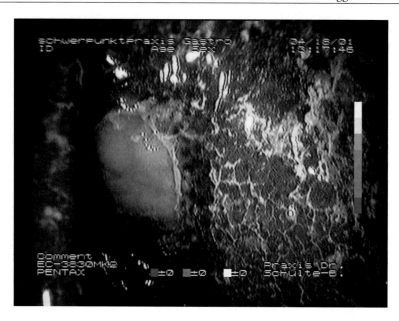

Fig. 5. A severe case of melanosis coli after prolonged use of stimulant laxatives.

sagrada (casanthranol), is 30 mg/d, while the usual daily dose of bisacodyl is 10–15 mg/d, and phenolphthalein (which is no longer sold in the U.S.) is 30–200 mg/d.

Stimulant laxatives, especially if used for acute constipation, cause abdominal cramping and tenesmus in 10% of patients *(17)*. Melanosis coli (Fig. 5) is a reversible black-brown discoloration of the colonic mucosa, which begins abruptly at the ileocecal valve and may progress distally to the dentate line. It is found frequently in patients who chronically use stimulant laxatives, especially anthraquinones. However, there is no present evidence that the presence of melanosis coli has any pathophysiological importance. In particular it is not a risk factor for colonic adenoma or carcinoma *(18)*.

Stimulant agents generally should not be prescribed longer than two continuous weeks. It is presently unclear whether chronic use of these substances can damage the enteric nerve system. It is well known that patients using these substances on a chronic basis may require increasing doses. Unfortunately, older patients may develop fecal incontinence while using stimulant laxatives. Allergic reactions, including Stevens-Johnson syndrome, have been described. These substances should not be used in pregnant women, as they may trigger uterus contractions.

There is a group of stimulant and irritant laxatives that we do not use in our clinical practice. Castor oil, obtained from the bean of the castor plant, *ricinus communis*, has been used since the time of the ancient Egyptians. It contains ricinoleic acid, has a terrible taste, and effects both secretion as well as motility. Castor oil causes cramping abdominal pain by a prokinetic effect on the small bowel. Bile acids, such as cholic acid (0.25 g three times daily) or chenodeoxycholic acid (0.25–0.5 g three times daily), reduce net absorption of water and electrolytes. These substances are quite expensive for use as a first line drug in treatment of constipation. We also do not use mineral oil routinely, because reflux of this material can cause lipid pneumonia. Available studies have shown minimal benefit of wetting agents or surfactants, such as docusate salts, in treatment of constipation. Docusate salts may also cause increased absorption of other drugs given concurrently.

5.2.4. PROKINETIC AGENTS

The fourth major class of laxatives are prokinetic agents or drugs that function as neurotransmitter agonists. These substances have potential use in patients with slow transit constipation, but may increase abdominal symptoms in patients with constipation related to an outlet obstruction. Bethanechol chloride is a muscarinic-cholinergic agonist that increases phasic contractions in human colon at a dose of 10–50 mg three times daily. Neostigmine bromide is an anticholinesterase agent that is rarely used due to the possible initiation of a cholinergic crisis. Misoprostol (600–2400 µg/d) induces an increase of colonic motility (usually noted as a side effect) and is effective in chronic refractory constipation. Similarly, the prokinetic side effect of colchicine has been used in these forms of constipation (0.6 mg three times daily).

Prucalopride is a new prokinetic drug not currently available in the U.S., which acts as a selective 5-hydroxytryptamine 4 agonist. Its effect is similar to cisapride, which has recently been withdrawn, and might replace this compound once there is sufficient proof of the safety of prucalopride. Erythromycin has been used as a prokinetic agent in the treatment of small bowel obstruction. However, it does not effect colonic motility adequately, perhaps because the number of motilin receptors that are stimulated by erythromycin decreases from proximal to distal in gastrointestinal tract. Finally, the opiate antagonist, naloxone HCl, has been used in idiopathic slow transit constipation. Its use has been limited by the necessity of parenteral administration and high cost.

5.2.5. SUPPOSITORIES AND ENEMAS

The fifth group of agents that are frequently used in treating constipation are suppositories and enemas. Bisacodyl, a known stimulant laxative, is commonly used in suppository form (10 mg) or in enema form (10 mg/30 mL). After rectal administration, it will initiate defecation within 15–60 min. Some patients will note cramping abdominal pain and a burning sensation in the rectum associated with mild proctitis has been observed.

Sorbitol, glycerol, and lactulose are commercially available in both suppository and enema form. These compounds function as rectal irritants (by dehydration of exposed mucosa) and rectal discomfort or a burning sensation has been reported. Carbon dioxide (CO_2-producing suppositories (a mixture of sodium bicarbonate and potassium bitartrate) distend the rectum with CO_2 and stimulate colorectal contractions. This mechanism may be beneficial in patients with chronic constipation and secondarily diminished rectal sensation of distension. We do not advise patients to use enemas at home without special training, due to the possibility of perforation of the anal canal or rectum by the enema tip.

5.3. Other and Unproven Therapies

There is little scientific evidence to support the widespread belief that increased water consumption, physical exercise, or abdominal massage are beneficial as primary therapy in patients with chronic constipation (19). It has been shown that water consumption has to be increased to more than 4 L daily before water intake will effect stool consistency. This is due to the large resorptive capacity of the small and large intestine.

Psychotherapy might be helpful in coping with the constipation predominant irritable bowel syndrome, but has not been shown to have an effect on intestinal transit (20,21). In children, behavioral techniques (bowel retraining), combined if necessary with fiber supplements and osmotic laxatives, improve bowel regularity in 50–75% (evidence level III or grade C).

It is claimed that probiotics, i.e., viable microbial supplements, might cause relief of constipation. There are double-blind studies with small numbers of patients with preparations containing *Escherichia coli* Nissle and lactobacilli (22). However, to date, there are no larger studies that prove a benefit of these substances in constipation. This is discussed in Chapter 10 in this text.

5.4. Combination Therapy and Herbal Preparations

We recommend that physicians use only one or two preparations from each main group of agents in treating constipation. This permits improved awareness of specific effects and potential side effects of different agents. There is no evidence that combinations of laxatives have an advantage over preparations containing a single ingredient. We discourage our patients from using herbal tea preparations and other "natural" laxative preparations, because the substances in these preparations are pharmacologically poorly defined, are not consistent in the amount of drug that is present, and may contain hepatotoxic alkaloids. Many herbal preparations contain anthraquinone compounds, whose prolonged use is not recommended.

5.5. Surgical Therapy

Surgical intervention in chronic constipation is a therapeutic option only for a select minority of patients refractory to conservative therapy (23). There is no role for surgery in patients with normal colorectal transit time (i.e., constipation predominant irritable bowel syndrome). Rectal outlet obstruction without a specific morphological change is also not an accepted indication for colonic resection therapy. Surgery is considered in outlet obstruction due to rectocele, rectal prolapse, volvulus, and intussusception. In very severe cases of slow transit constipation not responding to conservative therapy, total colectomy (usually with an ileorectal anastomosis) remains an option. If there is concomitant rectal outlet obstruction, this condition should be treated first. Pseudo-obstruction (if not evident) should be excluded by motility studies, including gastric emptying studies, oral-cecal transit studies, and antroduodenal manometry, before discussing a surgical option. A partial colectomy is only considered in patients with segmental megacolon or recurrent sigmoid intussusception. Studies completed since 1990 state that patient satisfaction after colonic resection for chronic constipation ranges between 80 and 97%. However, in 10–51% of patients, constipation is still present postoperatively, and anal incontinence is a relatively frequent postoperative complication. In summary, patients should be very carefully diagnosed and selected before considering operative therapy for chronic constipation. Thorough preoperative physiologic testing is mandatory for a successful outcome.

6. GENERAL MANAGEMENT OF THE CONSTIPATED PATIENT

In patients with chronic constipation who have constant symptoms for a long time (often for years) and who have no progression of their complaints or warning signs for an acute disease, such as weight loss, we initially recommend a high dietary fiber intake, as described (see Table 1). If the patient does not improve, we perform a laboratory evaluation and endoscopy, as set out in Subheading 4. If this evaluation provides a specific diagnosis, we treat the underlying disease.

In patients with constipation who have had a normal laboratory evaluation and endoscopy and have not improved with high fiber intake, we then proceed to a colonic transit study to determine the subtype of constipation.

In patients with outlet obstruction, we routinely advise a low residue diet, because stool that is not there does not have to be evacuated. As supplemental therapy, the regular use of glycerol or CO_2-producing suppositories (two to three mornings a week) may be beneficial in maintaining rectal evacuation. Specific causes of outlet obstruction should be treated (e.g., retraining of the use of the external sphincter by biofeedback in anismus). In addition, in patients with continued abdominal symptoms, we then recommend addition of an osmotic agent such as citrate of magnesia (30–120 mL at bedtime) or sorbitol 70% syrup (30–60 mL at bedtime). Some patients prefer the intermittent use citrate of magnesia (120–240 mL twice weekly).

In patients with normal transit constipation (probable irritable bowel syndrome), the main goal usually is relief of chronic abdominal pain. We initially try to determine whether pain relief occurs following colonic cleansing with either citrate of magnesia (120–240 mL) or PEG solution (2–4 L). If pain relief is satisfactory, we then begin stepwise drug treatment as described above for patients with outlet obstruction (except for the use of CO_2-producing suppositories, which have no role in normal transit constipation). Unfortunately, most individuals have continued abdominal pain following colonic cleansing. Therapies directed at hyperalgesia, such as antispasmodics (e.g., mebeverin), low dose tricyclic antidepressants, or newer drugs for treatment of the irritable bowel syndrome (such as serotonin antagonists) may be of help. Further treatment of these symptoms is described in more detail in Chapter 30 in this text.

In patients with slow transit constipation, we also advise a low residue diet. Drug therapy includes prokinetic agents and osmotic agents (preferably PEG electrolyte solutions). A small group of patients with slow transit constipation obtain relief from abdominal pain by colonic cleansing, but can not maintain colonic evacuation. These patients may obtain long-term improvement of their symptoms either by chronic use of a polymeric liquid diet. As described in Subheading 5.5, surgical therapy is a rare option for a very select group of patients.

7. SPECIAL SITUATIONS

7.1. Laxative and Enema Dependancy

After evacuation of the colon by using a stimulant laxative or enema, it may be several days before a spontaneous bowel movement occurs. The patient can assume that he is constipated, and a vicious cycle develops in which the patient becomes dependant on the daily use of a laxative or enema to induce defecation.

As additional problems that can develop in laxative dependancy, secondary hyperaldosteronism, steatorrhea, hypoalbuminemia, and osteomalacia have been described.

In patients with laxative dependency, our initial goals are to determine whether the patient has a treatable cause of constipation and to determine whether the patient has objective evidence for colorectal dysmotility. We complete the laboratory investigation described in Subheading 4 and initiate proper treatment if a specific diagnosis is made. Next, if the patient has an impaction, we obtain colonic cleansing with either the use of osmotic laxatives or the prolonged use of a polymeric liquid diet. Following disimpaction and in patients with no evidence for a fecal impaction, a colonic transit study is performed while the patient maintains a regular diet and avoids laxatives and enemas.

Patients with slow transit constipation or outlet obstruction are treated as described above. In the majority of patients who have normal transit constipation, we initially convert them from use of stimulant laxatives or enemas to osmotic agents or suppositories and we discuss initiation of the gastrocolonic response as described. It is very important at this stage to reassure the patient that there is no evidence for abnormal movement of solid material through the colon or rectum and to discuss the possible side-effects of continued use of stimulant laxatives or enemas. As a next step, we try to slowly increase fiber intake (up to 30 g of fiber daily), while we taper the intake of osmotic agents or suppositories. Laxative dependancy has not been well studied, but it appears that in about 50% of cases, it is possible to discontinue stimulant laxatives after introduction of a high fiber diet. In many cases, it is possible to convert a patient's stimulant laxative use to suppository use. In some patients, the believed need for routine use of stimulant laxatives and enemas can not be overcome, and we would then consider a psychiatric evaluation. In general, these patients have a great obsession about their bowel movements.

7.2. Pregnancy

There is no good data based on large studies concerning the prevalence of constipation in pregnancy, which may be due to the lack of a generally accepted definition and the subjective criteria used for assessment of bowel motions. Yet constipation is one of the most common gastrointestinal complaints in pregnancy (assumed prevalence between 11 and 38%, mostly in the last trimenon). Several factors add to cause constipation in pregnancy. Contractile activity of the smooth muscle may be inhibited by pregnancy hormones. Progesterone reduces contractility in all segments of the gastrointestinal tract by a change in the transepithelial calcium flux. Probably, progesterone can also inhibit motilin secretion (since motilin levels are reduced during pregnancy).

Patients presenting with constipation during pregnancy should initially receive a trial of 30 g of daily fiber intake. If this is not effective, lactulose or sorbitol may be used safely. Studies examining possible side effects of stimulant laxatives during pregnancy have been contradictory. Both the sennosides and bisacodyl have been examined for their embryonic and fetotoxic influences, and it is presently not clear whether they can be safely used in pregnancy. It has been suggested that castor oil can initiate uterine contractions and should not be used. Both bisacodyl and sennosides do appear in breast milk in the postpartum period, but the concentrations are so low that no side effects should be expected in breast-feeding babies. We do not recommend the regular use of enemas. Either bisacodyl or CO_2-producing suppositories should be safe in inducing rectal evacuation.

7.3. Spinal Cord Injury

Spinal cord injuries interrupt both afferent and efferent innervation of the anal sphincter. Constipation, similar to urinary bladder retention, commonly occurs shortly after the injury (so-called spinal shock). In a bowel rehabilitation program, recommendations include 30 g daily of fiber intake and to take advantage daily of the normal gastrocolonic response that occurs 20 min after breakfast. When beginning this bowel program, the spinal injury patient also has to initiate defecation by learning to apply digital rectal stimulation in combination with either bisacodyl or glycerol suppository or a CO_2-producing suppository (to induce rectal distension). Before beginning digital stimulation, feces present in the lower rectum should be removed digitally. A well-lubricated gloved finger should be inserted 2 to 3 cm into the rectum. A gentle circular motion toward the sacrum will relax the external anal sphincter, and stimulation of the autonomic nerves in the S2–S3 segment will initiate a rectal peristaltic reflex. After 1 to 2 min of digital stimulation, the suppository should be inserted as high above the sphincter as possible and held in place for 15 s. After waiting for 20 min, digitally stimulation is repeated for periods of 3 min every 5–10 min until defecation occurs. During this time, the patient should attempt to use Valsalva's manuever, if possible. Alternatively, the patient can lean forward in order to increase intra-abdominal pressure. If defecation is not achieved within 30 min, a second suppository may be inserted, and the above sequence may be repeated.

It is important to obtain regular evacuation of the rectum at least once every 3 d, because a stool-filled colon in these patients can induce bladder spasms with urinary incontinence and "autonomic hyperreflexia" in patients with T4–T6 or higher lesions. The symptoms of autonomic hyperreflexia are a rise in blood pressure, headache, and profuse sweating above the lesion. If routine evacuation is not obtained in these patients, fecal impaction can cause diarrhea by leakage of fecal fluid around a rectal impaction.

7.4. Cancer and Chemotherapy

Constipation is a common symptom of tumor patients that can considerably reduce quality of life. Possible causes are mechanical obstruction by tumor mass, analgesic therapy with opiates, use of serotonin antagonists as antiemetic drugs, and chemotherapy agents, such as vinblastine and vincristine.

Constipation is the most common and persistent side effect of opiate therapy. This is dose related. High dose opiate therapy inevitably leads to constipation. In contrast to the central effect of opiates in the peripheral effects responsible for constipation, there is no development of tolerance in prolonged use. The side effect of constipation is completely reversible if the treatment is discontinued. A laxative should routinely be given when analgesic therapy with opiates is begun. Controlled studies that compare different concomitant laxative therapies in opiate use do not exist to date.

Serotonin antagonists are potent antiemetic drugs. They frequently cause constipation (7–42% for ondansetrone, 2–26% for granisetrone, and approx 5% for tropisetrone). However, the constipation caused by serotonin antagonists usually resolves spontaneously within 2–3 d. Serotonin antagonists reduce the motility of the lower gastrointestinal tract and prolong colon transit time. They are, therefore, contraindicated in those patients with preexisting impairment of gastrointestinal motility or obstruction.

Most antineoplastic agents cause diarrhea. Chemotherapy with vinblastine or vincristine however, is associated with development of constipation. The vinca-alkaloids can damage afferent and efferent rectal innervation and can potentially damage the enteric nervous system. In principal, these effects are reversible, however this process can take a long time after discontinuation of the chemotherapy (up to several months). Stimulant laxatives may not be effective, and osmotic laxatives, such as lactulose, sorbitol, or PEG solution, are alternatives. Magnesium laxatives and sodium phosphate should be avoided due to possible magnesium retention or water and electrolyte depletion. Enemas or suppositories should not be used to avoid anal or rectal injury with resulting bleeding or infection. Fiber supplements may be helpful in patients complaining of difficulty initiating defecation or passage of hard feces.

7.5. Fecal Impaction

Fecal impaction, meaning large compacted masses of feces that cannot be passed by the patient and that obstruct the lumen of the bowel, is a serious complication of chronic constipation. It occurs mainly in institutionalized geriatric patients and in children. Painful anal disease may be a causative factor, other predisposing conditions include neurologic diseases and mechanical impediments. The presenting symptoms can be unspecific with abdominal pain, rectal discomfort, and paradoxical diarrhea caused by overflow, leading to soiling and anal incontinence. The impaction is found mostly in the rectum (70%), less often in the sigmoid region (20%), or more proximally. Fecoliths or fecolomas can lead to ulceration which can be complicated by bleeding or perforation with peritonitis. Urinary retention can be a further serious consequence. Diagnosis can often be made on physical examination if impacted stool is palpated digitally in a patient with a typical history. In an unclear situation, conventional transabdominal ultrasound can lead to the diagnosis. Sometimes sigmoidoscopy or a barium colon X-ray can clarify the situation. Treatment includes hydration, digital disimpaction (if necessary under systemic sedation), and enemas (given carefully to avoid damage to the intestinal wall) or endoscopic irrigation. Additionally, oral osmotic agents such as magnesium or PEG electrolyte solutions can be given. One should refrain from giving any oral medication that leads to increased intestinal gas, such as lactulose, due to the potential for dangerous distention of the bowel. Once the patient has been disimpacted, a regular small dose of osmotic agents, such as PEG electrolyte solutions, should be given to prevent recurrence of fecal impaction.

8. FUTURE DIRECTIONS

Proposing newer treatments for constipation would certainly be aided by additional information about the pathophysiology of these disorders. Outcomes research might aid in understanding whether our presently suggested classification system is actually of benefit in determining therapeutic options in proposed subsets of patients. The origin of constipation in most individuals remains unknown. There has yet been little genetic research in this area. One notable therapeutic trial was the use of recombinant human neurotrophic factor in the treatment of patients with constipation (24). This agent has been suggested as a means of increasing stool frequency in constipated patients. This effect was interpreted as evidence that exogenous neurotrophic factors could be used to stimulate gut motility in constipated individuals.

REFERENCES

1. Corazziari E, Talley NJ, Thompson WG, Whitehead WE. Rome II: a multinational consensus document on functional gastrointestinal disorders. *Gut*, **45(Suppl II)** (1999) 1–81.
2. Johanson JF. Geographic distribution of constipation in the United States. *Am. J. Gastroenterol.*, **93** (1998) 188–191.
3. Bassotti G, Iantorno G, Fiorella S, Bustos-Fernandez L, Bilder CR. Colonic motility in man: features in normal subjects and in patients with chronic idiopathic constipation. *Am. J. Gastroenterol.*, **94** (1999) 1760–1770.
4. Wald A. Evaluation and management of constipation. *Clin. Perspect. Gastroenterol.*, (1998) 106–115.
5. Ziegenhagen DJ, Tewinkel G, Kruis W, Herrmann F. Adding more fluid to wheat bran has no significant effects on intestinal functions in healthy subjects. *J. Clin. Gastroenterol.* **13** (1991) 525–530.
6. Kamm MA, Farthing MJG, Lennard-Jones JE, Perry LA, Chard T. Steroid hormone abnormalities in women with severe idiopathic constipation. *Gut*, **32** (1991) 80–84.
7. Mertz H, Naliboff B, Mayer E. Physiology of refractory chronic constipation. *Gastroenterology*, **94** (1999) 609–615.
8. Thompson WG, Longstreth GF, Drossman DA, Heaton KW, Irvine EJ, Müller-Lissner SA. Functional bowel disorders and functional abdominal pain. *Gut*, **45(Suppl 2)** (1999) 1143–1147.
9. Müller-Lissner S. Effect of wheat bran on weight of stool and gastrointestinal transit time: A meta analysis. *BMJ*, **296** (1988) 615–617.
10. Hinton JM, Lennard-Jones JE, Young AC. A new method for studying gut transit times using radiopaque markers. *Gut*, **10** (1969) 842–847.
11. Vaizey CJ, Kamm MA. Prospective assessment of the clinical value of anorectal investigations. *Digestion*, **61** (2000) 207–214.
12. Lienemann A. Radiological investigation of obstipation and outlet obstruction. *Zentralbl. Chir.*, **124** (1999) 768–774.
13. Camilleri M, Thompson WG, Fleshman JW. Clinical management of intractable constipation. *Ann. Intern. Med.*, **121** (1994) 520–528.
14. Andorsky R, Goldner F. Colonic lavage solution (PEG) as a treatment for chronic constipation: a double-blind, placebo controlled study. *Am. J. Gastroenterol.*, **85** (1991) 261–265.
15. Attar A, Lemann M, Ferguson A et al. Comparison of a low dose polyethylene glycol electrolyte solution with lactulose for the treatment of chronic constipation. *Gut*, **44** (1999) 226–230.
16. Dipalma JA, DeRidder PH, Orlando RC, Kolts BE, Cleveland MvB. A randomized placebo-controlled, multicenter study of the safety and efficacy of a new polyethylene glycol laxative. *Am. J. Gastroenterol.*, **95** (2000) 446–450.
17. Staumont G, Frexinos J, Fioramonti J, Bueno L. Sennosides and human colonic motility. *Pharmacology*, **36(Suppl 1)** (1988) 49–56.

18. Nusko G, Schneider B, Schneider I, Wittekind C, Hahn EG. Anthranoid laxative use is not a risk factor for colonic neoplasia: results of a prospective case control study. *Gut*, **46** (2000) 651–655.
19. Coenen C, Wegener M, Wedmann B, Schmidt G, Hoffmann S. Does physical exercise influence bowel transit time in healthy young men? *Am. J. Gastroenterol.*, **3** (1992) 292–295.
20. Drossman DA. Review article: an integrated approach to the irritable bowel syndrome. *Aliment. Pharmacol. Ther.*, **13(Suppl 2)** (1999) 3–14.
21. Drossman DA, Thompson WG. The irritable bowel syndrome: Review and a graduated multicomponent treatment approach. *Ann. Intern. Med.*, **116** (1992) 1009–1016.
22. Möllenbrink M, Bruckschen E. Treatment of chronic constipation with physiological *E. coli* bacteria. Results of a clinical trial on the efficacy and compatibility of microbiological therapy with the *E. coli* strain Nissle 1917. *Med. Klein.*, **89** (1994) 587–593.
23. von Flüe M. Surgery for idiopathic constipation: the modest role of successful surgery. *Schweiz. Med. Wochenschr.*, **130** (2000) 1766–1771.
24. Coulie B, Szarka LA, Camilleri M, et al. Recombinant human neurotrophic factors accelerate colonic transit and relieve constipation in humans. *Gastroenterology*, **119** (2000) 41–50.

28 Crohn's Disease

Amit G. Shah and Stephen B. Hanauer

CONTENTS

1. INTRODUCTION

The clinical and pathological description of Crohn's disease (CD) in 1932 described inflammation of the terminal ileum *(1)*. It was not until 1959, 100 yr after Samuel Wilks described ulcerative colitis (UC), that variants of CD were recognized to potentially, or exclusively, involve the colon *(2)*. Ileocolonic involvement was first described by Brooke in 1959 *(3)* and, 1 yr later, Lockhart-Mummery and Morson first described CD confined to the colon *(4)*.

We currently recognize a spectrum of idiopathic inflammatory bowel diseases (IBDs) with UC and CD being the most common and best-described variants. They are defined by the patterns of gastrointestinal tract involvement and extra-intestinal inflammatory sequelae. The idiopathic IBDs must be distinguished from colitis caused by infections, drugs, ischemia, radiation, immunologic, malignant, and systemic diseases *(5)*. Though initial presentations

From: *Colonic Diseases*
Edited by: T. R. Koch © Humana Press Inc., Totowa, NJ

overlap, and therapies are often similar, the distinction between colonic CD and UC is important in defining long-term therapy and outcome.

2. EPIDEMIOLOGY

Most epidemiological characteristics of UC and CD are similar. Both diseases are relatively common in developed countries and infrequent in countries with poor sanitation (6). In Western countries, the incidence of CD is approx 1–6 per 100,000 with a prevalence approximating 50 per 100,000 population. The most common initial presentation is between the second and third decades, with a smaller secondary peak between the sixth and seventh decades. The diseases can occur at any age, however, there may be a slight female preponderance to both diseases. Caucasians are the most commonly affected. Among ethnic groups, Ashkenazi Jews have a higher risk for IBD than other groups. There is, however, a rising incidence in Asians and Africans. In the United States, African Americans traditionally accounted for 20–50% of the IBD incidence of Caucasians, but this gap is narrowing (7).

The pattern of gastrointestinal tract involvement of CD has been studied in several series. Ileocolitis is the most common pattern occurring in approx 40% of patients, with ileitis or colitis alone occurring less frequently, approx 30 and 25%, respectively. The prospective National Crohn's Cooperative Study (NCCDS) documented ileocolitis in 55%, terminal ileal disease in 14%, 15% of patients with colonic only disease, and 3% with non-ileal small bowel sites (8). In a study of 615 CD patients from the Cleveland Clinic, 41% had ileocolitis, 27% had ileitis, 29% had colitis, and 3% had localized perianal involvement (9). In another review of 306 patients with CD, ileocolitis accounted for 26.5%, small bowel for 32.3%, colon alone in 39.9%, and perianal in 1.6% (10). Up to 42.4% of CD patients have symptomatic perianal disease (11). The location of the disease usually remains constant throughout its course, however, progression in extent may occur.

3. ETIOLOGY

CD remains an "idiopathic" IBD. Etiologic theories involve a combination of genetic and environmental influences leading to an over exuberant immunoinflammatory response to an, as yet, undetermined trigger. Genetics likely has a significant role, as family members of patients are affected between 20 and 40% of the time (12). When both parents are affected, the risk to offspring approaches 50%. Monozygotic twins have a concordance of up to 60% in CD compared with 20% in UC (13). In addition, the disease characteristics of age of onset and disease type (i.e., inflammatory, stenosing, or fistulizing) is more often concordant within families (14). Of interest, the concordance rate for CD confined to the colon may be less than for other extents (15), possibly related to misclassification of CD as UC in previous generations.

The most consistent potential genetic loci in IBD are present on chromosomes 1, 12, and 16 (16), with other possible loci on chromosomes 3, 6, 7, and X (17,18). In addition, there is an increased frequency of certain major histocompatibility complex (MHC) class I and II antigens in groups of patients with IBD (19). However, there seems to be significant genetic heterogeneity in that different ethnic groups display different MHC susceptibility and resistance markers (20).

Due to different incidence–prevalence numbers in IBD in first vs third world countries, much consideration has been given to dietary, environmental, bacterial flora, and lifestyle differences as explanations for the etiopathogenesis of IBD. Case-control studies suggest an association between IBD and ingestion of large amounts of refined sugar and possibly with unsaturated fats, although no definite dietary etiology has been identified (21). Early life events including lack of breastfeeding and in utero measles infection have been purported etiologies

(22,23). Environmental factors including climate, pollutants, animal contact, and occupation and stress have been considered, but none of these have been conclusively identified as etiologies. Previous history of surgical removal of immune system-associated organs, including tonsillectomy and appendectomy have also been loosely implicated in CD *(24)*. While appendectomy before the age of 20 seems to be protective for UC, there is no correlation between appendectomies and CD *(25)*. Use of oral contraceptives has also been implicated to slightly increase the risk of colonic CD *(26)*.

The strongest environmental–lifestyle association, to date, is smoking. It is enigmatic that cigarette smoking protects against UC, but is strongly associated with CD. This may, in fact, be a clue to different etiopathogeneses of the two diseases. Smoking adversely affects CD activity after surgery. In fact, it is an independent predictor for endoscopic, clinical, and surgical recurrence. It also predicts the need for immunosuppressive therapy in CD. Interestingly, colonic CD behaves much like UC with regards to smoking, in that CD patients who are smokers are less likely to have colonic CD *(27)*. It remains to be determined whether nicotine, or another component of cigarette smoke contributes to the protective or detrimental impacts of smoking on the course of IBD.

4. PATHOGENESIS

A series of animal models have been used to evaluate different components and types of intestinal inflammation although none, to date, replicates human CD. The cotton top tamarin (a new world monkey), under the stress of captivity, develops a colitis with features of human UC *(28,29)*. Animal models that more closely resemble CD include transgenic rats over-expressing human leukocyte antigen (HLA)-B27 or β_2-Microglobulin *(30,31)*. When these same rats are grown in a germ-free environment, the small and large intestine are spared. The requisite role of bacteria in development of colitis is consistent among multiple experimental models of IBD, including interleukin-2 (IL-2), IL-10, T cell receptor and transformation growth factor (TGF)-β knock-out mice. Therefore, the prevailing hypothesis propounds that IBD is initiated by environmental factors in a genetically susceptible host who then mounts a dysregulated immune response to a (potentially) commensal or pathogenic bacteria or bacterial component *(20)*.

The central role of T cells in the pathogenesis of CD has been shown in several models. IL-2 knock-outs crossed with B cell knock-outs develop colitis. However, when crossed with B and T cell knock-outs, they do not*(32)*. Furthermore, the addition of certain T cell subsets, such as CD45RB[high] T cells or T helper (Th)1 cells, to mice with severe combined immunodeficiency induces colitis that can be abrogated by administration of unfractionated CD4[+] T cells *(33,34)*.

Chronic inflammatory cells are a normal feature of the intestinal tract and function within the gut-associated lymphoid tissue. In IBD, however, there is an impaired ability to down-regulate mucosal inflammation compared to non-IBD patients. B cell populations are up-regulated as evidenced by increased immunoglobulin (Ig)G1 plasma cells in UC and IgG2-bearing plasma cells in CD *(35)*. In addition, IgA1 and IgA2 subsets are decreased in IBD *(36)*. T cells and macrophages also have an exaggerated response to antigen exposure in IBD. Once activated, they are important in recruiting nonspecific inflammatory cells, especially neutrophils, which are ultimately involved in tissue damage. IL-1, IL-6, and tumor necrosis factor-α (TNF-α) are increased in the mucosa but not the sera of patients with IBD. However, the balance of different cytokines differs in UC and CD, which likely accounts for differences in phenotypic expression. CD appears to have a predominantly Th1 cytokine profile, including interferon-γ (IFN-γ), IL-2, IL-12, and TNF-α *(20,37)*. Autoantibodies have been found that correspond to disease type but not severity. For example, perinuclear antineutrophil cytoplasmic antibodies (p-ANCAs) are prevalent in 80% of patients with UC *(38)*. However, p-ANCAs are also present in some patients with left-sided colonic CD *(39)*. Anti-*Saccharomyces cerevisiae* antibodies (ASCA) are more commonly found in patients with CD *(40)*. The role of these antibodies in disease pathogenesis is yet to be determined.

The final result of T cell, macrophage, and neutrophil activation is the production of cytokines, growth factors, antibodies, nitric oxide, proteases, and reactive oxygen species. The activation of the arachidonic acid pathway leads to prostaglandins, thromboxanes and lipo-oxygenases, and platelet activating factor. All of these contribute to tissue destruction and are potential targets for anti-inflammatory therapy.

5. DIAGNOSIS

Crohn's colitis may be difficult to distinguish from UC. Diarrhea, rectal bleeding, urgency, and/or tenesmus are symptoms common to both conditions. Features that may help separate the two include other clinical manifestations, endoscopic findings and possibly smoking status (see Table 1).

Perianal disease is a major distinguishing feature between Crohn's colitis and UC. Perianal symptoms and signs are distinctly uncommon in UC, so much so that their presence suggests CD. Perianal manifestations can be categorized as skin lesions, anal canal lesions, and fistulae. Perianal CD is most commonly associated with colonic rather than small bowel disease. The prospective NCCDS documented 46.7% of colonic CD patients to have perianal disease compared to 25.5% of small bowel only CD, with an intermediate value of 41.4% for ileocolonic CD *(42)*. Other studies have shown that in the setting of colonic disease, the risk of developing fistulae is approx 20%, with perianal fistulae being the most common type *(9,43)*.

Another distinguishing feature is rectal sparing, which is common in CD but rare in UC (except occasionally after topical treatment). The typical endoscopic features of focal, apht-hous, linear, and irregularly shaped ulcerations with intervening spared (normal) mucosa may be obscured by a diffuse, continuous pattern of colitis that is indistinguishable from UC in 10–20% of patients who are categorized as having an indeterminate colitis. Mucosal biopsies may demonstrate transmural disease, paradoxical deep lymphocytic inflammation with relative epithelial sparing, or granulomas. However, the histologic features may also be indeterminate, particularly in severe disease.

6. DIFFERENTIAL DIAGNOSIS

The differential diagnosis for diarrhea and rectal bleeding is extensive, but typically, the inflammatory nature of the symptoms is confirmed by the presence of fecal leukocytes. Inflammatory diarrheas can be further classified as infectious or noninfectious. Infectious colitis may be caused by invasive bacteria including *Salmonella*, *Shigella*, *Campylobacter*, and invasive and hemorrhagic *Escherichia coli*. These should be excluded by stool culture at the time of initial presentation with bloody diarrhea, fever and fecal leukocytes, and with new flare-ups of known IBD. Most of these are acute and self-limited as opposed to the more chronic and insidious presentation that is more typical of IBD. Colitis caused by *Clostridium difficile* or *Entamoeba histolytica* should also be excluded in the appropriate clinical situations. Noninfectious inflammatory diarrheas include those caused by IBD, microscopic colitis, radiation enterocolitis, and miscellaneous conditions including Behcet's syndrome, eosinophilic gastro-enteritis, graft vs host disease, Churg-Strauss, and Cronkhite-Canada syndrome *(44)*. Drug-induced colitis, particularly nonsteroidal anti-inflammatory drugs (NSAID)-induced colitis is more common than CD and can also mimic clinical and endoscopic features of IBD.

Table 1
Key Distinguishing Features of CD and UC

Feature	CD	UC
History:		
Smoking status	Smoker.	Nonsmoker or exsmoker.
Symptoms	Diarrhea, abdominal pain, weight loss, nausea, vomiting.	Rectal bleeding, cramps.
Physical examination	Perianal skin tags, fistulas, abscesses, abdominal mass.	Normal perianal findings, no abdominal mass.
Studies:		
Endoscopy	Rectal sparing; focal ulceration with normal intervening mucosa; aphthous, linear, or stellate ulcers; terminal ileum inflamed with aphthous or linear ulcers.	Rectal involvement; continuous superficial inflammation with granular, friable mucosa; terminal ileum normal or with backwash ileitis; periappendiceal red patch.
Radiology	Focal, asymmetric, transmural ulceration; strictures, inflammatory masses, fistulas; small bowel disease.	Diffuse, continuous superficial ulceration; ahaustral (lead pipe) colon; backwash ileitis.
Histology	Focal inflammation, aphthous ulcers, lymphoid aggregates, transmural inflammation, granulomas (15–30% of patients).	Diffuse, continuous, superficial inflammation; crypt architectural deformity.
Serology	ASCA positive (approx 30% of patients).	p-ANCA positive (60–80% of patients).

Adapted from ref. *41*.

The most important noninflammatory diarrhea in the differential of CD is irritable bowel syndrome, which is by far the most common cause of chronic alterations in bowel function and diarrhea. The presence of fecal leukocytes or occult blood excludes this diagnosis. Other noninflammatory diarrheas include medication and hormone-induced causes.

The differential diagnosis of frank or occult rectal bleeding includes hemorrhoids, diverticula, neoplasms, and ischemic colitis. The patient's age group often points to a specific etiology. Younger patients presenting with hematochezia often have hemorrhoids or anal fissures. The presence of perianal symptoms in a young individual should raise the suspicion of underlying CD that may not manifest subsequent clinical features for many years. Colonic adenomas and cancer must be considered in patients over 50 yr old. Ischemic colitis, often exacerbated by the use of NSAIDs or the presence of concomitant cardiac or vascular disease, also is a consideration in the elderly. Diverticular hemorrhage is usually profuse and painless. Endoscopic examination can help distinguish all of these conditions.

7. CLINICAL PRESENTATIONS

CD is diagnosed based on clinical, endoscopic, radiologic, and histologic criteria. There is no pathognomonic finding. The key history, physical, and laboratory findings help guide further workup. To date, there is no single reliable laboratory marker to assess disease activity, risk of recurrence, or responsiveness to specific therapies (*45,46*). An emerging possibility that requires further study is calprotectin, a neutrophilic calcium-binding protein. Calprotectin is measured in stool and has been reported to have a sensitivity and specificity of 90 and 83%, respectively, for active IBD, making it clinically feasible and useful *(47)*. However, this would not distinguish between UC and CD. In distinction to the more continuous superficial inflammation in UC, CD is more "focal" and is not necessarily limited to the colon. Because CD may affect portions of the gastrointestinal tract from mouth to anus, it has a greater spectrum of presentations than UC. Like UC, the location and pattern of inflammation tend to remain constant for an individual, but may progress *(48)*. The inflammation of CD may vary from a superficial inflammation, similar to that in UC, to transmural disease, with formation of fibrostenosing strictures, fistula, and inflammatory masses and abscesses *(49)*. Unlike UC, surgery for CD is generally not curative and, in fact, is often followed by recurrence at and proximal to surgical anastomoses *(50)*. However, total colectomy and end-ileostomy may be curative in some cases of CD confined to the colon.

CD can present with chronic symptoms that include: abdominal cramping, often postprandial; diarrhea; nocturnal bowel movements; rectal bleeding; anemia; and constitutional symptoms of fevers, night sweats and weight loss. Nausea and vomiting may accompany intestinal strictures with partial or complete small bowel obstructions. Transmural disease manifests as right lower quadrant masses or perianal skin tags, fistulas, or abscesses.

Ileocecal CD may mimic appendicitis acutely and often presents as right lower quadrant pain and tenderness, diarrhea with or without rectal bleeding, weight loss, fevers, chills, and night sweats.

CD confined to the colon can be divided into proctitis, distal colitis (distal to the splenic flexure), and extensive colitis (extending into and beyond the transverse colon). Patients with proctitis tend to have symptoms of rectal bleeding, urgency, and tenesmus, but often have a more benign course compared to those with more extensive colitis *(51)*. Patients with distal or left-sided colitis are more likely to have diarrhea and weight loss, accompanying symptoms of rectal bleeding, urgency, and tenesmus. They may also have fever and an inflammatory mass. Rarely, patients may present with colonic perforations. Extensive or total colitis more often induces diarrhea, with or without blood, depending on the severity of the disease. Weight loss and malaise are common. Obstructive features are less common in patients with colonic CD than those with small bowel disease. However, because of the transmural nature of CD, there may be associated serositis that induces abdominal pain and tenderness. If the disease is patchy or segmental, the distinction between CD and UC is not difficult. However, when the disease involves the entire colon, other features are relied upon. If a patient presents with perianal manifestations or involvement of other areas of the GI tract, distinction from UC is apparent *(52)*. Toxic megacolon and associated risk of perforation are complications of severe colitis associated with either form of IBD *(53,54)*.

Extraintestinal manifestations are more common in patients with colonic involvement in IBD than in patients with small bowel CD alone. Certain manifestations such as large joint arthritis, erythema nodosum and amyloidosis are more common in Crohn's colitis. Other eye (i.e. uveitis and iritis), joint (i.e. ankylosing spondylitis), skin (i.e. pyoderma gangrenosum) and oral manifestations are present in both UC and Crohn's colitis and are therefore not helpful in distinguishing the two *(55)*.

8. ENDOSCOPY IN DIAGNOSIS

Patients presenting with chronic diarrhea, rectal bleeding, and other symptoms consistent with IBD, including weight loss, abdominal pain, and rectal urgency, may be initially evaluated with an unprepped sigmoidoscopy on their very first visit. With active colitis, there is rarely significant stool in the involved lumen to impede the exam. This test may provide invaluable information and help distinguish the type of bowel disease, guiding early therapy. Colonoscopy is the best means of diagnosing colonic CD and should be performed when the patient is clinically able to tolerate the procedure. Aggressive colonoscopy is contraindicated in severe colitis, and endoscopy should be limited to sigmoidoscopy without prep and with minimal air insufflation. Rectal sparing and patchy or asymmetric involvement are signs of CD and contrast with the contiguous superficial erosions and granularity that begin in the rectum in UC *(56)*. Biopsies should be taken in endoscopically inflamed and uninvolved areas for pathologic analysis, as it is not unusual to identify histologic changes of CD in uninvolved rectum or colon *(57)*. Typical features of CD include aphthous, linear, serpiginous, and other irregularly shaped ulcerations. A study by Pera et al. *(56)* including 606 colonoscopies in 357 patients with UC, CD, or indeterminant colitis, found colonoscopy to be 89% accurate in diagnosis with 4% errors and 7% indeterminate interpretations, most often in the setting of severe inflammation. Findings of discontinuous disease, anal lesions, and cobblestoning (deep linear ulcerations that undermine patches of normal mucosal) were predictive of CD *(58)*. In contrast, erosions, micro-ulcers and granularity were more predictive of UC *(56)*. The ileocecal valve is often patulous in UC, whereas it may be deformed, strictured, and difficult to enter in CD. When possible, the terminal ileum should be intubated, visualized, and biopsied. The ileum is usually normal in UC, but may have "backwash ileitis" consisting of diffuse, continuous, superficial erosions. In CD, ileitis is manifest by lumenal narrowing and associated aphthous or linear ulceration. A patch of inflammation around the appendix ("peri-appendiceal" or "cecal" red patch) with otherwise normal appearing mucosa to the distal colon, while demonstrating "focality" in the colon, is more indicative of UC than CD.

Strictures are present more often in CD than in UC and may preclude evaluation of the proximal bowel. Inflammatory strictures are erythematous, friable, and ulcerated. Thin and short strictures characterize fibrotic strictures *(59)*. Dysplastic or malignant strictures are also more likely to be short, but typically occur in patients with disease of longer duration *(60)*. Biopsies should be obtained from the stricture edge and from within the stricture to rule out neoplasia. If unable to definitely enter the lesion, cytology brushings may be obtained *(59)*. Pseudopolyps arising from re-epithelialized granulation tissue can occur in both CD and UC. These do not have neoplastic potential, but may be difficult to distinguish from adenomatous polyps without biopsy.

9. RADIOLOGY IN DIAGNOSIS

Air contrast barium radiographs are an acceptable means of diagnosing colonic CD and defining intestinal complications such as strictures or fistulae. However, similar to endoscopic disease, radiographic changes do not correlate well with clinical severity. Patients with "burnt out", asymptomatic disease may have severe radiographic changes. Holdstock et al. compared findings on barium enema, colonoscopy, and histology and found that of 149 patients, 15% had total colitis by barium enema, 34% by colonoscopy, and 62% by histology *(61)*. These findings point out both that colonoscopy is more sensitive than barium enemia, and that histology is still the gold standard. Despite the decreased sensitivity of radiographic studies, they are reported to be 95% accurate in distinguishing CD and UC *(62)*. Barium contrast studies are more useful than endoscopy in assessing certain clinical questions. Specifically, single contrast barium studies are best at identifying fistulous tracts and strictures. Air insufflation combined with barium contrast, also called double-contrast, is superior at demonstrating mucosal detail, including granularity and ulceration, than single-contrast barium studies. Typical features of Crohn's colitis include patchy or right-sided only involvement or associated small bowel or perianal disease, with or without fistulous tracts. Other specific features of colonic Crohn's include aphthous, serpiginous, linear, and cobblestoning ulceration. Pseudodiverticula form proximal to strictures and represent the asymmetric mural involvement *(63)*. Similar to colonoscopic examinations, barium enemas are relatively contraindicated in severe colitis due to the risk of inducing toxic megacolon *(64,65)*. Barium sinography or "fistulograms" can be used for evaluation of fistulous tracts with cutaneous communications.

Plain films of the abdomen can demonstrate dilatation of the small and large bowel and air fluid levels, such as in partial or complete small bowel obstruction and toxic megacolon. Thumbprinting of the walls may also be seen, indicating ischemia. After plain films, ultrasound often is used as an early imaging modality in undiagnosed patients. It may help to rule out appendicitis in patients with right lower quadrant pain. Ultrasound can also visualize abscesses, and distended or thickened bowel loops, and may be able to differentiate CD from UC based upon the thickness of the colonic wall *(63)*.

Computed tomagraphy (CT) scan with oral and intravenous (IV) contrast provide additional and complementary information to barium studies. In particular, CT scanning can assess extra-colonic complications such as abscess, inflammatory mass, or ureteral obstruction. Magnetic resonance imaging (MRI) has been found to be useful in the assessment of perianal abscesses and fistulous tracts, especially those with complex communications to the pelvic floor and anal sphincter *(66)*.

Nuclear medicine-tagged leukocyte scanning may be helpful in distinguishing the patchy, segmental nature of Crohn's colitis from UC in a noninvasive way. Nuclear medicine scans will not help distinguish other causes of inflammation of the bowel from IBD *(63)*.

10. HISTOLOGY

Histology also contributes to the diagnosis of CD, but is often nonspecific in the absence of granulomas. Histological features are discussed in detail in Chapter 17. Other than the focal and asymmetric nature of the colonic involvement, the important distinguishing features of CD include: aphthous ulceration, transmural inflammation, serositis, microscopic fissuring and submucosal lymphedema, and fibrosis. In the absence of rare infectious causes, i.e., *Chlamydia trachomatis*, syphilis or lymphogranuloma venereum, non-caseating granulomas are essentially pathognomonic for Crohn's *(67)*; however, they are only present in approx 30–50% of biopsies and are not required for the diagnosis *(68)*. In addition, biopsies are useful to diagnose dysplasia or cancer in the setting of CD. Similar to patients with UC, the risk of dysplasia and/or cancer in CD is related to disease extent and duration. This necessitates entering patients with long-standing CD into similar surveillance colonoscopy programs to those recommended for UC. In a study of 259 patients with Crohn's colitis of 8 yr or longer, dysplasia or cancer was detected in 16% and was associated with age over 45 yr. Interestingly, despite a negative screening colonoscopy, progression to dysplasia or cancer was noted in 22% of patients by the fourth subsequent colonoscopy performed at 2-yr intervals *(69)*.

On gross exam (either at laparotomy or assessing resected specimens), the transmural nature of CD is appreciated with inflammatory changes from the mucosa to the serosa manifested by hyperemia of the serosa and "creeping" serosal or mesenteric fat. Submucosal fibrosis, deep fissuring, and fistulizing ulcerations are present with associated communicating tracts into the mesentery, bowel, and other organs, including bladder and vagina.

11. MEDICAL TREATMENT

Medical management is based on disease location (extent of colonic involvement and presence or absence of small bowel or perianal involvement in the case of CD) and severity of symptoms (remission, mild-moderate, moderate- severe, or severe-fulminant). Clinical remission refers to patients who are asymptomatic or who have responded to acute medical treatment without respect to endoscopic or radiographic findings. Patients who are steroid-dependent are not considered to be in remission. Mild–moderate CD defines patients that are ambulatory and tolerating an oral diet, but may have symptoms of diarrhea, bleeding, or crampy abdominal pain without dehydration, high fevers, abdominal tenderness, painful mass, obstruction, or significant weight loss. Moderate–severe disease is characterized by patients who have failed treatment for mild–moderate disease or those with more severe symptoms of loose stools, rectal bleeding, fever, abdominal cramps, pain or tenderness, intermittent nausea or vomiting (without obstruction), weight loss, or anemia. Severe–fulmi-nant disease applies to patients who have failed outpatient management with steroids or those presenting with high fever, persistent vomiting, intestinal obstruction, peritoneal signs, cachexia, or abdominal abscess *(70)*.

Prior to the initiation of medical therapy, factors that may be contributing to exacerbations of disease should be sought and corrected. These include concurrent medications such as NSAIDs or antibiotics, infections such as *C. difficile*, and changes in diet or lifestyle (includ-ing changes in smoking habits). In addition, manifestations of malnutrition, including caloric and nutrient deficiencies, anemia, and fluid and electrolyte imbalances, should be evaluated and treated. Malnutrition may be multifactorial and is most commonly caused by anorexia or the patient's attempt to avoid inducing symptoms. Often, an overly restrictive diet is self-imposed or encouraged by physicians. As there has been no clearly defined dietary etiology of CD, only foods that definitely correlate with symptoms should be avoided. In patients with previously diagnosed and treated disease, response to prior interventions is a critical deter-minant of subsequent therapy. The principles of management require a long-term approach to treatment, starting with therapy to induce clinical remissions followed by maintenance to prevent relapse. The current armamentarium includes conventional approaches with either mucosal anti-inflammatory properties (i.e., aminosalicylates) or systemic anti-inflammatory agents (i.e., corticosteroids). In contrast to treatment for UC, patients with mild–moderate CD often respond to antibiotic therapy. Immunomodulatory therapy with azathioprine (AZA) and 6-mercaptopurine (6-MP) has been useful in both UC and CD, whereas, methotrexate (MTX) has been more effective in CD. Most recently, anti-cytokine (anti-TNF) therapy has revolu-tionized the treatment of refractory CD (see Table 2).

The role of nutritional therapies such as total parenteral nutrition (TPN) and enteral nutrition as primary or adjunctive therapy remain controversial. While both disease activity and fistulae may respond to TPN, they typically recur with resumption of an oral diet *(72)*. Enteral feedings have been less efficacious than the combination of steroids and sulfasalazine and are, therefore, also not useful as primary therapy in most adults. However, enteral feedings with polymeric and elemental diets do have less inherent risks and are less expensive than TPN and, therefore, may be the preferred method of nutritional supplementation and adjunctive therapy, particu-larly in children wishing to avoid steroids *(72)*.

12. MILD–MODERATE CROHN'S COLITIS

Sulfasalazine has been efficacious for treatment of mild–moderate Crohn's colitis. It is inexpensive and tolerated by most patients. Unfortunately, the sulfapyridine moiety, a carrier for 5-aminosalicylic acid (5-ASA) delivery into the colon, is responsible for dose-related side effects (e.g., nausea, vomiting, anorexia, dyspepsia, and headaches) and hypersensitivity reac-tions that can include rash, fever, hemolytic anemia, agranulocytosis, and pancreatitis. The formulation of 5-ASA (mesalamine) compounds, without the sulfapyridine moiety, has allowed targeted delivery of the mucosally active mesalamine moiety directly to affected areas. Delayed

Table 2
Management of CD

Disease activity	Medication	Dose	Response range
Mild-Moderate	Sulfasalazine	3–6 g/d	38–62%
	5-ASA (mesalamine)	1.5–4.8 g/d	43–64%
	Metronidazole	10–20 mg/kg/d	67–95%
	Ciprofloxacin	1000–1500 mg/d	
Moderate–Severe	Corticosteroids	Prednisone 0.25–0.75 mg/kg/d orally (usual starting dose = 40 mg)	60–78%
		IV methylprednisolone 40–60 mg/d	
	Budesonide	9 mg/d	51–53%
Severe–Fulminant	Corticosteroids	Methylprednisolone 40–60 mg/d IV	60–78%
	Cyclosporin added to corticosteroids	2–5 mg/kg/d (usually 4 mg/kg/d)	60–80%
Fistulae	Metronidazole	20 mg/kg	Up to 95%
	Ciprofloxacin and metronidazole	1000–1500 mg ciprofloxacin 500–1500 mg metronidazole	86%
	6-Mercaptopurine (6-MP) or azathioprine (AZA)	1.5 mg/kg/d 6-MP or 2.5 mg/kg/d AZA	55%
	Infliximab	5 mg/kg at 0, 2, 6 wk	68%
	Cyclosporine	4 mg/kg/d IV followed by 6–8 mg/kg/d PO	88%
Maintenance	Sulfasalazine	1–3 g/d	62–87%
	5-ASA	1.5–3g/d	44–75%
	AZA/6-MP	2.5 mg/kg/d (AZA) or 1.5 mg/kg/d (6-MP)	54–100%
	Infliximab	5–10 mg/kg IV q 8 wk	53%
Steroid-dependent	Azathioprine	2.5 mg/kg/d	36–91%
	6-Mercaptopurine	1.5 mg/kg/d	36–91%
	Infliximab	5 mg/kg infusion—response for approx 8 wk	81%
	Methotrexate	25 mg/wk for 16 wk then 15 mg/wk	39–54%

Abbreviationa: IV, intravenously; PO, orally; q every.
Adapted, in part from ref. *71*.

pH-release formulations, such as Asacol, and sustained-release mesalamine, Pentasa, both deliver large proportions of mesalamine to the colon.

The National Cooperative and European Cooperative Crohn's Disease trials demonstrated the benefits of sulfasalazine for mild–moderate CD involving the colon. While sulfasalazine was not as efficacious as corticosteroid therapy, a significant number of patients could be treated without inducing steroid-related side effects. The NCCDS showed sulfasalazine at

1 g/15 kg/d for 17 wk to be superior to placebo in active Crohn's colitis. However, patients previously treated with steroids were less likely to respond to sulfasalazine. Mesalamine at over 3 g/d also has been shown to be effective in active CD *(73)*. Antibiotic therapy with metronidazole at 750 mg to 2 g/d or ciprofloxacin at 1 g/day has been shown to be comparable in efficacy to sulfasalazine in mild–moderate Crohn's colitis or ileocolitis *(74,75)*. In combination, ciprofloxacin and metronidazole, were comparable to methylprednisolone in efficacy in one trial *(76)*. In addition, evidence is mounting for the usefulness of these antibiotics to treat perianal disease *(77,78)*.However, despite theories for the potential of a mycobacterial etiology of CD, antimycobacterial therapies have not been proven useful *(79)*.

The U.S. Food and Drug Administration has recently approved a new corticosteroid, Budesonide, for the treatment of mild–moderate CD of the ileum and ascending colon. This corticosteroid has 90% first pass hepatic metabolism. The daily dose of 9 mg of Budesonide has been shown to be more effective than treatment with mesalamine, but this new corticosteroid is not approved for long-term maintenance therapy of CD.

13. MODERATE–SEVERE CROHN'S COLITIS

Patients with moderate–severe disease, and those who fail to respond to an aminosalicylate or antibiotic, are treated with oral corticosteroids, generally prescribed at a dose equivalent to 20–60 mg of prednisone/d. The usual starting dose is 40 mg/d until remission is achieved, with subsequent tapering by 5–10 mg/wk until 20 mg, followed by tapering by 2.5–5 mg/wk depending on the time required to induce remission. Recently, a rapidly metabolized "nonsystemic" steroid, budesonide, delivered as a controlled ileal release formulation, has been demonstrated to be nearly as efficacious as systemic steroids for patients with CD of the right colon. A dose ranging study found the 9 mg dose to be optimal, with 51% of patients given 9 mg daily for 8 wk achieving clinical remission with CD activity index (CDAI) of <150, compared to 20% of patients receiving placebo *(80)*. In another study, 53% of patients treated with budesonide over 10 wk achieved clinical remission vs 66% of patients treated with prednisolone, however the mean decrease in CDAI was from 275 to 175 in the budesonide group and 279 to 136 in the prednisolone group *(81)*. These studies also showed that budesonide did cause a significant suppression of the pituitary–adrenal axis, though not to the same extent as systemic corticosteroids *(81)*. In addition, budesonide delays time to relapse, but does not maintain remission at 1 yr *(82)*. For patients with systemic manifestations of CD, corticosteroids remain the benchmark therapy to induce clinical remissions, but have not been effective in maintenance of remission *(83)*.

Most recently, infliximab has been available for treatment of CD that has not responded to other medical therapies. In several trials, response rates of up to 80% have been observed with successful tapering of steroids. The ultimate positioning of infliximab for treatment of CD remains to be established. The clinical utility for treatment of fistulae, steroid-dependent disease, and maintenance of remission is discussed below.

14. SEVERE OR FULMINANT DISEASE

Failing outpatient therapy, patients require hospitalization to receive IV steroids at an equivalent dose to methylprednisolone 32–48 mg/d in divided doses or as a continuous infusion. In patients with abdominal tenderness or mass, steroids should be started after an abscess has been excluded with abdominal ultrasound or CT. Patients with significant malnutrition may require parenteral nutrition as a supplement or with bowel rest. As alluded to above, elemental diets have been used effectively as monotherapy in severe disease, but are not effective long-term and are logistically difficult for most patients. Patients with sepsis or signs of toxic megacolon should be treated with IV antibiotics and may require emergent colectomy. Patients responding to IV steroids should usually be started on immunomodulators before steroids are tapered because of their delayed efficacy.

When Crohn's colitis is not responsive to IV steroids within 5–7 d, cyclosporine (CSA) may be given in addition to steroids in an attempt to prevent colectomy. The calcineurin inhibitors CSA and tacrolimus (FK-506) selectively act on T cells in their role as immunosuppressants. Uncontrolled series have reported responses in 60–80% of patients when treated with IV CSA at 2–5 mg/kg/d as a continuous infusion (84). Monitoring for nephrotoxicity with or without hypertension and lowered seizure threshold, especially in the setting of low cholesterol levels, is important. Low dose oral CSA has been ineffective for maintenance (85,86). FK-506 has better absorption than CSA, even in diseased small bowel. In an open-label study of FK-506 in steroid refractory patients, there was a decline in CDAI in 11 of 13 patients, decrease in hospitalization and closure of fistulas in three of six patients. FK-506 was dosed at 0.1–0.2 mg/kg/d to achieve levels of 5–10 ng/mL (87).

15. MANAGEMENT OF FISTULIZING CD

Most of the medications used in CD have been tried for fistulizing disease, but have failed to demonstrate that sulfasalazine, mesalamine, or corticosteroids have any significant benefit. It has been proposed that corticosteroids may actually worsen outcomes, leading to the need for surgery or even death in the setting of fistula with abscess (88,89). In contrast, metronidazole, at a dose of 20 mg/kg has been efficacious in uncontrolled trials, with up to 95% partial response rate and 56% of patients with complete closure of fistulas (90). However, several trials have shown that fistulas reopen within 6 mo of stopping metronidazole. In addition, side effects limit long-term use. The combination of ciprofloxacin and metronidazole has also been useful. Therapy with 1000–1500 mg of ciprofloxacin combined with 500–1500 mg of metronidazole over 12 wk resulted in improvement in 9 of 14 patients, and three additional patients had complete healing. However, nine of these patients required ongoing therapy for durable responses (91).

The immunomodulators AZA and 6-MP have also been utilized to treat fistulizing CD. In one controlled trial 31% of patients had a complete response rate, and 24% had a partial response to 6-MP (92). In a follow-up study, five of seven patients who discontinued therapy had fistulas that reopened, but were successfully closed again with resumption of 6-MP at doses of 1.5 mg/kg (93). Data on the utility of MTX for fistulae has been published in abstract form and showed a closure rate of 25% and a partial response rate of 31% (94). A series of 16 patients treated with IV CSA showed a 44% complete closure rate and a 44% partial response rate with a mean time to response of only 7.4 d. Nine of ten patients that had not responded to immunomodulators responded to CSA, however many patients relapse when oral CSA is discontinued (95,96). Thus, CSA can be used as a means of rapid induction of fistula healing followed by long-term immunomodulator therapy. FK-506 has been used with limited success in closing fistulas, and a controlled series is underway.

In addition to its utility in active moderate–severe ileocolonic CD, infliximab has been found to be very beneficial in fistulizing CD. TNF-α up-regulates pro-inflammatory molecules including IL-1, nitric oxide, metalloproteinases, and adhesion molecules (97). Infliximab, a chimeric anti-TNF-α monoclonal IgG1 antibody, has the potential to bind and neutralize soluble TNF-α, induce lysis of TNF-α-expressing cells, and apoptosis of activated T cells (98,99). When treated with 5 mg/kg at 0, 2, and 6 wk, 55% of patients closed all their fistulas, and 68% of patients had a partial response compared to 13 and 26% in placebo-treated patients, respectively. Median time to response was 14 d, and duration of response was 3 mo, just as in active CD at other sites. Other anti-TNF therapies, including CDP-571 and thalidomide, have a more modest effect.

The general approach to fistulae involves an evaluation of whether associated abscess is present, which would require percutaneous or surgical drainage, the anatomy and type of fistula, internal or external, whether it is symptomatic, and the general state of the patient (including surgical candidacy). If no abscess is present, if the fistula drains externally, or if only a small internal fistula is present, antibiotic therapy with metronidazole with or without ciprofloxacin is a reasonable first line therapy. Failing antibiotics, immunomodulators or infliximab, either alone or in combination should be used next. CSA, with its inherent toxicities, and other experimental therapies may be tried. However, if fistulae remain symptomatic, surgery should be considered. Surgical therapy is especially important in perirectal fistula and abscesses. Setons placed to allow drainage as well as sphincter-saving surgery are important approaches.

16. MAINTENANCE OF REMISSION AND STEROID-SPARING THERAPIES

Although of potential benefit for maintaining remissions in patients responding to mesalamine *(100)*, for patients who require steroids for induction, aminosalicylates have not been effective in preventing relapse *(101)*. In contrast, patients whose symptoms increase as steroids are tapered (steroid-dependent) or in those who still do not achieve remission (steroid-refractory), the immunomodulators AZA and 6-MP are effective steroid-sparing and maintenance therapies *(102,103)*. However, the purine antimetabolites require up to 17 wk, or more, to obtain maximal clinical benefits *(104)*. AZA can be started at 50 mg/d and gradually increased, or immediately at 2–2.5 mg/kg/d. 6-MP, is started at 50 mg/d or dosed at 1–1.5 mg/kg/d. White blood counts should be monitored initially at 2-wk intervals and are used to adjust the dose to reduce the leukocyte count at or just above, 3–6000. Recently, the ability to monitor 6-MP metabolites has been used by some groups to guide dosing *(105)*. In any event, the complete blood count (CBC) should be monitored, at minimum, on a quarterly basis to avoid the potential of delayed leukopenia and the inherent risks of bone marrow suppression.

MTX has been shown to be effective for the treatment of steroid-dependent CD and as a maintenance agent for patients who have responded to MTX after steroids have been tapered. Treatment with 25 mg, either intramuscularly or subcutaneously/wk for 16 wk can be followed by 15 mg/wk for maintenance *(106,107)*. MTX has generally been found to be more efficacious when given parenterally, in contrast to oral formulations. Monitoring of blood counts and liver enzymes is required.

The development of an antibody to TNF-α, infliximab, has heralded a new era of targeted treatment in moderate and sometimes severe, steroid-dependent or refractory CD. A randomized controlled trial has shown that clinical response was maximal (81% of patients) at a dose of 5 mg/kg and that clinical remission occurred in 33% of patients compared to 4% of patients given placebo. The average duration of response after an initial infusion is variable between patients, but averages approx 8 wk. Retreatment of patients at 8-wk intervals with 10 mg/kg prolongs clinical remission to at least 44 wk in 53% of infliximab vs 20% of placebo-treated patients *(108)*. Concurrent immunomodulator therapy with AZA, 6-MP, or MTX seems to improve response *(109)* and protect against infusion reactions mediated by human antichimeric antibodies (HACA's) *(110,111)*. Retreatment at <12-wk intervals seems to prevent delayed hypersensitivity serum sickness-like reactions that occur in some patients. We have also demonstrated that infliximab therapy has long-term (12–24 mo) steroid-sparing benefits *(112)*. Infliximab has been associated with risks of opportunistic infections and tuberculosis, drug-induced lupus, and, rarely, demyelinating disorders *(111)*.

17. SURGICAL TREATMENT

The most common indications for surgery are disease refractory to medical therapy or medication side effects, including those due to steroid dependence. Up to two-thirds of patients with CD eventually require surgery at some point in their lives. Patients with unresponsive fulminant disease, failing 7–10 d of intensive inpatient management, are surgical candidates. Other reasons for surgery include intractable hemorrhage, perforation, or persistent or recurring obstruction or fistula causing malnutrition or decreased quality of life. Patients with abscesses that cannot be drained percutaneously also require surgical debridement.

Surgical therapy will be covered in more detail in Chapter 32 by Drs. Muldoon and Stryker.

18. INVESTIGATIONAL THERAPIES

As the complex interactions of the systemic and mucosal immune system in health and disease unfold, additional potential targets for therapy in IBD emerge. CDP-571 is an anti-TNF-α monoclonal antibody composed of 95% human and only 5% murine sequences, which may make it less immunogenic than infliximab. CDP-571 only neutralizes TNF-α, but does not fix complement or have antibody-mediated cytotoxicity .(110) Several preliminary studies of CDP-571 are promising for the treatment of chronically active and steroid-dependent CD *(113,114)*.

Thalidomide has had a resurgence as a potential therapy in several diseases, including CD. Thalidomide may be effective not only due to its anti-TNF-α and anti-IL-12 activity, but also due to its antiangiogenic and other properties *(115,116)*. Two preliminary open label studies found efficacy at daily doses of 50–100 mg and 200–300 mg given orally. More than 50% of patients responded by 4 wk and approx two-thirds by 12 wk *(117,118)*. Unfortunately, in addition to teratogenicity, sedation and neuropathy are limiting. Several derivatives of thalidomide with fewer side effects are being studied and are exciting potential therapies *(119)*.

Other cytokines that are potential targets for manipulation include IL-6, IL-11, and IL-12. Signaling caused by IL-6 binding to its receptor seems to trigger gene expression, which leads to resistance to apoptosis in T cells. This may account for disease chronicity and possibly refractoriness to therapy *(46)*. Neutralization of this IL-6 receptor interaction has been studied in several models and seems to suppress experimental colitis comparable to anti-TNF-α effects *(120)*. IL-11 has anti-inflammatory, mucosal protective, and thrombocytopoietic effects. Treatment with subcutaneous rhuIL-11 provided a 42% response rate in active CD in a placebo-controlled study *(121)*. IL-12 is involved in the Th1 pathway of inflammatory response and in IFN-γ production. An anti-IL-12 monoclonal antibody was useful in experimental colitis and may be useful in Crohn's colitis or UC *(122,123)*.

Attempts at broad inhibition of the inflammatory cascade involved in IBD could include blockade of antinuclear factor-κB (NF-κB). NF-κB controls transcription of genes encoding inflammatory cytokines including IL-1, TNF-α, IL-2, IL-6, IL-12, chemokines (IL-8), leukocyte adhesion molecules, and other inflammatory enzymes and acute phase proteins involved in IBD immune dysregulation *(124)*. Antisense oligonucleotide of NF-κB, both as a topical and IV therapy, has been used in experimental models to successfully decrease intestinal inflammation *(125)*.

Intercellular adhesion molecule 1(ICAM-1/CD54) and α_4-integrins are involved in leukocyte migration and activation and have been found to be up-regulated in inflamed CD mucosa *(126)*. A pilot trial of ISIS 2302, an antisense oligonucleotide capable of binding ICAM-1 mRNA, showed encouraging results in CD *(127)*. Antibodies to α_4-integrins are being tested as well.

Matrix metalloproteinases (MMPs) may act as the final common pathway by which T cell activation and cytokines cause intestinal tissue destruction. MMPs both degrade and remodel the extracellular matrix and are, therefore, involved in both wounding and healing in IBD *(128,129)* Modulation of these MMPs may be useful as a therapeutic option in IBD.

Novel methods of delivering drugs, including anti-inflammatory cytokines, antibodies and receptor antagonists to pro-inflammatory cytokines, and antisense oligonucleotides, to inflamed mucosa are being developed *(46,130)*. Viral vectors or bacterial plasmids could encode genes coding for these molecules, which could be delivered directly to the inflamed mucosa. Among others, IL-4 and IL-10 have been delivered by gene transfer, and have been found to be useful in experimental colitis *(131,132)*. These strategies would eliminate side effects due to systemic administration of drugs. In addition, smaller quantities could be used as first pass metabolism could be avoided.

With the knowledge that intestinal antigenic exposure, much of which is via intestinal microflora, has much to do in IBD pathogenesis, much effort is being devoted to understanding these interactions. Probiotic therapy, the delivery of beneficial microbial agents with the aim of altering the enteric flora or even delivering anti-inflammatory molecules, is a very promising area of IBD therapeutic research and is covered in Chapter 10.

Many other drugs, previously used for other diseases, have been, at times fortuitously and counter-intuitively, found to have properties that may make them useful in IBD. Despite being an anticoagulant, heparin, likely due to its anti-inflammatory effects on leukocytes and endothelial cells and epithelial reparative effects, is an interesting therapy for IBD *(133,134)*. Uncontrolled studies of unfractionated and low molecular weight heparins have shown efficacy in UC, and controlled trials are ongoing *(135–137)*. For similar reasons, heparin may be useful in Crohn's colitis as well *(138)*. Growth hormone, combined with a high protein diet, has been found in a short-term study to decrease CD activity and deserves further study *(139)*. Granulocyte colony-stimulating factor (G-CSF), despite increasing neutrophil number and delaying their apoptosis and despite the increased mucosal G-CSF in IBD, has been found to close refractory perianal fistulas *(140,141)*. Peroxisome proliferator-activated receptor (PPAR)-γ ligands used in diabetes, have been found to inhibit inflammation in colonic cells in vitro, seemingly by inhibition of NF-κB *(46,142)*.

19. FUTURE DIRECTIONS

The future of therapy for IBD and specifically Crohn's colitis is bright. As we continue to gain understanding of the etiology and pathogenesis of the diseases, we can more effectively target specific points along the inflammatory cascade. In addition, knowledge of genetic susceptibilities for subtypes of disease may allow targeted and prophylactic therapy. These strategies, along with further basic and clinical research, will undoubtedly bring great rewards in the management of IBD and demand our support. They will allow more effective and less toxic therapy for difficult and chronic IBDs, including Crohn's colitis.

REFERENCES

1. Crohn B, Ginzburg L, and Oppenheimer GD. Regional ileitis, a pathological and clinical entity. *JAMA,* **99** (1932) 1323–1329.
2. Wilks S. *Lectures on Pathological Anatomy.* 1st ed., Longman, et al. (eds.), Lindsay and Blakiston, Philadelphia, PA, 1859.
3. Brooke B. Granulomatous disease of the intestine. *Lancet,* **2** (1959) 745–749.
4. Lockhart-Mummery H, Morson B. Crohn's disease (regional enteritis) of the large intestine and its distinction from ulcerative colitis. *Gut,* **1** (1964) 87–105.
5. Surawicz C. Diagnosing colitis. *Contemp. Intern. Med.,* **3** (1991) 17.

62. Freeny PC. Crohn's disease and ulcerative colitis. Evaluation with double-contrast barium examination and endoscopy. *Postgrad. Med.*, **80** (1986) 139–156.

63. Kadell BM. Radiologic (radiographic) features of ulcerative colitis and Crohn's disease. In *Inflammatory Bowel Disease: From Bench to Bedside*. Targan SR, Shanahan F (eds.), Williams & Wilkinsk, Baltimore, MD, 1994, pp. 366–408.

64. Diner WC, Barnhard HJ. Toxic megacolon. *Semin. Roentgenol.*, **8** (1973) 433–436.

65. Halpert RD. Toxic dilatation of the colon. *Radiol. Clin. N. Am.*, **25** (1987) 147–155.

66. Jenss H, Starlinger M, Skaleij M. Magnetic resonance imaging in perianal Crohn's disease. *Lancet*, **340** (1992) 1286.

67. Surawicz CM. Differential diagnosis of colitis. In *Inflammatory Bowel Disease: From Bench to Bedside*. Targan S, Shanahan F (eds.), Williams & Wilkins, Baltimore, MD, 1994, pp. 409–428.

68. Hawk WA, Turnbull RB, Farmer RG. Regional enteritis of the colon. Distinctive features of the entity. *JAMA*, **201** (1967) 738–746.

69. Friedman S, Rubin PH, Bodian C, Goldstein E, Harpaz N, Present DH. Screening and surveillance colonoscopy in chronic crohn's colitis. *Gastroenterology*, **120** (2001) 820–826.

70. Hanauer SB, Sandborn W. Management of Crohn's disease in adults. *Am. J. Gastroenterol.*, **96** (2001) 635–643.

71. Stein RB, Hanauer SB. Medical therapy for inflammatory bowel disease. *Gastroenterol. Clin. N. Am.*, **28** (1999) 297–321.

72. Plevy SE, Targan SR. Specific management of Crohn's disease. In *Inflammatory Bowel Disease: From Bench to Bedside*. Targan S, Shanahan F (eds.), Williams & Wilkins, Baltimore, MD, 1994, pp. 582–609.

73. Greenfield SM, Punchard NA, Teare JP, Thompson RP. Review article: the mode of action of the aminosalicylates in inflammatory bowel disease. *Aliment. Pharmacol. Ther.*, **7** (1993) 369–383.

74. Ursing B, Alm T, Barany F, et al. A comparative study of metronidazole and sulfasalazine for active Crohn's disease: the cooperative Crohn's disease study in Sweden. II. Result. *Gastroenterology*, **83** (1982) 550–562.

75. Biancone L, Pallone F. Current treatment modalities in active Crohn's disease. *Ital. J. Gastroenterol. Hepatol.*, **31** (1999) 508–514.

76. Prantera C, Zannoni F, Scribano ML, et al. An antibiotic regimen for the treatment of active Crohn's disease: a randomized, controlled clinical trial of metronidazole plus ciprofloxacin. *Am. J. Gastroenterol.*, **91** (1996) 328–332.

77. Brandt LJ, Bernstein LH, Boley SJ, Frank MS. Metronidazole therapy for perineal Crohn's disease: a follow-up study. *Gastroenterology*, **83** (1982) 383–387.

78. Jakobovits J, Schuster MM. Metronidazole therapy for Crohn's disease and associated fistulae. *Am. J. Gastroenterol.*, **79** (1984) 533–540.

79. Borgaonkar M, MacIntosh D, Fardy J, Simms L. Anti-tuberculous therapy for maintaining remission of Crohn's disease. *Cochrane Database Syst. Rev.*, **2** (2000) CD000299.

80. Greenberg GR, Feagan BG, Martin F, et al. Oral budesonide for active Crohn's disease. Canadian Inflammatory Bowel Disease Study Group. *N. Engl. J. Med.*, **331** (1994) 836–841.

81. Rutgeerts P, Lofberg R, Malchaw H, et al. A comparison of budesonide with prednisolone for active Crohn's disease. *N. Engl. J. Med.*, **331** (1994) 842–845.

82. Greenberg GR, Feagan BG, Martin F, et al. Oral budesonide as maintenance treatment for Crohn's disease: a placebo-controlled, dose-ranging study. Canadian Inflammatory Bowel Disease Study Group. *Gastroenterology*, **110** (1996) 45–51.

83. Steinhart AH, Ewe K, Griffiths AM, Modigliani R, Thomsen OO. Corticosteroids for maintaining remission of Crohn's disease. *Cochrane Database Syst. Rev.*, **3** (2000) CD000301.

84. Sandborn W. A critical review of cyclosporine therapy in inflammatory bowel disease. *Inflamm. Bowel Dis.*, **1** (1995) 48–63.

85. Brynskov J, Freund L, Norby Rasmussen S, et al. Final report on a placebo-controlled, double-blind, randomized, multicentre trial of cyclosporin treatment in active chronic Crohn's disease. *Scand. J. Gastroenterol.*, **26** (1991) 689–695.

86. Feagan BG, McDonald JW, Rochon J, et al. Low-dose cyclosporine for the treatment of Crohn's disease. The Canadian Crohn's Relapse Prevention Trial Investigators. *N. Engl. J. Med.*, **330** (1994) 1846–1851.

87. Ierardi E, Principi M, Francavilla R, et al. Oral tacrolimus long-term therapy in patients with Crohn's disease and steroid resistance. *Aliment. Pharmacol. Ther.*, **15** (2001) 371–377.

88. Sparberg M, Kirsner JB. Long-term corticosteroid therapy for regional enteritis: an analysis of 58 courses in 54 patients. *Am. J. Dig. Dis.*, **11** (1966) 865–880.

89. Malchow H, Ewe K, Brandes JW, et al. European Cooperative Crohn's Disease Study (ECCDS): results of drug treatment. *Gastroenterology*, **86** (1984) 249–266.

90. Bernstein LH, Frank MS, Brandt LJ, Boley SJ. Healing of perineal Crohn's disease with metronidazole. *Gastroenterology*, **79** (1980) 599.

91. Solomon M, McLead RS, O'Connor BI, et. al. Combination ciprofloxacin and metronidazole in severe perianal Crohn's disease. *Can. J. Gastroenterol.*, **7** (1993) 571–573.

92. Present DH, Korelitz BI, Wisch N, Glass JL, Sachar DB, Pasternack BS. Treatment of Crohn's disease with 6-mercaptopurine. A long-term, randomized, double-blind study. *N. Engl. J. Med.*, **302** (1980) 981–987.

93. Korelitz BI, Present DH. Favorable effect of 6-mercaptopurine on fistulae of Crohn's disease. *Dig. Dis. Sci.*, **30** (1985) 58–64.

94. Mahadevan U, Marion J, Present D. The place of methotrexate in the treatment of refractory Crohn's disease (abstract). *Gastroenterology*, **112** (1997) A1031.

95. Present DH, Lichtiger S. Efficacy of cyclosporine in treatment of fistula of Crohn's disease. *Dig. Dis. Sci.*, **39** (1994) 374–380.

96. Egan LJ, Sandborn WJ, Tremaine WJ. Clinical outcome following treatment of refractory inflammatory and fistulizing Crohn's disease with intravenous cyclosporine. *Am. J. Gastroenterol.*, **93** (1998) 442–448.

97. Van Deventer SJ. Tumour necrosis factor and Crohn's disease. *Gut*, **40** (1997) 443–448.

98. Van Deventer SJ. Immunotherapy of Crohn's disease. *Scand. J. Immunol.*, **51** (2000) 18–22.

99. Present DH, Rutgeerts P, Targan S, et al., Infliximab for the treatment of fistulas in patients with Crohn's disease. *N. Engl. J. Med.*, **340** (1999) 1398–1405.

100. Hanauer SB, Krawitt EL, Robinson M, Rick GG, Safdi MA. Long-term management of Crohn's disease with mesalamine capsules (Pentasa). Pentasa Crohn's Disease Compassionate Use Study Group [see comments]. *Am. J. Gastroenterol.*, **88** (1993) 1343–1351.

101. Modigliani R, Colombel JF, Dupas JL, et al. Mesalamine in Crohn's disease with steroid-induced remission: effect on steroid withdrawal and remission maintenance, Groupe d'Etudes Therapeutiques des Affections Inflammatoires Digestives. *Gastroenterology*, **110** (1996) 688–693.

102. Korelitz B, Hanauer SB, et al. Postoperative prophylaxis with 6MP, 5-ASA or placebo in Crohn's disease: a 2 year multicenter trial. *Gastroenterology*, **114** (1998) A688.

103. Pearson DC, may GR, Fick G, Sutherland LR. Azathioprine for maintaining remission of Crohn's disease. *Cochrane Database Syst. Rev.*, **2** (2000) CD000067.

104. Sandborn W, Sutherland L, Pearson D, May G, Modigliani R, Prantera C. Azathioprine or 6-mercaptopurine for inducing remission of Crohn's disease. *Cochrane Database Syst. Rev.*, **2** (2000) CD000545.

105. Cuffari C, Theoret Y, Latour S, Seidman G. 6-Mercaptopurine metabolism in Crohn's disease: correlation with efficacy and toxicity. *Gut*, **39** (1996) 401–406.

106. Feagan BG, et al. A comparison of methotrexate with placebo for the maintenance of remission in Crohn's disease. North American Crohn's Study Group Investigators. *N. Engl. J. Med.*, **342** (2000) 1627–1632.

107. Feagan BG, Rochon J, Fedorak RN, et al. Methotrexate for the treatment of Crohn's disease. The North American Crohn's Study Group Investigators. *N. Engl. J. Med.*, **332** (1995) 292–297.

108. Targan SR, Hanauer SB, van Deventer SJ, et al. A short-term study of chimeric monoclonal antibody cA2 to tumor necrosis factor alpha for Crohn's disease. Crohn's Disease cA2 Study Group. *N. Engl. J. Med.*, **337** (1997) 1029–1035.

109. Rutgeerts P, D'Haens G, Targan S, et al. Efficacy and safety of retreatment with anti-tumor necrosis factor antibody (infliximab) to maintain remission in Crohn's disease. *Gastroenterology*, **117** (1999) 761–769.

110. Sandborn WJ, Hanauer SB. Antitumor necrosis factor therapy for inflammatory bowel disease: a review of agents, pharmacology, clinical results, and safety. *Inflamm. Bowel Dis.*, **5** (1999) 119–133.

111. Hanauer SB. Review article: safety of infliximab in clinical trials. *Aliment. Pharmacol. Ther.*, **13(Suppl 4)** (1999) 16–38.

112. Cohen RD, Tsang JF, Hanauer SB. Infliximab in Crohn's disease: first anniversary clinical experience. *Am. J. Gastroenterol.*, **95** (2000) 3469–3477.

113. Sandborn WJ, Feagan BG, hanauer SB, et al. An engineered human antibody to TNF (CDP571) for active Crohn's disease: a randomized double-blind placebo-controlled trial. *Gastroenterology*, **120** (2001) 1330–1338.

114. Stack WA, Mann SD, Roy AJ, et al. Randomised controlled trial of CDP571 antibody to tumour necrosis factor-alpha in Crohn's disease. *Lancet*, **349** (1997) 521–524.

115. Fishman SJ, Feins NR, D'Amoto RJ, Folkman J. Thalidomide for Crohn's disease. *Gastroenterology*, **119** (2000) 596.

116. Sands BE, Podolsky DK. New life in a sleeper: thalidomide and Crohn's disease. *Gastroenterology*, **117** (1999) 1485–1488.

117. Vasiliauskas EA, kam LY, Abreu-Martin MT, et al. An open-label pilot study of low-dose thalidomide in chronically active, steroid-dependent Crohn's disease. *Gastroenterology*, **117** (1999) 1278–1287.

118. Ehrenpreis ED, kane SV, Cohen LB, Cohen RD, Hanaver SB. Thalidomide therapy for patients with refractory Crohn's disease: an open-label trial. *Gastroenterology*, **117** (1999) 1271–1277.

119. Marriott JB, Westby M, Cookson S, et al. CC-3052: a water-soluble analog of thalidomide and potent inhibitor of activation-induced TNF-alpha production. *J. Immunol.*, **161** (1998) 4236–4243.

120. Atreya R, Mudter J, Finotto S, et al. Blockade of interleukin 6 trans signaling suppresses T-cell resistance against apoptosis in chronic intestinal inflammation: evidence in crohn disease and experimental colitis in vivo. *Nat. Med.*, **6** (2000) 583–588.

121. Sands BE, Bank S, Sninsky CA, et al. Preliminary evaluation of safety and activity of recombinant human interleukin 11 in patients with active Crohn's disease. *Gastroenterology*, **117** (1999) 58–64.

122. Neurath MF, Fuss I, Kelsall BL, Stuber E, Strober W. Antibodies to interleukin 12 abrogate established experimental colitis in mice. *J. Exp. Med.*, **182** (1995) 1281–1290.

123. Fuss IJ, Marth T, Neurath MF, Pearlstein GR, Jain A, Strober W. Anti-interleukin 12 treatment regulates apoptosis of Th1 T cells in experimental colitis in mice. *Gastroenterology*, **117** (1999) 1078–1088.

124. Schottelius AJ, Baldwin Jr AS. A role for transcription factor NF-kappa B in intestinal inflammation. *Int. J. Colorectal. Dis.*, **14** (1999) 18–28.

125. Neurath MF, Pettersson S, Meyer zum Buschenfelde KH, Strober W. Local administration of antisense phosphorothioate oligonucleotides to the p65 subunit of NF-kappa B abrogates established experimental colitis in mice. *Nat. Med.*, **2** (1996) 998–1004.

126. Salmi M, Jalkanen S. Molecules controlling lymphocyte migration to the gut. *Gut*, **45** (1999) 148–153.

127. Yacyshyn BR, Chevy WY, Goff J, et al. A placebo-controlled trial of ICAM-1 antisense oligonucleotide in the treatment of Crohn's disease. *Gastroenterology*, **114** (1998) 1133–1142.

128. Pender, S.L., et al., Suppression of T cell-mediated injury in human gut by interleukin 10: role of matrix metalloproteinases. *Gastroenterology*, **115** (1998) 573–583.

129. Pender SL, et al. A major role for matrix metalloproteinases in T cell injury in the gut. *J. Immunol.*, **158** (1997) 1582–1590.

130. Macdonald TT. Viral vectors expressing immunoregulatory cytokines to treat inflammatory bowel disease. *Gut*, **42** (1998) 460–461.

131. Hogaboam CM, Vallance BA, Kumar A, et al., Therapeutic effects of interleukin-4 gene transfer in experimental inflammatory bowel disease. *J. Clin. Invest.*, **100** (1997) 2766–2776.

132. Barbara G, Xing Z, Hogaboam CM, Gauldie J, Collins SM. Interleukin 10 gene transfer prevents experimental colitis in rats. *Gut*, **46** (2000) 344–349.

133. Korzenik JR. IBD: a vascular disorder? The case for heparin therapy. *Inflamm. Bowel Dis.*, **3** (1997) 87–94.

134. Day R, Forbes A. Heparin, cell adhesion, and pathogenesis of inflammatory bowel disease. *Lancet*, **354** (1999) 62–65.

135. Torkvist L, Thorlacius H, Sjoqvist U, et al., Low molecular weight heparin as adjuvant therapy in active ulcerative colitis. *Aliment. Pharmacol. Ther.*, **13** (1999) 1323–1328.

136. Gaffney PR, Doyle CT, Gaffney A, Hogan J, Hayes DP, Annis P. Paradoxical response to heparin in 10 patients with ulcerative colitis. *Am. J. Gastroenterol.*, **90** (1995) 220–223.

137. Evans RC, Wong VS, Morris AI, Rhodes JM. Treatment of corticosteroid-resistant ulcerative colitis with heparin— a report of 16 cases. *Aliment. Pharmacol. Ther.*, **11** (1997) 1037–1040.

138. Katz JA. Medical and surgical management of severe colitis. *Semin. Gastrointest. Dis.*, **11** (2000) 18–32.

139. Slonim AE, Bulone L, Damore MB, Goldberg T, Wingertzahn MA, McKinley MJ. A preliminary study of growth hormone therapy for Crohn's disease. *N. Engl. J. Med.*, **342** (2000) 1633–1637.

140. Ina K, Kusugami K, Hosokawa T, et al., Increased mucosal production of granulocyte colony-stimulating factor is related to a delay in neutrophil apoptosis in Inflammatory Bowel disease. *J. Gastroenterol. Hepatol.*, **14** (1999) 46–53.

141. Vaughan D, Drumm B. Treatment of fistulas with granulocyte colony-stimulating factor in a patient with Crohn's disease. *N. Engl. J. Med.*, **340** (1999) 239–240.

142. Su CG, Wen X, Bailey ST, et al. A novel therapy for colitis utilizing PPAR-gamma ligands to inhibit the epithelial inflammatory response. *J. Clin. Invest.*, **104** (1999) 383–389.

29

Ulcerative Colitis

Bret A. Lashner

CONTENTS

1. INTRODUCTION: EPIDEMIOLOGY

1.1. Incidence and Prevalence

Incident cases of ulcerative colitis are concentrated in the northern hemisphere, especially in the United States, Canada, Northern Europe, Scandinavia, and Israel. The annual incidence of ulcerative colitis ranges from 0.5–6.3/100,000 people depending on the region studied *(1,2)*. The peak age-specific incidence occurs near age 20, and a second smaller peak occurs near age 50. The prevalence of ulcerative colitis ranges from 10–70/100,000 people, but a study from Israel calculates prevalence as high as 167/100,000 people *(3)*. In the U.S., males and females are equally affected, but whites are at much higher risk of developing ulcerative colitis than nonwhites. In Leicester, United Kingdom, South Asian migrants acquire ulcerative colitis at rates of Europeans within the first generation, implying an environmental exposure is important in the pathogenesis of ulcerative colitis *(4)*. Further evidence for an environmental etiology for ulcerative colitis, especially from an exposure at a young age, is the striking variability in mortality among birth cohorts *(5)*.

1.2. Genetic Susceptibility

A genetic predisposition exists for ulcerative colitis. In Israel, Ashkenazi Jews (Eastern European background) have up to six times the risk of Sephardi Jews (Spanish, African, and Middle Eastern backgrounds) despite having similar environmental exposures. Up to 20% of ulcerative colitis patients have a first- or second-degree family member affected with inflammatory bowel disease. The relative risk for a first-degree relative of an ulcerative colitis patient to develop ulcerative colitis is 5.1 *(6)*. The development of ulcerative colitis in spouses is rare. Ulcerative colitis patients with human leukocyte antigen (HLA)-B27 are at risk for developing ankylosing spondylitis or uveitis *(1)*. It is not likely that an environmental agent is the only cause of ulcerative colitis.

From: *Colonic Diseases*
Edited by: T. R. Koch © Humana Press Inc., Totowa, NJ

Perinuclear antineutrophil cytoplasmic antibodies (p-ANCAs) are seen in up to 75% of patients with ulcerative colitis in the U.S. and are very specific for disease *(7)*. Jewish ulcerative colitis patients with primary sclerosing cholangitis have a particularly high rate of p-ANCA positivity. The difference in p-ANCA positivity between ulcerative colitis and Crohn's disease patients make it useful in establishing the diagnosis in the 10% of cases classified as indeterminate colitis. Also, p-ANCAs are associated with chronic pouchitis occurring after total proctocolectomy and ileal pouch–anal anastomosis *(8)*. p-ANCAs were found in 100% of patients with chronic pouchitis, 50% of patients with a pouch but no pouchitis, and 70% of ulcerative colitis patients who had colectomy with ileostomy.

1.3. Environmental Factors

Current adult smokers are less likely than community-based nonsmoking controls to develop ulcerative colitis; former smokers are more likely than controls to develop ulcerative colitis *(9,10)*. Furthermore, former smokers are more likely than never smokers to have severely active disease at the time of diagnosis and be diagnosed at a young age *(11)*. Passive smoking exposure in nonsmoking children increases the risk of ulcerative colitis compared to community-based controls *(12)*. Nicotine, either as chewing gum or a transdermal patch, has been used to treat some nonsmoking ulcerative colitis patients, especially former smokers *(13,14)*. The mechanism of this effect is unknown. Nicotine addiction can be avoided if therapy lasts <8 wk, and maintenance therapy with nicotine patches is not useful *(15)*.

Other possible risk factors for the development of ulcerative colitis are oral contraceptive use, dietary composition, and appendectomy. Three cohort studies have shown a harmful effect of oral contraceptive use on the development of ulcerative colitis, but these findings could not be supported by a case-control studies of incident cases and community-based controls *(16)*. A case-control study demonstrated that high intake of mono- and polyunsaturated fat, as well as vitamin B_6, has been shown to be associated with the development of ulcerative colitis *(17)*. A meta- analysis of 13 case-control studies involving 2770 ulcerative colitis patients showed that appendectomy reduced the risk of developing ulcerative colitis by 69% *(18)*. The reason for this consistent protective effect remains elusive.

2. DIAGNOSIS

2.1. Signs and Symptoms

Typically, ulcerative colitis patients present with rectal bleeding, diarrhea, tenesmus, and abdominal pain. The most commonly used criteria for disease severity assessment of mild, moderate, and severe disease was developed in 1955 by Truelove and Witts (Table 1) *(19)*. Patients with fulminate or toxic colitis usually have more than 10 bowel movements per day, continuous bleeding, abdominal distention and tenderness, radiologic evidence of edema and possibly dilatation, and require transfusions. Since patients with moderate disease according to Truelove and Witts' criteria may have a wide range of symptoms, such a classification is inadequate for clinical trials where objective and sensitive measures of disease activity are required. A combination of endoscopic, histologic, and symptom scores usually is preferred for clinical trials. Objective measures of disease activity in ulcerative colitis, such as indium-labeled white blood cell scanning and fecal α-1-antitrypsin determinations are not sufficiently sensitive or specific to be used in clinical trials.

2.2. Endoscopic Appearances

Active disease in ulcerative colitis is characterized by superficial ulcerations, friability, a distorted mucosal vascular pattern, and exudate. Patients with mildly active disease have

Table 1
Truelove and Witts' Criteria for Assessing Disease Activity
in Ulcerative Colitis (16)

	Mild activity	Severe activity
Daily bowel movements	<5	5
Hematochezia	Small amounts	Large amounts
Temperature	<37.5°C	37.5°C
Pulse	<90/min	90/min
Sedimentation rate	<30 mm/h	30 mm/h
Hemoglobin	>10 g%	10 g%

Patients with some, but not all 6 of the above criteria for severe activity have moderately active disease.

friability, a distorted vascular pattern, and few superficial ulcerations. Patients with moderately active disease often have more ulcerations and worse friability. Patients with severely active disease often have exudate, deep ulcers, and friability that result in spontaneous bleeding. Typical distribution of disease is continuous disease from the rectum proximally. However, patients with partially treated ulcerative colitis may have discontinuous or patchy involvement (20). Histologic features include disease limited to the mucosa and submucosa, mucin depletion, ulcerations, exudate, and crypt abscesses. Ulcerative colitis can be differentiated from Crohn's disease endoscopically by the latter's rectal sparing, discrete "punched-out" or serpiginous ulcerations, aphthoid ulcers (small erosions with no surrounding erythema), cobblestone appearance, and skip areas.

Patients with quiescent disease often demonstrate areas of previous involvement with a distorted vascular pattern and granularity or no abnormality whatsoever. Histology of quiescent disease could show branched crypts, crypt atrophy, and mild expansion of cellular elements in the lamina propria. Chronic changes of ulcerative colitis could include granularity, loss of a mucosal vascular pattern, loss of haustrae with tubularization of the colon, effacement of the ileocecal valve, mucosal bridging, strictures, and pseudopolyps. Pseudopolyps, or inflammatory polyps, are polypoid structures that have only inflammatory cells and no dysplastic epithelium. Mucosal bridges develop from deep connecting ulcers of severely active inflammation. These fragile mucosal bridges may cause bleeding in the absence of an acute flare of ulcerative colitis. True colonic strictures in ulcerative colitis more often than not are neoplastic.

It has been suggested that estimating wall thickness with magnetic resonance imaging with the negative superparamagnetic oral contrast agent ferumoxil is comparable to endoscopy in assessing activity of ulcerative colitis (21).

2.3. Differential Diagnosis

The diagnosis of ulcerative colitis is confirmed with typical endoscopic features, negative stool cultures, and the exclusion of reasonable alternatives in the differential diagnosis. The most common diagnoses that mimic ulcerative colitis are infectious colitides or acute self-limited colitis. The principal diagnoses in the differential diagnosis are listed in Table 2. Ischemic bowel disease and diverticulitis should be excluded before inflammatory bowel disease can be initially diagnosed in a patient older than 50 yr (22).

Table 2
Principal Alternatives in the Differential Diagnosis
of Inflammatory Bowel Disease that may
Mimic Ulcerative Colitis, Crohn's Disease, or Both

Ulcerative colitis	Crohn's Disease	Both
Infectious colitis	Appendicitis	Diverticulitis
Antibiotic-associated colitis	Scleroderma	Diarrhea of AIDS
Amyloidosis	Bacterial overgrowth	Ischemic colitis
Solitary rectal ulcer syndrome	Bowel tuberculosis	Radiation enteropathy
Large bowel cancer	Small bowel cancer	Irritable bowel syndrome
Lymphocytic colitis	Carcinoid tumors	
Collagenous colitis	Celiac sprue	
Behcet's disease	Oral contraceptive colitis	
	Endometriosis	
	Lymphoma	
	Postsurgical adhesions	

AIDS, acquired immunodeficiency syndrome.

3. COMPLICATIONS

3.1. Disease Progression

The principal determinant of prognosis in ulcerative colitis patients is extent of disease. In the largest reported series of 1116 ulcerative colitis patients, 46% had endoscopic assessment of proctosigmoiditis, 17% had left-sided disease (to the splenic flexure), and 37% had pancolitis at presentation (23). Patients with pancolitis at onset of disease were more likely to develop toxic megacolon, refractory symptoms, malignancy, extraintestinal manifestations, and to require surgery. Over time, though, more than half of patients with limited disease advanced to more extensive disease. Therefore, repeated examinations may be necessary to confirm that disease has not advanced proximally, thereby altering prognosis.

3.2. Extraintestinal Manifestations

Cholestatic liver disease is the most common hepatic abnormality of inflammatory bowel disease and is approximately three times more common in ulcerative colitis patients than in Crohn's disease patients (24). Approximately 5% of ulcerative colitis patients will develop cholestasis, most commonly pericholangitis. Only 1 to 2% of ulcerative colitis patients will develop primary sclerosing cholangitis, a cholestatic liver disease diagnosed by the appearance of extrahepatic and intrahepatic strictures on a cholangiogram. Pericholangitis usually does not progress to cirrhosis, but primary sclerosing cholangitis patients can develop worsening biliary obstruction and secondary biliary cirrhosis that may require liver transplantation. Rarely, primary sclerosing cholangitis patients will develop cholangiocarcinoma. Cholestatic liver disease in ulcerative colitis is a risk factor for colorectal cancer and dysplasia (25). Treatment of bowel symptoms, even total proctocolectomy, does not influence the course of cholestatic liver disease. Fatty infiltration of the liver, chronic active hepatitis, amyloidosis, and drug-induced disease (from steroids, azathioprine, 6-mercaptopurine, or sulfasalazine) are other reported hepatic manifestations of inflammatory bowel disease.

Erythema nodosum, present in up to 3% of patients, is characterized by raised tender erythematous nodules, typically appearing on the extremities. Pyoderma gangrenosum, a rare ulcerating and necrotic lesion, is seen with both Crohn's disease and ulcerative colitis and represents an extraintestinal manifestation of vasculitis. Healing is prolonged and usually requires immunosuppressive therapy with steroids, 6-mercaptopurine or azathioprine, oral antibiotics for superinfection, and steroid injections for indurated margins. Cyclosporine has been successful in cases refractory to steroids, azathioprine, and/or 6-mercaptopurine.

Arthritis of inflammatory bowel disease is usually seronegative, mono- or pauciarticular, and asymmetric. The large joints are most often affected, and there is no synovial destruction. Arthritis more often affects females, exhibits no subcutaneous nodules, and correlates with disease activity. Axial arthritis, either ankylosing spondylitis or sacroiliitis, is related to HLA-B27, does not correlate with disease activity, and may be progressive and severe.

Ocular symptoms and signs of inflammatory bowel disease include blurred vision, eye pain, photophobia, inflammatory cells in the anterior chamber, and keratitic precipitates. Patients with uveitis often have HLA-B27, whereas patients with episcleritis and iritis usually do not.

Cerebrovascular accidents and other thromboembolic events can result from hypercoagulability secondary to chronic inflammation or other inherited syndromes such as factor V Leiden mutation. Precautions for deep vein thrombosis and pulmonary embolism may be necessary when there is inflammation in proximity to pelvic veins.

3.3. Colorectal Cancer

Over the course of the disease, colorectal cancer is expected to occur in approx 6% and be the cause of death in approx 3% of ulcerative colitis patients with extensive disease. Colorectal cancer incidence and mortality rates seem to be decreasing and are approaching the rates of populations unaffected by inflammatory bowel disease (26). Still, the risk of colorectal cancer in ulcerative colitis patients is elevated and has been estimated to be over four times what is expected among age- and sex-matched controls (27).

The colorectal cancer risk in ulcerative colitis increases with increasing extent and duration of disease, older age at symptom onset, and cholestatic liver disease (28). High-risk patients, such as those with disease proximal to the splenic flexure of more than 7 yr, should be enrolled in surveillance programs where colonoscopies with multiple biopsies are performed every 1–3 yr, depending on the patient's individual risk. The screening interval should decrease as the duration of disease increases (29). Total proctocolectomy is often recommended if either low-grade dysplasia, high-grade dysplasia, or cancer is detected (30). While these recommendations have not universally reduced cancer-related mortality, have not been recommended by all gastroenterologists, and are not predicted in a Markov model to improve cancer-related survival, cancer surveillance for ulcerative colitis patients has become the standard-of-care and must be offered to eligible patients (28,31,32). Surveillance of lower-risk patients (those with left-sided disease or disease of less than 7 yr) should be discouraged, because it is not likely to be cost-effective and is not yet standard-of-care (28).

Research is being done to better understand the biology of cancer and to determine whether intermediate markers of malignancy provide a more objective, accurate, sensitive, specific, and clinically useful marker than dysplasia. Candidate markers include DNA aneuploidy detected by flow cytometry and suppressor gene (particularly p53) mutations and loss of heterozygosity detected either immunohistochemically or with polymerase chain reaction techniques (33–35).

Distinguishing a dysplasia-associated lesion or mass, the so-called DALM lesion, from an adenoma or a pseudopolyp may be impossible, but is vital in determining appropriate therapy. Typically, DALMs are elevated and have the nodular appearance of a sessile adenoma (36). DALMs are thought to carry a poor prognosis and should prompt consideration for colectomy. Recently, this advice has been challenged, since two series of patients with DALMs did not have colectomy and did not develop cancer *(37,38)*. Still, to be safe, polypoid lesions with dysplasia in an area never affected with colitis in patients over age 50 yr are the only lesions that should be considered adenomas and should be treated with polypectomy. Polypoid lesions with dysplasia in an area previously affected with colitis or in a younger person should be considered DALMs and be treated with colectomy *(39)*. Patients with a stricture that cannot be traversed or adequately biopsied should have a colectomy as a result of the high risk of cancer or dysplasia in the stricture *(40)*.

4. MEDICAL MANAGEMENT

4.1. Supportive and Dietary Therapy

Therapy for patients with a mild or moderate disease flare should include supportive therapy with fluids, anticholinergics, and antidiarrheals. However, antidiarrheals and anticholinergics in patients with severely active disease could precipitate a toxic dilatation of the colon. Supportive therapy allows the naturally remitting feature of the ulcerative colitis to occur. Indeed, approximately one-third of patients given placebo in randomized clinical trials achieve remission. Diet recommendations should include a multivitamin supplement. Complete bowel rest with total parenteral nutrition is not effective primary therapy for ulcerative colitis patients.

Dietary supplements may be helpful. Eicosopentenoic acid (fish oil) competes with arachidonic acid for metabolism by lipoxygenase to produce leukotriene B_5, a much less potent proinflammatory cytokine than the arachidonic acid metabolite leukotriene B_4. High oral doses of fish oil can treat ulcerative colitis and enable patients to reduce steroid intake *(41,42)*. However, the extremely high dose causes odoriferous side effects, which limits the use of such therapy.

Short-chain fatty acids (acetate, butyrate, and proprionate), which are products of the colonic bacterial metabolism of dietary fiber, are fuel sources preferred by colonocytes over glucose and ketone bodies. Short-chain fatty acid enemas may be useful in patients with moderately active proctosigmoiditis, especially those refractory to more conventional therapy *(43,44)*. Oral butyrate coated in a pH-dependent soluble polymer targeted for colonic delivery when combined with oral 5-aminosalicylic acid (5ASA) improves symptoms in ulcerative colitis better than 5ASA alone *(45)*.

Administration of a nonpathogenic strain of *Escherichia coli* was as effective as 5ASA in maintaining remission in patients with ulcerative colitis *(46)*. Such a finding suggests that favorably altering the colonic flora with a probiotic may negate the "pro-inflammatory" effects of as yet unidentified pathogenic bacteria.

4.2. Aminosalicylates

For the past 50 yr, sulfasalazine, the combination of sulfapyridine and 5ASA, has been the most commonly used medication for ulcerative colitis. 5ASA is the therapeutically active ingredient that is released when colonic bacteria cleave a diazo bond with sulfapyridine. 5ASA interferes with both the cyclo-oxygenase and lipoxygenase pathways of arachidonic acid metabolism, as well as free-radical scavenging. Sulfasalazine, given in divided doses of 2–4 g/d, usually is helpful for treating mildly to moderately active ulcerative colitis and for maintaining remission *(47)*. Sulfasalazine is a competitive inhibitor of folic acid absorption and an oral supplement of folic acid is needed in patients so treated *(48)*.

Up to half of patients are allergic to or intolerant of sulfasalazine especially at high doses, primarily to sulfapyridine. 5ASA can be delivered directly to these patients with similar effectiveness by using newer, but more expensive, topical (Rowasa® enemas, Solvay, Marietta, GA) and oral preparations (olsalazine [Dipentum®, Pharmacia and Upjohn, Norwalk, CT], resin-coated mesalamine [Asacol®, Procter & Gambel, Cincinnati, OH], and ethylcellulose-coated 5ASA beads [Pentasa®, Shire, Florence, KY]). Olsalazine consists of two 5-ASA molecules linked by a diazo bond that requires cleavage from colonic bacteria. Although effective, a secretory diarrhea in more than 10% of patients limits its usefulness (49). The frequency of diarrhea from Dipentum can be diminished by taking the medication with food. All of these compounds can both induce and maintain remission.

Balsalazide (Colazide®, Salix, Raleigh, NC) is 5ASA attached via a diazo bond to an inert carrier molecule and is now available in the United States. Balasalazide has been shown to be more effective, and better tolerated, than Asacol in inducing remission in patients with ulcerative colitis (50).

The combination of oral 5ASA and topical 5ASA is more effective in treating ulcerative colitis patients, even those with pancolitis, than either 5ASA agent alone. Also, topical 5ASA often is more effective than topical steroids and should be used as first-line therapy in patients with ulcerative proctitis or proctosigmoiditis.

4.3. Corticosteroids

Oral, intravenous, or topical corticosteroids are very effective for treating active ulcerative colitis through inhibition of phospholipase A_2 and the subsequent decrease in the levels of leukotrienes. There is no difference in outcome if steroids are given on a continuous basis or given as "pulse" therapy (51). Prolonged prednisone administration, though, is limited by adverse effects, and therefore, it is not useful for maintenance therapy. Steroid analogs that are metabolized and inactivated by the liver during the first pass may be useful by acting locally before hepatic inactivation occurs, thereby producing fewer side effects. Budesonide, a steroid analog, is 90% inactivated by the liver during the first pass. The compound is modified by packaging with both ethylcellulose beads and eudrigit-L, ensuring small bowel and colonic effects before it is absorbed and inactivated. Budesonide has fewer adverse effects than prednisone (52,53). Since adrenal suppression does occur with budesonide, long-term use for maintenance is not recommend.

4.4. Immunosuppressives

6-Mercaptopurine and its S-imidazole precursor, azathioprine, are purine analogs that interfere with DNA replication of rapidly dividing cells, such as lymphocytes and macrophages. These drugs are safe and effective, have different adverse effects from corticosteroids, and can be considered "steroid-sparing." Approximately 10% of patients require discontinuation for reversible marrow suppression, about 3% will experience acute pancreatitis, and 1% will develop allergy characterized by abdominal pain, fever, and rash. Both azathioprine and 6-mercaptopurine at daily doses of 50–100 mg are effective maintenance therapy in ulcerative colitis, enabling patients to avoid long-term use of corticosteroids (54,55). The duration of therapy, before a clinical response is observed, can be 3 mo or longer. Because of this delay in response, adjusting the dose according to response may not be appropriate. Some have suggested that the dose of immunosuppressives be increased until mild leukopenia (white blood cell counts between 3000–5000 cells/fL) develops, since patients treated to leukopenia have a faster and more complete response (56). Metabolite levels of 6-thioguanine, the active metabolite, and 6-methylmercaptopurine, the toxic metabolite, can be determined to identify the dose that will find the narrow window between toxicity and effectiveness (57).

Cyclosporine is a cyclic polypeptide that is used extensively as an immunosuppressive agent in organ transplantation. It inhibits interleukin (IL)-2 gene transcription and, thereby, reduces activation of lymphocytes, mostly T helper cells. Cyclosporine binds to lipoproteins and requires bile salts for absorption. It is metabolized and inactivated by the hepatic cytochrome p450 system, and levels will be affected by drugs that induce cytochrome p450 activity. Nephrotoxicity, hepatotoxicity, hypertrichosis, gingival hyperplasia, tremors, parasthesias, seizures, and lymphoproliferative disorders are the most common adverse effects. High dose intravenous cyclosporine can initiate a quick response and successfully delay colectomy in up to 80% of patients with severely active ulcerative colitis (58). The long-term success of avoiding a colectomy is 50% or less. Responders, though, have a superior quality-of-life than patients who require surgery (59). Once remission is induced with IV cyclosporine, patients should be maintained on oral cyclosporine for at least 6 mo as prednisone is tapered and azathioprine or 6-mercaptopurine becomes effective (60).

Biologic therapies, such as infliximab (a mouse–human chimeric antibody to tumor necrosis factor) and the anti-inflammatory cytokines IL-10 and IL-11 have not been approved for ulcerative colitis patients.

4.5. Treatment of Pouchitis

Appoximately one-third of patients with ulcerative colitis and extensive disease will require total colectomy, mostly for toxic colitis, toxic megacolon, excessive bleeding, intractability of disease despite maximal medical therapy, and steroid dependence. A few, approx 10% of patients needing colectomy, will have surgery for colorectal cancer, dysplasia detected on a screening examination, or colonic stricture that cannot be adequately examined colonoscopically for malignancy. Total colectomy rids the patient of all bowel complications of ulcerative colitis.

The most important advance in the surgery for ulcerative colitis patients has been total proctocolectomy with ileal pouch–anal anastomosis. This surgery is indicated for patients under age 70 yr with adequate sphincter tone who have no neoplastic disease of the distal rectum. Quality-of-life measures are excellent following surgery. However, within 5 yr of surgery, approx 40% of patients will develop acute pouchitis (61). Typical symptoms of pouchitis are diarrhea, urgency, occasional incontinence, and rarely, fever. Endoscopically and histologically, pouchitis does not appear to be different from ileitis with ulcerations, friability, loss of vascular pattern, occasional exudate, and, on biopsy, an expansion of the lamina propria with mononuclear cells, mostly neutrophils (62). Even though there is bacterial overgrowth in all pouches, more than 90% of episodes of acute pouchitis respond to metronidazole. Pouchitis that is unresponsive to metronidazole may respond to a second antibiotic such as ciprofloxacin or topical administration of 5ASA, steroids, or glutamine (63). Other complications of the ileal pouch–anal anastomoses procedure include solitary ulcer and, rarely, dysplasia (64). The risk of cancer in a pouch is so low that surveillance is not required.

5. FUTURE INNOVATIONS

In the coming years, advances in the fields of genetic susceptibility, cancer surveillance, and treatment options are likely to greatly improve the lives of ulcerative colitis patients. Investigators are getting closer to identifying the genetic mutations that are responsible for the development of ulcerative colitis. Once identified, transfer of wild-type genes or replacement of defective protein products may actually cure the disease. For cancer surveillance, research is centering on markers that predict a poor prognosis that can be used along with dysplasia to more accurately identify patients who would benefit from total proctocolectomy. Pharmaceutical companies are concentrating on blocking selective pathways in the inflammatory process without the myriad of adverse effects from the available nonspecific anti-inflammatory agents.

In all, there are likely to be major breakthroughs ahead in the understanding and treatment of ulcerative colitis.

REFERENCES

1. Sandler RS. Epidemiology of inflammatory bowel disease. In *Inflammatory Bowel Disease: From Bench to Bedside*. Targan SR, Shanahan F (eds.), Williams & Wilkins, Baltimore, MD, 1994.
2. Loftus EV Jr., Silverstein MD, Sandborn WJ, Tremaine WJ, Harmsen WS, Zinsmeister AR. Ulcerative colitis in Olmsted County, Minnesota, 1940–1993: incidence, prevalence, and survival. *Gut*, **46** (2000) 336–343.
3. Niv Y, Abuksis G, Fraser GM. Epidemiology of ulcerative colitis in Israel: a survey of Israeli kibbutz settlements. *Am. J. Gastroenterol.*, **95** (2000) 693–698.
4. Carr I, Mayberry JF. The effects of migration on ulcerative colitis: a three-year prospective study among Europeans and first- and second-generation South Asians in Leicester (1991-1994). *Am. J. Gastroenterol.*, **94** (1999) 2918–2922.
5. Delco F, Sonnenberg A. Birth-cohort phenomenon in the time trends of mortality from ulcerative colitis. *Am. J. Epidemiol.*, **150** (1999) 359–366.
6. Orholm M, Fonager K, Sorensen HT. Risk of ulcerative colitis and Crohn's disease among offspring of patients with chronic inflammatory bowel disease. *Am. J. Gastroenterol.*, **94** (1999) 3236–3238.
7. Yang H, Rotter JI, Toyoda H, et al. Ulcerative colitis: a genetically heterogenous disorder defined by genetic (HLA class II) and subclinical (antineutrophil cytoplasmic antibodies) markers. *J. Clin. Invest.*, **92** (1993) 1080–1084.
8. Sandborn WJ, Landers CJ, Tremaine WJ, Targan SR. Antineutrophil cytoplasmic antibody correlates with chronic pouchitis after ileal pouch-anal anastomosis. *Am. J. Gastroenterol.*, **90** (1995) 740–747.
9. Boyko EJ, Koepsell TD, Perera DR, Inui TS. Risk of ulcerative colitis among former and current cigarette smokers. *N. Engl. J. Med.*, **316** (1987) 707–710.
10. Reif S, Lavy A, Keter D, et al. Lask of association between smoking and Crohn's disease but the usual association with ulcerative colitis in Jewish patients in Israel: a multicenter study. *Am. J. Gastroenterol.*, **95** (2000) 474–478.
11. Riegler G, Tartaglione MT, Carratu R, et al. Age-related clinical severity at diagnosis in 1705 patients with ulcerative colitis: a study by GISC. *Dig. Dis. Sci.*, **45** (2000) 462–465.
12. Lashner BA, Shaheen MJ, Hanauer SB, Kirschner BS. Passive smoking is associated with an increased risk of developing inflammatory bowel disease in children. *Am. J. Gastroenterol.*, **88** (1993) 336–359.
13. Lashner BA, Hanauer SB, Silverstein MD. Testing nicotine gum for ulcerative colitis patients: experience with single-patient trials. *Dig. Dis. Sci.* **35** (1990) 827–832.
14. Pullan RD, Rhodes J, Ganesh S, et al. Transdermal nicotine for active ulcerative colitis. *N. Engl. J. Med.* **330** (1994) 811–815.
15. Thomas GAO, Rhodes J, Mani V, et al. Transdermal nicotine as maintenance therapy for ulcerative colitis. *N. Engl. J. Med.*, **332** (1995) 988–992.
16. Lashner BA, Kane SV, Hanauer SB. Lack of association between oral contraceptives and ulcerative colitis. *Gastroenterology*, **99** (1990) 1032–1036.
17. Geerling BJ, Bagnelie PC, Badart-Smook A, Russel MG, Stockbrugger RW, Brummer RJ. Diet as a risk factor the development of ulcerative colitis. *Am. J. Gastroenterol.*, **95** (2000) 1008–1013.
18. Koutroubakis IE, Vlachinikolis IG. Appendectomy and the development of ulcerative colitis: results of a metaanalysis of published case-control studies. *Am. J. Gastroenterol.*, **95** (2000) 171–176.
19. Truelove SC, Witts LJ. Cortisone in ulcerative colitis: final report on a therapeutic trial. *BMJ*, **2** (1955) 1041–1048.
20. Kim B, Barnet JL, Kleen CG, Appelman HD. Endoscopic and histological patchiness in treated ulcerative colitis. *Am. J. Gastroenterol.*, **94** (1999) 3258–3262.
21. D'Arienzo A, Scaglione G, Vicinanza G, et al. Magnetic resonance imaging with ferumoxil, a negative superparamagnetic oral contrast agent in the evaluation of ulcerative colitis. *Am. J. Gastroenterol.*, **95** (2000) 720–724.
22. Lashner BA, Kirsner JB. Inflammatory bowel disease in older people. *Clin. Geriatr. Med.*, **7** (1991) 287–299.
23. Farmer RG, Easley KA, Rankin GB. Clinical patterns, natural history, and progression of ulcerative colitis: a long-term follow-up of 1,116 patients. *Dig. Dis. Sci.*, **38** (1993) 1137–1146.
24. Ponsioen CI, Tytgat GN. Primary sclerosing cholangitis: a clinical review. *Am. J. Gastroenterol.*, **93** (1998) 515–523
25. Shetty K, Rybicki L, Brzezinski A, Carey WD, Lashner BA. The risk of cancer or dysplasia in ulcerative colitis patients with primary sclerosing cholangitis. *Am. J. Gastroenterol.*, **94** (1999) 1643–1649.

26. Langholz E, Munkholm P, Davidsen M, Binder V. Colorectal cancer risk and mortality in patients with ulcerative colitis. *Gastroenterology*, **103** (1992) 1444–1451.

27. Karlen P, Lofberg R, Brostrom O, Leijonmarck CE, Hellers G, Persson PG. Increased risk of cancer in ulcerative colitis: a population-based cohort study. *Am. J. Gastroenterol.*, **94** (1999) 1047–1092.

28. Lashner BA. Recommendations for colorectal cancer surveillance in ulcerative colitis: a review of research from a single university-based surveillance program. *Am. J. Gastroenterol.*, **87** (1992) 168–175.

29. Lashner BA, Hanauer SB, Silverstein MD. Optimal timing of colonoscopy to screen for cancer in ulcerative colitis. *Ann. Intern. Med.*, **108** (1988) 274–278.

30. Provenzale D, Kowdley KV, Arora S, Wong JB. Prophylactic colectomy for surveillance for chronic ulcerative colitis? A decision analysis. *Gastroenterology*, **109** (1995) 1188–1196.

31. Eaden JA, Ward BA, Mayberry JF. How gastroenterologists screen for colonic cancer in ulcerative colitis: an analysis of performance. *Gastrointest. Endosc.*, **51** (2000) 123–128.

32. Delco F, Sonnenberg A. A decision analysis of surveillance for colorectal cancer in ulcerative colitis. *Gut*, **46** (2000) 500–506.

33. Rubin CE, Haggitt RC, Burma GC, et al. DNA aneuploidy in colonic biopsies predicts future development of dysplasia in ulcerative colitis. *Gastroenterology*, **103** (1992) 1611–1620.

34. Brentnall TA, Crispin DA, Rabinovitch PS, et al. Mutations in *p53* gene: an early marker of neoplastic progression in ulcerative colitis. *Gastroenterology*, **107** (1994) 369–378.

35. Lashner BA, Shapiro BD, Husain A, Goldblum JR. Evaluation of the usefulness of testing for p53 mutations in colorectal cancer surveillance for ulcerative colitis. *Am. J. Gastroenterol.*, **94** (1999) 456–462.

36. Blackstone MO, Riddell RH, Rogers BHG, Levin B. Dysplasia-associated lesion or mass (DALM) detected by colonoscopy in long-standing ulcerative colitis: an indication for colectomy. *Gastroenterology*, **80** (1981) 366–374.

37. Engelsgjred M, Farraye FA, Odze RD. Polypectomy may be adequate treatment for adenoma-like dysplastic lesions in chronic ulcerative colitis. *Gastroenterology*, **117** (1999) 1288–1294.

38. Rubin PH, Friedman S, Harpaz N, et al. Colonoscopic polypectomy in chronic colitis: conservative management after endoscopic resection of dysplastic polyps. *Gastroenterology*, **117** (1999) 1295–1300.

39. Odze RD. Adenomas and adenoma-like DALMs in chronic ulcerative colitis: a clinical, pathological, and molecular review. *Am. J. Gastroenterol.*, **94** (1999) 1746–1750.

40. Lashner BA, Turner BC, Bostwick DG, Frank PH, Hanauer SB. Dyspalsia and cancer complicating strictures in ulcerative colitis. *Dig. Dis. Sci.*, **35** (1990) 349–352.

41. Stenson WF, Cort D, Rodgers J, et al. Dietary supplementation with fish oil in ulcerative colitis. *Ann. Intern. Med.*, **116** (1992) 609–614.

42. Belluzzi A, Boschi S, Brignola C, Munarini A, Cariani G, Miglio F. Polyunsaturated fatty acids and inflammatory bowel disease. *Am. J. Clin. Nutr.* **71** (2000) 339S–342S.

43. Sheppach W. Sommer H, Kirschner T, et al. Effect of butyrate enemas on the colonic mucosa in distal ulcerative colitis. *Gastroenterology*, **116** (1992) 609–614.

44. Breuer RI, Soergel KH, Lashner BA, et al. Short chain fatty acid rectal irrigation for left-sided ulcerative colitis: a randomized placebo-controlled trial. *Gut*, **40** (1997) 485–491.

45. Vernia P, Monteleone G, Grandinetti G, et al. Combined oral sodium butyrate and mesalazine treatment compared to oral mesalazine alone in ulcerative colitis: randomized, double-blind, placebo-controlled pilot study. *Dig. Dis. Sci.*, **45** (2000) 976–981.

46. Rembacken BJ, Snelling AM, Hawkey PM, Chalmers DM, Axon AT. Non-pathogenic *Escherichia coli* versus mesalazine for the treatment of ulcerative colitis: a randomized trial. *Lancet*, **354** (1999) 635–639.

47. Brzezinski A, Rankin GB, Seidner DL, Lashner BA. 5-Aminosalicylic acid in inflammatory bowel disease: old and new preparations. *Cleve. Clin. J. Med.*, **62** (1995) 317–323.

48. Lashner BA. Red blood cell folate is associated with the development of dysplasia and cancer in ulcerative colitis. *J. Cancer Res. Clin. Oncol.* **119** (1993) 549–554.

49. Meyers S, Sachar DB, Present DH, Janowitz HD. Olsalazine sodium in the treatment of ulcerative colitis among patients intolerant of sulfasalazine: a prospective, randomized, placebo-controlled, double-blind, dose-ranging clinical trial. *Gastroenterology*, **93** (1987) 1255–1262.

50. Green JR, Lobo AJ, Holdsworth CD, et al. Balsalazide is more effective and better tolerated than mesalamine in the treatment of acute ulcerative colitis. *Gastroenterology*, **114** (1998) 15–22.

51. Oshitani N, Matsumoto T, Jinno Y, et al. Prediction of short-term outcome for patients with active ulcerative colitis. *Dig. Dis. Sci.*, **45** (2000) 982–986.

52. Rutgeerts P, Lofberg R, Malchow H, et al. A comparison of budesonide with prednisolone for active Crohn's disease. *N. Engl. J. Med.*, **331** (1994) 842–845.

53. Greenberg GR, Feagan BG, Martin F, et al. Oral budesonide for active Crohn's disease. *N. Engl. J. Med.*, **331** (1994) 836–841.

54. Present DH. 6-mercaptopurine and other immunosuppressive agents in the treatment of Crohn's disease and ulcerative colitis. *Gastroenterol. Clin. N. Am.*, **18** (1989) 57–72.

55. Hawthorne AB, Logan RFA, Hawkey CJ. Randomized controlled trial of azathioprine withdrawal in ulcerative colitis. *BMJ*, **305** (1992) 20–22.

56. Colonna T, Korelitz BI. The role of leukopenia in the 6-mercaptopurine-induced remission of refractory Crohn's disease. *Am. J. Gastroenterol.*, **89** (1994) 362–366.

57. Dubinsky MC, Lamothe S, Yang HY, et al. Pharmacogenomics and metabolite measurement for 6-mercaptopurine therapy in inflammatory bowel disease. *Gastroenterology*, **118** (2000) 705–713.

58. Lichtiger S, Present DH, Kornbluth A, et al. Cyclosporine in severe ulcerative colitis refractory to steroid therapy. *N. Engl. J. Med.*, **330** (1994) 1841–1845.

59. Cohen RD, Brodsky AL, Hanauer SB. A comparison of the quality of life in patients with severe ulcerative colitis after total colectomy versus medical treatment with intravenous cyclosporine. *Inflamm. Bowel Dis.*, **5** (1999) 1–10.

60. Kornbluth A, Present DH, Lichtiger S, Hanauer S. Cyclosporine for severe ulcerative colitis: a users guide. *Am. J. Gastroenterol.*, **92** (1997) 1424–1428.

61. Michelassi F, Stella M, Block GE. Prospective assessment of functional results after ileal J pouch-anal restorative proctocolectomy. *Arch. Surg.*, **128** (1993) 889–895.

62. Sandborn WJ, Tremaine WJ, Batts KP, Pemberton JH, Phillips SF. Pouchitis after ileal pouch-anal anastomosis: a pouchitis disease activity index. *Mayo Clin. Proc.*, **69** (1994) 409–415.

63. Wischmeyer P, Pemberton JH, Phillips SF. Chronic pouchitis after ileal pouch-anal anastomosis: response to butyrate and glutamine suppositories in a pilot study. *Mayo Clin. Proc.*, **68** (1993) 978–981.

64. Santos MC, Thompson JS. Late complications of the ileal pouch-anal anastomosis. *Am. J. Gastroenterol.* **88** (1993) 3–10.

30 Irritable Bowel Syndrome

Michael Camilleri

Contents

1. INTRODUCTION

Irritable bowel syndrome (IBS) is a common and important disorder. This chapter focuses on the definitions, epidemiology, natural history and pathophysiology of IBS, as these are essential to understand strategies for optimal management and a discussion of conventional and newer treatments of IBS.

1.1. IBS Definition

IBS is defined as "a functional bowel disorder in which abdominal pain is associated with defecation or a change in bowel habit, with features of disordered defecation and distention" *(1)*. The consensus definition and criteria for IBS have been formalized in the "Rome criteria", which are based on Manning's criteria (Table 1). The specificity of the symptoms alone is relatively poor. Specificity is enhanced by the inclusion of limited tests to exclude organic disease *(2,3)*. Thus, IBS is a disorder that can be diagnosed positively on the basis of a series of symptom criteria and limited evaluation to exclude organic disease *(4–6)*.

1.2. Epidemiology, Natural History, and Economic Impact of IBS

1.2.1. PREVALENCE DATA

The prevalence data from questionnaire studies *(7,8)* range around 10–20% in random samples of the population. The precise incidence of IBS is unclear, but it has been estimated at almost 1%/yr.

From: *Colonic Diseases*
Edited by: T. R. Koch © Humana Press Inc., Totowa, NJ

Table 1
Criteria for IBS

Rome II Criteria for IBS	Manning criteria for IBS
At least 12 wk or more, which need not be consecutive, in the previous 12 mo of abdominal pain or discomfort that has two out of three features: 1. Relief with defecation; and/or 2. Onset associated with a change in the frequency of stool; and/or 3. Onset associated with a change in form (appearance) of stool.	1. Pain relieved by defecation. 2. More frequent stools at the onset to pain. 3. Looser stools at the onset of pain. 4. Visible abdominal distention. 5. Passage of mucus. 6. Sensation of incomplete evacuation.

1.2.2. SYMPTOM SUBGROUPS

The symptom subgroups, based on the predominant bowel habit such as constipation-predominant, diarrhea-predominant, and IBS with alternating bowel movements, have equal prevalence rates (5.2 per 100) in epidemiological studies in Olmsted County, Minnesota (8), although clinical samples show a different distribution, possibly reflecting regional research expertise or interest. The gender ratio in these subgroups is similar, except in constipation-predominant IBS, which is more common in women (8). The female preponderance is more apparent in clinical samples (3 to 4:1) relative to those with symptoms who did not seek medical attention (<2:1) identified by mailed questionnaires. In the United States Householder study, 11.6% had IBS, 3.6% had functional constipation, and 1.8% had functional diarrhea (7). The prevalence of IBS is lower in the elderly. Traditionally, IBS is not diagnosed in those patients presenting with the symptom complex for the first time after the age of 60 yr.

1.2.3. NATURAL HISTORY OF IBS

IBS is a chronic disease whose course is extremely variable in the general population. While functional gastrointestinal symptoms are common in middle-aged persons, the overall prevalence in a community sample appears relatively stable over 12–20 mo. This is because there is a substantial degree of "turnover," because many people's symptoms fluctuate over time, and they, therefore, move in and out of the IBS cohort (8). IBS is a "safe" diagnosis. It is seldom that a patient followed with such a diagnosis turns out to suffer from serious organic disease; and the time-honored clinical strategy to reassure the patient that the diagnosis is benign without significant risk of missing an organic disease is well justified.

Fluctuation of symptoms often results in seeking of further health care. Repetitive investigations serve merely to reinforce the illness behavior. On the other hand, it is equally important that physicians not attribute to IBS those symptoms that do not "fit" the usual syndrome in the individual patient or symptoms that do not conform with the broader characteristics of the symptom complex embodied in the Manning or Rome criteria. The development of rectal bleeding, anemia, and a high erythrocyte sedimentation rate were significant negative predictive factors for IBS in Kruis et al. study of IBS (2) and constitute "alarm" features that are easy to elicit in the evaluation of IBS patients presenting with GI symptoms. Similarly, in the presence of rectal bleeding (which was not an independent significant predictor in Kruis's study), further investigation is mandatory.

1.2.4. IMPACT OF IBS

It is estimated that only 10–25% of IBS patients seek medical care; however, the illness has an enormous economic impact. In the United States alone, the latter is estimated at $25 billion

Table 2
Pathophysiological Mechanisms Contributing to IBS

Pathophysiology of IBS: a biopsychosocial disorder

Altered motility and enhanced visceral perception.
Approximately 50% of IBS patients have psychological symptoms at time of presentation.
The role of physical and sexual abuse in the development of IBS is controversial.
Up to a third (range 7–31%) of IBS presenters recall an antecedent gastroenteritis.

Proposed mechanisms contributing to IBS

Abnormal motility.
Heightened visceral perception: peripheral or central.
Psychological distress.
Intraluminal factors irritating small bowel or colon.
Lactose, other sugars,
Bile acids, short-chain fatty acids, and
Food allergens.
Postinfectious neuroimmune modulation of gut functions.

Interaction between different mechanisms may occur in individual patients. Reproduced from Camilleri (38).

annually through direct costs in healthcare utilization and indirect costs through absenteeism from work. In countries with socialized medicine, direct charges are lower, but this expenditure may still account for 0.5% of healthcare budgets (data reviewed in ref. 9).

Patients with IBS undergo more surgical procedures, including hysterectomy, cystoscopy, and appendectomy. IBS accounts for 2.4–3.5 million physician visits in the United States annually, making it the most common diagnosis in gastroenterology practice (about 28% of all patients), while accounting for 12% of primary care visits. Annually, there are 2.2 million medication prescriptions for IBS patients in the United States. Hence, direct costs are high, even in the managed care era (10). Patients with IBS have three times more absenteeism from work and report reduced quality of life.

2. MECHANISMS OF IBS

Symptoms in IBS have a physiological basis, but there is no single physiological mechanism responsible for symptoms of IBS. Table 2 and Fig. 1 summarize the pathophysiological mechanisms that appear to contribute to IBS. These individual mechanisms are not mutually exclusive. IBS is considered a biopsychosocial disorder resulting from a combination of three interacting mechanisms: psychosocial factors, altered motility (literature summarized in Table 3), and transit, which may reflect severity of bowel dysfunction and increased sensitivity (literature summarized in Table 4) of the intestine or colon.

There are preliminary data suggesting a genetic contribution to functional bowel disorders that require further validation. Gastrointestinal hypersensitivity and anorectal dysfunction have been extensively studied and are so frequently associated with the syndrome that they are reasonable targets for therapy. It has been hypothesized that altered peripheral functioning of visceral afferents (recruitment of silent nociceptors, increased excitability of dorsal horn neurons) and/or the central processing of afferent information are important in the altered somatovisceral sensation and motor dysfunction in patients with functional bowel disease. Vagal nerve dysfunction and abnormal sympathetic adrenergic function have been respec-

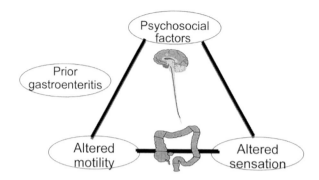

Fig. 1. Mechanisms involved in IBS. Adapted from ref. 5.

Table 3
Alterations in Bowel Motility in IBS

Psychological and physical stress increase colonic contractions.

Diarrhea-predominant IBS:
- Prominent colonic contractile response to feeding.
- Increased number of fast colonic and propagated contractions increased with diarrhea and decreased in constipation-predominant IBS.
- Accelerated whole gut transit; faster ascending and transverse colon emptying is positively correlated with stool weight.

Constipation-predominant IBS:
- Decreased number of fast colonic and propagated contractions in constipation-predominant IBS.
- Idiopathic constipation and normal anorectal and pelvic floor function: delay in whole gut transit, and rate of ascending and transverse colon emptying.
- Rectal and colonic compliance and tone are normal, although few reports suggest minor abnormalities in constipation of unclear clinical significance.

Pain-predominant IBS:
- "Clustered" contractions in the jejunum, and ileal-propagated giant contractions during episodes of abdominal colic are not pathognomonic for IBS. Sensory abnormalities accompany postprandial motor dysfunctions.

Reproduced from Camilleri *(38)*.

Table 4
Enhanced Visceral Perception in IBS

Diarrhea-predominant IBS:
- Lower thresholds for sensation of gas, stool, discomfort, and urgency by progressive rectal balloon distention, accompanied by excessive reflex contractile activity in the rectum.

Constipation-predominant IBS:
- Discomfort at greater distention volumes (reduced sensitivity) than in health; others report rectal or sigmoid hypersensitivity. Normal or increased thresholds for somatic pain stimuli.
- Increased visceral perception in patients with pain-predominant IBS on rectosigmoid, ileal and anorectal balloon distention; normal bowel compliance.

Reproduced from Camilleri *(38)*.

tively demonstrated in subgroups of patients with constipation- and diarrhea-predominant IBS. Sample references of the motor and sensory disorders in IBS are indicated in refs. *11–14*.

2.1. Stress and Emotions

Stress and emotions affect gastrointestinal function and cause symptoms to a greater degree in IBS patients compared to healthy controls *(15–17)*. Psychological symptoms, which are more common in patients with IBS, include somatization, anxiety, hostility, phobia, and paranoia. Identification of this co-morbidity and somatization is key to optimizing patient management. IBS patients seen in medical clinics show elevated scales of depression, anxiety, somatization, and neuroticism. At the time of presentation to gastroenterologists, almost half of the IBS patients demonstrate one or more of these symptoms. Since psychosocial symptoms modulate experience of somatic symptoms, they contribute to the greater illness behavior, doctor consultations, and reduced coping capability that are so common among IBS patients. Life event stressors and hypochondriasis are important determinants of the patients with postinfectious diarrhea who develop the full picture of IBS at 3 mo.

2.2. Abuse

The role of physical and sexual abuse in the development of the psychosocial factors that are manifested by patients with functional gastrointestinal disease is controversial. If identified, abuse requires specific and expert care. Psychopathology or psychological distress is manifest particularly in patients presenting to the clinic and in those with history of abuse.

2.3. Infectious Gastroenteritis

Persisting neuroimmune interactions following infectious gastroenteritis might result in continuing sensorimotor dysfunction *(18)*. Infectious diarrhea precedes the onset of IBS symptoms in 7–30% of patients in different series. Certain toxins appear to be more likely associated with long-term symptoms in patients with prior *Campylobacter* enteritis. Microscopic inflammatory changes, such as infiltration of the enteric nervous system may contribute to the development of IBS. Gwee et al. *(18)* have shown that about a quarter of patients with infectious diarrhea IBS continue to experience symptoms after 3 mo. However, these patients were admitted to their local hospital, suggesting they suffered a severe form of diarrhea, raising questions about the generalizability of the observation. In fact, the community diarrhea-based study in Nottingham, United Kingdom, suggests that less than 10% of patients with acute diarrhea went on to develop IBS. From the study of Gwee et al. *(18)*, it appears that the "mind" plays a greater role than "matter" since life event stress and hypochondriasis are predictive factors in the persistence of IBS. In contrast, physiological parameters, such as whole gut transit time and sensory thresholds are not different in patients with or without IBS symptoms at 3 mo after an episode of "infectious" diarrhea. Recent data *(19)* also suggest that postinfectious IBS is associated with an increased number of lymphocytes in the lamina propria of colonic biopsies, increased number of serotonin- and peptide YY (PYY)-containing enteroendocrine cells in the mucosa, and increased mucosal permeability of small sugars when compared to noninfectious IBS and controls.

2.4. Carbohydrate Intolerance

Carbohydrate intolerance may contribute to the symptoms of IBS. Lactose intolerance has a higher prevalence among Hispanic and African-Americans, whereas fructose and sorbitol intolerance are more prevalent among people of Northern European extraction. The clinical effect of lactose intolerance is also dependent on the total carbohydrate load, since exposure

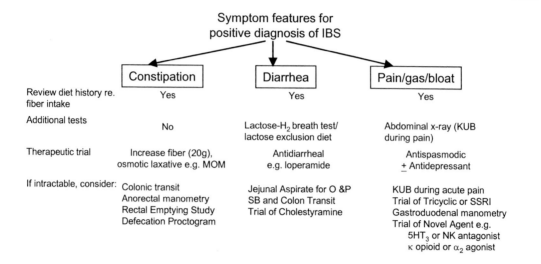

Fig. 2. Algorithm for management of IBS based on predominant symptom. Adapted from ref. *37.*

to the equivalent of an 8-oz glass of milk per day does not appear to cause symptoms. Gas formation as a result of maldigestion in the small intestine and subsequent metabolism in the colon accounts for bloating *(20)*; formation of osmotically active metabolites leads to diarrhea.

Measurements of intestinal gas have not always correlated with symptoms, but gas dynamics may be important in IBS *(21,22).*

Experimental data suggest that food allergens may also be important in IBS. One clinical trial showed that 40% of patients with IBS persistently improved with dietary exclusions. The role of dietary exclusion is still controversial, though there is evidence that the greater rate (though not the quantity) of gas excretion in IBS patients can be reduced by exclusion diets, and this parallels improvement in symptoms.

The ileum of patients with IBS is excessively sensitive to the secretory effects of perfused bile acids. Recent studies also emphasized the interaction between gas retention and other cofactors, particularly in the constipation-predominant IBS patients. This has led to experimental use of colonic prokinetics as a means to enhance gas clearance and has shown that gas clearance was increased.

3. MANAGEMENT OF IBS

3.1. Diagnosis

Identification of symptoms consistent with the syndrome, thorough physical exam, and careful search for psychosocial factors, stress, possibly physical and sexual abuse, and exclusion of organic diseases that have similar clinical presentations *(6,7,23)* are the bases for optimal diagnosis (Fig. 2). Diagnostic tests may aid the identification of the underlying mechanism in patients who do not respond to empiric trials; by definition, tests should follow. Establishing an effective doctor-patient relationship and sizing up the patient's agenda are crucial to effective patient management.

3.1.1. LIMITED SERIES OF INITIAL INVESTIGATIONS

A limited series of initial investigations is necessary to exclude organic structural, metabolic, or infectious diseases *(6,7).* These include hematology and chemistry tests; stool examination for occult blood, ova, and parasites (in those with diarrhea-predominance); flexible sigmoidoscopy; and, in those over 40 yr of age or with a family history of colon polyps or cancer, a complete colonic evaluation.

3.1.2. MORE SPECIALIZED INVESTIGATION

Formal studies have assessed the role of more specialized investigation. Ultrasound or computed tomography (CT) of the abdomen and pelvis and rectal biopsy provide little incremental value to the simpler work-up proposed for IBS. However, rectal biopsy may be appropriate to exclude lymphocytic, microscopic, or collagenous colitis in some patients with painless diarrhea. The controversy of flexible sigmoidoscopy vs colonoscopy as a screening test for organic disease is still unresolved; one approach is to use American Cancer Society or the World Health Organization (WHO) criteria to select the endoscopic procedure dictated for screening for colon cancer in patients with suspected IBS.

3.1.3. PELVIC FLOOR DYSFUNCTION

Pelvic floor dysfunction is a discrete disorder and may present with symptoms consistent with constipation-predominant IBS: constipation, sense of incomplete evacuation, and secondary abdominal pain *(24)*.

3.1.4. THERAPEUTIC TRIALS

A therapeutic trial is an extension of the diagnostic process, and should be pursued for at least 4 wk, particularly when it involves antidepressants *(25)*.

3.1.5. ADDITIONAL DIAGNOSTIC TESTS

Additional diagnostic tests (Fig. 1) may be required if the therapeutic trial fails *(5)*. The most appropriate test will depend on the predominant symptom in the individual patient and the previous therapeutic trials undertaken. In patients with predominant constipation, colonic transit and tests of the stool evacuation process are indicated when a trial of fiber and osmotic laxative fails. In patients with predominant diarrhea or pain-gas-bloat symptoms, a more detailed dietary history may identify factors that may be aggravating or even causing those symptoms. Among those with predominant diarrhea, a lactose-, fructose-, or sorbitol-exclusion diet should be included in the therapeutic trial. Among patients with predominant pain-gas-bloat, a plain abdominal radiograph during an acute episode of pain provides some reassurance that there is no mechanical obstruction. Thereafter, a therapeutic trial with a smooth muscle relaxant (discussed below) is reasonable, although effectiveness of this group of drugs in IBS is controversial.

4. CONVENTIONAL THERAPIES FOR IBS

Effective management requires an effective doctor–patient relationship and attention to the art of healing, in addition to the science of modern medicine. Initial treatment of IBS is summarized in Table 5.

4.1. Role of Fiber in Treatment of IBS

In constipation-predominant IBS patients, fiber (20–30 g/d) accelerates colonic or oro-anal transit *(26)*, and this is associated with increased stool weight and percentage of unformed stools. As a group, constipation-predominant IBS patients do not consume less dietary fiber than control subjects. It is often postulated that fiber may decrease intracolonic pressures and, thereby, reduce pain, since it is recognized that wall tension is one of the factors that contributes to visceral pain. Fiber reduces bile salt concentrations in the colon, and it has been

Table 5
Initial Treatment: The Therapeutic Trial

Reassurance and an effective doctor–patient relationship.

Diarrhea:
- Antidiarrheal agents such as diphenoxylate or loperamide (e.g., 2 mg as-needed up to 4/d).

Diarrhea and pain:
- Tricyclic antidepressants, such as desipramine, 50 mg three times daily, or amitriptyline, 10–25 mg twice daily significantly relieve diarrhea and associated pain.

Constipation:
- Dietary fiber supplementation (20 g/d).
- Osmotic laxatives, such as a magnesium salt, lactulose, or polyethylene glycol are usually efficacious.

Pain:
- Antispasmodics for pain on an as-needed basis; effectiveness unclear.

Reproduced from Camilleri *(38)*.

speculated that this indirectly reduces colonic contractile activity. However, symptom relief was not associated with changes in rectosigmoid motility.

Fiber alleviates pain in children with idiopathic chronic abdominal pain and simple constipation in adults *(27)*. There have been few randomized or mechanistic studies of fiber in patients with IBS. Francis and Whorwell *(28)* reported exacerbation of symptoms at the start of treatment; symptom aggravation persisted long-term, particularly with citrus fruits.

In practice, many patients complain of bloating with higher doses of fiber. Bran is reported to be no better than placebo in relief of overall IBS symptoms and may possibly be worse than a normal diet for some symptoms of IBS from intraluminal distention by bowel gas produced by bacterial fermentation of fiber. Fiber may induce bloating by increasing residue loading and bacterial fermentation without accelerating the onward movement of the increased residue.

4.2. Loperamide and Antidiarrheal Agents in IBS

Diarrhea-predominant IBS is associated with acceleration of small bowel and proximal colonic transit and responds to opioids *(29)*. Most prefer to use loperamide over diphenoxylate which contains atropine and may induce side effects that may be dangerous, particularly in the elderly, e.g., bladder dysfunction, glaucoma, tachycardia. Loperamide (2–4 mg, up to four times daily), which is a synthetic opioid, decreases intestinal transit, enhances intestinal water and ion absorption, and increases anal sphincter tone at rest *(29)*. One study also showed reduced intensity of pain associated with improved stool consistency and reduced frequency of defecation *(30)*. However, the patients treated with loperamide also experienced increased nightly abdominal pain *(30)*. Symptoms of patients with constipation-predominant IBS given loperamide are not improved.

4.2.1. CHOLESTYRAMINE

Cholestyramine is considered a third-line treatment in IBS with predominant diarrhea, because of poor palatability and low patient compliance. The rationale for its use is based on the documentation of bile acid malabsorption in some patients with functional, typically painless, diarrhea that mimics IBS with diarrhea.

4.3. Smooth Muscle Relaxants in IBS

In clinical practice, antispasmodics and anticholinergic agents are best used on an as-needed basis up to two times per day for acute attacks of pain, distention, or bloating *(31,32)*. Agents such as dicyclomine or mebeverine seem to retain efficacy when used on an as needed basis, but become less effective with chronic use. Clidinium is no longer available as a separate drug and is combined with the benzodiazepine, chlorodiazepoxide. While these drugs have generally fallen out of favor, it remains to be conclusively demonstrated that the newer medications (discussed in Subheading 5.1) are actually superior for pain in IBS in head-to-head comparisons. This has been demonstrated in a phase III trial of alosetron vs mebeverine (discussed in Subheading 5.1).

4.4. Psychotrophic Agents used in IBS

To date, psychotrophic agents of the tricyclic group have been used effectively in patients with diarrhea and pain-predominant IBS *(6,25)*. However, there is increasing interest in the potential application of selective serotonin (5-HT) reuptake inhibitors (SSRIs), which tend not to cause constipation and may even induce diarrhea in some patients. One uncontrolled study supports the efficacy of SSRIs in treating patients with IBS.

Tricyclic agents (e.g., amitriptyline, imipramine, doxepin) are now frequently used to treat patients with IBS, particularly those with more severe or refractory symptoms, impaired daily function, and associated depression or panic attacks. Initially, their use was based on the fact that a high proportion of patients with IBS reported significant depression *(31,32)*. Antidepressants have neuromodulatory and analgesic properties, which may benefit patients independently of the psychotrophic effects of the drugs. It appears that the clinical effects of agents, such as amitryptiline, result from their central actions. Thus, amitryptiline has no significant effects on esophageal and rectal sensory thresholds and compliance in healthy subjects; and in the functional upper gastrointestinal disorder, nonulcer dyspepsia, clinical benefit seemed to be associated with better sleep rather than changes in gastric sensitivity.

Neuromodulatory effects may occur sooner and with lower dosages in IBS patients than for the treatment of depression (e.g., 10–25 mg amitryptiline or 50 mg desipramine). Because antidepressants must be used on a continual rather than an as-needed basis, they are generally reserved for patients having frequently recurrent or continual symptoms. A 2- to 3-mo trial is usually needed before excluding a therapeutic benefit.

The placebo-controlled trials of antidepressants in IBS have been summarized elsewhere *(6)*. In two large studies *(31,32)*, trimipramine decreased abdominal pain, nausea, and depression, but did not alter stool frequency. The beneficial effect seems to be greater in those with abdominal pain and diarrhea. For example, desipramine improved abdominal pain and diarrhea while, in an earlier study that combined patients with either diarrhea or constipation, there was no significant benefit for desipramine over placebo. Nortriptyline in combination with fluphenazine reduced abdominal pain and diarrhea in two studies. SSRIs, which may cause diarrhea, are currently the focus of prospective studies in IBS.

4.5. Hypnotherapy and Other Psychological Treatments

Hypnotherapy or psychotherapy may be effective in IBS *(6)*, but they are generally less easily available to the practicing physician. Factors indicating a favorable response to psychotherapy include predominance of diarrhea and pain, association of IBS with overt psychiatric symptoms, and intermittent pain exacerbated by stress. In contrast, patients with constant abdominal pain do poorly with psychotherapy or hypnotherapy. In a systematic review of the literature, Talley et al. *(33)* concluded that the efficacy of psychological treatment for IBS has

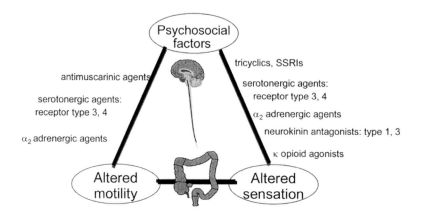

Fig. 3. Pharmacological approaches to correction of sensory, motor, and psychological disturbances in IBS. Adapted from ref. *5*.

not been established because of methodological inadequacy. While eight studies reported psychological treatment superior to control therapy, five failed to detect a significant effect.

4.6. Alternative Therapies in IBS

Efficacy of alternative therapies has been difficult to ascertain in view of the lack of controlled trials; however, a first parallel-group placebo-controlled 16-wk trial of alternative medicine has recently been reported. In this study, individualized or conventional Chinese herbal medicines significantly improved bowel symptom scores, global symptoms, and reduced IBS-related interference with life relative to placebo, which was administered in a capsule and was designed to taste, smell, and look similar to a Chinese herb formula *(34)*. An intriguing result is that patients receiving individualized Chinese herbal medicine continued to report benefit beyond the actual treatment period *(34)*.

5. NOVEL AND EXPERIMENTAL MEDICATIONS FOR IBS

The availability of agents with visceral analgesic and sensorimotor modulatory properties has stimulated much interest in the field of IBS therapy (Fig. 3). These agents include the κ-opioid agonist, fedotozine, other 5-HT$_3$ and 5-HT$_4$ antagonists, other serotonergic agents, and neurokinin antagonists, some of which are now becoming available for routine clinical usage.

5.1. 5-HT3 Antagonist, Alosetron

Alosetron hydrochloride, a selective 5-HT$_3$ antagonist, is effective in relieving pain, normalizing bowel frequency, and reducing urgency in diarrhea-predominant female IBS patients *(35)*. 5-HT$_3$ receptors are extensively distributed on enteric motor neurons and in peripheral afferents and central locations, such as the vomiting center. Antagonism of these receptors reduces visceral pain, colonic transit, and small intestinal secretion.

In large placebo-controlled trials, alosetron was more effective than placebo in inducing adequate relief of pain and discomfort, and improvement in bowel frequency, consistency and urgency in women with diarrhea-predominant IBS (Fig. 4). Another study compared alosetron (1 mg twice daily) to mebeverine, an antispasmodic approved in Europe for treatment of IBS, and showed similar results over the active comparator *(36)*.

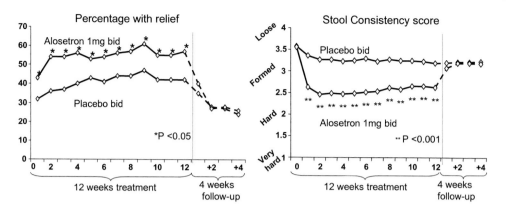

Fig. 4. Effect of alosetron and placebo on adequate relief of pain and stool consistency seen in female patients with diarrhea-predominant IBS. Note the rapid onset of symptom relief and persistence of effect until cessation of medication (vertical line at 12 wk). Reproduced with permission from ref. *35.*

The beneficial response for pain and bowel dysfunction was observed within 1–4 wk of beginning therapy and was sustained throughout the duration of the trial. Benefit was observed only in female patients with diarrhea-predominant IBS symptoms, and further studies in males are awaited.

The most common adverse event with alosetron treatment is constipation compared to placebo (28 vs 5%). Acute ischemic colitis was estimated to occur in 0.1–1% of patients. The cases reported resolved after several days to weeks without sequelae. Risk factors were not identified. This class of drugs should be discontinued in patients who experience rectal bleeding or a sudden worsening of pain or significant constipation. The drug, alosetron, was withdrawn from the market after the observation of complications from constipation that developed during treatment with alosetron. Other medications in this class are ondansetron, granisetron, tropisetron, and cilansetron. The former three are approved for treatment of chemotherapy-induced emesis. The latter is undergoing further study.

5.2. Novel Partial or Full 5-HT₄ Agonists

New partial or full 5-HT$_4$ agonists appear promising in the treatment of constipation or constipation-predominant IBS and are in phase III trials.

5.2.1. Tegaserod

The partial agonist, tegaserod, was recently shown to enhance peristalsis in an in vitro model, at least in part by stimulating the intrinsic primary afferent neuron, thereby activating excitatory and inhibitory intrinsic neurons that result in peristalsis. Tegaserod may also stimulate motility via a systemic action, since it increases small bowel and colonic contractions after intravenous administration in the dog. It reduces visceral afferent firing during rectal distention and reduces abdominal contractions in response to noxious rectal distention, a pseudo-affective model of visceral pain. Tegaserod reduces visceral afferents firing during noxious rectal distention in animal studies.

Tegaserod results in global relief of IBS symptoms in females with constipation-predominant IBS. The more effective dose of tegaserod is 6 mg twice daily. The drug is significantly effective with approx 15% advantage over placebo in females and in those with documented constipation during the baseline run-in period.

Tegaserod also appeared to reduce daily pain score, bloating score, and to normalize frequency and consistency of bowel movements. Tegaserod appears quite safe. No serious adverse events reported in the clinical trials program and in the cohort treated in open evaluation for over 6 mo. The medication was approved for prescription to patients (female) with IBS whose predominant bowel dysfunction is constipation.

5.2.2. PRUCALOPRIDE

The full $5\text{-}HT_4$ agonist, prucalopride, induces strong contractions in the proximal colon in vivo in dogs and accelerates colonic transit in healthy participants and, most importantly, in patients with functional constipation. Prucalopride induced a significant increase in the number of spontaneous and complete bowel movements in phase II trials of patients with functional constipation which, in clinical practice, overlaps with constipation-predominant IBS patients. The effects of prucalopride on abdominal pain have not been thoroughly assessed, and hence, further studies are needed. However, phase III clinical trials are currently on hold while a more thorough evaluation of potential intestinal carcinogenicity in animal species is completed.

5.2.3. OTHER INVESTIGATIONAL AGENTS AND NEW APPROACHES

Other investigational agents and new approaches that are currently being explored in phase II studies include: newer type 3 antimuscarinic agents; cholecystokinin antagonists; the α_2-adrenergic agonist, clonidine; a $5\text{-}HT_1$ agonist, buspirone; and an SSRI, citalopram. Clonidine has been shown to enhance rectal compliance in health and in IBS. Formal trials of its clinical efficacy are awaited. Buspirone reduces gastric and colonic responses to volume distentions and may, similarly, have potential in functional disorders. Buspirone's anxiolytic activity may impact on the symptomatic benefits demonstrated in a small clinical trial. Citalopram reduces colonic sensation to volume distension and inhibits the colonic motor response to feeding.

5.2.4. NEUROKININ ANTAGONISTS AND κ-OPIOID AGONISTS

Neurokinin antagonists also have therapeutic potential in IBS. Three types of receptor antagonists have been developed and confer benefit through their effects on smooth muscle, intrinsic excitatory neurons, and visceral afferents. Fedotozine and other κ-opioid agents, such as asimadoline, require further study to determine whether a peripheral κ-opioid approach might significantly reduce pain and discomfort in IBS. Pharmacodynamic studies need to be performed to clarify the subgroups of IBS patients most likely to respond to these agents.

6. SUMMARY AND CONCLUSION

Management of IBS involves positive diagnosis, limited exclusion of organic disease, reassurance, and selection of symptom-relieving medications. Insights into enteric neuroscience and the brain–gut axis have led to the development of novel therapies. It is anticipated that the role of infection and the neurotransmitters involved in visceral pain will be clarified and will enhance the management of patients with IBS.

ACKNOWLEDGMENTS

This work was supported in part by grants RO1-DK54681-04 and K24-DK02638-02 (Dr. M. Camilleri) from the National Institutes of Health. I wish to thank Mrs. Cindy Stanislav for excellent secretarial assistance.

REFERENCES

1. Drossman DA, Corazziari E, Talley NJ, Thompson WG, Whitehead WE. Rome II: A multinational consensus document on functional gastrointestinal disorders. *Gut*, **45** (1999) 1–81.
2. Kruis W, Thieme C, Weinzierl M, Schussler P, Holl J, Paulus W. A diagnostic score for the irritable bowel syndrome. Its value in the exclusion of organic disease. *Gastroenterology*, **87** (1984) 1–7.
3. Vanner SJ, Depew WT, Paterson WG, DaCosta LR, Groll AG, Simon JB, Djurfeldt M. Predictive value of the Rome criteria for diagnosing the irritable bowel syndrome. *Am. J. Gastroenterol.*, **94** (1999) 1912–1917.
4. Manning AP, Thompson WG, Heaton KW, Morris AF. Towards a positive diagnosis of the irritable bowel. *BMJ*, **2** (1978) 653–654.
5. Camilleri M, Choi MG. Review article: irritable bowel syndrome. *Aliment. Pharmacol. Ther.*, **11** (1997) 3–15.
6. Drossman DA, Whitehead WE, Camilleri M. Irritable Bowel Syndrome: A technical review for practice guideline development. *Gastroenterology*, **112** (1997) 2120–2137.
7. Drossman DA, Li Z, Andruzzi E, et al. U.S. householder survey of functional gastrointestinal disorders. *Dig. Dis. Sci.*, **38** (1993) 1569–1580.
8. Talley NJ, Zinsmeister AR, Melton LJ. Irritable bowel syndrome in a community: symptom subgroups, risk factors and health care utilization. *Am. J. Epidemiol.*, **142** (1995) 76–83.
9. Camilleri M, Williams DE. Economic burden of irritable bowel syndrome reappraised with strategies to control expenditures. *Pharmacoeconomics*, **4** (2000) 331–338.
10. Longstreth GF. Irritable bowel syndrome. Diagnosis in the managed care era. *Dig. Dis. Sci.*, **42** (1997) 1105–1111.
11. Bazzocchi G, Ellis J, Villaneuva-Meyer J, et al. Postprandial colonic transit and motor activity in chronic constipation. *Gastroenterology*, **98** (1990) 686–693.
12. Cann PA, Read NW, Brown C, Hobson N, Holdsworth CD. Irritable bowel syndrome: relationship of disorders in the transit of a single solid meal to symptom patterns. *Gut*, **24** (1983) 405–411.
13. Vassallo M, Camilleri M, Phillips SF, Brown ML, Chapman NJ, Thomforde GM. Transit through the proximal colon influences stool weight in the irritable bowel syndrome. *Gastroenterology*, **102** (1992) 102–108.
14. Ritchie J. Pain from distension of the pelvic colon by inflating a balloon in the irritable bowel syndrome. *Gut*, **14** (1973) 125–132.
15. Whitehead WE, Crowell MD, Robinson JC, Heller BR, Schuster MM. Effects of stressful life events on bowel symptoms: subjects with irritable bowel syndrome compared with subjects without bowel dysfunction. *Gut*, **33** (1992) 825–830.
16. Young SJ, Alpers DH, Norland CC, Woodruff RA Jr. Psychiatric illness and the irritable bowel syndrome. Practical implications for the primary physician. *Gastroenterology*, **70** (1976) 162–166.
17. Alpers DH. Editorial: why should psychotherapy be a useful approach to management of patients with non-ulcer dyspepsia? *Gastroenterology*, **119** (2000) 869–871.
18. Gwee KA, Leong YL, Graham C, et al. The role of psychological and biological factors in postinfective gut dysfunction. *Gut*, **44** (1999) 400–406.
19. Spiller RC, Jenkins D, Thornley JP, et al. Increased rectal mucosal enteroendocrine cells, T lymphocytes, and increased gut permeability following acute *Campylobacter* enteritis and in post-dysenteric irritable bowel syndrome. *Gut*, **47** (2000) 804–811.
20. Haderstorfer B, Psycholgin D, Whitehead WE, Schuster MM. Intestinal gas production from bacterial fermentation of undigested carbohydrate in irritable bowel syndrome. *Am. J. Gastroenterol.*, **84** (1989) 375–378.
21. Serra J, Azpiroz F, Malagelada J-R. Intestinal gas dynamics and tolerance in humans. *Gastroenterology*, **115** (1998) 542–550.
22. Serra J, Azpiroz F, Malagelada J-R. Impaired transit and tolerance of intestinal gas in the irritable bowel syndrome. *Gut*, **48** (2001) 14–19.
23. Drossman DA. Diagnosing and treating patients with refractory functional gastrointestinal disorders. *Ann. Intern. Med.*, **123** (1995) 688–697.
24. Camilleri M, Thompson WG, Fleshman JW, Pemberton JH. Clinical management of intractable constipation. *Ann. Intern. Med.*, **121** (1994) 520–528.
25. Clouse RE, Lustman PJ, Geisman RA, Alpers DH. Antidepressant therapy in 138 patients with irritable bowel syndrome: a five-year clinical experience. *Aliment. Pharmacol. Ther.*, **8** (1994) 409–416.
26. Cann PA, Read NW, Holdsworth CD. What is the benefit of coarse wheat bran in patients with irritable bowel syndrome? *Gut*, **25** (1984) 168–173.
27. Voderholzer WA, Schatke W, Muhldorfer BE, Klauser AG, Birkner B, Muller-Lissner SA. Clinical response to dietary fiber treatment of chronic constipation. *Am. J. Gastroenterol.*, **92** (1997) 95–98.
28. Francis CY, Whorwell PJ. Bran and irritable bowel syndrome: time for reappraisal. *Lancet*, **344** (1994) 39–40.

29. Cann PA, Read NW, Holdsworth CD, Barends D. Role of loperamide and placebo in management of irritable bowel syndrome. *Dig. Dis. Sci.*, **29** (1984) 239–247.
30. Efskind PS, Bernklev T, Vatn MH. A double-blind, placebo-controlled trial with loperamide in irritable bowel syndrome. *Scand. J. Gastroenterol.*, **31** (1996) 463–468.
31. Greenbaum DS, Mayle JE, Vanegeren LE, et al. The effects of desipramine on IBS compared with atropine and placebo. *Dig. Dis. Sci.*, **32** (1987) 257–266.
32. Ritchie JA, Truelove SC. Comparison of various treatments for irritable bowel syndrome. *BMJ*, **281** (1980) 1317–1319.
33. Talley NJ, Owen BK, Boyce P, Paterson K. Psychological treatments for irritable bowel syndrome: a critique of controlled treatment trials. *Am. J. Gastroenterol.*, **91** (1996) 277–283.
34. Bensoussan A, Talley NJ, Hing M, Menzies R, Guo A, Ngu M. Treatment of the irritable bowel syndrome with Chinese herbal medicine: a randomised controlled trial. *JAMA*, **280** (1998) 1585–1589.
35. Camilleri, M, Northcutt, AR, Kong, S, et al. Efficacy and safety of alosetron in women with irritable bowel syndrome: a randomised, placebo-controlled trial. *Lancet*, **355** (2000) 1035.
36. Jones, RH, Holtmann, G, Rodrigo, L, et al. Alosetron relieves pain and improves bowel function compared with mebeverine in female nonconstipated irritable bowel syndrome patients. *Aliment. Pharmacol. Ther.*, **13** (1999) 1419–1427.
37. Camilleri M, Prather CM. The irritable bowel syndrome: mechanisms and a practical approach to management. *Ann. Intern. Med.*, **116** (1992) 1001–1008.
38. Camilleri M. Management of the irritable bowel syndrome. *Gastroenterology*, **129** (2001) 652–668.

31 Ischemic Colitis

Peter Grübel and David R. Cave

CONTENTS

1. INTRODUCTION

Ischemic colitis is the most frequent form of mesenteric ischemia, and it predominantly affects the elderly. There are two principal forms: 85% of patients show a nongangrenous type, and 15% develop transmural necrosis *(1)*.

Nongangrenous ischemia is usually transient and resolves without sequelae. Only a minority of patients suffers from chronic damage presenting either as persistent segmental colitis or stricture.

The etiologies are numerous Table 1, but often ischemic colitis develops insidiously, and no specific cause can be identified.

The diagnosis and treatment of patients can be challenging, since it often occurs in a debilitated patient population with multiple medical problems.

From: *Colonic Diseases*
Edited by: T. R. Koch © Humana Press Inc., Totowa, NJ

Table 1
Causes of Ischemic Colitis

Major vascular occlusion

- Mesenteric artery thrombosis *(1)*
- Cholesterol emboli *(72)*
- Aortic dissection *(74)*
- Arterial embolus *(71)*
- Colectomy with IMA ligation *(73)*
- Aortic reconstruction *(75)*

Mesenteric venous thrombosis

- Coagulopathy *(76)*
- Portal hypertension *(78)*
- Lymphocytic phlebitis *(77)*
- Pancreatitis *(79)*

Small vessel disease

- Diabetes *(80)*
- Rheumatoid arthritis *(82)*
- Vasculitis *(84)*
- Antiphospholipid antibodies *(86)*
- Takayasu's arthritis *(88)*
- Anticentromere antibodies *(90)*
- Amyloidosis *(81)*
- Radiation *(83)*
- Polyarthritis nodosa *(85)*
- Lupus erythematosus *(87)*
- Wegener's granulomatosis *(89)*
- Buerger's disease *(91)*

Shock

- Cardiac failure *(92)*
- Pancreatitis *(93)*
- Hemodialysis *(64)*
- Anaphylaxis *(94)*

Mechanical obstruction

- Strangulated hernia *(95)*
- Adhesion *(97)*
- Fecal impaction or pseudo-obstruction *(99)*
- Colon cancer *(96)*
- Rectal prolapse *(98)*

Blood dyscrasia

- Coagulopathy *(100)*
- Sickle cell disease *(101)*

Iatrogenic

- Surgical
- Cardiopulmonary bypass *(60)*
- Colonoscopy *(103)*
- Aortoiliac reconstruction *(53)*
- Renal transplant *(102)*
- Barium enema *(104)*

Drugs

- Alosetron *(105)*
- Diuretics *(107)*
- Estrogens *(109)*
- NSAID's *(111)*
- Digitalis *(106)*
- Cocaine *(108)*
- Danazol *(110)*
- Vasoactive substances *(112)*

Others

- Long distance running *(113)*
- Dialysis *(65)*
- Spontaneous in young adults *(115)*
- Neurogenic *(114)*
- Infections
  (cytomegalovirus [CMV], *E. coli* O157:H7) *(116)*

2. BLOOD SUPPLY OF THE COLON

Except for the rare individual anatomic variation, the colon has a specific vascular arrangement *(2)*. The superior mesenteric artery (SMA) and inferior mesenteric artery (IMA) both supply blood to the colon (Fig. 1A). The SMA arises from the aorta, about 1 cm below the celiac axis at the level of L1–2. It supplies the entire small intestine except for the superior part of the duodenum. The SMA has four main branches: the inferior pancreaticoduodenal, middle colic, right colic, and the ileocolic arteries. In general, the ileocolic artery supplies the terminal ileum, cecum, appendix, and proximal ascending colon, whereas a portion of the ascending colon and hepatic flexure receive blood from the right colic artery. The middle colic artery supplies the proximal transverse colon.

The IMA arises from the aorta about 3 cm proximal to the aortic bifurcation at about L3 and branches into the left colic, which supplies the distal transverse colon and splenic flexure, the sigmoid arteries, which supply the sigmoid and descending colon, and the superior rectal artery, which supplies a large part of the rectum. The inferior rectal arteries, derived from the internal pudendal arteries, and the small and inconsistent middle rectal arteries, derived from the internal iliac arteries, also supply the rectum.

An abundant collateral blood supply exists between the SMA and IMA and the IMA and internal iliac arteries. The arcades of the SMA and IMA interconnect at the base and border of the mesentery. The connection at the base of the mesentery is called the Arc of Riolan, whereas the connection along the mesenteric border is known as the marginal artery of Drummond. Collateral flow between the IMA and iliac arties occurs via the superior and middle–inferior rectal vessels. Since the rectum has a dual blood supply from the IMA and iliac arteries, ischemic damage of the rectum is rare. The collateral pathways protect against ischemia during mesenteric occlusion, and open immediately when a mesenteric artery is occluded. Despite the presence of collaterals, the colon vasculature has two weak points. Narrow terminal branches of the SMA supply the splenic flexure, and narrow terminal branches of the IMA supply the rectosigmoid junction. These two watershed areas are the most vulnerable to develop ischemia during systemic hypotension. This vulnerability is enhanced by the quite common and clinically unapparent occlusion of the IMA.

The veins parallel the arteries. The superior mesenteric vein (SMV) drains the small intestine, cecum, ascending, and transverse colon via the jejunal, ileal, ileocolic, right colic, and middle colic veins. The inferior mesenteric vein (IMV) drains the descending colon through the left colic, the sigmoid through the sigmoid, and the rectum through the superior rectal vein. The IMV fuses with the splenic vein, which then joins the SMV to form the portal vein.

3. PATHOPHYSIOLOGY

Colonic ischemia is usually the result of a sudden and mostly temporary reduction in blood flow that is insufficient to meet the metabolic demands of discrete regions of the colon. Blood flow may be compromised by changes in the systemic circulation or by anatomic or functional changes in the local mesenteric vasculature Table 1. Occasionally, a specific cause may be recognized, but usually, no clear cause for the ischemia is identified.

Depending largely on food ingestion, the splanchnic vascular bed receives between 10 and 35% of the cardiac output. The intestinal vasculature has a very high capillary density and much higher capillary permeability than most other vascular circuits. Since the intestinal venous outflow has to also perfuse the liver via portal vein, the venous blood pressure and mean hydrostatic capillary pressures are higher in the intestine than in other vascular beds. Intestinal oxygen extraction is normally low, which allows for the provision of sufficient oxygen to the

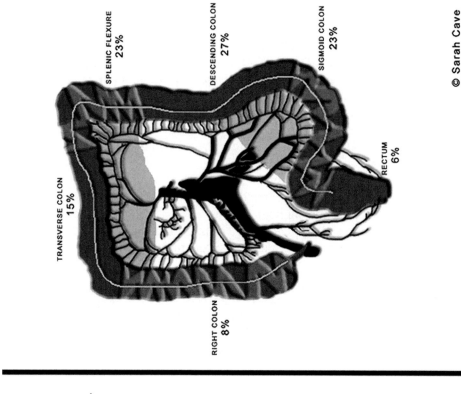

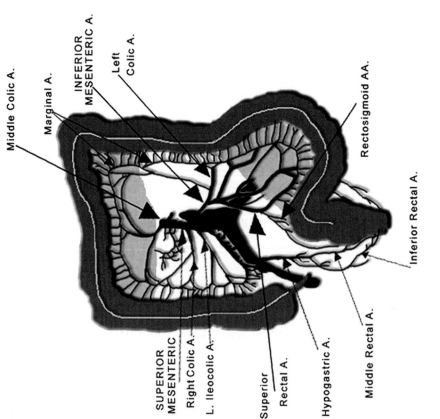

Fig. 1. (A) Arterial blood supply to the colon. (B) Anatomic distribution of ischemic colitis with reference to the arterial blood supply.

liver. As gut blood flow reduces, tissue extraction of oxygen increases reciprocally to maintain intestinal oxygen supply sufficient. Intestinal blood flow has to be reduced by at least 50% from the normal fasting level to affect oxygen extraction *(3)*.

The splanchnic vessels respond vigorously to vasoactive substances, which accounts in part for the occurrence of vasospasm and nonocclusive ischemia *(2)*. Vasospasm occurs also as a homeostatic response to systemic hypotension to facilitate the redirection of flow from the gut to brain and heart. This can overwhelm the normal autoregulation of intestinal perfusion. Usually, the intestinal vascular bed autoregulates its blood flow over a wide pressure range. In contrast to tissue like skeletal muscle, autoregulation prevails over external central control mediated via sympathetic vasoconstrictor nerve stimulation. Experiments indicated that perfusion pressure has to be reduced to approx 30 mmHg or mesenteric mean arterial pressure to 45 mmHg to cause injury *(4)*.

Ischemic tissue injury has a hypoxic, as well as a reperfusion, component. The hypoxic component causes detectable injury in the superficial part of the mucosa within 1 h. Prolonged severe ischemia causes necrosis of the epithelium and mucous layer. The serosa and muscularis propria are the least susceptible to the effects of ischemia. If there is no rapid resolution of the ischemia, transmural infarction can be seen within 8–16 h *(5)*. The reperfusion component of intestinal injury is mainly seen following partial ischemia. Initiated by an increased release of oxygen free radicals, other toxic byproducts of ischemic injury, and neutrophil activation, reperfusion injury may lead to multisystem organ failure *(6)*.

4. ACUTE ISCHEMIC COLITIS

Generally, the clinical presentation varies with the degree of severity of the condition. Three progressive clinical stages have been described *(7,8)*:

1. Hyperactive phase. Soon after occlusion or hypoperfusion, severe pain is dominating with frequent passage of bloody loose stools. Blood loss is usually low without need for transfusion. Characteristically, there is a discrepancy between the severe pain and abdominal exam, with pain being out of proportion to the physical findings and often poorly localized. More than 80% of all patients show only mucosal and submucosal injury, with resolution of symptoms with conservative measures, and no long-term sequelae.

2. Paralytic phase. The pain usually diminishes, becoming more continuous and diffuse. The abdomen becomes more tender and distended with no bowel sounds as an ileus develops.

3. Shock phase. Massive fluid shifts may occur, with protein, blood, and electrolytes leaking through a necrotic mucosa. Severe fluid balance alterations dominate, and irreversible shock may develop. Fortunately, this most severe form affects only 10–20% of patients necessitating rapid surgical intervention.

All parts of the colon may be affected by ischemia, but the left colon is most commonly involved in more than 75% of cases (Fig. 1B). Ischemia secondary to low flow state (nonocclusive mesenteric ischemia) often affects the right colon and the watershed areas of splenic flexure or rectosigmoid junction *(9)*.

5. DIAGNOSIS

The mainstay of diagnosis remains an appropriate history and physical exam in conjunction with a high index of suspicion followed by radiological and/or endoscopic studies. Frequently, the clinical diagnosis is difficult to make, in an unconscious patient in an ICU *(10)*.

Invasive studies with angiography or laparoscopy are rarely needed, but may be of value in special situations when the diagnosis is unclear or there is a need to follow patients after ischemic bowel surgery. Magnetic Resonance Angiography and duplex sonography are recent technological innovations that provide noninvasive vascular imaging in patients with suspected proximal arterial mesenteric vessel or mesenteric venous disease. They are hardly ever required in the work-up of suspected colonic ischemia. Stool cultures for *Salmonella*, *Shigella*, *Campylobacter*, *Yersinia*, and *Escherichia coli* 0157:H7 should be obtained if diarrhea is a prominent feature. Stools should be examined for ova and parasites if the history is suggestive of amoebiasis.

The differential diagnosis includes infectious colitis, inflammatory bowel disease, pseudomembraneous colitis, diverticulitis, and colon carcinoma.

5.1. Laboratory Tests

There are no specific laboratory markers for ischemia, although an increased serum lactate, lactate dehydrogenase (LDH), creatine phosphokinase (CPK), amylase, or serum acidosis may indicate advanced tissue damage. The white blood count may be markedly elevated, but is obviously nonspecific.

6. RADIOLOGY

6.1. Plain Abdominal Film

This frequently shows nonspecific findings. In one series of 23 cases, specific signs, such as thumbprinting from submucosal edema and hemorrhage could be identified in only 30% of patients with mesenteric infarction *(11)*. In another study, patients with a normal plain abdominal X-ray (KUB) appeared to have a lower mortality rate of 29%, whereas mortality rate was 78% in those with an abnormal KUB *(12)*.

6.2. Computer-Assisted Tomography (Abdominal)

If there are no signs of peritonitis and plain abdominal films are unrevealing, a computed tomography (CT) is frequently obtained. Scans may be fully normal in early ischemic colitis and show specific findings in only one-third of patients with proven mesenteric infarction *(11,13)*. Typical but not pathognomonic findings are thickening of the bowel wall in a segmental pattern with pneumatosis and gas in the mesenteric veins in the terminal stage *(14)*.

7. COLONOSCOPY

If the diagnosis is still unclear, colonoscopy should be performed within 48 h, unless peritonitis and radiological evidence of perforation are demonstrated. Colonoscopy is preferable to contrast enemas, since it is more sensitive in detecting mucosal lesions, allows for biopsy, and does not preclude angiography. Overdistension and high intraluminal pressures of the colon should be avoided during colonoscopy, since it may aggravate ischemic damage. We would recommend that the procedure be terminated once the diagnosis is made in order to minimize the risk of perforation.

In the acute setting, a pale mucosa with petechial bleeding is a sign of mild ischemia. Hemorrhagic nodules may be seen representing submucosal bleeding; these are the equivalent to "thumbprints" detected on radiological studies. More severe disease is distinguished by darker mucosa and hemorrhagic ulcerations (Fig. 2A,B). Segmental distribution, abrupt transition between injured and noninjured mucosa, rectal sparing, and rapid resolution on serial endoscopy favor ischemia rather than inflammatory bowel disease or an infectious colitis. Biopsies taken from affected areas may show nonspecific changes, such as hemorrhage, crypt destruction, capillary thrombosis, granulation tissue with crypt abscesses, and pseudopolyps, which may mimic Crohn's disease *(15,16)*.

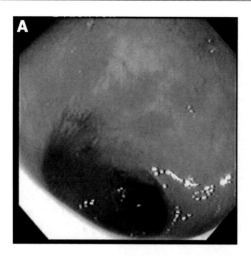
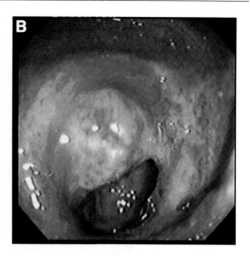

Fig. 2. (A) Acute ischemic colitis in the sigmoid. The photograph is at the edge of the involved lesion and shows a patchy distribution of erythema with early pseudomembrane formation over the more hemorrhagic lesion. (B) Acute ischemic colitis in the sigmoid colon of the same patient as panel 2A, showing hemorrhagic changes in the mucosa edema and mucosal necrosis.

In the chronic phase of ischemic colitis, mucosal atrophy and areas of granulation tissue with or without a fibrinous pseudomembrane may be found. Biopsy of a postischemic stricture is marked by extensive transmural fibrosis and mucosal atrophy.

8. BARIUM ENEMA

Abnormalities on barium enema are typically segmental and transient. Thumbprinting is the most diagnostic finding in a double-contrast study. It is seen early in the course of the disease and usually resolves or is replaced within 1 or 2 wk by an acute ulcerative pattern (17). In a series of 40 patients with nongangrenous ischemia, 75% had thumbprinting (Fig. 3), and 60% showed longitudinal ulcers (18).

9. MESENTERIC ANGIOGRAPHY

Is rarely helpful in ischemic colitis. In most cases, colonic blood flow has already returned to normal by the time of symptom onset. In addition, ischemic colon vessels are mostly involved at the arteriolar level, whereas mesenteric vessels and arcades are often patent. However IMA occlusion is a frequent finding particularly in the elderly and is usually preexistent and clinically silent.

However, angiography may be indicated if the clinical exam cannot exclude acute small intestinal mesenteric ischemia. Angiography has also been shown to perform slightly better than CT in the diagnosis of mesenteric infarction. In one study, 14 of 16 angiography studies (sensitivity 87.5%) and 18 of 22 CT examinations (sensitivity 82%) were correct in the diagnosis of mesenteric infarction (19).

Angiography has its limitations. First, it is not readily available. Second, patients with ischemic colitis frequently suffer from co-morbid conditions, such as cardiac and renal failure, making contrast injection (60–100 mL) hazardous. Third, these patients are frequently markedly dehydrated and acidotic. These abnormalities require correction before angiography can be performed.

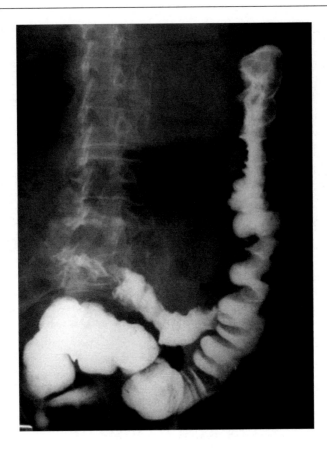

Fig. 3. Barium enema in a patient with sigmoid ischemic colitis demonstrating mucosal edema of "thumbprinting" (black-filled arrows).

10. DUPLEX SONOGRAPHY

Is an evolving noninvasive technique to identify patients with high grade stenosis of the proximal celiac axis, SMA, and IMA. However, significant stenotic vessel changes occur in many asymptomatic patients and do not necessarily indicate mesenteric ischemia *(20,21)*. Increase in flow velocity, poststenotic turbulence, and collateral vessels suggest significant arterial stenosis. Absence of arterial flow in the thickened wall of the ischemic colon may be indicative of more severe colitis *(22)*.

11. LAPAROSCOPY

This technique may be an important diagnostic tool, particular in the elderly patient with co-morbid diseases with poor tolerance to laparotomy *(23)*. Laparoscopy may also be useful for a second look inspection to assess the viability of the remaining bowel and integrity of the anastomosis after surgery for ischemic bowel *(24)*.

The procedure can be carried out under local anesthesia with light intravenous sedation. During laparoscopy, only the serosal surface of the bowel can be inspected, and the bowel cannot be palpated. These are drawbacks, since the external surface of the gut may appear normal in early or mild ischemia. In a more progressive phase, dark peritoneal fluid may be present. The ischemic bowel may display edema, patchy hemorrhages, frank gangrenes, or perforation.

A concern specific to to laparoscopy is the effect of pneumoperitoneum on mesenteric blood flow. Kleinhaus et al. showed in an animal model that mesenteric blood flow was reduced by more than 70% to baseline when the intraperitoneal pressure was more than 20 mmHg. In addition, a pronounced drop in femoral artery pressures was observed *(25)*. It is, therefore, prudent that intraperitoneal pressure should not exceed 10–15 mmHg in a patient with mesenteric ischemia.

12. TREATMENT

Once the diagnostic workup does not suggest gangrene or perforation, the patient may be managed conservatively. Generally, parenteral fluids are administered, and the bowel is placed at rest. If an ileus is present, nasogastric suction is instituted. Broad-spectrum antibiotics are generally recommended.

Cardiorespiratory function is optimized, and medications that may contribute to colonic ischemia, such as vasopressors, are withdrawn if possible. Vital signs and abdominal findings are carefully monitored. Serial radiological or colonoscopic examinations are indicated in patients with slow clinical recovery and who are at risk of developing colonic infarction.

So far, there are no proven pharmacological agents to show superior outcome by augmenting colonic perfusion or tissue oxygenation. If angiography has been used, and there is a nonocclusive cause for the colonic ischemia, the catheter can be used for local infusion of papaverine (30–60 mg/h). If there are no signs of infarction, papaverine infusion is continued for at least 24 h in an attempt to resolve vasoconstriction. However, the therapeutic benefit of papaverine is unproven. In one animal study, papaverine increased SMA flow *(26)*, whereas in another it not only failed to increase collateral flow but decreased flow caused by vasodilatation in the nonischemic bed (steal phenomenon) *(27)*.

Most patients improve within 1 or 2 d with complete clinical and radiological resolution within 1 to 2 wk. More severe ischemia causes ulceration and inflammation, which may develop into a segmental ulcerating colitis or stricture. These lesions may be asymptomatic, however they should be followed to document either healing or the development of persistent colitis or stricture.

Nongangrenous colitis shows a low mortality of 6% and a very low recurrence rate *(28)*.

13. COLONIC INFARCTION

Manifests clinically as sepsis, peritonitis, free intra -abdominal air, or extensive gangrene visualized endoscopically, mandating urgent laparotomy and segmental bowel resection. The colonoscopy should not be completed if severe colitis is encountered. The bowel should not be cleansed in preparation for surgery, because bowel preps can precipitate perforation or toxic dilatation of the colon.

Right-sided colonic ischemia and necrosis can be treated with right hemicolectomy and primary anastomosis. If perforation is associated with peritonitis, a resection with terminal ileostomy and colonic mucocutaneous fistula should be performed *(29)*.

Patients with left-sided colonic involvement should undergo colon resection with proximal stoma and distal mucous fistula or Hartmann's procedure. Resection with primary anastomosis faces the problem of the solid feces filled colon. Antegrade intra-operative colonic irrigation has been attempted in such situation, but has shown to have significant peri-operative mortality in 8% of patients, anastomotic leak in 7% of patients and wound infection in 3% of patients *(30)*. When the rectum is involved, a mucocutaneous fistula of the distal stump or a Hartmann's procedure should be performed.

Ostomy closure following the Hartmann's procedure is more difficult and time-consuming than ostomy closure after loop colostomy, divided colostomy, or divided ileostomy-colostomy. Ostomy closure should be delayed for 4–6 mo, although frequently, the patient never proceeds to reversal because of co-morbid conditions. Mortality and morbidity rates for reversal of the Hartmann's procedure are mainly extrapolations obtained from cancer and diverticulosis surgery with mortality of 0%, morbidity of 30%, and anastomotic stricture rate of 9% *(31)*.

The rare fulminating-type of colonic ischemia involving most of the colon and rectum requires colectomy with terminal ileostomy *(32)*.

The value for a second look laparotomy after surgery for intestinal ischemia is well established, however there are no clearly established guidelines. Regardless of the origin, arterial or venous, revascularization procedure, and unrelated to the type, anastomosis or stoma creation, a second look operation should be made based on the findings during the first operation as well as clinical exam and should be performed within 12–24 h to ensure bowel viability *(29)*.

14. OUTCOMES FOR TRANSMURAL INFARCTION

The overall picture remains bleak.

Guivarc'h et al. reported their experience with 88 surgical cases of ischemic colitis *(33)*. Gangrene with 17 perforations occurred in 76 cases, strictures in 6, and spontaneous resolution in 6 cases. Colon resection was required in 77 patients. Morbidity was 53% in cases with perforated gangrene and 28% without perforation.

Longo et al. determined the outcome of 43 patients with ischemic colitis, comparing patients with segmental disease with those with total colonic ischemia *(34)*. Segmental colitis was present in 31 of 43 patients (72%), and 11 of these 31 (35%) were successfully managed nonoperatively. Two of the nonsurgically treated developed strictures that necessitated late segmental resection. Sixteen (51%) of these 31 patients with segmental colitis underwent early resection and 4 (12%) required surgery after failed initial conservative therapy. Nine (75%) of 12 patients treated by resection and stoma underwent eventual stoma closure. None of the nonoperatively treated patients died, whereas the 30-d mortality rate in those that required surgery was 22%.

All 12 patients with total colonic ischemia required surgery, and 9 of these 12 patients (75%) died.

The same author assessed the prognosis for 31 patients requiring colonic resection for nonocclusive mesenteric ischemia (NOMI) *(28)*. Segmental resection was performed on 24 (77%) and abdominal colectomy on 7 (23%) patients. Second look laparotomy in 8 patients (26%) revealed further ischemia in 2 (20%). Enteric continuity was reestablished in 14 (45%) patients. Seventeen (55%) of the 31 cases had significant complications, such as sepsis, respiratory failure or dep vein thrombosis (DVT). Overall mortality was 29%. No patient developed recurrent ischemia (mean follow-up of 5.3 yr).

15. MESENTERIC VEIN THROMBOSIS

This condition rarely involves the colon, and almost always involves the small intestine in the jejunoileal bowel *(35)*. It has to be treated with thrombectomy or thrombolysis, however experience is limited with these interventions *(36–39)*.

Once the diagnosis is made, immediate anticoagulation is advocated since re-canalization occurred in 25 of 27 patients given anticoagulation and neither of the 2 patients not given anticoagulation *(40)*. Intravenous anticoagulation with heparin should be maintained even intraoperatively and in the early postoperative phase to prevent rethrombosis. CT or MRA can be used to monitor patients until recanalization occurs. Patients who have had an episode of acute mesenteric vein thrombosis and do not have a contraindication to antico-agulation should be anticoagulated with warfarin for 3–6 mo or lifelong, if there is a coagulopathy or cardiac source *(41)*.

In one retrospective study of 53 patients with acute mesenteric thrombosis, 58% of patients had to undergo bowel resection *(42)*. Recurrent mesenteric venous thrombosis occurred in 36%, and the 30-d mortality was 27%.

16. AORTOILIAC SURGERY

A special risk for ischemic colitis is seen with aorto-iliac reconstructive surgery with an incidence of up to 7% of patients *(43)*. After repair of ruptured abdominal aneurysms, the incidence of transmural infarction is 7% in patients who survive the operation *(44)*. Ischemic bowel changes seen on colonoscopy can be as high as 60% of such cases.

Several factors contribute to bowel ischemia, which almost always affects the left colon, including loss of collaterals, embolization, traction of the vessels with surgical instruments, hematoma within the mesocolon, and hypotension. Independent risk factors for the occurrence of intestinal ischemia are age, renal disease, prior colectomy (because of collateral interruption), emergency surgery, experience of the surgeon, aorto-bifemoral bypass, cross-clamping time, and ligation of both iliac arteries *(45)*.

Important preventive steps are: (i) to have at least one internal iliac artery perfused, (ii) IMA reimplanatation if retrograde filling of the SMA from the IMA has been demonstrated. Others have recommended the use of intraoperative Laser Doppler flowmetry to assess colonic blood flow *(46)*, intravenous administration of fluorescein to help predict who might benefit from colonic revascularization or immediate colectomy *(47)*, or intramural pH measurements by endoluminal tonometry to determine luminal $_pCO_2$, which are correlated with pH and colonic wall $_pCO_2$ values *(48,49)*. However, the lack of a universally accepted method is a testament to the inadequacies associated with each method.

A novel and less invasive therapy of abdominal aortic aneurysm is endovascular treatment with stent-grafts. However, intestinal ischemia of the left colon related to the procedure has been reported *(50,51)*. Acute mesenteric artery obstruction is the principal cause of ischemic colitis, initiated by either arterial rupture on graft deployment, graft thrombosis, migration of the prosthesis, or peripheral embolization *(52)*.

Early recognition of postoperative ischemic colitis is important. Passage of bloody stools in the early postoperative period, unexplained failure to improve, fever, leucocytosis, or thrombocytopenia should raise suspicion of ischemia. The majority of lesions are within the reach of sigmoidoscopy in this context *(53,54)*. Patients treated conservatively may undergo sigmoidoscopy/colonoscopy every other day to assess the status of the ischemia. Disappointingly, endoscopy might not separate transmural from the clinically less important mucosal ischemia and had no impact on mortality in any of the prospective series published *(55)*. Diagnostic laparotomy may be an alternative if there is diagnostic suspicion of ischemia, and is not associated with significant morbidity or mortality. Ultimately, early laparotomy using the Hartmann's procedure or colectomy is the only way to decrease mortality once ischemic colitis has occurred. Primary anastomosis is contraindicated, because it may result in leakage and contamination of the aortic graft *(56)*.

Patients with colon necrosis who are conservatively treated will invariably die, whereas colectomy lowers mortality rates to 66–90% *(44,53)*. In one large series of 2137 patients undergoing abdominal aortic reconstruction, overt intestinal ischemia occurred in 1% of patients, mainly in the colon *(57)*. Fifty percent of those patients required resection. Overall mortality was 25%, but rose to 50% if resection was needed.

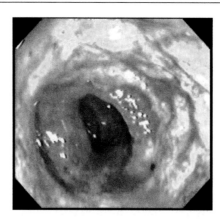

Fig. 4. Chronic ischemic colitis with pseudomembranes still present, in conjuction with an ischemic stricture in the descending colon.

17. CARDIOPULMONARY BYPASS

Colonic ischemia after cardiopulmonary bypass is an uncommon (0.2%) but lethal complication with a mortality rate of up to 85% *(58,59)*. Risk factors include older age, a positive history of gastrointestinal disease, re-operative valve surgery, and severe postoperative low cardiac output. In addition to the low flow state of bypass perfusion, the procedure exposes the patient's blood to foreign surfaces, which may lead to coagulopathy, microemboli, alterations in cells and proteins, release of vasoactive substances, and activation of the complement cascade. Long bypass times, the use postoperative inotropic agents, and the use of the intra-aortic balloon pump act as cumulative insults *(60)*.

There is often a reluctance to submit these patients to major abdominal surgery following cardiac surgery. Surgical intervention, however, is not associated with significant increase in mortality and may be life-saving in patients who are poorly able to compensate for hemodynamic instabilities associated with untreated colonic ischemia *(61)*.

18. CHRONIC RENAL FAILURE REQUIRING HEMODIALYSIS

Mesenteric infarction is the most common cause of acute abdomen in the hemodialysis population and is responsible for 9% of the deaths in the dialysis population *(62)*. In many cases, the right colon is injured by nonocclusive mesenteric ischemia (NOMI) *(63–65)*. Arteriosclerosis, diabetes, and hemodialysis-induced hypotension are the main inciting factors for NOMI development *(66)*.

A retrospective review of 29 of 1370 long-term hemodialysis patients who developed NOMI showed that the majority of patients experienced abdominal pain more than 24 h before admission. Sixteen patients (55%) had ischemia of the small bowel, all underwent laparotomy, and nine (56%) died. Thirteen patients (45%) had ischemia of the colon and were managed nonoperatively; four (31%) of them died. Overall mortality rate for NOMI was 45% *(66)*.

19. CHRONIC ISCHEMIC COLITIS

About 20% of patients develop chronic colitis from irreversible ischemic injury *(67)*. Clinically, these patients present either with recurrent bacteremia, persistent sepsis, asymptomatic colonic stricture (Fig. 4), bloody diarrhea, weight loss from protein losing enteropathy, or abdominal pain *(67)*.

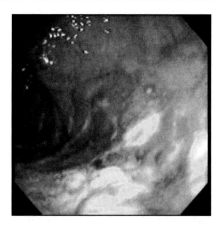

Fig. 5. Chronic ischemic colitis in the transverse colon. The lower portion of the photograph shows a yellow pseudomembrane clearly demarcated from the normal mucosa, which is in the upper half of the image.

Recurrent episodes of bacteremia or sepsis in patients with unhealed areas of segmental colitis are indications for segmental colon resection (Fig. 5). If misdiagnosed as inflammatory bowel disease, patients will poorly respond to immunosuppressive therapy with an increased risk of perforation on steroids.

Ischemic strictures that produce no symptoms should be observed. In contrast to malignant strictures, barium enema typically demonstrates a smooth and tapered stricture that lacks overhanging edges. Some strictures will return to normal within 12–24 mo without specific therapy. If symptoms of obstruction develop, segmental resection is adequate *(68)*. Endoscopic dilatation *(69)* or stenting *(70)* may be alternatives, albeit unproven ones.

REFERENCES

1. Greenwald DA, Brandt LJ. Colonic ischemia. *J. Clin. Gastroenterol.*, **27** (1998) 122–128.
2. Rosenblum JD, Boyle CM, Schwartz LB. The mesenteric circulation. Anatomy and physiology. *Surg. Clin. N. Am.*, **77** (1997) 289–306.
3. Bulkley GB, Kvietys PR, Parks DA, Perry MA, Granger DN. Relationship of blood flow and oxygen consumption to ischemic injury in the canine small intestine. *Gastroenterology*, **89** (1985) 852–857.
4. Haglund U, Bergqvist D. Intestinal ischemia—the basics. *Langenbecks. Arch. Surg.*, **384** (1999) 233–238.
5. Haglund U, Bulkley GB, Granger DN. On the pathophysiology of intestinal ischemic injury. Clinical review. *Acta Chir. Scand.*, **153** (1987) 321–324.
6. Granger DN, Rutili G, McCord JM. Superoxide radicals in feline intestinal ischemia. *Gastroenterology*, **81** (1981) 22–29.
7. Boley S.J., Brandt L.F. Ischemic disorders of the intestines. *Curr. Prob. Surg.*, **15** (1978) 1–85.
8. Hunter GC, Guernsey JM. Mesenteric ischemia. *Med. Clin. N. Am.*, **72** (1988) 1091–1115.
9. Gandhi SK, Hanson MM, Vernava AM, Kaminski DL, Longo WE. Ischemic colitis. *Dis. Colon Rectum*, **39** (1996) 88–100.
10. Dorudi S, Lamont PM. Intestinal ischaemia in the unconscious intensive care unit patient. *Ann. R. Coll. Surg. Engl.*, **74** (1992) 356–359.
11. Smerud MJ, Johnson CD, Stephens DH. Diagnosis of bowel infarction: a comparison of plain films and CT scans in 23 cases. *Am. J. Roentgenol.*, **154** (1990) 99–103.
12. Ritz JP, Runkel N, Berger G, Buhr HJ. (Prognostic factors in mesenteric infarct) Prognosefaktoren des Mesenterialinfarktes. *Zentralbl. Chir.*, **122** (1997) 332–338.
13. Alpern MB, Glazer GM, Francis IR. Ischemic or infarcted bowel: CT findings. *Radiology*, **166** (1988) 149–152.

14. Balthazar EJ, Yen BC, Gordon RB. Ischemic colitis: CT evaluation of 54 cases. *Radiology*, **211** (1999) 381–388.
15. Mitsudo S, Brandt LJ. Pathology of intestinal ischemia. *Surg. Clin. N. Am.*, **72** (1992) 43–63.
16. Price AB. Ischaemic colitis. *Curr. Top. Pathol.*, **81** (1990) 229–246.
17. Wolf EL, Sprayregen S, Bakal CW. Radiology in intestinal ischemia. Plain film, contrast, and other imaging studies. *Surg. Clin. N. Am.*, **72** (1992) 107–124.
18. Iida M, Matsui T, Fuchigami T, Iwashita A, Yao T, Fujishima M. Ischemic colitis: serial changes in double-contrast barium enema examination. *Radiology*, **159** (1986) 337–341.
19. Klein HM, Lensing R, Klosterhalfen B, Tons C, Gunther RW. Diagnostic imaging of mesenteric infarction. *Radiology*, **197** (1995) 79–82.
20. Roobottom CA, Dubbins PA. Significant disease of the celiac and superior mesenteric arteries in asymptomatic patients: predictive value of Doppler sonography. *Am. J. Roentgenol.*, **161** (1993) 985–988.
21. Nicoloff AD, Williamson WK, Moneta GL, Taylor LM, Porter JM. Duplex ultrasonography in evaluation of splanchnic artery stenosis. *Surg. Clin. N. Am.*, **77** (1997) 339–355.
22. Danse EM, Van Beers BE, Jamart J, et al. Prognosis of ischemic colitis: comparison of color doppler sonography with early clinical and laboratory findings. *Am. J. Roentgenol.*, **175** (2000) 1151–1154.
23. Zamir G, Reissman P. Diagnostic laparoscopy in mesenteric ischemia. *Surg. Endosc.*, **12** (1998) 390–393.
24. Slutzki S, Halpern Z, Negri M, Kais H, Halevy A. The laparoscopic second look for ischemic bowel disease. *Surg. Endosc.*, **10** (1996) 729–731.
25. Kleinhaus S, Sammartano R, Boley SJ. Effects of laparoscopy on mesenteric blood flow. *Arch. Surg.*, **113** (1978) 867–869.
26. Williams RA, Wilson SE. Effect of intra-arterial vasodilators on blood flow in ischemic dog colon. *Arch. Surg.*, **115** (1980) 602–605.
27. Bulkley GB, Womack WA, Downey JM, Kvietys PR, Granger DN. Collateral blood flow in segmental intestinal ischemia: effects of vasoactive agents. *Surgery*, **100** (1986) 157–166.
28. Longo WE, Ballantyne GH, Gusberg RJ. Ischemic colitis: patterns and prognosis. *Dis. Colon Rectum*, **35** (1992) 726–730.
29. Hanisch E, Schmandra TC, Encke A. Surgical strategies—anastomosis or stoma, a second look — when and why? *Langenbecks. Arch. Surg.*, **384** (1999) 239–242.
30. Koruth NM, Krukowski ZH, Youngson GG, et al. Intra-operative colonic irrigation in the management of left-sided large bowel emergencies. *Br. J. Surg.*, **72** (1985) 708–711.
31. Mosdell DM, Doberneck RC. Morbidity and mortality of ostomy closure. *Am. J. Surg.*, **162** (1991) 633–636.
32. Welch GH, Shearer MG, Imrie CW, Anderson JR, Gilmour DG. Total colonic ischemia. *Dis. Colon Rectum*, **29** (1986) 410–412.
33. Guivarc'h M, Roullet-Audy JC, Mosnier H, Boche O. [Ischemic colitis. A surgical series of 88 cases] Colites ischemiques. Une serie chirurgicale de 88 cas. *J. Chir. (Paris.)*, **134** (1997) 103–108.
34. Longo WE, Ward D, Vernava AM, Kaminski DL. Outcome of patients with total colonic ischemia. *Dis. Colon Rectum*, **40** (1997) 1448–1454.
35. Clavien PA, Durig M, Harder F. Venous mesenteric infarction: a particular entity. *Br. J. Surg.*, **75** (1988) 252–255.
36. Hassan HA, Raufman JP. Mesenteric venous thrombosis. *South. Med. J.*, **92** (1999) 558–562.
37. Ryu R, Lin TC, Kumpe D, et al. Percutaneous mesenteric venous thrombectomy and thrombolysis: successful treatment followed by liver transplantation. *Liver Transpl. Surg.*, **4** (1998) 222–225.
38. Eldrup-Jorgensen J, Hawkins RE, Bredenberg CE. Abdominal vascular catastrophes. *Surg. Clin. N. Am.*, **77** (1997) 1305–1320.
39. Rhee RY, Gloviczki P. Mesenteric venous thrombosis. *Surg. Clin. N. Am.*, **77** (1997) 327–338.
40. Condat B, Pessione F, Helene DM, Hillaire S, Valla D. Recent portal or mesenteric venous thrombosis: increased recognition and frequent recanalization on anticoagulant therapy. *Hepatology*, **32** (2000) 466–470.
41. Anonymous. American Gastroenterological Association Medical Position Statement: guidelines on intestinal ischemia [published erratum appears in *Gastroenterology*, **119** (2000) 280–1]. *Gastroenterology*, **118** (2000) 951–953.
42. Rhee RY, Gloviczki P, Mendonca CT, et al. Mesenteric venous thrombosis: still a lethal disease in the 1990s. *J. Vasc. Surg.*, **20** (1994) 688–697.
43. Hagihara PF, Ernst CB, Griffen WOJ. Incidence of ischemic colitis following abdominal aortic reconstruction. *Surg. Gynecol. Obstet.*, **149** (1979) 571–573.
44. Longo WE, Lee TC, Barnett MG, et al. Ischemic colitis complicating abdominal aortic aneurysm surgery in the U.S. veteran. *J. Surg. Res.*, **60** (1996) 351–354.

45. Bjorck M, Troeng T, Bergqvist D. Risk factors for intestinal ischaemia after aortoiliac surgery: a combined cohort and case-control study of 2824 operations. *Eur. J. Vasc. Endovasc. Surg.*, **13** (1997) 531–539.

46. Redaelli CA, Schilling MK, Carrel TP. Intraoperative assessment of intestinal viability by laser Doppler flowmetry for surgery of ruptured abdominal aortic aneurysms. *World J. Surg.*, **22** (1998) 283–289.

47. Bergman RT, Gloviczki P, Welch TJ, et al. The role of intravenous fluorescein in the detection of colon ischemia during aortic reconstruction. *Ann. Vasc. Surg.*, **6** (1992) 74–79.

48. Schiedler MG, Cutler BS, Fiddian-Green RG. Sigmoid intramural pH for prediction of ischemic colitis during aortic surgery. A comparison with risk factors and inferior mesenteric artery stump pressures. *Arch. Surg.*, **122** (1987) 881–886.

49. Bjorck M, Lindberg F, Broman G, Bergqvist D. pHi monitoring of the sigmoid colon after aortoiliac surgery. A five-year prospective study [In Process Citation]. *Eur. J. Vasc. Endovasc. Surg.*, **20** (2000) 273–280.

50. Jaeger HJ, Mathias KD, Gissler HM, Neumann G, Walther LD. Rectum and sigmoid colon necrosis due to cholesterol embolization after implantation of an aortic stent-graft. *J. Vasc. Interv. Radiol.*, **10** (1999) 751–755.

51. Madhavan P, McDonnell CO, Dowd MO, et al. Suprarenal mycotic aneurysm exclusion using a stent with a partial autologous covering [In Process Citation]. *J. Endovasc. Ther.*, **7** 2000. 404–409.

52. D'Ayala M, Hollier LH, Marin ML. Endovascular grafting for abdominal aortic aneurysms. *Surg. Clin. N. Am.*, **78** (1998) 845–862.

53. Van Damme H, Creemers E, Limet R. Ischaemic colitis following aortoiliac surgery. *Acta Chir. Belg.*, **100** (2000) 21–27.

54. Brandt CP, Piotrowski JJ, Alexander JJ. Flexible sigmoidoscopy. A reliable determinant of colonic ischemia following ruptured abdominal aortic aneurysm. *Surg. Endosc.*, **11** (1997) 113–115.

55. Houe T, Thorboll JE, Sigild U, Liisberg-Larsen O, Schroeder TV. Can colonoscopy diagnose transmural ischaemic colitis after abdominal aortic surgery? An evidence-based approach. *Eur. J. Vasc. Endovasc. Surg.*, **19** (2000) 304–307.

56. Betzler M. (Surgical technical guidelines in intestinal ischemia) Chirurgisch-technische Leitlinien bei intestinaler Ischamie. *Chirurg.*, **69** (1998) 1–7.

57. Brewster DC, Franklin DP, Cambria RP, et al. Intestinal ischemia complicating abdominal aortic surgery [see comments]. *Surgery*, **109** (1991) 447–454.

58. Tsiotos GG, Mullany CJ, Zietlow S, van Heerden JA. Abdominal complications following cardiac surgery. *Am. J. Surg.*, **167** (1994) 553–557.

59. Simic O, Strathausen S, Hess W, Ostermeyer J. Incidence and prognosis of abdominal complications after cardiopulmonary bypass. *Cardiovasc. Surg.*, **7** (1999) 419–424.

60. Zacharias A, Schwann TA, Parenteau GL, et al. Predictors of gastrointestinal complications in cardiac surgery [In Process Citation]. *Tex. Heart Inst. J.*, **27** (2000) 93–99.

61. Huddy SP, Joyce WP, Pepper JR. Gastrointestinal complications in 4473 patients who underwent cardiopulmonary bypass surgery. *Br. J. Surg.*, **78** (1991) 293–296.

62. Bender JS, Ratner LE, Magnuson TH, Zenilman ME. Acute abdomen in the hemodialysis patient population. *Surgery*, **117** (1995) 494–497.

63. Flobert C, Cellier C, Berger A, et al. Right colonic involvement is associated with severe forms of ischemic colitis and occurs frequently in patients with chronic renal failure requiring hemodialysis. *Am. J. Gastroenterol.*, **95** (2000) 195–198.

64. Han SY, Kwon YJ, Shin JH, Pyo HJ, Kim AR. Nonocclusive mesenteric ischemia in a patient on maintenance hemodialysis. *Korean J. Intern. Med.*, **15** (2000) 81–84.

65. Hung KH, Lee CT, Lam KK, et al. Ischemic bowel disease in chronic dialysis patients. *Chang. Keng. I. Hsueh. Tsa. Chih.*, **22** (1999) 82–87.

66. John AS, Tuerff SD, Kerstein MD. Nonocclusive mesenteric infarction in hemodialysis patients. *J. Am. Coll. Surg.*, **190** (2000) 84–88.

67. Cappell MS. Intestinal (mesenteric) vasculopathy. II. Ischemic colitis and chronic mesenteric ischemia. *Gastroenterol. Clin. N. Am.*, **27** (1998) 827–860, vi.

68. Simi M, Pietroletti R, Navarra L, Leardi S. Bowel stricture due to ischemic colitis: report of three cases requiring surgery. *Hepatogastroenterology*, **42** (1995) 279–281.

69. Oz MC, Forde KA. Endoscopic alternatives in the management of colonic strictures. *Surgery*, **108** (1990) 513–519.

70. Profili S, Bifulco V, Meloni GB, Demelas L, Niolu P, Manzoni MA. [A case of ischemic stenosis of the colon-sigmoid treated with self-expandable uncoated metallic prosthesis] Su un caso di stenosi ischemica del colon-sigma ricanalizzata mediante protesi metallica autoespansibile non rivestita. *Radiol. Med. (Torino.)*, **91** (1996) 665–667.

71. Elian N, Tabbi-Annani D, Goarin JP, Barrat C, Vayre P. [Thrombus floating in the thoracic aorta revealed by mesenteric ischemia (letter).] Thrombus flottant dans l'aorte thoracique revele par une ischemie mesenterique. *J. Chir. (Paris.)*, **133** (1996) 146–147.

72. Smith FC, Boon A, Shearman CP, Downing R. Spontaneous cholesterol embolisation: a rare cause of bowel infarction. *Eur. J. Vasc. Surg.*, **5** (1991) 581–582.

73. Dworkin MJ, Allen-Mersh TG. Effect of inferior mesenteric artery ligation on blood flow in the marginal artery-dependent sigmoid colon. *J. Am. Coll. Surg.*, **183** (1996) 357–360.

74. Wang N, Wong DT, Rivera JL, Bansal RC, Gundry SR. Repair of acute descending aortic dissection complicated by visceral ischemia. *Ann. Thorac. Surg.*, **68** (1999) 1067–1068.

75. Jarvinen O, Laurikka J, Salenius JP, Lepantalo M. Mesenteric infarction after aortoiliac surgery on the basis of 1752 operations from the National Vascular Registry. *World J. Surg.*, **23** (1999) 243–247.

76. Bonariol L, Virgilio C, Tiso E, et al. Spontaneous superior mesenteric vein thrombosis (SMVT) in primary protein S deficiency. A case report and review of the literature. *Chir. Ital.*, **52** (2000) 183–190.

77. Rademaker J. Veno-occlusive disease of the colon—CT findings. *Eur. Radiol.*, **8** (1998) 1420–1421.

78. Witte CL, Brewer ML, Witte MH, Pond GB. Protean manifestations of pylethrombosis. A review of thirty-four patients. *Ann. Surg.*, **202** (1985) 191–202.

79. Kukora JS. Extensive colonic necrosis complicating acute pancreatitis. *Surgery*, **97** (1985) 290–293.

80. Nagai T, Tomizawa T, Monden T, Mori M. Diabetes mellitus accompanied by nonocclusive colonic ischemia. *Intern. Med.*, **37** (1998) 454–456.

81. Zahn DG, Goerttler K. [Intestinal arteriosclerosis. Pathomorphological findings, localization and occurrence] Uber die Sklerose der Eingeweidearterien. Pathomorphologische Befunde, Lokalisation und Haufigkeit. *Arch. Kreislaufforsch.*, **64** (1971) 235–272.

82. Okuda Y, Takasugi K, Imai A, et al. [Two cases of rheumatoid arthritis complicated with vasculitis-induced ischemic enterocolitis]. *Ryumachi.*, **30** (1990) 403–407,408.

83. Israeli D, Dardik H, Wolodiger F, Silvestri F, Scherl B, Chessler R. Pelvic radiation therapy as a risk factor for ischemic colitis complicating abdominal aortic reconstruction. *J. Vasc. Surg.*, **23** (1996) 706–709.

84. Ha HK, Lee SH, Rha SE, et al. Radiologic features of vasculitis involving the gastrointestinal tract. *Radiographics*, **20** (2000) 779–794.

85. Wood MK, Read DR, Kraft AR, Barreta TM. A rare cause of ischemic colitis: polyarteritis nodosa. *Dis. Colon Rectum*, **22** (1979) 428–433.

86. Lee HJ, Park JW, Chang JC: Mesenteric and portal venous obstruction associated with primary antiphospholipid antibody syndrome [see comments]. *J. Gastroenterol. Hepatol.*, **12** (1997) 822–826.

87. Byun JY, Ha HK, Yu SY, et al. CT features of systemic lupus erythematosus in patients with acute abdominal pain: emphasis on ischemic bowel disease. *Radiology*, **211** (1999) 203–209.

88. Vega SJ, Barajas MJ, Torres AM. [Ischemic colitis as manifestation of Takayasu arteritis] Colitis isquemica como manifestacion de arteritis de Takayasu. *Gastroenterol. Hepatol.*, **18** (1995) 326–329.

89. Storesund B, Gran JT, Koldingsnes W. Severe intestinal involvement in Wegener's granulomatosis: report of two cases and review of the literature [see comments]. *Br. J. Rheumatol.*, **37** (1998) 387–390.

90. Kitamura T, Kubo M, Nakanishi T, et al. Phlebosclerosis of the colon with positive anti-centromere antibody [see comments]. *Intern. Med.*, **38** (1999) 416–421.

91. Guay A, Janower ML, Bain RW, McCready FJ. A case of Buerger's disease causing ischemic colitis with perforation in a young male. *Am. J. Med. Sci.*, **271** (1976) 239–234.

92. Bailey RW, Bulkley GB, Hamilton SR, Morris JB, Smith GW. Pathogenesis of nonocclusive ischemic colitis. *Ann. Surg.*, **203** (1986) 590–599.

93. Aldridge MC, Francis ND, Glazer G, Dudley HA. Colonic complications of severe acute pancreatitis. *Br. J. Surg.*, **76** (1989) 362–367.

94. Travis S, Davies DR, Creamer B. Acute colorectal ischaemia after anaphylactoid shock. *Gut*, **32** (1991) 443–446.

95. Carlin MS, Manashil GB. Ischemic colitis proximal to incarcerating left inguinal hernia. *Am. J. Gastroenterol.*, **59** (1973) 547–550.

96. Halligan MS, Saunders BP, Thomas BM, Phillips RK. Ischaemic colitis in association with sigmoid carcinoma: a report of two cases. *Clin. Radiol.*, **49** (1994) 183–184.

97. Vinci R, Angelelli G, Stabile IA, Gaballo A, Rotondo A. [Vascular complications in intestinal obstructions. The role of computed tomography.] Complicazioni vascolari nelle occlusioni intestinali. Ruolo della Tomografia Computerizzata. *Radiol. Med. (Torino).*, **98** (1999) 157–161.

98. Kawarada Y, Satinsky S, Matsumoto T. Ischemic colitis following rectal prolapse. *Surgery*, **76** (1974) 340–343.

99. Senati E, Coen LD. Massive gangrene of the colon—a complication of fecal impaction. Report of a case. *Dis. Colon Rectum*, **32** (1989) 146–148.

100. Iwakiri R, Fujimoto K, Hirano M, Hisatsugu T, Nojiri I, Sakemi T. Snake-strike—induced ischemic colitis with colonic stricture complicated by disseminated intravascular coagulation. *South. Med. J.*, **88** (1995) 1084–1085.

101. Gage TP, Gagnier JM. Ischemic colitis complicating sickle cell crisis. *Gastroenterology*, **84** (1983) 171–174.

102. Lao A, Bach D. Colonic complications in renal transplant recipients. *Dis. Colon Rectum*, **31** (1988) 130–133.

103. Rice E, DiBaise JK, Quigley EM. Superior mesenteric artery thrombosis after colonoscopy. *Gastrointest. Endosc.*, **50** (1999) 706–707.

104. Williams SM, Harned RK. Recognition and prevention of barium enema complications. *Curr. Probl. Diagn. Radiol.*, **20** (1991) 123–151.

105. Anonymous. Irritable bowel syndrome. New treatment drug on the market. *Harv. Health Lett.*, **25** (2000) 7.

106. Levinsky RA, Lewis RM, Bynum TE, Hanley HG. Digoxin induced intestinal vasoconstriction. The effects of proximal arterial stenosis and glucagon administration. *Circulation*, **52** (1975) 130–136.

107. Sharefkin JB, Silen W. Diuretic agents: inciting factor in nonocclusive mesenteric infarction? *JAMA*, **229** (1974) 1451–1453.

108. Freudenberger RS, Cappell MS, Hutt DA. Intestinal infarction after intravenous cocaine administration. *Ann. Intern. Med.*, **113** (1990) 715–716.

109. Barcewicz PA, Welch JP: Ischemic colitis in young adult patients. *Dis. Colon Rectum*, **23** (1980) 109–114.

110. Miyata T, Tamechika Y, Torisu M. Ischemic colitis in a 33-year-old woman on danazol treatment for endometriosis. *Am. J. Gastroenterol.*, **83** (1988) 1420–1423.

111. Carratu R, Parisi P, Agozzino A. Segmental ischemic colitis associated with nonsteroidal antiinflammatory drugs. *J. Clin. Gastroenterol.*, **16** (1993) 31–34.

112. Roberts C, Maddison FE. Partial mesenteric arterial occlusion with subsequent ischemic bowel damage due to pitressin infusion. *Am. J. Roentgenol.*, **126** (1976) 829–831.

113. Kam LW, Pease WE, Thompson PD. Exercise-related mesenteric infarction. *Am. J. Gastroenterol.*, **89** (1994) 1899–1900.

114. Woodward JM, Sanders DS, Keighley MR, Allan RN. Ischaemic enterocolitis complicating idiopathic dysautonomia. *Gut*, **43** (1998) 285–287.

115. Matsumoto T, Iida M, Kimura Y, Nanbu T, Fujishima M. Clinical features in young adult patients with ischaemic colitis. *J. Gastroenterol. Hepatol.*, **9** (1994) 572–575.

116. Ailani RK, Simms R, Caracioni AA, West BC. Extensive mesenteric inflammatory veno-occlusive disease of unknown etiology after primary cytomegalovirus infection: first case. *Am. J. Gastroenterol.*, **92** (1997) 1216–1218.

32 Surgical Treatments for Colonic Diseases

Joseph P. Muldoon and Steven J. Stryker

CONTENTS

1. INTRODUCTION

Historically, surgery for colonic diseases was characterized by the challenge of curing life-threatening intestinal ailments, while minimizing perioperative morbidity and mortality. Over the past 60 years, adjuncts have made colonic resection much less daunting, including broad-spectrum antibiotics, blood transfusions, advances in anastomotic techniques, and increasing understanding of nutritional and critical care concepts. With this progress and the resultant decrease in morbidity and mortality, attention is currently directed toward a new major focus, that being preservation of function. The ensuing sections will highlight the efforts to balance adequate disease extirpation and maintenance of quality of life.

2. CROHN'S DISEASE

2.1. Introduction

Surgery for Crohn's disease is often complex and varies with the site involved. Because the disease can frequently involve the small bowel, colon, rectum, and/or anus, a thorough evaluation or staging of the disease extent and severity must be made preoperatively before surgical therapy is undertaken. Previous resections and the attendant loss of absorptive surface are not an uncommon scenario in patients with Crohn's disease, making preoperative planning even more imperative in order to minimize unnecessary loss of functioning small bowel.

2.2. Nutritional Considerations

Malnutrition or malabsorption is not uncommon in patients with Crohn's disease. This may manifest as weight loss, anemia, hypoproteinemia, and/or specific vitamin deficiencies. Underlying origins for these findings include the presence of early satiety, postprandial abdominal pain, anorexia, decreased small bowel absorptive area, protein losing enteropathy, and drug–nutrient interactions inhibiting nutrient absorbtion and utilization. Increased energy expenditure caused by chronic inflammation and low-grade sepsis exacerbates these

From: *Colonic Diseases*
Edited by: T. R. Koch © Humana Press Inc., Totowa, NJ

problems. There is an inverse relationship between postoperative complications and concentrations of serum albumin and total iron binding capacity *(1)*. Specific nutritional deficiencies should be corrected preoperatively, if possible, and monitored postoperatively.

2.3. Indications for Surgery

Surgery for Crohn's disease is reserved for disabling symptoms not manageable by other less invasive means. Common indications for surgery of small bowel Crohn's disease include recurrent partial bowel obstruction, abscess, or symptomatic fistula. For colonic Crohn's disease, diarrhea, tenesmus, toxic colitis, and perianal disease are the most common indications for surgery. Extraintestinal manifestations of Crohn's disease are not usually a primary indication for surgery, but may contribute to the decision to proceed. Peripheral arthropathy, but not liver disease, may respond well to colectomy in patients with active colitis.

2.4. Technical Considerations

Intestinal resection in Crohn's disease should be conservative, in that the margin of healthy tissue surrounding the diseased segment removed should be minimal. Most surgeons recommend a minimum 2-cm margin from areas of overt disease *(2)*. The margins are usually determined by gross examination at surgery. Although visual inspection is often adequate for determining the extent of disease, palpation of the mesenteric margin may be helpful in more subtle cases. The mesentery of diseased bowel is invariably thickened on palpation, and finding an area of normal thickness is a sensitive indicator of the limit of disease. Obtaining microscopically clear margins, using intraoperative frozen section pathology, has not been found to reduce recurrent rates and is not recommended for most resections *(3)*.

2.5. Operative Options

When operative intervention is necessary, resection is the procedure of choice. Resection is preferable to bypass or exclusion because: (i) symptomatic recurrence rates are lowest with this operation; (ii) pathologic diagnosis is obtained; (iii) the septic focus is removed; and (iv) while the risk of carcinoma formation in the bypassed or excluded segment is small, surveillance of these segments is often not possible postoperatively.

There are specific circumstances in which bypass is an acceptable operation in Crohn's disease. It is the recommended treatment for patients with gastroduodenal Crohn's disease who are symptomatic, since resection of the duodenum would warrant an unnecessarily radical extirpation. In addition, when the inflammatory mass or phlegmon is firmly adherent to the iliac vessels or other retroperitoneal structures, bypass may be the safest alternative. Often, the surgeon can return after several months of bypass to attempt resection of the hopefully less-adherent mass.

Patients who present with chronic obstructive symptoms secondary to stricture often require resection, especially if the disease is primarily in the small bowel. Some patients having short segment disease or multiple strictures in the small bowel may be a candidate for intestinal strictureplasty, a surgical technique that widens the intestinal lumen, without requiring resection. Strictureplasty was first performed in 1961 by Brian Brooke. By using this technique, it may be possible to preserve small bowel length and absorptive surface area. Large series have reported the efficacy and safety of this procedure *(4)*.

Indications for strictureplasty have been outlined in a review by Tjandra and Fazio *(5)* and include: (i) previous extensive small bowel resection; (ii) rapid recurrence of symptoms (within 12 mo of previous resection); (iii) evidence of short bowel syndrome; (iv) presence of fibrotic strictures; and (v) diffuse or multiple symptomatic strictures. Absolute and relative contraindications to this surgical intervention include: (i) patients with free perforation; (ii) the presence of fistula or inflammatory phlegmon at the intended site; (iii) multiple adjacent strictures within a short segment of bowel; (iv) severe malnutrition (albumin levels <20 g/L); and (v) strictures longer than 30 cm.

Intestinal fistulas are a common finding in Crohn's disease. Enteroenteral, enterovesical, and enterocutaneous fistulas occur with the greatest frequency. When asymptomatic, enteroenteral fistulas are often not treated surgically. Symptomatic fistulas that fail medical treatment, however, will require resection of the diseased segment of bowel. When resection is performed, only the diseased portion of intestine (origin of fistula) needs to be removed, while the secondarily involved structure or "innocent bystander" organ can be repaired and left in place.

Perforation is not uncommon in Crohn's disease, but most commonly is a local phenomenon with phlegmon formation and abscess. Initial treatment, in these cases, is intravenous antibiotics and bowel rest. In the absence of abscess formation, clinical improvement is frequently seen, and surgery can often be avoided. If a well-defined abscess has formed, however, percutaneous drainage by radiologic means is often required. A fistula often results, frequently requiring an elective surgical resection in the ensuing weeks.

Free perforation secondary to Crohn's disease requires urgent exploration and resection of the affected segment. Stomas formation should be considered if there is perforation of the distal colon, if there is significant soiling of the peritoneal cavity, or if the patient is septic or malnourished.

Massive hemorrhage can occur in Crohn's disease. If the distribution of the Crohn's disease is limited, early surgical intervention is warranted. If the disease is multifocal or if the percise site of hemorrhage is in doubt, evaluation to establish the site of bleeding should proceed in the standard fashion with the use of endoscopy, bleeding scan, and/or visceral angiography. The majority of these patients will require surgery. The sudden onset of major hemorrhage typically originates in the terminal ileum and ileocolonic resection is the most frequently performed surgical procedure in these patients.

Finally, laparoscopic intestinal resection is being used with increasing frequency in the surgical management of Crohn's disease. The theoretical advantages include less pain, shorter hospitalization, an earlier return to work, and a better cosmetic result. While uncontrolled series seem to justify its use, laparoscopic intestinal resection for Crohn's disease has not yet been investigated in a randomized controlled fashion (6). Similarly, patient selection for this procedure varies widely from center to center and remains controversial.

2.6. Crohn's Colitis

Colonic involvement in Crohn's disease occurs in 20–45% of patients. Differentiating Crohn's colitis from ulcerative colitis can sometimes be difficult. There are clinical features suggestive of Crohn's colitis, including: (i) rectal sparing; (ii) apthous ulcers; (iii) areas of disease separated by "skip areas" of normal mucosa; (iv) presence of ileal disease; (v) presence of perianal disease with features typical of Crohn's disease; and (vi) internal fistulas to small bowel, bladder, or vagina. Up to two-thirds of patients with colonic disease will have extensive involvement, but 25–50% will have rectal sparing. In less than 10% of patients with Crohn's colitis, a segmental pattern will be observed (7).

Patients with Crohn's colitis may require emergency surgical intervention on rare occasions. Indications include severe colitis with sepsis, toxic megacolon, massive lower gastrointestinal bleeding, acute colonic obstruction, or perforation. For acute toxic colitis, a brief trial of aggressive medical treatment should initially be instituted with close observation. If the patient's clinical picture does not stabilize or improve over 12–24 h, surgical intervention is necessary. Surgical options include abdominal colectomy with ileostomy and rectal preservation, proctocolectomy with permanent ileostomy, and, less commonly, diverting ileostomy without resection. Simple diverting ileostomy may initially improve the patient's symptoms, but does not reliably prevent perforation. Proctocolectomy in the emergent setting carries high morbidity and mortality rates and, therefore, is not commonly performed. Most surgeons perform abdominal colectomy with Hartmann closure of the rectum and end ileostomy. This treatment removes the inflamed colon and diverts the fecal stream, while avoiding the increased morbidity of removing the rectum.

The most common indication for surgery in the elective setting is medical intractability of disease. Other indications include cancer arising in the colitic colon, obstruction, internal fistulas, and perianal disease. Diverting ileostomy alone is rarely performed in the elective setting for Crohn's colitis. This does not treat the underlying problem, and it has been demonstrated that only a small percentage of these patients go on to have intestinal continuity restored.

Segmental colectomy can be performed for patients with Crohn's colitis. Ideal candidates are those with short segments of disease and rectal sparing. The remaining colon should otherwise be normal in appearance. The most common indication is a localized stricture confined to the colon. Recurrence rates after segmental resection for Crohn's colitis range from 20–68% in reported series (8,9). Despite high recurrent rates, segmental resection may allow for better bowel function and avoidance of a stoma for several years.

Some patients have disease limited to the rectum or rectosigmoid. Treatment options for these patients include abdominoperineal resection with end colostomy or proctocolectomy with ileostomy. Lockhart-Mummery and Ritchie reported a series of 24 patients who underwent abdominoperineal resection (APR) for Crohn's disease. The cumulative recurrence rate was 6% at 5 yr and 11% at 10 yr (10). Most clinicians would argue that the quality of life in a patient with an end colostomy is superior to that with an ileostomy. Recurrences involving the stoma can be treated by repeat segmental resection or completion colectomy and ileostomy, depending on the extent of colonic disease.

For patients with rectal sparing, abdominal colectomy with ileorectal anastamosis can be performed. Patients should have normal rectal mucosa with a distensible rectal ampulla and adequate small bowel length to consider this operation. Patients with active perianal disease are poor candidates for this operation. The average patient will have four to seven bowel movements per day after this operation. Recurrence rates are high and this is usually a temporary solution. Longo et al. (11) reviewed 131 patients undergoing ileorectal anastamosis after colectomy for Crohn's disease. Anastomotic leak occurred in four patients, and 13 patients with a protective stoma never underwent closure. Of the 118 remaining patients, 65% had recurrent disease. However, 61% of the patients retained a functioning ileorectal anastomosis after a mean follow-up of 9.2 yr (11).

Total abdominal colectomy with ileostomy and Hartmann closure of the rectum is sometimes performed in the elective setting despite rectal involvement. This may be considered for patients in their child-bearing years to decrease the likelihood of postoperative impotence and infertility. Approximately 50% of these patients will require completion proctectomy within 10 yr. Patients more likely to require proctectomy include those with perianal disease at initial operation. If the rectum remains in place, endoscopic surveillance is mandatory in view of the increased risk of malignant degeneration.

2.7. Perianal Crohn's Disease

Perianal disease is a frequent manifestation of Crohn's disease. Perianal symptoms are the presenting sign of the disease in up to 15% of patients. Anal Crohn's disease is most commonly seen in patients who have colonic manifestations, but is also seen in patients with disease limited to the small bowel. Manifestations of perianal Crohn's disease include severe fissuring or ulceration of the anal canal, fistulas and abscesses, anal strictures, rectovaginal fistula, and large edematous skin tags. Surgery for perianal Crohn's disease is aimed at reducing local sepsis and pain, while avoiding unnecessarily aggressive surgical procedures, which may impair continence.

3. ULCERATIVE COLITIS

3.1. Introduction

The type of surgical procedure recommended for ulcerative colitis is based on the following principles: (i) the rectum is almost invariably involved in the disease process, with the rest of the colon being affected in a continuous fashion from the rectum proximally to a variable extent; (ii) the small intestine is not involved in the disease process and rare instances of "backwash ileitis" do not alter the surgical decisions; medical treatment is the primary therapy for patients with ulcerative colitis; and (iii) the anal canal has only musosal–submucosal involvement, with sparing of the distal anoderm and underlying sphincter complex.

3.2. Indications for Surgery

The most common indication for surgery for ulcerative colitis is intractability of disease. Patients who have persistent bloody diarrhea, anemia, abdominal pain, and/or tenesmus despite medical treatment, or have become dependant on corticosteroids to maintain remission, should be considered for operation. The introduction of the ileoanal pouch procedure has increased patient acceptance of surgery by obviating the need for permanent ileostomy.

Patients who present with fulminant colitis need to be aggressively resuscitated with fluids and electrolytes and have their medical therapy optimized. If there is continued deterioration clinically over the next 24 h or no significant improvement in the ensuing 5–7 d while receiving intensive medical therapy, surgical intervention is warranted (12,13).

Fulminant colitis not responding to medical therapy may rapidly progress to toxic megacolon, a rare but life threatening complication of ulcerative colitis. Precipitating factors in the development of toxic megacolon include antidiarrheal agents, belladonna alkaloids, opiate narcotics, and barium enema. With aggressive medical treatment, more than half of these patients can avoid emergency surgery. These patients may ultimately require colectomy, but patients fare better when this is performed under elective conditions (14).

Uncontrolled hemorrhage secondary to ulcerative colitis is rare, with a reported incidence of 0.2–4.5%. Robert et al. reported that 10% of the emergency colectomies performed for patients with ulcerative colitis were performed for massive bleeding (15).

Precancerous changes within the colitic colon or frank carcinoma itself is another major indication for colectomy. The risk of colorectal carcinoma complicating ulcerative colitis increases after 10 yr in patients with pancolitis, rising 1 to 2%/yr. Colonoscopy at intervals of 18–24 mo beyond the tenth year of disease has been recommended as a strategy to attempt to identify precancerous changes. Random biopsies should be obtained from each area of the colon looking for the presence of mucosal dysplasia. Abnormal appearing areas must also be biopsied. The presence of dysplasia represents a risk factor for the formation of cancer and these patients should be encouraged to undergo proctocolectomy. Patients with frank carcinoma obviously should undergo immediate colonic resection.

3.3. Surgical Options

3.3.1. TOTAL ABDOMINAL COLECTOMY WITH ILEOSTOMY
AND HARTMANN CLOSURE OF THE RECTUM OR ILEORECTAL ANASTOMOSIS

In the emergent setting, total abdominal colectomy with ileostomy and Hartmann closure of the rectum is the procedure of choice. Though not a curative procedure, it allows for removal of the majority of disease with less morbidity and lower mortality rates than proctocolectomy with ileostomy. Later, after the patient has recovered and is nutritionally replete, several options are available to deal with the retained defunctionalized rectum. If the rectum has minimal active disease and exhibits normal distensibility, ileorectal anastomosis remains an option. In carefully selected patients, functional results after ileorectal anastomosis are fair, with patients having 6–10 bowel movements per day. Recrudescence of disease in the remaining rectum may worsen the outcome. Satisfactory results were reported in up to 55% of patients with 5- to 17-yr follow-up at the Mayo Clinic *(16)*. In those patients with retained rectum, yearly surveillance proctoscopy with biopsies must be remembered due to the increased risk of rectal cancer. With the advent of ileoanal pouch surgery, ileorectal anastomosis is rarely used today for the surgical management of ulcerative colitis.

3.3.2. PROCTOCOLECTOMY WITH ILEOSTOMY

Historically, proctocolectomy with ileostomy was the operation of choice for patients with ulcerative colitis unresponsive to medical therapy. Advantages for this procedure include: (i) removal of all diseased bowel or at risk bowel (i.e., curative); (ii) elimination of the need for chronic medications; (iii) elimination of the colon cancer risk; and (iv) the performance of a one-stage procedure in the elective setting. The need for a permanent ileostomy, however, makes this option less desirable. Nonetheless, proctocolectomy with ileostomy is still a reasonable option in patients with a sphincter damaged by prior surgery or sepsis, or in elderly high risk individuals who are deemed too frail for complex continence-preserving techniques.

3.3.3. CONTINENT ILEOSTOMY

Creation of a continent ileostomy, a procedure championed by Kock in the 1960s and 1970s, was an attempt to provide those patients requiring ileostomy more control of bowel function and to remove the need for an external appliance. An intestinal pouch with valve and conduit is created from terminal ileum to act as a reservoir for stool. The pouch is continent and emptied using a catheter. Initial enthusiasm for this technique has waned because of a high rate of complications associated with the continent ileostomy. Significant early postoperative complications occurred in as many as 23% of patients. In one study *(17)*, late complications, primarily valve dysfunction, requiring revision surgery occurred in 53% of patients.

3.3.4. ILEAL POUCH-ANAL ANASTOMOSIS

Restoring intestinal continuity and maintaining anal sphincter function after proctocolectomy for ulcerative colitis was thought by many to be an unattainable goal. Poor functional results and septic complications from anastomotic leaks complicated initial attempts at ileoanal anastomosis. In 1978, Parks and Nicholls published their series showing that modifications of this operation made this a viable option for patients with ulcerative colitis *(18)*. Proctocolectomy with ileostomy was the operation of choice through the 1970s. The decade of the 1980s saw the ileal pouch–anal anastomosis (IPAA) increasingly gain acceptance. Currently, it is the surgical procedure of choice for most patients with ulcerative colitis.

Proctocolectomy with IPAA is a complex surgical procedure with the potential for considerable perioperative morbidity. Patients ideally suited for proctocolectomy with immediate ileal pouch reconstruction are in good overall health. When patients have severe colitis and associated malnutrition or sepsis, abdominal colectomy with ileostomy, a more expeditious procedure, may be prudent until the patient recovers sufficiently. Performing IPAA in the acutely ill patient has been shown to increase the risk of pelvic sepsis and anastomotic leak rates significantly *(19)*. During early experience with this operation, proper patient selection was thought to be important, and the procedure was only offered to young patients with mildly or moderately active disease. With increased experience, it is now performed in most age groups. It is important that patients have good anal sphincter function because stool consistency is typically liquid or semisolid. Postoperatively, patients usually have four to six bowel movements per day, typically without urgency. Formation of an ileal reservoir allows storage of stool prior to evacuation. Several techniques of pouch construction have been used over the years. A J-shaped pouch is the most common configuration used today. Pouch length should be 15–20 cm to allow for adequate storage. The pouch is anastomosed to the anal canal either at or just above the dentate line after removal of all diseased mucosa.

4. RECTAL CANCER

4.1. Introduction

Rectal cancer was diagnosed in approx 37,000 people in the U. S. in 2001 *(20)*. The surgeon's approach to rectal cancer continues to evolve, as new technologies have allowed for better preoperative staging and improved surgical decision making. The approach to middle third and distal rectal cancers has changed significantly, with the current emphasis on sphincter preservation, when appropriate. The use of preoperative combined modality chemotherapy and radiation to downstage the tumor is gaining acceptance in an effort to improve sphincter preservation and decrease local recurrence.

4.2. Evaluation

Physical exam begins with a general exam to evaluate for concurrent illnesses and to look for evidence of metastatic disease such as jaundice, lymphadenopathy, hepatomegaly, or ascites. A thorough evaluation of the anorectum should be performed. Digital examination is especially helpful in low cancers for evaluating the relationship of the tumor to the anal sphincter, texture of the tumor, and whether or not fixation to adjacent structures is present. Rigid proctosigmoidoscopy provides a more precise measurement of location above the anal verge than flexible endoscopy.

Because synchronous colon cancer is reported in up to 6% of patients with colorectal cancer, all patients require full evaluation of the colon by colonoscopy or barium enema if possible. Patients with obstructing or near obstructing lesions sometimes cannot be evaluated with these tests initially.

Blood tests important in the evaluation include complete blood count, serum electrolytes, and liver function tests, including serum bilirubin, alkaline phosphatase, aspartate aminotransferase (AST), and alanine aminotransferase (ALT). Serum carcinoembrionic antigen levels should be drawn preoperatively. All patients should undergo a computed tomography (CT) scan of the abdomen and pelvis and chest X-ray to rule out locally advanced or metastatic disease. Other tests used in the preoperative evaluation of rectal cancer may include endorectal ultrasound, magnetic resonance imaging (MRI) or position emission tomography (PET) scan.

4.3. COMPUTED TOMOGRAPHY

CT of the abdomen and pelvis should be performed on all patients with rectal cancer, preoperatively, looking for evidence of metastatic disease and to evaluate the extent of local disease. It is considered accurate in the diagnosis of liver metastases, especially those >1.5 cm. Studies by Williams et al. *(21)* demonstrated 97% accuracy, when assessed at laparotomy, for hepatic metastases >1.5 cm. This accuracy drops off significantly, however, when the lesions are <1.5 cm. New helical CT scanners allow for biphasic and triphasic intravenous contrast evaluations of the liver. Evaluation of the liver is performed during the arterial contrast and venous contrast phases, thereby optimizing the sensitivity of the test. If suspicious hepatic lesions are identified, biopsy can also be performed with CT or ultrasound guidance to confirm the diagnosis in appropriate cases.

The accuracy of an abdominal CT scan for evaluation of local disease, including depth of rectal wall penetration (T stage) and presence of lymph node metastases, is not as good (33–83%). Shank et al. *(22)* prospectively evaluated the accuracy of preoperative local–regional staging. When separate radiologists staged the tumors by abdominal CT scan alone, interobserver agreement was only 37%. Indeed when the same observer studied the same subject twice at different times, the agreement between readings was only 51%. Overall agreement with Duke's stage was only 33%. The inability to accurately diagnose lymph node metastases has also been demonstrated by several studies *(23,24)*. Patients who are being considered for sphincter preserving operations, especially local resection, should undergo further testing including endorectal ultrasound.

4.4. Endorectal Ultrasound

To assess the extent of local disease preoperatively, endorectal ultrasound is the most accurate and cost-effective modality. Using a 7.5–10 MHz transducer, excellent visualization of the layers of the rectal wall can be obtained. Depth of rectal wall penetration can accurately be predicted in 85–90% of patients when the test is performed by an experienced operator *(25)*. Evaluation of lymph nodes is less impressive, but is superior to abdominal CT and MRI scanning. Hildebrant et al. *(26)* demonstrated accuracy in diagnosing lymph node metastases in 72% of individuals vs lymph node inflammation with a specificity of 83%. Because there is often difficulty in interpretation, conservative judgment of lymph node disease is appropriate *(27)*.

Proper technique and operator experience are the keys to reliable preoperative staging. Use of a proctoscope for precise placement of the probe is recommended. It should be noted that this modality is much less accurate in determining the extent of rectal wall involvement with viable tumor if the patient has undergone preoperative radiation therapy.

4.5. Magnetic Resonance Imaging

MRI with the use of endorectal surface coil is being examined as a modality for preoperative evaluation of local disease. It appears that this method is accurate in estimating rectal wall penetration. Limitations in its ability to diagnose lymph node metastases make it no better, at this time, than abdominal CT scanning. Limited availability of this test and expense of the highly specialized coil make endorectal ultrasound a more viable option at the present time.

4.6. Management

The optimal management of patients with rectal cancer requires a team approach, which includes surgeon, radiation oncologist, and medical oncologist. After an appropriate preoperative work-up, the treatment plan best suited to the individual patient can be implemented. Surgery remains the mainstay in the treatment of rectal cancer and in early cancers may be the only treatment that is needed. While the primary goal of treatment is the cure of the patient, sphincter preservation is also very desirable, if possible. The use of preoperative combined modality radiation and chemotherapy can often achieve both goals and is most appropriate for Stage II and Stage III rectal cancers *(28)*.

4.7. Operative Management

The location and stage of the tumor determine the operative management of rectal cancer. For ease of discussion, the rectum will be divided into thirds. The rectum 12–16 cm from the anal verge is the upper third, 7–12 cm is the middle third, and <7 cm represents the distal third of the rectum. Rectal cancer involving the upper third of the rectum, at or just above the peritoneal reflection, is best treated by low anterior resection in the majority of cases. Cancers of the mid and distal rectum are more difficult to treat because of their proximity to the anal sphincter and the technical difficulties posed by the narrow confines of the pelvis.

4.8. Operative Procedures

4.8.1. Abdominoperineal Resection (APR)

APR has long been considered the gold standard for treatment of rectal cancers below 10 cm. This idea is being challenged by many surgeons who are demonstrating that sphincter preservation can be achieved on tumors <10 cm from the anal verge with equal oncologic efficacy *(29,30)*. APR remains an important operation in selected patients with rectal cancers. Rectal cancer involving the levator muscles or sphincter muscles is an absolute indication for APR. Patients with poor sphincter function and marginal continence preoperatively, and patients who are bedridden or otherwise nonambulatory, are usually best treated by APR as well.

4.8.2. Low Anterior Resection with Anal Sphincter Preservation

Low anterior resection (LAR) has largely replaced APR as the primary surgical approach to rectal cancer. To justify the use of sphincter preserving operations for low rectal cancers, oncologic principles of the operation must not be compromised, morbidity must be kept to a minimum, and the functional result must be consistent with a reasonably good quality of life.

The goal of resection is removal of all local disease. Better understanding of pelvic anatomy and routes of tumor spread in rectal cancer have guided present recommendations for resection margins. Local recurrence may be minimized by appropriate emphasis on adequate lateral resection margins, including partial mesorectal excision for tumors of the upper one-third of the rectum, and total mesorectal excision for tumors of the middle and distal thirds of the rectum. Autonomic nerve preservation during pelvic dissection is also increasingly recognized as an invaluable technique for minimizing postoperative bladder and sexual dysfunction. Surgical stapling devices have largely supplanted handsewn suture techniques for low pelvic anastomoses. These staplers are easier to use and result in a more secure anastomosis deep in the pelvis. Finally, selected use of temporary proximal fecal diversion may also minimize morbidity in the low-lying high risk anastomosis.

When the tumor is located in the mid to distal rectum, achieving a satisfactory distal margin of clearance may require creation of an anastomosis at or within the anal canal. Coloanal anastomosis is ideally suited for this situation, where the sigmoid or descending colon is mobilized sufficiently to allow anastomosis at the level of the anal sphincter. At this extremely low level, stapled anastomosis is still a consideration, but a handsewn endoanal anastomosis may be necessary. Temporary proximal diverting stoma is almost always utilized with coloanal reconstruction. In recent years, a colonic J-shaped reservoir has been incorporated into coloanal reconstruction to enhance postoperative function.

4.8.3. Functional Results of LAR or Coloanal Anastomosis

Although anal sphincter preserving techniques are possible in the majority of patients with rectal cancers, the functional outcome of these procedures can vary widely and is often initially less than ideal. Stool frequency and incontinence to varying degrees result in significant morbidity and patient frustration. Several authors have demonstrated that functional outcome worsens with the more distal anastomosis (31). The reason for the worsened functional results is the decreased capacity of the rectal remnant and, to a lesser extent, reduced resting anal pressures identified after these operations. Functional results gradually improve over the initial 9 mo following surgery. This improvement may, in part, be due to increased rectal capacity over time. As previously mentioned, the functional results of these low anastomoses appear to be improved by the construction of a colonic J-shaped pouch (32,33).

4.8.4. Local Excision for Rectal Cancer

A small percentage of cancers involving the lower rectum are amenable to local excision via a variety of approaches. Retrospective investigation of this possibility was done by Morson et al. (34), and this question has recently been studied prospectively by Bleday et al. (35)and Ota et al. (36). This operative modality is appropriate for a select group, comprising approx 5–15% of patients with rectal cancer. Good results are dependent on accurate patient selection. Several factors, including T stage, presence of lymph node metastases, tumor size, and histological characteristics of the tumor, must be considered.

Patients with rectal cancer confined to the mucosa and submucosa (T_1) that are completely excised with adequate lateral and deep surgical margins require no further treatment. Those undergoing local resection for lesions involving but not through the muscularis propria (T_2) should be offered radiation with chemotherapy, while patients found to have transmural extension (T_3) on pathologic examination of the locally excised lesion should be urged to undergo a formal resection (LAR, coloanal anastomosis, or APR). Retrospective pathology studies report an incidence of lymph node metastases in up to 20% of patients with T_2 tumors. Local failure rates reported by Minsky et al. (37) after local resection and radiation averaged 3% (for T_1), 10% (T_2), and 24% (T_3). In the Bleday et al. study (35), recurrence was associated with positive margins following resection, or lymphatic invasion. Forty-eight patients were studied (T_1, 21 patients, T_2, 21 patients, and T_3, 5 patients) with an overall recurrence rate of 8%.

The techniques used for local excision of rectal tumors include transanal, transsphincteric, and transcoccygeal approaches. The approach used is dependent upon tumor location, body habitus, and physician experience. The transanal approach is the approach used in the majority of patients. With adequate anesthesia and the available anal retractors, most tumors of the lower rectum can be resected transanally. Using this approach also minimizes the likelihood of complications such as fistula and incontinence, which are more commonly seen after the transcoccygeal and transsphincteric approaches.

4.8.5. Transanal Endoscopic Microsurgery

Transanal endoscopic microsurgery (TEM) is a form of minimal access surgery, performed through a transanal route, utilizing specialized instruments and stereoscopic optics. It follows the same principles and indications as the more traditional transanal surgery described above. The benefit of this technology is that it extends the boundaries of the traditional procedures to the level of the rectosigmoid region. The principles of traditional local transanal resection should be followed. The improved visibility of TEM, however, allows more precise delineation of margins and allows enhanced suture placement at more proximal locations within the rectum. Advanced training in TEM techniques, expense of these highly specialized instruments, and the relative small percentage of rectal cancers amenable to local resection, limit the availability of TEM to only a few surgeons in a given medical community.

REFERENCES

1. Lindor KD, Fleming CR, Ilstrup DM. Preoperative nutritional status and other factors that influence surgical outcome in patients with Crohn's disease. *Mayo Clin. Proc.*, **60** (1985) 393–396.
2. Fazio VW, Marchetti F, Church JM, et al. Effect of resection margins on the recurrance of Crohn's disease in the small bowel. A randomized controlled trial. *Ann. Surg.* **224** (1996) 563–573.
3. Chardavayne R, Flint GW, Pollack S, Wise L. Factors affecting recurrence following resection for Crohn's disease. *Dis. Colon Rectum*, **29** (1986) 495–499.
4. Hurst RD, Michelassi F. Strictureplasty for Crohn's disease: techniques and long term results. *World J. Surg.* **22** (1998) 359–363.
5. Tjandra JJ, Fazio VW. Techniques of strictureplasty. *Perspect. Colon Rectal Surg.*, **5** (1992) 189–198.
6. Alabaz O; Iroatulam AJ; Nessim A; Weiss EG; Nogueras JJ; Wexner SD. Comparison of laparoscopically assisted and conventional ileocolic resection for Crohn's disease. *Eur. J. Surg.*, **166** (2000) 213–217.
7. Goligher JC. Surgical treatment of Crohn's disease affecting mainly or entirely the large bowel. *World J. Surg.*, **12** (1988) 186.
8. Prabhakar LP, Laramee C, Nelson H, et al. Avoid a stoma: Role for segmental or abdominal colectomy in Crohn's colitis. *Dis. Colon Rectum*, **40** (1997) 71–78.
9. Allan A, Andrews H, Hilton CJ, et al. Segmental colonic resection is appropriate operation for short skip lesions due to Crohn's disease of the colon. *World J. Surg.*, **13** (1989) 611–616.
10. Lockhart-Mummery HE, Ritchie JK. Surgical treatment: large intestine. In *Inflammatory Bowel Disease*. 1st ed. Allan RN, Keighley MRB, Alexander-Williams J, et al. (eds.), Churchill Livingstone, Edinburgh, UK, 1993, pp. 462–468.
11. Longo WE, Oakley JR, Lavery IC, et al. Outcome of ileorectal anastomosis for Crohn's colitis. *Dis. Colon Rectum*, **35** (1992) 1066–1071.
12. Hawley PR. Emergency surgery for ulcerative colitis. *World J. Surg.* **12** (1988) 169–173.
13. Albrechstein D, Bergan A, Nygaard K, et al. Urgent surgery for ulcerative colitis: Early colectomy in 132 patients. *World J. Surg.*, **5** (1981) 607–615.
14. Grant CS, Dozios RR. Toxic megacolon: Ultimate fate of patients after successful medical management. *Amer. J. Surg.*, **147** (1984) 106–110.
15. Robert JH, Sachar DB, Aufses AH, et al. Management of severe hemorrhage in ulcerative colitis. *Amer. J. Surg.*, **147** (1990) 106–110.
16. Farnell MB, van Heerden JA, Beart RW, et al. Rectal preservation in nonspecific inflammatory disease of the colon. *Ann. Surg.*, **192** (1980) 249–253.
17. Vernava AM, Goldberg SM. Is the Kock pouch still a viable option? *Int. J. Colorectal Dis.*, **3** (1988) 135–138.
18. Parks AG, Nicholls RJ. Proctocolectomy without ileostomy for ulcerative colitis. *Br. J. Med.*, **2** (1978) 85–88.
19. Hayvaert G, Penninckx F, Filez L, et al. Restorative proctocolectomy in elective emergency cases of ulcerative colitis. *Int. J. Colorectal Dis.*, **9** (1994) 73–76.
20. Parker SL, Tong T, Bolden S, Wingo PA. Cancer statistics 1997. *CA Cancer J. Clin.*, **47** (1997) 5–27.
21. Williams NS, Durdey P, Quirk P. Pre-operative staging of rectal neoplasm and its impact on clinical management. *Br. J. Surg.*, **72** (1985) 868–874.
22. Shank B, Dershaw DD, Caravelli J, et al. A prospective study of the accuracy of preoperative computed tomographic staging of patients with biopsy-proven rectal carcinoma. *Dis. Colon Rectum*, **33** (1990) 285–290.
23. Freenz PC, Marks WM, Ryan JA, et al. Colorectal carcinoma evaluation with CT: Preoperative staging and detection of postoperative recurrence. *Radiology*, **158** (1986) 347–353.
24. Kramann B, Hildebrant U. Computed tomography versus endosonography in the staging of rectal carcinoma: a comparative study. *Int. J. Colon Dis.*, **1** (1986) 216–218.
25. Deen K, Madoff R, Belemonte C, et al. Preoperative staging of rectal neoplasms with endorectal ultrasonography. *Semin. Colon Rectal Surg.*, **6** (1995) 78–85.
26. Hildebrant U, Klein T, Feifel G, et al. Endosonography of pararectal lymph nodes: in vitro and in vivo evaluation. *Dis. Colon Rectum*, **33** (1990) 863–868.
27. Orrom WJ, Wong WD, Rothenberger DA, et al. Endorectal ultrasound in the preoperative staging of rectal tumors: a learning experience. *Dis. Colon Rectum*, **33** (1990) 654–659.

28. Stryker SJ, Kiel KD, Rademaker A, Shaw JM, Ujiki GT, Poticha SM. Preoperative "Chemoradiation" for stages II and III rectal carcinoma. *Arch. Surg.*, **131** (1996) 514–519.
29. Heald RJ, Ryall RDH. Recurrence and survival after total mesorectal excision for rectal cancer. *Lancet*, **1** (1986) 1479–1482.
30. Lasson ALL, Ekelund GR, Lindstrom CG. Recurrence risks after stapled anastamosis for rectal carcinoma. *Acta Chir. Scand.*, **150** (1984) 85–89.
31. Lewis WG, Martin IG, Williamson MER, et al. Why do some patients experience poor functional results after resection of the rectum for carcinoma? *Dis. Colon Rectum*, **38** (1995) 259–263.
32. Ho YH, Tan M, Seow-Choen F. Prospective randomized controlled study of clinical function and anorectal physiology after low anterior resection: comparison of a straight and colonic J pouch anastamosis. *Br. J. Surg.*, **83** (1996) 978–980.
33. Parc R, Tiret E, Frileux P, et al. Resection and colo-anal anastamosis with colonic reservior for rectal carcinoma. *Br. J. Surg.*, **73** (1986) 139–141.
34. Morson BC, Bussey HJ, Samoorian S. Policy of local excision for early cancer of the colorectum. *Gut*, **18** (1977) 1045–1050.
35. Bleday R, Breen E, Jessup JM, et al. Prospective evaluation of local excision for small rectal cancers. *Dis. Colon Rectum*, **40** (1997) 388–392.
36. Ota DM, Skibber J, Rich TA. M.D. Anderson cancer center experience with local excision and multimodality therapy for rectal cancer. *Surg. Oncol. Clin. N. Am.*, **1** (1992) 147–152.
37. Minsky B, Cohen A, Enker W, et al. Preoperative 5 fluouracil, low dose leukovorin, and concurrent radiation therapy for rectal cancer. *Cancer*, **73** (1994) 273–280.

33 Anorectal Disorders

Mohammed M. H. Kalan and Bruce A. Orkin

CONTENTS

INTRODUCTION

Anorectal disorders are extremely common, and well over 50% of the population will be afflicted by one or more during a lifetime. Although hemorrhoids are typically blamed for virtually any anorectal complaint, other disorders are just as common. Appropriate treatment is based on identification of the correct diagnosis. In this chapter we will review the common benign anorectal problems the practitioner is likely to encounter including hemorrhoids, fissures, abscesses and fistulae, pruritus ani, hypertrophied anal papillae, and skin tags.

2. HEMORRHOIDS

Hemorrhoidal vessels—veins and arteries—are the normal vascular plexes that surround the anal canal. The internal hemorrhoidal vessels lie in the submucosal connective tissue above the dentate line, while the external hemorrhoidal vessels lie in the subcutaneous position below the dentate line in the lower anal canal and around the anal verge. Bundles of the internal hemorrhoidal vessels, with their surrounding smooth muscle and connective tissue, create the internal "anal cushions," which are felt to contribute to fine apposition of the anorectal ring. When these vessels become dilated and the surrounding connective tissue degenerates, these bundles enlarge. They may slide down, or prolapse, with the passage of stool and often bleed. These are symptomatic internal hemorrhoids.

Hemorrhoids are a common complaint and are often wrongly blamed by patients for virtually any anorectal symptom. The mere presence of hemorrhoids does not constitute an indication for treatment, irrespective of size. Only symptomatic hemorrhoids require treatment. Definitive diagnosis is by inspection and anoscopy. Sigmoidoscopy is necessary to rule out

From: *Colonic Diseases*
Edited by: T. R. Koch © Humana Press Inc., Totowa, NJ

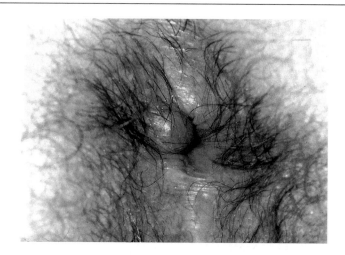

Fig. 1. Thrombosed external hemorrhoid.

other rectal pathology, and colonoscopy (or barium enema) may be required in higher risk cases. Two common varieties are encountered: external and internal hemorrhoids.

External hemorrhoids are located below the dentate line and are covered by squamous epithelium. These usually present with significant pain when they are acutely thrombosed (Fig. 1). Bleeding is unusual, but may occur when the skin overlying the thrombosis ulcerates. A history of straining or recent labor and delivery may be forthcoming. Local examination reveals a tender, bluish lump at the anal verge. Management depends upon severity of symptoms and time of presentation. Most patients feel better by the fourth or fifth day after symptom onset. In the first few days when symptoms are acute, excision of the thrombosed vessel with a small wedge of skin may be performed under local anesthesia. The wound is left to heal secondarily. This is usually an office procedure, which results in instant relief of pain. Incision and clot extraction alone is not recommended, as it often results in incomplete resolution of pain, persistent bleeding, and recurrence. If the patient's symptoms are improving spontaneously, analgesics, stool softeners, and warm tub baths are sufficient. Suppositories and topical agents are not useful.

Internal hemorrhoids are dilated vessels of the internal hemorrhoidal plexus, located above the dentate line and covered by transitional and columnar epithelium. Common symptoms include painless bright red bleeding at the end of defecation and prolapsing tissue (Fig. 2). The patient may complain of blood coating the stool, dripping or squirting into the toilet bowl, or simply seen on the toilet paper. Major hemorrhage and anemia are rare and, if found, should prompt further investigation before ascribing them to hemorrhoids. Pain usually suggests a complication such as thrombosis or, more likely, an associated condition such as a fissure. Chronic prolapse predisposes patients to pruritus and perianal discomfort as a result of mucous and fecal irritation of the perineum. Four grades of severity are commonly described based on the extent of prolapse: (i) first degree do not prolapse, but are dilated and may bleed; (ii) second degree prolapse with bowel movements and reduce spontaneously; (iii) third degree prolapse and requires manual reduction; and (iv) fourth degree are chronically prolapsed.

The majority of patients with hemorrhoids are treated without surgery. Patient symptoms may often be controlled by a regime of a high fiber diet, stool bulking agents, and fluids. Mild symptoms may respond to dietary measures alone. Office procedures, such as rubber band

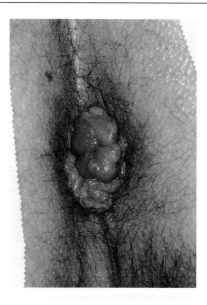

Fig. 2. Prolapsing internal hemorrhoid.

ligation, infrared coagulation, or sclerotherapy, may be used for persistent bleeding from first, second, and selected cases of third degree hemorrhoids. Rubber band ligation is quick, easy, and relatively painless if performed correctly. Generally, only one column is treated initially, but if it is well-tolerated, two ligations may be performed at the next visit. The most common complication is bleeding, so aspirin and NSAIDs are to be avoided for 10 d before and after treatment. The most significant reported complication is perianal sepsis, which may result in death; fortunately, this is extremely rare. Rubber band ligation works well for larger bulbous internal hemorrhoids, while infrared coagulation and sclerotherapy are appropriate treatment for smaller bleeding hemorrhoids. Treatment with lasers is expensive and unnecessary. Topical agents are mentioned only to be condemned. Steroid medications do not address the underlying pathology, as these are not inflammatory conditions and prolonged use may result in thinning of the tissues and poor healing. Hemorrhoidectomy is required in fewer than 10% of patients with symptomatic hemorrhoids and is reserved for patients with large third and fourth degree internal hemorrhoids. The operation is performed in the prone jackknife or the lithotomy position, in an outpatient setting. Recurrence rates are only 2–5 % and may be managed either conservatively or, rarely, with repeat surgery. Emergency hemorrhoidectomy is necessary in the presence of incarcerated prolapse, strangulation and necrosis (Fig. 3). Prolapse and thrombosis occurring during delivery may be treated operatively in the immediate postpartum period. Immunosuppressed patients are at somewhat higher risk of local complications, but may be offered surgery as needed.

3. ANAL FISSURE

An anal fissure is a linear tear in the skin of the lower anal canal. Fissures are extremely common and may often cause pain that seems out of proportion to their appearance. Both sexes are equally affected. In men, the vast majority of fissures occur in the posterior midline, while 10% or more of fissures in females occur in the anterior midline. Lateral or multiple fissures

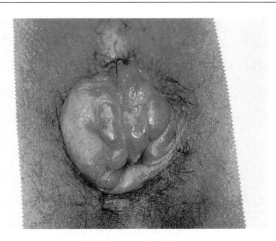

Fig. 3. Prolapsed thrombosed incarcerated hemorrhoids.

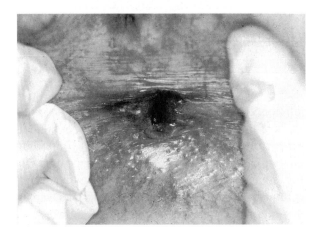

Fig. 4. A chronic fissure *in ano* with fibrotic edges and a small skin tag. The hypertrophied anal papilla above at the dentate line may be seen with an anoscope.

are relatively uncommon and may be associated with trauma, Crohn's disease, and human immunodeficiency virus (HIV) infection. Most fissures are associated with a history of constipation and passage of a hard stool, but explosive diarrhea may also be a cause. A tight anal sphincter may be the cause in a minority of mostly younger patients. Fissures may be classified as acute and chronic.

Acute fissures are painful and often bleed. The pain is sharp and can be severe, generally beginning with a bowel movement and lasting for minutes to hours. The pain is often described as cutting or tearing. Once the painful episode subsides, the patient may experience little or no discomfort, until the next bowel movement. Bleeding is bright red and usually seen on the toilet paper or streaking the stools. Diagnosis is usually made by inspection alone. Gentle separation of the buttocks reveals the fissure, associated spasm of the orifice. Chronic fissures may typically be found in association with the classical triad of a skin tag at the anal verge below the fissure (the "sentinel pile") and a hypertrophied anal papilla at the dentate line above (Fig. 4). Digital examination and proctoscopy may cause severe pain and will often be resisted by the patient. Therefore, further evaluation may need to be deferred for several weeks (but not forgotten). Treatment is usually conservative. Compliance with a 6–8 wk regimen of bowel management, including a high fiber diet, fluids, fiber supplements, and stool softeners, combined with warm tub baths and analgesics results in healing of the acute fissure in well over 90% of cases. Local steroid creams and suppositories play no role in the management of fissures.

Symptoms of a chronic anal fissure are similar to those of the acute variety, but may be intermittent in nature. Bleeding may not be a major symptom in the presence of extensive scarring. Examination typically reveals the classical triad: the fissure itself with its indurated edges, the sentinel pile, and a hypertrophied papilla at the dentate line. Many of these patients still exhibit poor bowel habits, and they will respond to the same conservative approach as used for acute fissures. This is successful in 60–70% of patients. Most who fail, do so because they have an elevated internal sphincter resting pressure, which may be confirmed by manometry testing. Measures recently advocated for persistent fissures include topical 0.2% nitropaste (often limited by headaches) or nifedipine and botulinum toxin (Botox) injection. These are not yet proven or standard of care, and results are quite variable. Manual anal dilatation has been generally abandoned because of its uncontrolled and variable results and complications (tearing of the sphincter in several locations and incontinence). Fissurectomy is rarely necessary and recurrence is common afterwards because of the failure to address the underlying problem. Lateral internal sphincterotomy is the standard approach to the patient with a persistent fissure and high resting pressures. The procedure may be performed in the office using local anesthetic or in the operating suite. The lower one half of the internal anal sphincter is divided sharply, resulting in a "give" and a palpable relaxation of the anal canal. This leads to healing of nearly 95% of persistent chronic fissures. The major risk is fecal incontinence, minor (gas or diarrhea) in 5–10% of patients and major (loss of solid stool) in 1 to 2% of patients. An incomplete internal sphincterotomy may be a cause of recurrence.

4. ANORECTAL ABSCESS

Anorectal abscesses are felt to usually occur due to occlusion of one of the intersphincteric anal glands that drain into the dentate line crypts. Feces, trauma, and inflammatory disorders are the most frequent causes of occlusion. The bacteria that normally live in the glands and along the ducts multiply. If the dust is open they shed into the lumen and stool. If not, they accumulate and develop into an abscess. This is known as the "cryptoglandular theory of perirectal sepsis." Once the infection is established, manifestations depend upon direction of spread. Caudal spread presents as a perianal abscess. Lateral spread across the external sphincter results in an ischiorectal fossa abscess. These are the two most common varieties of abscesses. Cephalad extension is uncommon and may cause a supralevator or high intermuscular abscess. These may be more difficult to diagnose since, although the patient complains of pain, little is seen on external exam and internal exam may be impossible. Therefore, a high degree of suspicion must be maintained. Circumferential spread may result in a "horseshoe" abscess.

Patients usually present with a several day history of increasing pain and an increasing swelling or tender mass in the perianal region. Systemic manifestations of sepsis, such as fever, chills, or sweats, are uncommon. Deep rectal pain and dysuria may indicate a high site of sepsis. A history of similar symptoms in the past may be forthcoming. Examination may reveal an erythematous and indurated mass, which is very tender and may be fluctuant. A high fistula may be bereft of external findings, but may be suspected if there is fullness and tenderness on digital rectal exam.

Treatment of an anorectal abscess is prompt incision and drainage of the pus. Deep curettage is not necessary in the ambulatory setting. The vast majority of patients are treated in the clinic or emergency room, reserving operative treatment for high, extensive or recurrent abscesses. Antibiotics alone are never indicated once the diagnosis is made. Postoperative antibiotics may be helpful when there is extensive cellulitis or deep-seated infections and in patients with diabetes or compromised immune systems. Patients are placed on a bowel management program of tub baths, oral analgesics, and dressing changes twice a day. Most improve immediately and resolve quickly. Recurrence as a new abscess or a chronic fistula occurs in about 50% of patients, due to persistence of the internal opening at the dentate line in most cases.

5. FISTULA IN ANO

Fistulae are the chronic manifestation of perianal sepsis while abscesses represent the acute process. Nearly all fistulae are preceded by an anorectal abscess. A fistula is a tract that communicates two surfaces lined by epithelium. A simple anorectal fistula runs between the dentate line and the perianal skin and comprises nearly 95% of all cases encountered in practice. The internal opening of such a fistula arises from a crypt at the dentate line. The remainder are complex fistulae, with the internal opening being above the anorectal ring. These may be due to Crohn's disease, diverticular disease, HIV, or other unusual infections, malignancy, radiation, trauma, or iatrogenic injury.

Patients typically complain of persistent perianal soreness, swelling or a lump. Sometimes the abscess will rupture spontaneously with a bloody or purulent discharge followed by temporary relief of symptoms. Local examination reveals the external opening of the fistula on the perianal skin (Fig. 5). It may be surround by heaped up skin and be mistaken for a tag, wart or other lesion. Gently probing of the opening will often reveal the true nature of the lesion, but vigorous attempts to probe the length of the tract often causes severe pain and is not necessary. Digital exam of the anal canal and anoscopy with gentle probing may identify the internal opening in half of patients, but failure to find it in the office does not preclude its presence.

The treatment of all varieties of fistulae is surgery. The aim of surgery is to achieve healing of the fistula, without significant damage to the anorectal sphincter complex. For the purpose of treatment plans, fistulae may be divided into low, mid and high complex varieties. Low fistulae, which involve <30–40% of the sphincter are easily treated with a primary fistulotomy, by simply dividing the tissues from the skin to a probe in the tract, curetting the base, and trimming the lateral edges (Fig. 6). Healing is by secondary intention with twice-daily washing and packing. Mid level fistulae, involving 40–70% of the vertical length of the sphincter including the external sphincter, are treated with a staged approach to reduce the risk of incontinence. The lower tract and cavity outside of the sphincters are incised, unroofed, and curetted. A "seton" (silastic band or thick nonabsorbable suture) is placed through the transsphincteric portion of the tract to control it and encourage scar formation, while the rest of the wound is allowed to heal (Fig. 7). Wound cares are performed twice daily. A second operation is performed 2 to 3 mo later after the lateral wound has healed in, leaving a short often lowered trans-sphincteric tract. The remaining portion of the tract and muscle is divided, often using local anesthetic in the office. Occasionally, the seton will work itself through. High or complex fistulae require an individualized approach, depending on the underlying disorder and findings. One or more setons are often placed and, in selected cases, an advancement flap repair may be performed subsequently. Fibrin glue, which has recently become commercially available, has been used either alone or in addition to an internal repair with good results in 50–70% of cases.

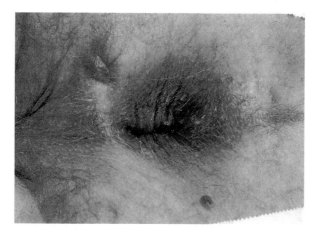

Fig. 5. An external fistula opening with heaped up edges. Probing reveals the true nature of the lesion.

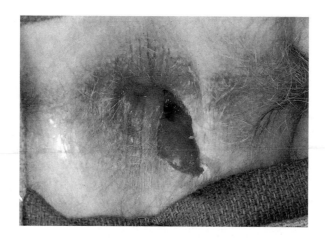

Fig. 6. The operative wound after a primary fistulotomy.

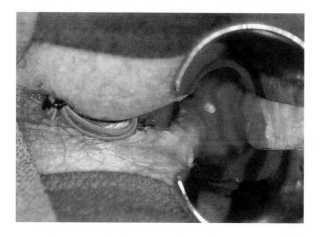

Fig. 7. A seton made from a Silastic vessel loop and a no. 1 silk suture.

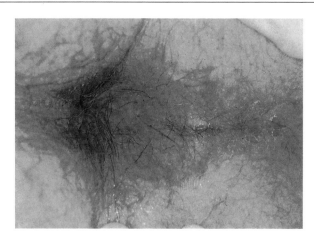

Fig. 8. Moderately severe pruritus ani with symmetrical erythema.

6. PRURITUS ANI

Pruritus ani is an extremely common condition that is often poorly understood and, at times, may be difficult to manage. Pruritus ani is simply perianal irritation and itching. These symptoms are often wrongly attributed to hemorrhoids. Most patients are men who complain of insidious onset of excessive itching and burning in the perianal region. The vast majority are due to particles of stool or sweat left on the perianal skin and subsequent attempts to wipe clean with rough dry toilet paper. This may grind the particles into the skin, setting up a further reaction. The paper also often flakes apart, leaving additional material on the skin, contributing to the condition. A myriad of conditions such as diabetes, infections including pinworms, anorectal disorders, vaginal discharge, antibiotic use, local steroid use, and anal intercourse may also be at fault. Hemorrhoidal prolapse may deposit stool or mucous on the perianal skin and result in secondary pruritus. Poor general and anal hygiene and stress are often contributory factors. Physical exam is variable and may reveal essentially normal appearing skin to a friable erythematous appearance to a severely ulcerated, weeping, or lichenified perianal skin (Fig. 8). The findings are symmetrical and may not correlate with the severity of the symptoms. An effort should be made to locate and treat specific anorectal disorders as well as systemic illnesses that may cause pruritus.

Management of idiopathic pruritus ani aims at reassurance and maintaining a dry and clean perianal skin at all times. Aggressive shaving of hairs, medicated soaps, local application of steroids and topical analgesics should be discouraged. Unscented baby wipes are soothing and assist in cleaning. The patient is encouraged to cleanse after every bowel movement followed by careful drying of the skin, possible with a hair dryer on low power and low heat. A small opened gauze or cotton from a cotton roll may be tucked into the anal cleft to help absorb sweat, decrease friction, and keep the area dry. A variety of foods may cause irritation is some patients. Common culprits include citrus fruits, coffee–caffeine, tea, sodas, alcohol, chocolates, and dairy or tomato products. If local cares do not suffice, a program of diet limitation with gradual reintroduction of these items may demonstrate the offending agent. Perseverance and a sympathetic, reassuring attitude is needed to treat this often recurring disorder that causes much misery and frustration to the patient.

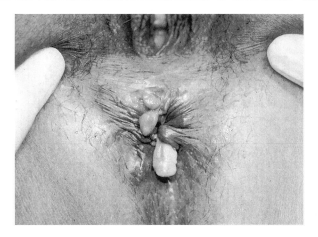

Fig. 9. A female patient with an anterior skin tag (top) and a posterior prolapsing hypertrophied anal papilla (bottom).

7. HYPERTROPHIED ANAL PAPILLA

This term refers to enlargement of the anal papillae at the dentate line. They are much more common than generally appreciated. The majority are asymptomatic, are discovered incidentally during endoscopic or digital exams, and are not associated with any identifiable cause. The rest may be associated with a chronic anal fissure as part of the classical triad of a sentinel skin tag, the fissure, and the hypertrophied anal papilla. When asymptomatic, no specific treatment is required. They are often mistaken for hemorrhoids or polyps on retroflexed view during colonoscopy. Attempts at biopsy or "polypectomy" result in severe pain, since they are covered by innervated skin. Occasionally, enlargement may be to the point that the papilla prolapses externally and is felt as a mass (Fig. 9). It may then be simply excised.

8. SKIN TAGS

Skin tags are probably the most common findings on anorectal examination. Fifty percent of the population has one or more skin tags. They arise from the anal verge and range from small raised bits of skin to large floppy lobes (Fig. 9). They are commonly and incorrectly labeled external hemorrhoids, but they do not have the dilated hemorrhoidal blood vessels that distinguish that entity. They develop for a variety of reasons or, seemingly, for no reason at all. Many are the residual, stretched-out skin remaining after resolution of a thrombosed external hemorrhoid. They may be the lower manifestation of a chronic fissure, as noted above. They may represent the lower end of a prolapsing internal hemorrhoid. They are often found in patients with Crohn's disease as bluish edematous tags. The patient may be asymptomatic or complain of soreness or pruritus ani, since they may interfere with adequate cleansing following a bowel movement. Symptomatic external skin tags may be easily excised in the office, under local anesthesia or may be removed during procedures from other anorectal disorders. Usually, they are innocent bystanders and may be left alone.

INDEX